Recent Advances in Closed-Loop Neurophysiology

Recent Advances in Closed-Loop Neurophysiology

Editor: George Morris

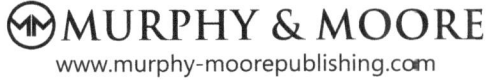

MURPHY & MOORE
www.murphy-moorepublishing.com

www.murphy-moorepublishing.com

⊗ MURPHY & MOORE

Cataloging-in-Publication Data

Recent advances in closed-loop neurophysiology / edited by George Morris.
    p. cm.
Includes bibliographical references and index.
ISBN 978-1-63987-474-3
1. Neurophysiology. 2. Neurobiology. 3. Physiology. I. Morris, George.
QP353 .R43 2022
612.809--dc23

Murphy & Moore Publishing,
1 Rockefeller Plaza,
New York City, NY 10020, USA

ISBN 978-1-63987-474-3 (Hardback)

Contents

Permissions

List of Contributors

Index

Preface

The branch of study which focuses on the nerve cells as well as the manner in which they transmit and receive information is termed as neurophysiology. There are various methods of research within this field, a few of which are using patch clamp, extracellular single-unit recording, and voltage clamp for electrophysiological recording. Close loop neurophysiology is one of the approaches to the study of neural systems wherein the neural behavior and activity is recorded and used to deliver a real time activity-dependent stimulation. This approach considers the brain to be a set of loops which is interacting with itself as well as with the environment in a relational fashion. This book explores all the important aspects of closed-loop neurophysiology in the present day scenario. It strives to provide a fair idea about this discipline and to help develop a better understanding of the latest advances within this field. The book is appropriate for students seeking detailed information in this area as well as for experts.

Significant researches are present in this book. Intensive efforts have been employed by authors to make this book an outstanding discourse. This book contains the enlightening chapters which have been written on the basis of significant researches done by the experts.

Finally, I would also like to thank all the members involved in this book for being a team and meeting all the deadlines for the submission of their respective works. I would also like to thank my friends and family for being supportive in my efforts.

Editor

Restoration of motor function following spinal cord injury via optimal control of intraspinal microstimulation: toward a next generation closed-loop neural prosthesis

Peter J. Grahn[1], Grant W. Mallory[2], B. Michael Berry[1], Jan T. Hachmann[2], Darlene A. Lobel[3] and J. Luis Lujan[2,4] *

[1] Mayo Clinic College of Medicine, Mayo Clinic, Rochester, MN, USA
[2] Department of Neurologic Surgery, Mayo Clinic, Rochester, MN, USA
[3] Department of Neurosurgery, Cleveland Clinic, Cleveland, OH, USA
[4] Department of Physiology and Biomedical Engineering, Mayo Clinic, Rochester, MN, USA

Edited by:
Mitsuhiro Hayashibe, University of Montpellier, France

Reviewed by:
Ken Yoshida, Indiana University-Purdue University Indianapolis, USA
Lee Fisher, Univeristy of Pittsburgh, USA

*Correspondence:
J. Luis Lujan, Departments of Neurologic Surgery and Physiology and Biomedical Engineering, Mayo Clinic, 200 First Street SW, Rochester, MN 55905, USA
e-mail: luis.lujan@mayo.edu

Movement is planned and coordinated by the brain and carried out by contracting muscles acting on specific joints. Motor commands initiated in the brain travel through descending pathways in the spinal cord to effector motor neurons before reaching target muscles. Damage to these pathways by spinal cord injury (SCI) can result in paralysis below the injury level. However, the planning and coordination centers of the brain, as well as peripheral nerves and the muscles that they act upon, remain functional. Neuroprosthetic devices can restore motor function following SCI by direct electrical stimulation of the neuromuscular system. Unfortunately, conventional neuroprosthetic techniques are limited by a myriad of factors that include, but are not limited to, a lack of characterization of non-linear input/output system dynamics, mechanical coupling, limited number of degrees of freedom, high power consumption, large device size, and rapid onset of muscle fatigue. Wireless multi-channel closed-loop neuroprostheses that integrate command signals from the brain with sensor-based feedback from the environment and the system's state offer the possibility of increasing device performance, ultimately improving quality of life for people with SCI. In this manuscript, we review neuroprosthetic technology for improving functional restoration following SCI and describe brain-machine interfaces suitable for control of neuroprosthetic systems with multiple degrees of freedom. Additionally, we discuss novel stimulation paradigms that can improve synergy with higher planning centers and improve fatigue-resistant activation of paralyzed muscles. In the near future, integration of these technologies will provide SCI survivors with versatile closed-loop neuroprosthetic systems for restoring function to paralyzed muscles.

Keywords: spinal cord injury, brain machine interface, closed-loop control, feedback control, neuroprosthetics, sensors, implantable systems

INTRODUCTION

Approximately 300,000 individuals in the United States, and more than 2.5 million individuals worldwide, are affected by traumatic spinal cord injury (SCI) (National Spinal Cord Injury Statistical Center, 2013). Overall health-care related cumulative costs are estimated to exceed $9 billion annually in the United States alone (DeVivo, 2012). In 2010, 36.5% of SCI resulted from motor vehicle accidents, 28.5% from falls, 14% from violence (including gunshot wounds), 9% from sports accidents, and 11% from other incidences not reported in detail (National Spinal Cord Injury Statistical Center, 2013). The demographic profile has changed over the last 40 years to involve older aged individuals. However, males still comprise the majority of injuries (Sekhon and Fehlings, 2001; DeVivo, 2012; Lenehan et al., 2012; National Spinal Cord Injury Statistical Center, 2013).

Traumatic SCI can occur when an excessive load to the spinal column is transmitted (directly or indirectly) to the spinal cord (Rowland, 1991; Watson et al., 2009). Damage to the spinal cord begins at the moment of injury, when displaced fragments of bone, disc material, or ligaments typically cause bruises or tears to spinal cord tissue (McDonald and Sadowsky, 2002). However, paralysis has been observed with no radiographic evidence of damage to the spinal cord or vertebral column (Pang and Wilberger, 1982; Mirovsky et al., 2005; Mahajan et al., 2013). Regardless of the injury mechanism, SCI involves permanent sensorimotor and autonomic deficits (Scivoletto et al., 2014), with long term complications including muscle atrophy and increased risk of cardiovascular disease (Phillips et al., 1998; Chen et al., 1999).

Most spinal cord injuries do not completely sever the spinal cord (Marino et al., 2003; National Institute of Neurological Disorders and Stroke, 2013). Instead, key pathways necessary for signal transmission between the brain and the rest of the body are disrupted. Spinal cord injuries can be classified as complete and incomplete injuries (Marino et al., 2003). Complete injuries are indicated by a total lack of sensory and motor function below the level of injury. In contrast, the ability to convey messages to or from the brain is not completely lost in cases of incomplete injury. That is, limited sensation and movement remain below the level of injury. Although SCI interrupts connections between the brain and effector muscles, key planning, coordination, and effector centers above and below the injury remain intact (Krajl et al., 1986; Triolo et al., 1996; Jilge et al., 2004; Minassian et al., 2004; Fisher et al., 2008, 2009; Yanagisawa et al., 2011; Wang et al., 2013; Collinger et al., 2014). Functional electrical stimulation (FES) is a form of therapy that applies external currents into intact neuromuscular circuitry below the level of injury, activating intact neural components to cause muscle contractions that can lead to restoration of motor function (Jackson and Zimmermann, 2012).

This manuscript reviews current therapeutic applications of electrical stimulation of the spine for providing functional coordination of muscle contraction and restoring function to paralyzed muscles. Additionally, this manuscript describes the development of neurostimulation technologies and control strategies, combining brain signals, optimal control algorithms, and emerging FES strategies to develop a clinically-translatable FES system that optimizes restoration of neurologic function following SCI (**Figure 1**).

ELECTRICAL STIMULATION OF EXCITABLE TISSUE

The use of electrical stimulation for investigating the function of the nervous system began with the Italian physician and scientist Luigi Galvani (Galvani and Aldini, 1792). Galvani discovered that nerves and muscles are electrically excitable, and was able to evoke muscle contractions in frog legs by stimulating them with brief jolts of electricity, produced by static generators (Hambrecht, 1992). Since then, it has been well established that nerve cells

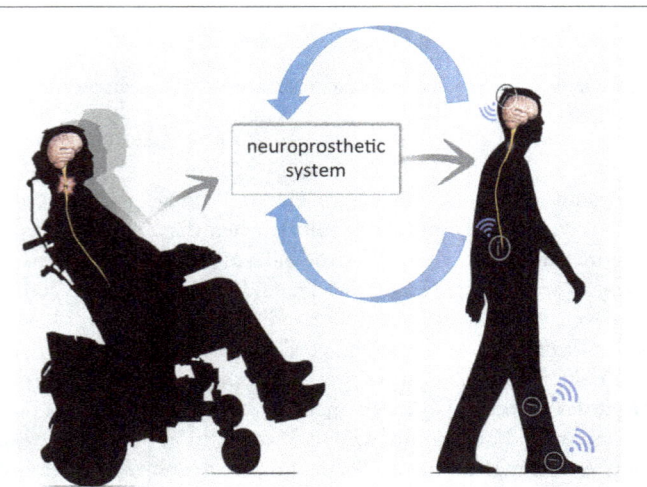

FIGURE 1 | Neuroprosthetic system. The neuroprosthetic system is capable of interpreting volitional movement signals from the brain, integrating these commands with sensor feedback (e.g., joint angle, limb velocity, etc.) and, delivering appropriate commands into intact neural circuitry below the level of injury.

can be activated using electrical currents delivered into neural tissue via stimulating electrodes (Glenn et al., 1976; Branner et al., 2001; Brill et al., 2009; Kilgore et al., 2009; Kent and Grill, 2013; Nishimura et al., 2013). Active nerve cells fire electrical impulses, also known as action potentials, that travel along the nerve axon and propagate across neuromuscular junctions via neurotransmitter signaling (Bean, 2007; Meriney and Dittrich, 2013). In turn, this signaling mechanism causes muscle fibers connected to nerve fibers (i.e., motor unit) to contract (Hughes et al., 2006).

ELECTRICALLY EVOKED MUSCLE ACTIVATION

The strength of stimulation-evoked muscle contractions can be controlled by varying the frequency, amplitude, and pulsewidth of the external stimuli (Grobelnik, 1973; Kralj et al., 1988; Kralj and Bajd, 1989; Bhadra and Peckham, 1997). At low frequencies, individual muscle twitches are evoked with each stimulus pulse. At higher frequencies, responses to individual stimuli fuse and muscles respond with smooth contractions. Higher stimulus frequencies produce stronger muscle contractions, but also increase the rate of muscle fatigue (Tanae et al., 1973; McDonnall et al., 2004; Bamford, 2005). Activation of motor units can be achieved using different stimulation modalities: transcutaneous stimulation, percutaneous stimulation, intramuscular stimulation, peripheral nerve stimulation, and spinal stimulation.

TRANSCUTANEOUS STIMULATION

Transcutaneous stimulation, also known as surface stimulation, relies on stimulating electrodes placed on the skin surface directly over the muscle motor points (i.e., locations that produce an optimal balance between contraction strength and stimulation amplitude) (Hirokawa et al., 1990; Scremin et al., 1999; Mangold et al., 2005). This non-invasive, reversible, and inexpensive technique has been successfully used in locomotion and hand grasp systems (Kralj and Bajd, 1989; Popovic et al., 2005). However, transcutaneous muscle stimulation has multiple practical limitations. Specifically, the skin offers a high resistance compared to muscle tissue (Bîrlea et al., 2014). For this reason, higher stimulation currents (>30 mA) are required to achieve desired motor responses using surface stimulation (Triolo et al., 2001; Lujan and Crago, 2009). Additionally, the limited degree of selectivity can lead to activation of antagonist muscle groups or an inability to selectively activate deep muscle groups (Schmit and Mortimer, 1997; Triolo et al., 2001). Furthermore, current spread due to suboptimal electrode placement and limited stimulation specificity can result in pain (Niddam et al., 2001).

PERCUTANEOUS STIMULATION

Percutaneous stimulation systems rely on intramuscular needle electrodes that pass through the skin and stimulate target muscles (Caldwell and Reswick, 1975; Stanic et al., 1978; Malezic et al., 1984; Marsolais and Kobetic, 1986; Bogataj et al., 1989). This allows activation of deep muscles and provides isolated, selective, and repeatable muscle contractions. Percutaneous stimulation requires lower stimulation intensities compared to transcutaneous stimulation. However, increased risks of infection, lead breakage, and movement restrictions limit the use of percutaneous stimulation outside of a laboratory environment (Knutson et al., 2002).

IMPLANTED INTRAMUSCULAR AND PERIPHERAL NERVE STIMULATION

Implanted neurostimulation systems are associated with electrical current delivery via both intramuscular and nerve cuff electrodes (Rabischong and Ohanna, 1992; Peckham et al., 2002; Guiraud et al., 2006). As the name implies, intramuscular stimulation relies on electrodes implanted directly into the muscle (Crago et al., 1980; Hobby et al., 2001; Peckham et al., 2001, 2002; Peckham and Knutson, 2005; Kilgore et al., 2008). Peripheral nerve stimulation relies on electrode cuffs that are surgically placed around nerves innervating target muscles (Stein et al., 1975; Hoffer et al., 1996; Strange and Hoffer, 1999; Sinkjaer, 2000; Branner et al., 2001; Brill et al., 2009; Fisher et al., 2009; Polasek et al., 2009). Although capable of evoking strong, selective, and repeatable muscle activation, intramuscular and nerve cuff stimulation techniques often recruit the largest and most fatigable motor units first, resulting in early fatigue onset (Popovic et al., 2002). Discontinuous activation of muscle compartments and interleaved frequency stimulation have both been reported to delay fatigue onset (Boom et al., 1993; McDonnall et al., 2004). Saigal et al. demonstrated fatigue-resistant stepping in a spinalized cat by stimulating the lumbrosacral cord via interleaved stimulation (Saigal et al., 2004). Interleaved stimulation reduces muscle fatigue by decreasing the stimulation frequency (Mushahwar and Horch, 1997; Tai et al., 2000). The asynchronous nature of interleaved stimulation is designed to evoke fused contractions despite a lack of tetanic firing in individual motor units. However, the limited number of controllable degrees of freedom, high power consumption, and other technological and practical limitations have restricted the widespread application of electrical stimulation therapy outside research environments (Peckham and Knutson, 2005; Ragnarsson, 2008; Creasey and Craggs, 2012).

SPINAL CORD STIMULATION

Direct stimulation of the spinal cord may be advantageous over conventional FES techniques as spinal stimulation provides an opportunity to directly activate higher level circuitry, which oversees and coordinates motor function (Minassian et al., 2004, 2007; Bamford, 2005; Gerasimenko et al., 2008; Bamford and Mushahwar, 2011; Holinski et al., 2011; van den Brand et al., 2012; Angeli et al., 2014). Two modalities of spinal stimulation have been described: epidural and intraspinal stimulation.

In epidural stimulation, stimulating electrodes are placed directly over the spinal cord (Lavrov et al., 2008; Hachmann et al., 2013). Two recent studies reported that neuromodulation of spinal circuitry via epidural stimulation, combined with intense physical rehabilitation, was capable of allowing individuals with incomplete and complete SCI to process conceptual, auditory and visual feedback to regain voluntary control of paralyzed muscles for short durations of time. Results of these studies suggest some degree of residual connectivity through the area of SCI (Harkema et al., 2011; Angeli et al., 2014). These studies, although promising, require using rigorous patient selection and replication in larger patient populations.

In intraspinal microstimulation (ISMS), stimulating electrodes are implanted within the ventral gray matter of the spinal cord (Bamford and Mushahwar, 2011). ISMS is hypothesized to directly activate alpha motor neurons, preferentially activating fatigue resistant muscle fibers (Gorman, 2000; Bamford, 2005). Several studies have highlighted the potential of ISMS to restore bladder and respiratory function, as well as upper and lower extremity function in animal models (Mushahwar and Horch, 2000a,b; Mushahwar et al., 2002; Moritz et al., 2007; Bamford et al., 2010; Bamford and Mushahwar, 2011; Nishimura et al., 2013; Sunshine et al., 2013).

INTRASPINAL MICROSTIMULATION (ISMS)

Intraspinal stimulation has been extensively used to study the effects of electrical stimulation on the central nervous system, as well as synaptic delays and network interconnections across spinal pathways (Renshaw, 1946; Jankowska and Roberts, 1972a,b; Gustafsson and Jankowska, 1976). More recently, ISMS has been used to investigate the organization of motor circuitry within the spinal cord in amphibious, rodent, and feline animal models (Bizzi et al., 1991; Giszter et al., 1993; Tresch and Bizzi, 1999; Lemay et al., 2001, 2009; Saltiel et al., 2001; Lemay and Grill, 2004).

Similarly, over the past 15 years, ISMS has been used to investigate restoration of motor function in spinalized and anesthetized rodents and cats (Mushahwar et al., 2002; Bamford, 2005; Pikov et al., 2007; Yakovenko et al., 2007; Holinski et al., 2011; Kasten et al., 2013; Sunshine et al., 2013). Work performed by Lau et al. demonstrated that ISMS is capable of producing standing in cats for over 20 min (Lau et al., 2007). The lower stimulation amplitudes associated with intraspinal stimulation (in the order of a few microamperes) are believed to be, at least in part, responsible for the longer periods of muscle contraction observed (Bamford, 2005). Other studies suggest that the fatigue resistance observed with ISMS techniques is the result of preferential activation of type I slow-twitch fatigue-resistant motor fibers (Mushahwar, 2000; Mushahwar and Horch, 2000a; Saigal et al., 2004; Bamford, 2005; Nishimura et al., 2013). Moreover, Bamford et al. showed ISMS recruitment of up to 44% fatigue-resistant muscle fibers compared to less than 1% fatigue-resistant muscle fibers recruited using peripheral nerve cuff stimulation (Caldwell and Reswick, 1975; Marsolais and Kobetic, 1986; Bamford, 2005). As such, when combined with interleaved stimulation, ISMS has been associated with further decrease in muscle fatigue (Rack and Westbury, 1969; McDonnall et al., 2004; Lau et al., 2007; Mushahwar et al., 2007).

The close proximity of spinal motor centers to higher control centers responsible for controlling motor function, together with the improved fatigue response, make ISMS an excellent alternative for restoring locomotor function in individuals with SCI (Etlin et al., 2014; Guertin, 2014). However, before spinal or other electrical stimulation technology can be clinically used to optimally improve quality of life for individuals with SCI, appropriate stimulation control paradigms must be established.

OPTIMAL CONTROL PARADIGMS

Electrical stimulation systems have been previously used to assist respiratory function (Kaneyuki et al., 1977; Gorman, 2000; Posluszny et al., 2014), hand grasp (Avestruz et al., 2008; Skarpaas and Morrell, 2009; Rosin et al., 2011; Gan et al., 2012; Basu et al., 2013; Grant and Lowery, 2013), locomotion (Behrend et al., 2009), as well as bladder and bowel function (Lee et al., 2004; Shon et al., 2010a,b; MacDonald et al., 2013) in patients with SCI. These FES systems have relied on a variety of control strategies, ranging from linear models to adaptive controllers, but all aimed at enhancing stimulation-evoked functional responses. Many neuroprosthetic control systems rely on feedforward configurations (Moro et al., 1999; Molinuevo et al., 2000), in which controller output depends only on user inputs (e.g., stimulus parameters). These controllers have fast response times, but do not make corrections if the target and actual outputs differ (Lee et al., 2009). Furthermore, these controllers will not alter their response in the face of unexpected internal or external perturbations (Blaha and Phillips, 1996; Lee et al., 2006). However, the highly non-linear nature of muscle responses, coupled with environmental perturbations found in activities of daily living, require that optimal neuroprosthetic control paradigms rely on feedback signals. Feedback-based control systems continuously monitor musculoskeletal system outputs and adjust stimulation parameters if the stimulation-evoked musculoskeletal system outputs (e.g., limb position, force) differ from the desired outputs (Lujan and Crago, 2009; Griessenauer et al., 2010; Chang et al., 2012). This guarantees the system can respond to and compensate for unforeseen perturbations. Feedback control has been previously used for control of hand grasp (Lujan and Crago, 2009), standing posture (Fraix et al., 2006; Rosin et al., 2011), and locomotion (Roham et al., 2007; Takmakov et al., 2010; Fitzgerald, 2014) in SCI individuals. Simple feedback control can be improved by using adaptive systems (Karniel and Inbar, 2000; Kobravi and Erfanian, 2012). Adaptive algorithms modify controller behavior in response to changes in the system and the environment (Chizek et al., 1988; Narendra, 1990; Narendra and Parthasarathy, 1990; Teixeira et al., 1991; Kostov et al., 1995; Davoodi and Andrews, 1998, 1999; Jonić et al., 1999; Abbas and Riener, 2001).

Studies have demonstrated the ability of neural networks to successfully control motor neuroprostheses, both in paraplegic (Riess and Abbas, 1999, 2000, 2001; Nataraj et al., 2013) and tetraplegic individuals (Fujita et al., 1998; Lujan and Crago, 2009). Artificial neural networks (ANNs) can model static and dynamic non-linear systems (Durfee, 1989; Funahashi, 1989; Hornik et al., 1989; Chakraborty et al., 1992; Barron, 1993; Lan et al., 1994; Piche, 1994; Graupe and Kordylewski, 1995; Hassoun, 1995; Kostov et al., 1995; Chang et al., 1996; Chen et al., 1997; Demuth and Beale, 2000). Additionally, ANNs can generalize from experimental input/output data, eliminating the need for analytical models of the system (Funahashi, 1989; Hornik et al., 1989; Graupe and Kordylewski, 1995; Hassoun, 1995; Narendra, 1996; Demuth and Beale, 2000). Furthermore, ANNs are less sensitive to noise and easily implemented in hardware (Narendra, 1996). Moreover, ANN-based controllers allow changes to the controller without requiring changes in data collection or controller training methods. Backpropagation neural networks have been used to model the non-linear relationship between stimulus intensity and stimulation-evoked responses (Fujita et al., 1998; Lujan and Crago, 2009). Additionally, ANNs have been successfully used to create inverse dynamic models of musculoskeletal systems for neuroprosthetic control (Chang et al., 1997; Yoshida et al., 2002). These models are particularly useful for learning the characteristics of electrically-activated muscles in coupled multi-joint systems acted upon by redundant muscles (Adamczyk and Crago, 1997, 2000; Lujan and Crago, 2009).

Thus, optimal neuroprosthetic control systems should rely on a combination of non-linear feedforward and feedback techniques in order to pre-emptively reduce the amount of error in real-time while minimizing time delays inherent to feedback control systems. Development of such optimal closed-loop neuroprosthetic controllers will require high-quality sensors that can withstand daily use under a wide range of daily life activities.

FEEDBACK SIGNALS FOR OPTIMAL CONTROL OF NEURAL PROSTHESES

Neuroprosthetic systems with feedback control are capable of identifying, decoding, and extracting features from appropriate input signals in order to respond to unforeseen perturbations and changes in the environment (Bhadra et al., 2002; Dominici et al., 2012; Holinski et al., 2013). However, optimal feedback modulation for clinical application will require fully implantable smart sensors that provide consistent and reliable chronic information to the control system (Shih et al., 2012; Peckham and Kilgore, 2013). There is already a wide range of sensors that can detect and measure information about the system and its environment. The most commonly used sensors include electrophysiological sensors, chemical sensors, force transducers, and magnetic sensors. Electrophysiological sensors measure potential differences generated by muscle (i.e., myoelectric signals) and neural tissue (e.g., electroencephalogram, electrocorticogram, electroneurogram) (Leuthardt et al., 2004; Müller-Putz et al., 2005; Holinski et al., 2013). These sensors can monitor muscle state and evaluate expected muscle responses. In turn, this allows adaptation of stimulation parameters in the presence of muscle fatigue (Hayashibe et al., 2011; Zhang et al., 2013). Chemical sensors (e.g., carbon fiber microelectrodes coupled to fast scan cyclic voltammetry devices) can detect changes in stimulation-evoked analytes (e.g., neurotransmitters) (Bledsoe et al., 2009; Chang et al., 2012) that can be used to modulate stimulation levels. Force transducers (e.g., piezoelectric devices, accelerometers) can be used to detect changes in limb position, ground reaction forces, heel strike, and other events that are critical for event detection and optimal control of stimulation (Tan et al., 2004). Magnetic sensors detect changes in magnetic fields and can be used to detect limb position and orientation (Bhadra et al., 2002; Tan et al., 2004). However, having reliable sensors is not enough to develop an optimal feedback controller. In order for the signals measured by these sensors to be of clinical use, they must be properly decoded and integrated with both existing and novel neuroprosthetic control systems (Shadmehr et al., 2010). This will most likely happen in the way of a brain machine interface.

Restoration of motor function following spinal cord injury via optimal control of intraspinal...

5

BRAIN MACHINE INTERFACES

Brain machine interfaces (BMI) are neural interface systems that can record, analyze, and decode brain signals (Wang et al., 2010) to infer volitional intent, which in turn can be used to control limb movement and assistive devices (**Figure 2**) (Leuthardt et al., 2004; Hochberg et al., 2006; Schwartz et al., 2006; Miller et al., 2010; Carmena, 2012; Fifer et al., 2012). Brain commands may be recorded using sensors located on the scalp (electroencephalogram), the surface of the brain (electrocorticogram), or the brain parenchyma using intracortical electrodes that record activity from single neurons (single unit recording) or groups of neurons (local field potentials) (**Figure 3**). Electroencephalographic recordings offer a non-invasive recording technique that is safe and easy to implement. However, controlling multiple degrees of freedom with electroencephalographic signals has proven difficult due to challenges with extracting and classifying individual signal features as well as an inherent low spatial resolution (Yang et al., 2011). Single unit recordings and local field potentials offer excellent signal resolution, but are highly invasive (Buzsáki et al., 2012). Single unit recordings capture the activity of distinct neurons. The high spatial and temporal resolution provided by single unit recordings allows for precise measurements of neuronal spikes (Buzsáki et al., 2012). The downfall to single unit recordings is a difficulty isolating specific neural activity due to crosstalk from neighboring cells (Bai and Wise, 2001). Furthermore, single unit recordings can be biased toward activity from larger neurons adjacent to the intended neuron (Buzsáki et al., 1983). Finally, electrode migration, immune responses (e.g., glial scarring), and disruption of surrounding neural tissue interfere with signal quality and limit reliable single unit activity to acute recording conditions (Carter and Houk, 1993; Polikov et al., 2005). Local field potentials reflect a weighted average of integrative processes and associations between cells that can be detected over

longer distances through extracellular space (Logothetis, 2003a,b; Andersen et al., 2004; Bronte-Stewart et al., 2009; Buzsáki et al., 2012; Rosa et al., 2012). Unfortunately, the longer recording range of local field potential techniques is associated with decreased spatial resolution. Electrocorticogram presents a good balance between risks and benefits, as it provides good spatiotemporal resolution without damaging underlying cortical tissue (Leuthardt et al., 2004; Wilson et al., 2006; Schalk et al., 2008; Moran, 2010; Slutzky et al., 2010).

Extracted brain signals must undergo filtering to remove movement artifacts and electrical noise before they can be used by a BMI and neuroprosthetic controller to generate motor commands (Kowalski et al., 2013). Filtered signals must be analyzed using classifiers and signal processing algorithms that identify unique features or signatures (Kowalski et al., 2013). In turn, these features are mapped to specific functions and/or degrees of freedom that control neuroprosthetic systems and assistive devices (Pfurtscheller et al., 2003; Musallam et al., 2004; Müller-Putz et al., 2005; Jackson et al., 2006; Moritz et al., 2008; Daly et al., 2009; Chadwick et al., 2011).

Pioneering work by Georgopoulos et al. used single unit recordings to establish a high degree of correlation between arm movement and cortical activity within a non-human primate (Georgopoulos et al., 1986). Subsequently, several studies in non-human primates and SCI-survivors have demonstrated stable, chronic, intracortical recordings using microelectrode arrays such as the Utah and Michigan arrays (Wessberg et al., 2000; Serruya et al., 2002; Taylor et al., 2002; Pfurtscheller et al., 2003; Suner et al., 2005; Cheung, 2007; Cheung et al., 2007; Moritz et al., 2008; Langhals and Kipke, 2009; Sharma et al., 2010, 2011; Do et al., 2011; Hochberg et al., 2012). Cortical signatures can be identified from their spatial, temporal, and frequency-dependent features (Nicolas-Alonso and Gomez-Gil, 2012). However, BMI

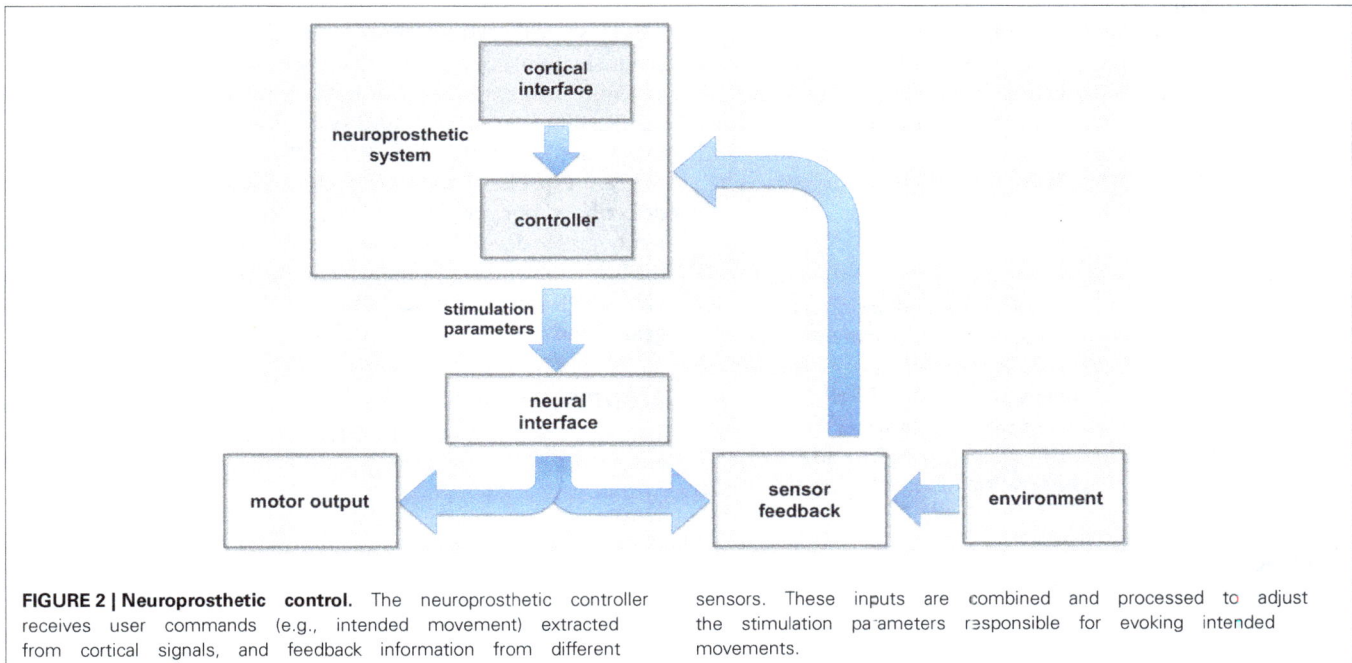

FIGURE 2 | Neuroprosthetic control. The neuroprosthetic controller receives user commands (e.g., intended movement) extracted from cortical signals, and feedback information from different sensors. These inputs are combined and processed to adjust the stimulation parameters responsible for evoking intended movements.

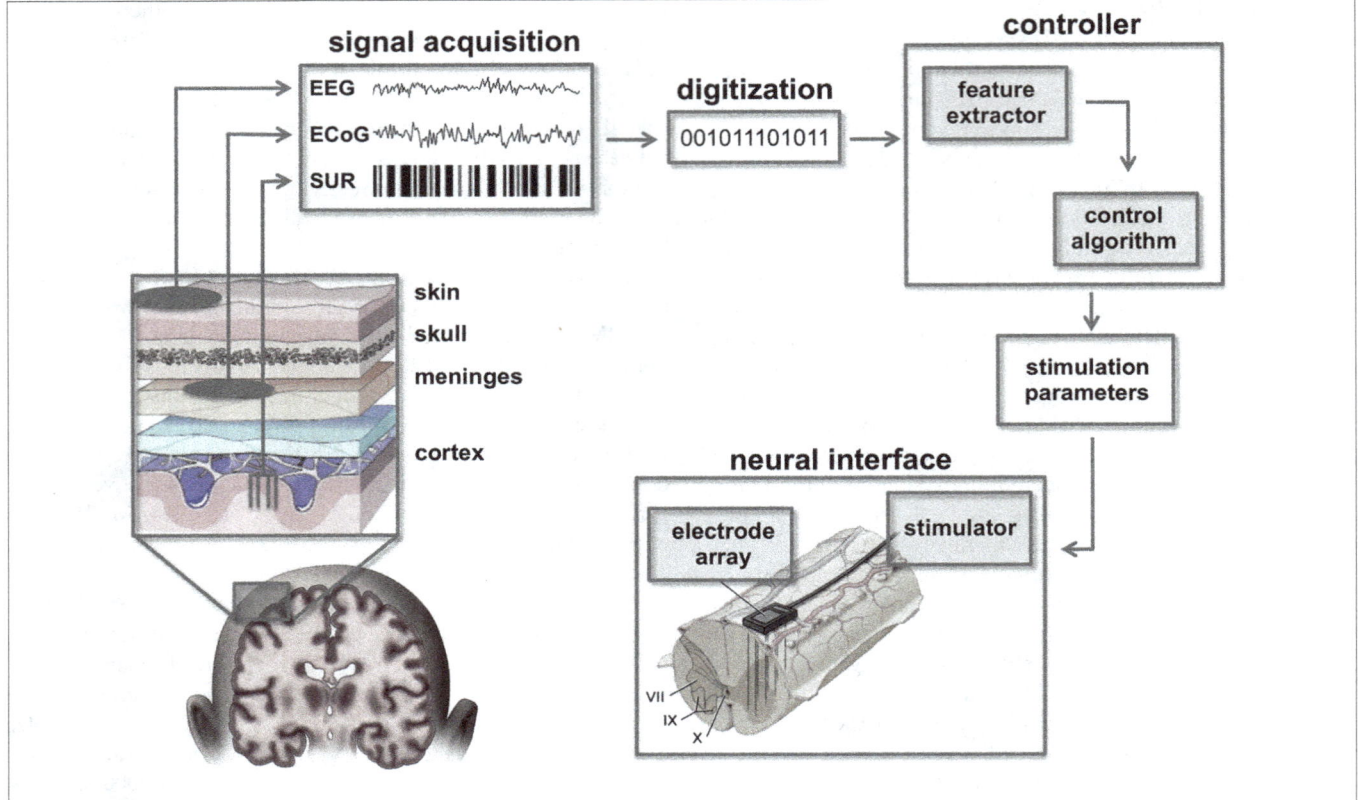

FIGURE 3 | Cortico-spinal neuroprostheses. Command signals from the brain can be extracted using a variety of brain signal recording techniques such as single unit recordings (SUR), electrocorticographic signals (ECoG), or electroencephalographic signals (EEG). Raw signals must be digitized and filtered to extract essential features that can be classified by the controller in order to calculate appropriate stimulation parameters. In turn, these parameters are used by a neural interface to activate spinal circuitry below the level of injury. Figure adapted from Smart Draw LifeART Collection Images and Lobel and Lee (2014).

application to complex neuroprosthetic control has been limited due to the difficulty of extracting sufficient numbers of unique signatures for control of systems with multiple degrees of freedom (Shih et al., 2012). Ongoing efforts in decoding algorithms, together with advances in neural training techniques such as motor imagery, have recently improved feature extraction, allowing SCI survivors to control complex movements using BMI (Wang et al., 2009, 2013; Chao et al., 2010; Yanagisawa et al., 2011).

CONCLUSIONS

Recent advances in the fields of BMIs and electrical stimulation therapy provide a promising outlook for patients with SCI. However, it is clear that successful restoration of independence for SCI survivors requires integration of selective electrical stimulation techniques, feedback control, and optimal control algorithms. As is the case in normal human neurophysiology, selective muscle activation as well as integration of force feedback, balance, proprioception, and reduction of muscle fatigue are all critical for motor function. Therefore, next-generation closed-loop neuroprosthetic systems must integrate fully implantable multi-channel stimulators and feedback sensors with adaptive control systems. Furthermore, control algorithms must be designed for seamless integration with BMI systems and real-time processing, integration, and transmission of feedback control signals. Devices that are capable of coupling such novel stimulation, intention detection, proprioceptive sensing, and control algorithms are currently under development, with clinical translation just beyond the horizon. Ultimately, these technologies will provide SCI survivors with increased independence in daily life, improved overall health, and enhanced quality of life.

ACKNOWLEDGMENTS

This work was supported by NIH R21 NS087320, The Grainger Foundation, and a gift from Louise Chapman.

REFERENCES

Abbas, J. J., and Riener, R. (2001). Using mathematical models and advanced control systems techniques to enhance neuroprosthesis function. *Neuromodulation* 4, 187–195. doi: 10.1046/j.1525-1403.2001.00187.x

Adamczyk, M. M., and Crago, P. E. (1997). "Integrated hand/wrist control in a neu-roprosthesis for individuals with tetraplegia," in *19th International Conference of IEEE EMBS* (Chicago, IL).

Adamczyk, M. M., and Crago, P. E. (2000). Simulated feedforward neural network coordination of hand grasp and wrist angle in a neuroprosthesis. *IEEE Trans.*

Rehabil. Eng. 8, 297–304. doi: 10.1109/86.867871

Andersen, R. A., Musallam, S., and Pesaran, B. (2004). Selecting the signals for a brain–machine interface. *Curr. Opin. Neurobiol.* 14, 720–726. doi: 10.1016/j.conb.2004.10.005

Angeli, C. A., Edgerton, V. R., Gerasimenko, Y. P., and Harkema, S. J. (2014). Altering spinal cord excitability enables voluntary movements after chronic complete paralysis in humans. *Brain* 137, 1394–1409. doi: 10.1093/brain/awu038

Avestruz, A.-T., Santa, W., Carlson, D., Jensen, R., Stanslaski, S., Helfenstine, A., et al. (2008). A 5 uW/channel spectral analysis IC for chronic bidirec-tional brain-machine interfaces. *IEEE J. Solid-State Circuits* 43, 3006–3024. doi: 10.1109/JSSC.2008.2006460

Bai, Q., and Wise, K. D. (2001). Single-unit neural recording with active microelec-trode arrays. *IEEE Trans. Biomed. Eng.* 48, 911–920. doi: 10.1109/10.936367

Bamford, J. A. (2005). Intraspinal microstimulation preferentially recruits fatigue-resistant muscle fibres and generates gradual force in rat. *J. Physiol.* 569, 873–884. doi: 10.1113/jphysiol.2005.094516

Bamford, J. A., and Mushahwar, V. K. (2011). Intraspinal microstimulation for the recovery of function following spinal cord injury. *Prog. Brain Res.* 227–239. doi: 10.1016/B978-0-444-53815-4.00004-2

Bamford, J. A., Todd, K. G., and Mushahwar, V. K. (2010). The effects of intraspinal microstimulation on spinal cord tissue in the rat. *Biomaterials* 31, 5552–5563. doi: 10.1016/j.biomaterials.2010.03.051

Barron, A. R. (1993). Universal approximation bounds for superpositions of a sigmoidal function. *IEEE Trans. Inform. Theory* 39, 930–945. doi: 10.1109/18.256500

Basu, I., Graupe, D., Tuninetti, D., Shukla, P., Slavin, K. V., Metman, L. V., et al. (2013). Pathological tremor prediction using surface electromyogram and accel-eration: potential use in "ON-OFF" demand driven deep brain stimulator design. *J. Neural Eng.* 10:036019. doi: 10.1088/1741-2560/10/3/036019

Bean, B. P. (2007). The action potential in mammalian central neurons. *Nat. Rev. Neurosci.* 8, 451–465. doi: 10.1038/nrn2148

Behrend, C. E., Cassim, S. M., and Pallone, M. J. (2009). Toward feed-back controlled deep brain stimulation: dynamics of glutamate release in the subthalamic nucleus in rats. *J. Neurosci. Methods.* 180, 278–289. doi: 10.1016/j.jneumeth.2009.04.001

Bhadra, N., and Peckham, P. H. (1997). Peripheral nerve stimulation for restoration of motor function. *J. Clin. Neurophysiol.* 14, 378–393. doi: 10.1097/00004691-199709000-00004

Bhadra, N., Peckham, P. H., and Keith, M. W. (2002). Implementation of an implantable joint-angle transducer. *J. Rehabil. Res. Dev.* 39, 411–422.

Bîrlea, S. I., Breen, P. P., Corley, G. J., Bîrlea, N. M., Quondamatteo, F., and ÓLaighin, G. (2014). Changes in the electrical properties of the electrode-skin-underlying tissue composite during a week-long programme of neuro-muscular electrical stimulation. *Physiol. Meas.* 35, 231–252. doi: 10.1088/0967-3334/35/2/231

Bizzi, E., Mussa-Ivaldi, F. A., and Giszter, S. (1991). Computations underlying the execution of movement: a biological perspective. *Science* 253, 287–291. doi: 10.1126/science.1857964

Blaha, C. D., and Phillips, A. G. (1996). A critical assessment of electrochemical procedures applied to the measurement of dopamine and its metabolites dur-ing drug-induced and species-typical behaviours. *Behav. Pharmacol.* 7, 675–708. doi: 10.1097/00008877-199611000-00004

Bledsoe, J. M., Kimble, C. J., Covey, D. P., Blaha, C. D., Agnesi, F., Mohseni, P., et al. (2009). Development of the wireless instantaneous neurotransmit-ter concentration system for intraoperative neurochemical monitoring using fast-scan cyclic voltammetry. *J. Neurosurg.* 111, 712–723. doi: 10.3171/2009.3.JNS081348

Bogataj, U., Gros, N., Malezic, M., Kelih, B., Kljajiæ, M., and Acimoviæ, R. (1989). Restoration of gait during two to three weeks of therapy with multichannel electrical stimulation. *Phys. Ther.* 69, 319–327.

Boom, H. B., Mulder, A. J., and Veltink, P. H. (1993). Fatigue during functional neuromuscular stimulation. *Prog. Brain Res.* 97, 409–418. doi: 10.1016/S0079-6123(08)62300-6

Branner, A., Stein, R. B., and Normann, R. A. (2001). Selective stimulation of cat sciatic nerve using an array of varying-length microelectrodes. *J. Neurophysiol.* 85, 1585–1594.

Brill, N., Polasek, K., Oby, E., Ethier, C., Miller. L., and Tyler, D. (2009). Nerve cuff stimulation and the effect of fascicular organization for hand grasp in non-human primates. *Conf. Proc. IEEE Eng. Med. Biol. Soc.* 2009, 1557–1560 doi: 10.1109/IEMBS.2009.5332395

Bronte-Stewart, H., Barberini, C., Koop, M. M., Hill, B. C., Henderson, J. M., and Wingeier, B. (2009). The STN beta-band profile in Parkinson's disease is station-ary and shows prolonged attenuation after deep brain stimulation. *Exp. Neurol.* 215, 20–28. doi: 10.1016/j.expneurol.2008.09.008

Buzsáki, G., Anastassiou, C. A., and Koch, C. (2012). The origin of extracellu-lar fields and currents—EEG, ECoG, LFP and spikes. *Nat. Rev. Neurosci.* 13, 407–420. doi: 10.1038/nrn3241

Buzsáki, G., Leung, L. W., and Vanderwolf, C. H. (1983). Cellular bases of hip-pocampal EEG in the behaving rat. *Brain Res.* 287, 139–171. doi: 10.1016/0165-0173(83)90037-1

Caldwell, C. W., and Reswick, J. B. (1975). A percutaneous wire electrode for chronic research use. *IEEE Trans. Biomed. Eng.* 22, 429–432. doi: 10.1109/TBME.1975.324516

Carmena, J. (2012). Becoming bionic: the new brain-machine interfaces that exploit plasticity of the brain may allow people to control prosthetic devices in a natural way. *IEEE Spectr.* 24–29. doi: 10.1109/MSPEC.2012.615860

Carter, R. R., and Houk, J. C. (1993). Multiple single-unit recordings from the CNS using thin-film electrode arrays. *IEEE Trans. Rehab. Eng.* 1, 175–184. doi: 10.1109/86.279266

Chadwick, E. K., Blana, D., Simeral, J. D., Lambrecht, J., Kim, S P., Cornwell, A. S., et al. (2011). Continuous neuronal ensemble control of simulated arm reaching by a human with tetraplegia. *J. Neural Eng.* 8:034003. doi: 10.1088/1741-2560/8/3/034003

Chakraborty, K., Mehrotra, K., Mohan, C. K., and Ranka, S. (1992). Forecasting the behavior of multivariate time series using neural networks. *Neural Netw.* 5, 961–970. doi: 10.1016/S0893-6080(05)80092-9

Chang, G. C., Liao, G. D., Luh, J. J., Lai, J. S., Cheng, C K., and Kuo, T. S. (1996). "Application of neural network-based controller for the knee-joint position control with quadriceps stimulation," in *IEEE* (Amsterdam), 455–456.

Chang, G. C., Luh, J. J. Liao, G. D., Lai, J. S., Cheng, C. K., Kuo, B. L., et al. (1997). A neuro-control system for the knee joint position control with quadriceps stimulation. *IEEE Trans. Rehabil. Eng.* 5, 2–11. doi: 10.1109/86.559344

Chang, S.-Y., Kim, I., Marsh, M. P., Jang, D. P., Hwang, S.-C., Van Gompel, J. J., et al. (2012). Wireless fast-scan cyclic voltammetry to monitor adenosine in patients with essential tremor during deep brain stimulation. *Mayo Clin. Proc.* 87, 760–765. doi: 10.1016/j.mayocp.2012.05.006

Chao, Z. C., Nagasaka, Y., and Fujii, N. (2010). Long-term asynchronous decoding of arm motion using electrocorticographic signals in monkeys. *Front. Neuroeng.* 3:3. doi: 10.3389/fneng.2010.00003

Chen, D., Apple, D. F., Hudson, L. M., and Bode, R. (1999). Medical complications during acute rehabilitation following spinal cord injury—current experience of the Model Systems. *Arch. Phys. Med. Rehabil.* 80, 1397–1401.

Chen, J. J., Yu, N. Y., Huang, D. G., Ann, B. T., and Chang, G. C. (1997). Applying fuzzy logic to control cycling movement induced by functional electrical stimu-lation. *IEEE Trans. Rehabil. Eng.* 5, 158–169. doi: 10.1109/86.593285

Cheung, K. C. (2007). Implantable microscale neural interfaces. *Biomed. Microdevices* 9, 923–938. doi: 10.1007/s10544-006-9045-z

Cheung, K. C., Renaud, P., Tanila, H., and Djupsund, K. (2007). Flexible polyimide microelectrode array for *in vivo* recordings and current source density analysis. *Biosens. Bioelectron.* 22, 1783–1790. doi: 10.1016/j.bios.2006.08.035

Chizek, H. J., Kobetic, R., and Marsolais, E. B. (1988). *Control of Functional Neuromuscular Stimulation Systems for Standing and Locomotion in Paraplegics.* Washington, DC: IEEE.

Collinger, J. L., Vinjamuri, R., Degenhart, A. D., Weber, D. J., Sudre, G. P., Boninger, L., et al. (2014). Motor-related brain activity during action observation: a neural substrate for electrocorticographic brain-computer interfaces after spinal cord injury. *Front. Integr. Neurosci.* 8:17. doi: 10.3389/fnint.2014.00017

Crago, P. E., Peckham, P. H., and Thrope, G. B. (1980). Modulation of muscle force by recruitment during intramuscular stimulation. *IEEE Trans. Biomed. Eng.* 27, 679–684. doi: 10.1109/TBME.1980.326592

Creasey, G. H., and Craggs, M. D. (2012). Functional electrical stimulation for bladder, bowel, and sexual function. *Handb.*

Clin. Neurol. 109, 247–257. doi: 10.1016/B978-0-444-52137-8.00015-2

Daly, J. J., Cheng, R., Rogers, J., Litinas, K., Hrovat, K., and Dohring, M. (2009). Feasibility of a new application of noninvasive Brain Computer Interface (BCI): a case study of training for recovery of volitional motor control after stroke. *J. Neurol. Phys. Ther.* 33, 203–211. doi: 10.1097/NPT.0b013e3181c1fc0b

Davoodi, R., and Andrews, B. J. (1998). Computer simulation of FES standing up in paraplegia: a self-adaptive fuzzy controller with reinforcement learning. *IEEE Trans. Rehabil. Eng.* 6, 151–161. doi: 10.1109/86.681180

Davoodi, R., and Andrews, B. J. (1999). Optimal control of FES-assisted standing up in paraplegia using genetic algorithms. *Med. Eng. Phys.* 21, 609–617. doi: 10.1016/S1350-4533(99)00093-4

Demuth, H., and Beale, M. (2000). *Neural Network Toolbox: For Use with MATLAB.* Natick, MA: The Mathworks, Inc.

DeVivo, M. J. (2012). Epidemiology of traumatic spinal cord injury: trends and future implications. *Spinal Cord* 50, 365–372. doi: 10.1038/sc.2011.178

Do, A. H., Wang, P. T., King, C. E., Abiri, A., and Nenadic, Z. (2011). Brain-computer interface controlled functional electrical stimulation sys-tem for ankle movement. *J. Neuroeng. Rehabil.* 8:49. doi: 10.1186/1743-0003-8-49

Dominici, N., Keller, U., Vallery, H., Friedli, L., van den Brand, R., Starkey, M. L., et al. (2012). Versatile robotic interface to evaluate, enable and train loco-motion and balance after neuromotor disorders. *Nat. Med.* 18, 1142–1147. doi: 10.1038/nm.2845

Durfee, W. K. (1989). Task-based methods for evaluating electrically stimulated antagonist muscle controllers. *IEEE Trans. Biomed. Eng.* 36, 309–321. doi: 10.1109/10.19852

Etlin, A., Finkel, E., Cherniak, M., Lev-Tov, A., and Anglister, L. (2014). The motor output of hindlimb innervating segments of the spinal cord is modulated by cholinergic activation of rostrally projecting sacral relay neurons. *J. Mol. Neurosci.* 53, 517–524. doi: 10.1007/s12031-014-0351-2

Fifer, M. S., Acharya, S., Benz, H. L., Mollazadeh, M., Crone, N. E., and Thakor, V. (2012).

Toward electrocorticographic control of a dexterous upper limb prosthesis: building brain-machine interfaces. *IEEE Pulse* 3, 38–42. doi: 10.1109/MPUL.2011.2175636

Fisher, L. E., Miller, M. E., Bailey, S. N., Davis, J. A., Anderson, J. S., Rhode, L., et al. (2008). Standing after spinal cord injury with four-contact nerve-cuff electrodes for quadriceps stimulation. *IEEE Trans. Neural Syst. Rehabil. Eng.* 16, 473–478. doi: 10.1109/TNSRE.2008.2003390

Fisher, L. E., Tyler, D. J., Anderson, J. S., and Triolo, R. J. (2009). Chronic stability and selectivity of four-contact spiral nerve-cuff electrodes in stimu-lating the human femoral nerve. *J. Neural Eng.* 6:046010. doi: 10.1088/1741-2560/6/4/046010

Fitzgerald, P. J. (2014). Is elevated norepinephrine an etiological factor in some cases of Parkinson's disease? *Med. Hypotheses* 82, 462–469. doi: 10.1016/j.mehy.2014.01.026

Fraix, V., Houeto, J.-L., Lagrange, C., Le Pen, C., Krystkowiak, P., Guehl, D., et al. (2006). Clinical and economic results of bilateral subthalamic nucleus stimu-lation in Parkinson's disease. *J. Neurol. Neurosurg. Psychiatr.* 77, 443–449. doi: 10.1136/jnnp.2005.077677

Fujita, K., Shiga, K., and Takahashi, H. (1998). "Learning control of hand posture with neural network in FES for hemiplegics," in *IEEE* (Hong Kong), 2588–2589. Funahashi, K.-I. (1989). On the approximate realization of continuous map-pings by neural networks. *Neural Netw.* 2, 183–192. doi: 10.1016/0893-6080(89)90003-8

Galvani, L., and Aldini, G. (1792). *De Viribus Electricitatis in Motu Musculari Commentarius.* Bologna: Ex typographia Instituti Scientiarum.

Gan, L. S., Ravid, E., Kowalczewski, J. A., Olson, J. L., Morhart, M., and Prochazka, A. (2012). First permanent implant of nerve stimulation leads activated by surface electrodes, enabling hand grasp and release: the stim-ulus router neuroprosthesis. *Neurorehabil. Neural Repair* 26, 335–343. doi: 10.1177/1545968311420443

Georgopoulos, A. P., Schwartz, A. B., and Kettner, R. E. (1986). Neuronal popula-tion coding of movement direction. *Science* 233, 1416–1419. doi: 10.1126/sci-ence.3749885

Gerasimenko, Y., Roy, R. R., and Edgerton, V. R. (2008). Epidural stimulation: com-parison of

the spinal circuits that generate and control locomotion in rats, cats and humans. *Exp. Neurol.* 209, 417–425. doi: 10.1016/j.expneurol.2007.07.015

Giszter, S. F., Mussa-Ivaldi, F. A., and Bizzi, E. (1993). Convergent force fields organized in the frog's spinal cord. *J. Neurosci.* 13, 467–491.

Glenn, W. W., Holcomb, W. G., Shaw, R. K., Hogan, J. F., and Holschuh, K. R. (1976). Long-term ventilatory support by diaphragm pacing in quadriplegia. *Ann. Surg.* 183, 566–577. doi: 10.1097/00000658-197605000-00014

Gorman, P. H. (2000). An update on functional electrical stimulation after spinal cord injury. *Neurorehabil. Neural Repair* 14, 251–263.

Grant, P. F., and Lowery, M. M. (2013). Simulation of cortico-basal ganglia oscilla-tions and their suppression by closed loop deep brain stimulation. *IEEE Trans. Neural Syst. Rehabil. Eng.* 21, 584–594. doi: 10.1109/TNSRE.2012.2202403

Graupe, D., and Kordylewski, H. (1995). Artificial neural network control of FES in paraplegics for patient responsive ambulation. *IEEE Trans. Biomed. Eng.* 42, 699–707. doi: 10.1109/10.391169

Griessenauer, C. J., Chang, S.-Y., Tye, S. J., Kimble, C. J., Bennet, K. E., Garris, P. A., et al. (2010). Wireless Instantaneous neurotransmitter con-centration system: electrochemical monitoring of serotonin using fast-scan cyclic voltammetry-a proof-of-principle study. *J. Neurosurg.* 113, 656–665. doi: 10.3171/2010.3.JNS091627

Grobelnik, S. (1973). Functional electrical stimulation—a new hope for paraplegic patients? *Bull. Prosthet. Res.* 75–102.

Guertin, P. A. (2014). Preclinical evidence supporting the clinical development of central pattern generator-modulating therapies for chronic spinal cord-injured patients. *Front. Hum. Neurosci.* 8:272. doi: 10.3389/fnhum.2014.00272

Guiraud, D., Stieglitz, T., Koch, K. P., Divoux, J.-L., and Rabischong, P. (2006). An implantable neuroprosthesis for standing and walking in paraplegia: 5-year patient follow-up. *J. Neural Eng.* 3, 268–275. doi: 10.1088/1741-2560/3/4/003

Gustafsson, B., and Jankowska, E. (1976). Direct and indirect activation of nerve cells by electrical pulses applied extracellularly. *J. Physiol.* 258, 33–61.

Hachmann, J. T., Jeong, J. H., Grahn, P. J., Mallory, G. W., Evertz, L. Q., Bieber, A. J., et al. (2013). Large animal model for development of functional restoration paradigms using epidural and intraspinal stimulation. *PLoS ONE* 8:e81443. doi: 10.1371/journal.pone.0081443

Hambrecht, F. T. (1992). "A brief history of neural prostheses for motor control of paralyzed extremeties," in *Neural Prostheses: Replacing Motor Function After Disease or Disability*, eds R. B. Stein, P. H. Peckham and D. Popović (Oxford, UK: Oxford University Press), 3–14.

Harkema, S., Gerasimenko, Y., Hodes, J., Burdick, J., Angeli, C., Chen, Y., et al. (2011). Effect of epidural stimulation of the lumbosacral spinal cord on volun-tary movement, standing, and assisted stepping after motor complete paraple-gia: a case study. *Lancet* 377, 1938–1947. doi: 10.1016/S0140-6736(11)60547-3

Hassoun, M. H. (1995). *Fundamentals of Artificial Neural Networks.* Google Books. Hayashibe, M., Zhang, Q., Guiraud, D., and Fattal, C. (2011). Evoked EMG-based torque prediction under muscle fatigue in implanted neural stimulation. *J. Neural Eng.* 8:064001. doi: 10.1088/1741-2560/8/6/064001

Hirokawa, S., Grimm, M., Le, T., Solomonow, M., Baratte, R. V., Shoji, H., et al. (1990). Energy consumption in paraplegic ambulation using the reciprocat-ing gait orthosis and electric stimulation of the thigh muscles. *Arch. Phys. Med. Rehabil.* 71, 687–694.

Hobby, J., Taylor, P. N., and Esnouf, J. (2001). Restoration of tetraplegic hand function by use of the neurocontrol freehand system. *J. Hand Surg. Br.* 26, 459–464. doi: 10.1054/jhsb.2001.0587

Hochberg, L. R., Bacher, D., Jarosiewicz, B., Masse, N. Y., Simeral, J. D., Vogel, J., et al. (2012). Reach and grasp by people with tetraplegia using a neurally controlled robotic arm. *Nature* 485, 372–375. doi: 10.1038/nature11076

Hochberg, L. R., Serruya, M. D., Friehs, G. M., Mukand, J. A., Saleh, M., Caplan, A. H., et al. (2006). Neuronal ensemble control of prosthetic devices by a human with tetraplegia. *Nature* 442, 164–171. doi: 10.1038/nature04970

Hoffer, J. A., Stein, R. B., Haugland, M. K., Sinkjaer, T., Durfee, W. K., Schwartz, A. B., et al. (1996). Neural signals for command control and feedback in functional neuromuscular stimulation: a review. *J. Rehabil. Res. Dev.* 33, 145–157.

Holinski, B. J., Everaert, D. G., Mushahwar, V. K., and Stein, R. B. (2013). Real-time control of walking using recordings from dorsal root ganglia. *J. Neural Eng.* 10:056008. doi: 10.1088/1741-2560/10/5/056008

Holinski, B. J., Mazurek, K. A., Everaert, D. G. K., Stein, R. B., and Mushahwar, V. K. (2011). Restoring stepping after spinal cord injury using intraspinal microstim-ulation and novel control strategies. *Conf. Proc. IEEE Eng. Med. Biol. Soc.* 2011, 5798–5801. doi: 10.1109/IEMBS.2011.6091435

Hornik, K., Stinchcombe, M., and White, H. (1989). Multilayer feedforward net-works are universal approximators. *Neural Netw.* 2, 359–366. doi: 10.1016/0893-6080(89)90020-8

Hughes, B. W., Kusner, L. L., and Kaminski, H. J. (2006). Molecular architecture of theneuromuscular junction. *Muscle Nerve* 33, 445–461. doi: 10.1002/mus.20440

Jackson, A., Mavoori, J., and Fetz, E. E. (2006). Long-term motor cortex plas-ticity induced by an electronic neural implant. *Nature* 444, 56–60. doi: 10.1038/nature05226

Jackson, A., and Zimmermann, J. B. (2012). Neural interfaces for the brain and spinal cord—restoring motor function. *Nat. Rev. Neurol.* 8, 690–699. doi: 10.1038/nrneurol.2012.219

Jankowska, E., and Roberts, W. J. (1972a). An electrophysiological demonstration of the axonal projections of single spinal interneurons in the cat. *J. Physiol.* 222, 597–622.

Jankowska, E., and Roberts, W. J. (1972b). Synaptic actions of single interneurones mediating reciprocal Ia inhibition of motorneurones. *J. Physiol.* 222, 623–642.

Jilge, B., Minassian, K., Rattay, F., Pinter, M. M., Gerstenbrand, F., Binder, H., et al. (2004). Initiating extension of the lower limbs in subjects with complete spinal cord injury by epidural lumbar cord stimulation. *Exp. Brain Res.* 154, 308–326. doi: 10.1007/s00221-003-1666-3

Jonić, S., Janković, T., Gajiœ, V., and Popović, D. (1999). Three machine learning techniques for automatic determination of rules to control locomotion. *IEEE Trans. Biomed. Eng.* 46, 300–310. doi: 10.1109/10.748983

Kaneyuki, T., Hogan, J. F., Glenn, W., and Holcomb, W. G. (1977). Diaphragm pacing. Evaluation of current waveforms for effective ventilation. *J. Thorac. Cardiovasc. Surg.* 74, 109–115.

Karniel, A., and Inbar, G. F. (2000). Human motor control: learning to control a time-varying, nonlinear, many-to-one system. *IEEE Trans. Syst. Man Cybern.* 30, 1–11. doi: 10.1109/5326.827449

Kasten, M. R., Sunshine, M. D., Secrist, E. S., Horner, P. J., and Moritz, C. T. (2013). Therapeutic intraspinal microstimulation improves forelimb function after cervical contusion injury. *J. Neural Eng.* 10:044001. doi: 10.1088/1741-2560/10/4/044001

Kent, A. R., and Grill, W. M. (2013). Model-based analysis and design of nerve cuff electrodes for restoring bladder function by selective stimulation of the pudendal nerve. *J. Neural Eng.* 10:036010. doi: 10.1088/1741-2560/10/3/036010

Kilgore, K. L., Hoyen, H. A., Bryden, A. M., Hart, R. L., Keith, M. W., and Peckham, P. H. (2008). An implanted upper-extremity neuroprosthesis using myoelectric control. *J. Hand Surg. Am.* 33, 539–550. doi: 10.1016/j.jhsa.2008.01.007

Kilgore, K. L., Peckham, P., and Keith, M. W. (2009). Twenty year experience with implanted neuroprostheses. *Conf. Proc. IEEE Eng. Med. Biol. Soc.* 2009, 7212–7215. doi: 10.1109/IEMBS.2009.5335272

Knutson, J. S., Naples, G. G., Peckham, P. H., and Keith, M. W. (2002). Electrode fracture rates and occurrences of infection and granuloma associated with percutaneous intramuscular electrodes in upper-limb functional electrical stim-ulation applications. *J. Rehabil. Res. Dev.* 39, 671–683.

Kobravi, H.-R., and Erfanian, A. (2012). A decentralized adaptive fuzzy robust strategy for control of upright standing posture in paraplegia using functional electrical stimulation. *Med. Eng. Phys.* 34, 28–37. doi: 10.1016/j.medengphy.2011.06.013

Kostov, A., Andrews, B. J., Popović, D. B., Stein, R. B., and Armstrong, W. W. (1995). Machine learning in control of functional electrical stimulation sys-tems for locomotion. *IEEE Trans. Biomed. Eng.* 42, 541–551. doi: 10.1109/10.387193

Kowalski, K. C., He, B. D., and Srinivasan, L. (2013). Dynamic analysis of naive adaptive brain-machine interfaces. *Neural Comput.* 25, 2373–2420. doi: 10.1162/NECO_a_00484

Krajl, A., Bajd, T., Turk, R., and Benko, H. (1986). Posture switching for prolonging functional electrical stimulation standing in paraplegic patients. *Paraplegia* 24, 221–230. doi: 10.1038/sc.1986.31

Kralj, A., Bajd, T., and Turk, R. (1988). Enhancement of gait restoration in spinal injured patients by functional electrical stimulation. *Clin. Orthop. Relat. Res.* 233, 34. doi: 10.1097/00003086-198808000-00006

Kralj, A. R., and Bajd, T. (1989). *Functional Electrical Stimulation: Standing and Walking After Spinal Cord Injury.* Google Books.

Lan, N., Feng, H. Q., and Crago, P. E. (1994). Neural network generation of muscle stimulation patterns for control of arm movements. *IEEE Trans. Rehab. Eng.* 2, 213–224. doi: 10.1109/86.340877

Langhals, N. B., and Kipke, D. R. (2009). Validation of a novel three-dimensional electrode array within auditory cortex. *Conf. Proc. IEEE Eng. Med. Biol. Soc.* 2009, 2066–2069. doi: 10.1109/IEMBS.2009.5333958

Lau, B., Guevremont, L., and Mushahwar, V. K. (2007). Strategies for generating prolonged functional standing using intramuscular stimulation or intraspinal microstimulation. *IEEE Trans. Neural Syst. Rehabil. Eng.* 15, 273–285. doi: 10.1109/TNSRE.2007.897030

Lavrov, I., Courtine, G., Dy, C. J., van den Brand, R., Fong, A. J., Gerasimenko, Y., et al. (2008). Facilitation of stepping with epidural stimu-lation in spinal rats: role of sensory input. *J. Neurosci.* 28, 7774–7780. doi: 10.1523/JNEUROSCI.1069-08.2008

Lee, K. H., Blaha, C. D., Garris, P. A., Mohseni, P., Horne, A. E., Bennet, K. E., et al. (2009). Evolution of deep brain stimulation: human electrometer and smart devices supporting the next generation of therapy. *Neuromodulation* 12, 85–103. doi: 10.1111/j.1525-1403.2009.00199.x

Lee, K. H., Blaha, C. D., Harris, B. T., Cooper, S., Hitti, F. L., Leiter, J. C., et al. (2006). Dopamine efflux in the rat striatum evoked by electrical stimulation of the subthalamic nucleus: potential mechanism of action in Parkinson's disease. *Eur. J. Neurosci.* 23, 1005–1014. doi: 10.1111/j.1460-9568.2006.04638.x

Lee, K. H., Chang, S.-Y., Roberts, D. W., and Kim, U. (2004). Neurotransmitter release from high-frequency stimulation of the subthalamic nucleus. *J. Neurosurg.* 101, 511–517. doi: 10.3171/jns.2004.101.3.0511

Lemay, M. A., Galagan, J. E., Hogan, N., and Bizzi, E. (2001). Modulation and vectorial summation of the spinalized frog's hindlimb end-point force produced by intraspinal electrical stimulation of the cord. *IEEE Trans. Neural Syst. Rehabil. Eng.* 9, 12–23. doi: 10.1109/7333.918272

Lemay, M. A., Grasse, D., and Grill, W. M. (2009). Hindlimb Endpoint forces predict movement direction evoked by intraspinal microstimulation in cats. *IEEE Trans. Neural Syst. Rehabil. Eng.* 17, 379–389. doi: 10.1109/TNSRE.2009.2023295

Lemay, M. A., and Grill, W. M. (2004). Modularity of motor output evoked by intraspinal microstimulation in cats. *J. Neurophysiol.* 91, 502–514. doi: 10.1152/jn.00235.2003

Lenehan, B., Street, J., Kwon, B. K., Noonan, V., Zhang, H., Fisher, C. G., et al. (2012). The epidemiology of traumatic spinal cord injury in British Columbia, Canada. *Spine* 37, 321–329. doi: 10.1097/BRS.0b013e31822e5ff8

Leuthardt, E. C., Schalk, G., Wolpaw, J. R., Ojemann, J. G., and Moran, D. W. (2004). A brain-computer interface using electrocorticographic signals in humans. *J. Neural Eng.* 1, 63–71. doi: 10.1088/1741-2560/1/2/001

Lobel, D. A., and Lee, K. H. (2014). Brain machine interface and limb reanimation technologies: restoring function after spinal cord injury through development of a bypass system. *Mayo Clin. Proc.* 89, 708–714. doi: 10.1016/j.mayocp.2014.02.003

Logothetis, N. K. (2003a). MR imaging in the non-human primate: studies of function and of dynamic connectivity. *Curr. Opin. Neurobiol.* 13, 630–642. doi: 10.1016/j.conb.2003.09.017

Logothetis, N. K. (2003b). The underpinnings of the BOLD functional magnetic resonance imaging signal. *J. Neurosci.* 23, 3963–3971.

Lujan, J. L., and Crago, P. E. (2009). Automated optimal coordination of multiple-DOF neuromuscular actions in feedforward neuroprostheses. *IEEE Trans. Biomed. Eng.* 56, 179–187. doi: 10.1109/TBME.2008.2002159

MacDonald, A. A., Monchi, O., Seergobin, K. N., Ganjavi, H., Tamjeedi, R., and MacDonald, P. A. (2013). Parkinson's disease duration determines effect of dopaminergic therapy on ventral striatum function. *Mov. Disord.* 28, 153–160. doi: 10.1002/mds.25152

Mahajan, P., Jaffe, D. M., Olsen, C. S., Leonard, J. R., Nigrovic, L. E., Rogers, A. J., et al. (2013). Spinal cord injury without radiologic abnormality in chil-dren imaged with magnetic resonance imaging. *J. Trauma Acute Care Surg.* 75, 843–847. doi: 10.1097/TA.0b013e3182a74abd

Malezic, M., Stanic, U., Kljajić, M., Acimović, R., Krajnik, J., Gros, N., et al. (1984). Multichannel electrical stimulation of gait in motor disabled patients. *Orthopedics* 7, 1187–1195.

Mangold, S., Keller, T., Curt, A., and Dietz, V. (2005). Transcutaneous functional electrical stimulation for grasping in subjects with cervical spinal cord injury. *Spinal Cord* 43, 1–13. doi: 10.1038/sj.sc.3101644

Marino, R. J., Barros, T., Biering-Sorensen, F., Burns, S. P., Donovan, W. H., Graves, D. E., et al. (2003). International standards for neurological classification of spinal cord injury. *J. Spinal Cord Med.* 26(Suppl. 1), S50–S56.

Marsolais, E. B., and Kobetic, R. (1986). Implantation techniques and experience with percutaneous intramuscular electrodes in the lower extremities. *J. Rehabil. Res. Dev.* 23, 1–8.

McDonald, J. W., and Sadowsky, C. (2002). Spinal-cord injury. *Lancet* 359, 417–425. doi: 10.1016/S0140-6736(02)07603-1

McDonnall, D., Clark, G. A., and Normann, R. A. (2004). Interleaved, multisite electrical stimulation of cat sciatic nerve produces fatigue-resistant, ripple-free motor responses. *IEEE Trans. Neural Syst. Rehabil. Eng.* 12, 208–215. doi: 10.1109/TNSRE.2004.828425

Meriney, S. D., and Dittrich, M. (2013). Organization and function of transmitter release sites at the neuromuscular junction. *J. Physiol.* 591, 3159–3165. doi: 10.1113/jphysiol.2012.248625

Miller, K. J., Schalk, G., Fetz, E. E., den Nijs, M., Ojemann, J. G., and Rao, R. P. N. (2010). Cortical activity during motor execution, motor imagery, and imagery-based online feedback. *Proc. Natl. Acad. Sci. U.S.A.* 107, 4430–4435. doi: 10.1073/pnas.0913697107

Minassian, K., Jilge, B., Rattay, F., Pinter, M. M., Binder, H., Gerstenbrand, F., et al. (2004). Stepping-like movements in humans with complete spinal

cord injury induced by epidural stimulation of the lumbar cord: electromyographic study of compound muscle action potentials. *Spinal Cord* 42, 401–416. doi: 10.1038/sj.sc.3101615

Minassian, K., Persy, I., Rattay, F., Pinter, M. M., Kern, H., and Dimitrijevic, M. R. (2007). Human lumbar cord circuitries can be activated by extrinsic tonic input to generate locomotor-like activity. *Hum. Mov. Sci.* 26, 275–295. doi: 10.1016/j.humov.2007.01.005

Mirovsky, Y., Shalmon, E., Blankstein, A., and Halperin, N. (2005). Complete para-plegia following gunshot injury without direct trauma to the cord. *Spine* 30, 2436–2438. doi: 10.1097/01.brs.0000184588.54710.61

Molinuevo, J. L., Valldeoriola, F., Tolosa, E., Rumia, J., Valls-Sole, J., Roldan, H., et al. (2000). Levodopa withdrawal after bilateral subthalamic nucleus stimulation in advanced Parkinson disease. *Arch. Neurol.* 57, 983–988. doi: 10.1001/archneur.57.7.983

Moran, D. (2010). Evolution of brain–computer interface: action potentials, local field potentials and electrocorticograms. *Curr. Opin. Neurobiol.* 20, 741–745. doi: 10.1016/j.conb.2010.09.010

Moritz, C. T., Lucas, T. H., Perlmutter, S. I., and Fetz, E. E. (2007). Forelimb move-ments and muscle responses evoked by microstimulation of cervical spinal cord in sedated monkeys. *J. Neurophysiol.* 97, 110–120. doi: 10.1152/jn.00414.2006

Moritz, C. T., Perlmutter, S. I., and Fetz, E. E. (2008). Direct control of paralysed muscles by cortical neurons. *Nature* 456, 639–642. doi: 10.1038/nature07418

Moro, E., Scerrati, M., Romito, L. M., Roselli, R., Tonali, P., and Albanese, A. (1999). Chronic subthalamic nucleus stimulation reduces medication requirements in Parkinson's disease. *Neurology* 53, 85–90. doi: 10.1212/WNL.53.1.85

Müller-Putz, G. R., Scherer, R., Pfurtscheller, G., and Rupp, R. (2005). EEG-based neuroprosthesis control: a step towards clinical practice. *Neurosci. Lett.* 382, 169–174. doi: 10.1016/j.neulet.2005.03.021

Musallam, S., Corneil, B. D., Greger, B., Scherberger, H., and Andersen, R. A. (2004). Cognitive control signals for neural prosthetics. *Science* 305, 258–262. doi: 10.1126/science.1097938

Mushahwar, V. (2000). Spinal cord microstimulation generates

functional limb movements in chronically implanted cats. *Exp. Neurol.* 163, 422–429. doi: 10.1006/exnr.2000.7381

Mushahwar, V. K., Gillard, D. M., Gauthier, M. J. A., and Prochazka, A. (2002). Intraspinal micro stimulation generates locomotor-like and feedback-controlled movements. *IEEE Trans. Neural Syst. Rehabil. Eng.* 10, 68–81. doi: 10.1109/TNSRE.2002.1021588

Mushahwar, V. K., and Horch, K. W. (1997). Proposed specifications for a lumbar spinal cord electrode array for control of lower extremities in paraplegia. *IEEE Trans. Rehabil. Eng.* 5, 237–243. doi: 10.1109/86.623015

Mushahwar, V. K., and Horch, K. W. (2000a). Muscle recruitment through electrical stimulation of the lumbo-sacral spinal cord. *IEEE Trans. Rehabil. Eng.* 8, 22–29. doi: 10.1109/86.830945

Mushahwar, V. K., and Horch, K. W. (2000b). Selective activation of muscle groups in the feline hindlimb through electrical microstimulation of the ventral lumbo-sacral spinal cord. *IEEE Trans. Rehabil. Eng.* 8, 11–21. doi: 10.1109/86.830944

Mushahwar, V. K., Jacobs, P. L., Normann, R. A., Triolo, R. J., and Kleitman, N. (2007). New functional electrical stimulation approaches to standing and walking. *J. Neural Eng.* 4, S181–S197. doi: 10.1088/1741-2560/4/3/S05

Narendra, K. S. (1990). *Neural Networks for Control.*—Google Books. Narendra, K. S. (1996). Neural networks for control theory and practice. *Proc. IEEE* 84, 1385–1406. doi: 10.1109/5.537106

Narendra, K. S., and Parthasarathy, K. (1990). Identification and control of dynam-ical systems using neural networks. *IEEE Trans. Neural Netw.* 1, 4–27. doi: 10.1109/72.80202

Nataraj, R., Audu, M. L., and Triolo, R. J. (2013). Center of mass acceleration feedback control of standing balance by functional neuromuscular stimulation against external postural perturbations. *IEEE Trans. Biomed. Eng.* 60, 10–19. doi: 10.1109/TBME.2012.2218601

National Institute of Neurological Disorders and Stroke. (2013). *National Institute of Neurological Disorders and Stroke.* National Institutes of Health. Available online at: http://www.ninds.nih.gov/disorders/sci/detail_sci.htm (Accessed May 30, 2014).

National Spinal Cord Injury Statistical Center. (2013). Spinal cord injury

facts and figures at a glance. *J. Spinal Cord Med.* 36, 1–2. doi: 10.1179/1079026813Z.00000000 0136

Nicolas-Alonso, L. F., and Gomez-Gil, J. (2012). Brain computer interfaces, a review. *Sensors (Basel)* 12, 1211–1279. doi: 10.3390/s120201211

Niddam, D. M., Graven-Nielsen, T., Arendt-Nielsen, L., and Chen, A. C. (2001). Non-painful and painful surface and intramuscular electrical stimulation at the thenar and hypothenar sites: differential cerebral dynamics of early to late latency SEPs. *Brain Topogr.* 13, 283–292. doi: 10.1023/A:1011180713285

Nishimura, Y., Perlmutter, S. I., and Fetz, E. E. (2013). Restoration of upper limb movement via artificial corticospinal and musculospinal connections in a monkey with spinal cord injury. *Front. Neural Circuits* 7, 1–9. doi: 10.3389/fncir.2013.00057

Pang, D., and Wilberger, J. E. (1982). Spinal cord injury without radio-graphic abnormalities in children. *J. Neurosurg.* 57, 114–129. doi: 10.3171/jns.1982.57.1.0114

Peckham, P. H., Keith, M. W., Kilgore, K. L., Grill, J. H., Wuolle, K. S., Thrope, G. B., et al. (2001). Efficacy of an implanted neuroprosthesis for restoring hand grasp in tetraplegia: a multicenter study. *Arch. Phys. Med. Rehabil.* 82, 1380–1388. doi: 10.1053/apmr.2001.25910

Peckham, P. H., and Kilgore, K. L. (2013). Challenges and opportunities in restoring function after paralysis. *IEEE Trans. Biomed. Eng.* 60, 602–609. doi: 10.1109/TBME.2013.2245128

Peckham, P. H., Kilgore, K. L., Keith, M. W., and Bryden, A. M. (2002). An advanced neuroprosthesis for restoration of hand and upper arm con-trol using an implantable controller. *J. Hand Surg. Am.* 27, 265–276. doi: 10.1053/jhsu.2002.30919

Peckham, P. H., and Knutson, J. S. (2005). Functional electrical stimulation for neuromuscular applications. *Annu. Rev. Biomed. Eng.* 7, 327–360. doi: 10.1146/annurev.bioeng.6.040803.140103

Pfurtscheller, G., Müller, G. R., Pfurtscheller, J., Gerner, H. J., and Rupp, R. (2003). "Thought"—control of functional electrical stimulation to restore hand grasp in a patient with tetraplegia. *Neurosci. Lett.* 351, 33–36. doi: 10.1016/S0304-3940(03)00947-9

Phillips, W. T., Kiratli, B. J., Sarkarati, M., Weraarchakul, G., Myers, J., Franklin, B. A., et al. (1998). Effect of spinal cord injury on the heart and cardiovascular fitness. *Curr. Probl. Cardiol.* 23, 641–716. doi: 10.1016/S0146-2806(98)80003-0 Piche, S. W. (1994). Steepest descent algorithms for neural network controllers and filters. *IEEE Trans. Neural Netw.* 5, 198–212. doi: 10.1109/72.279185

Pikov, V., Bullara, L., and McCreery, D. B. (2007). Intraspinal stimulation for blad-der voiding in cats before and after chronic spinal cord injury. *J. Neural Eng.* 4, 356–368. doi: 10.1088/1741-2560/4/4/002

Polasek, K. H., Schiefer, M. A., Pinault, G. C. J., Triolo, R. J., and Tyler, D. J. (2009). Intraoperative evaluation of the spiral nerve cuff electrode on the femoral nerve trunk. *J. Neural Eng.* 6:066005. doi: 10.1088/1741-2560/6/6/066005

Polikov, V. S., Tresco, P. A., and Reichert, W. M. (2005). Response of brain tissue to chronically implanted neural electrodes. *J. Neurosci. Methods* 148, 1–18. doi: 10.1016/j.jneumeth.2005.08.015

Popović, M. R., Popović, D. B., and Keller, T. (2002). Neuroprostheses for grasping. *Neurol. Res.* 24, 443–452. doi: 10.1179/016164102101200311

Popovic, M. R., Thrasher, T. A., Adams, M. E., Takes, V., Zivanovic, V., and Tonack, M. I. (2005). Functional electrical therapy: retraining grasping in spinal cord injury. *Spinal Cord* 44, 143–151. doi: 10.1038/sj.sc.3101822

Posluszny, J. A. Jr., Onders, R., Kerwin, A. J., Weinstein, M. S., Stein, D. M., Knight, J., et al. (2014). Multicenter review of diaphragm pacing in spinal cord injury. *J. Trauma Acute Care Surg.* 76, 303–310. doi: 10.1097/TA.0000000000000112

Rabischong, E., and Ohanna, F. (1992). Effects of functional electrical stimulation (FES) on evoked muscular output in paraplegic quadriceps muscle. *Paraplegia* 30, 467–473. doi: 10.1038/sc.1992.100

Rack, P. M., and Westbury, D. R. (1969). The effects of length and stimulus rate on tension in the isometric cat soleus muscle. *J. Physiol.* 204, 443–460.

Ragnarsson, K. T. (2008). Functional electrical stimulation after spinal cord injury: current use, therapeutic effects and future directions. *Spinal Cord* 46, 255–274. doi: 10.1038/sj.sc.3102091

Renshaw, B. (1946). Interaction of nerve impulses in the gray matter as a mecha-nism in central inhibition. *Fed. Proc.* 5:86.

Riess, J., and Abbas, J. J. (2000). Adaptive neural network control of cyclic move-ments using functional neuromuscular stimulation. *IEEE Trans. Rehabil. Eng.* 8, 42–52. doi: 10.1109/86.830948

Riess, J., and Abbas, J. J. (2001). Adaptive control of cyclic movements as muscles fatigue using functional neuromuscular stimulation. *IEEE Trans. Neural Syst. Rehabil. Eng.* 9, 326–330. doi: 10.1109/7333.948462

Riess, J. A., and Abbas, J. J. (1999). "Control of cyclic movements as muscles fatigue using functional neuromuscular stimulation," in *IEEE* (Atlanta, GA), 659.

Roham, M., Halpern, J. M., Martin, H. B., Chiel, H. J., and Mohseni, P. (2007). Diamond microelectrodes and CMOS microelectronics for wireless transmis-sion of fast-scan cyclic voltammetry. *Conf. Proc. IEEE Eng. Med. Biol. Soc.* 2007, 6044–6047.

Rosa, M., Giannicola, G., Marceglia, S., Fumagalli, M., Barbieri, S., and Priori, A. (2012). *Neurophysiology of Deep Brain Stimulation*, 1st Edn. Oxford, UK: Elsevier Inc.

Rosin, B., Slovik, M., Mitelman, R., Rivlin-Etzion, M., Haber, S. N., Israel, Z., et al. (2011). Closed-loop deep brain stimulationis superior in ameliorating parkinsonism. *Neuron* 72, 370–384. doi: 10.1016/j.neuron.2011.08.023

Rowland, L. P. (1991). "Clinical syndromes of the spinal cord and brain stem," in *Principles of Neural Science*, eds E. Kandel, J. Schwartz, and T. Jessell (East Norwalk, CT: Appleton & Lange), 711–731.

Saigal, R., Renzi, C., and Mushahwar, V. K. (2004). Intraspinal microstimulation generates functional movements after spinal-cord injury. *IEEE Trans. Neural Syst. Rehabil. Eng.* 12, 430–440. doi: 10.1109/TNSRE.2004.837754

Saltiel, P., Wyler-Duda, K., D'Avella, A., Tresch, M. C., and Bizzi, E. (2001). Muscle synergies encoded within the spinal cord: evidence from focal intraspinal NMDA iontophoresis in the frog. *J. Neurophysiol.* 85, 605–619.

Schalk, G., Miller, K. J., Anderson, N. R., Wilson, J. A., Smyth, M. D., Ojemann, J. G., et al. (2008). Two-dimensional movement control using electrocorticographic signals in humans. *J. Neural Eng.* 5, 75–84. doi: 10.1088/1741-2560/5/1/008

Schmit, B. D., and Mortimer, J. T. (1997). The tissue response to epimysial elec-trodes for diaphragm pacing in dogs. *IEEE Trans. Biomed. Eng.* 44, 921–930. doi: 10.1109/10.634644

Schwartz, A. B., Cui, X. T., Weber, D. J., and Moran, D. W. (2006). Brain-controlled interfaces: movement restoration with neural prosthetics. *Neuron* 52, 205–220. doi: 10.1016/j.neuron.2006.09.019

Scivoletto, G., Tamburella, F., Laurenza, L., Torre, M., and Molinari, M. (2014). Who is going to walk? A review of the factors influencing walking recovery after spinal cord injury. *Front. Hum. Neurosci.* 8:141. doi: 10.3389/fnhum.2014.00141

Scremin, A. E., Kurta, L., Gentili, A., and Wiseman, B. (1999). Increasing mus-cle mass in spinal cord injured persons with a functional electrical stimulation exercise program. *Arch. Phys. Med. Rehabil.* 80, 1531–1536. doi: 10.1016/s0003-9993(99)90326-X

Sekhon, L. H., and Fehlings, M. G. (2001). Epidemiology, demographics, and pathophysiology of acute spinal cord injury. *Spine* 26, S2–S12. doi: 10.1097/00007632-200112151-00002

Serruya, M. D., Hatsopoulos, N. G., Paninski, L., Fellows, M. R., and Donoghue, J. P. (2002). Instant neural control of a movement signal. *Nature* 416, 141–142. doi: 10.1038/416141a

Shadmehr, R., Smith, M. A., and Krakauer, J. W. (2010). Error correction, sensory prediction, and adaptation in motor control. *Annu. Rev. Neurosci.* 33, 89–108. doi: 10.1146/annurev-neuro-060909-153135

Sharma, A., Rieth, L., Tathireddy, P., Harrison, R., Oppermann, H., Klein, M., et al. (2011). Long term *in vitro* functional stability and recording longevity of fully integrated wireless neural interfaces based on the Utah Slant Electrode Array. *J. Neural Eng.* 8:045004. doi: 10.1088/1741-2560/8/4/045004

Sharma, A., Rieth, L., Tathireddy, P., Harrison, R., and Solzbacher, F. (2010). Long term *in vitro* stability of fully integrated wireless neural interfaces based on Utah slant electrode array. *Appl. Phys. Lett.* 96, 73702. doi: 10.1063/1.3318251

Shih, J. J., Krusienski, D. J., and Wolpaw, J. R. (2012). Brain-computer interfaces in medicine. *Mayo Clinic Proc.* 87, 268–279. doi: 10.1016/j.mayocp.2011.12.008

Shon, Y.-M., Chang, S.-Y., Tye, S. J., Kimble, C. J., Bennet, K. E., Blaha, C. D., et al. (2010a). Comonitoring of adenosine and dopamine using the wireless instanta-neous neurotransmitter concentration system: proof of principle. *J. Neurosurg.* 112, 539–548. doi: 10.3171/2009.7.JNS09787

Shon, Y.-M., Lee, K. H., Goerss, S. J., Kim, I. Y., Kimble, C., Van Gompel, J. J., et al. (2010b). High frequency stimulation of the subthalamic nucleus evokes striatal dopamine release in a large animal model of human DBS neurosurgery. *Neurosci. Lett.* 475, 136–140. doi: 10.1016/j.neulet.2010.03.060

Sinkjaer, T. (2000). Integrating sensory nerve signals into neural prosthesis devices. *Neuromodulation* 3, 34–41. doi: 10.1046/j.1525-1403.2000.00035.x

Skarpaas, T. L., and Morrell, M. J. (2009). Intracranial stimulation therapy for epilepsy. *Neurotherapeutics* 6, 238–243. doi: 10.1016/j.nurt.2009.01.022

Slutzky, M. W., Jordan, L. R., Krieg, T., Chen, M., Mogul, D. J., and Miller, L. E. (2010). Optimal spacing of surface electrode arrays for brain-machine interface applications. *J. Neural Eng.* 7:26004. doi: 10.1088/1741-2560/7/2/026004

Stanic, U., Acimović-Janezic, R., Gros, N., Trnkoczy, A., Bajd, T., and Kljajić, M. (1978). Multichannel electrical stimulation for correction of hemiplegic gait. Methodology and preliminary results. *Scand. J. Rehabil. Med.* 10, 75–92.

Stein, R. B., Charles, D., Davis, L., Jhamandas, J., Mannard, A., and Nichols, T. R. (1975). Principles underlying new methods for chronic neural recording. *Can. J. Neurol. Sci.* 2, 235–244.

Strange, K. D., and Hoffer, J. A. (1999). Restoration of use of paralyzed limb muscles using sensory nerve signals for state control of FES-assisted walking. *IEEE Trans. Rehabil. Eng.* 7, 289–300. doi: 10.1109/86.788466

Suner, S., Fellows, M. R., Vargas-Irwin, C., Nakata, G. K., and Donoghue, J. P. (2005). Reliability of signals from a chronically implanted, silicon-based elec-trode array in non-human primate primary motor cortex. *IEEE Trans. Neural Syst. Rehabil. Eng.* 13, 524–541. doi: 10.1109/TNSRE.2005.857687

Sunshine, M. D., Cho, F. S., Lockwood, D. R., Fechko, A. S., Kasten, M. R., and Moritz, C. T. (2013). Cervical intraspinal microstimulation evokes robust forelimb movements before and after injury. *J. Neural Eng.* 10:036001. doi: 10.1088/1741-2560/10/3/036001

Tai, C., Booth, A. M., Robinson, C. J., de Groat, W. C., and Roppolo, J. R. (2000). Multimicroelectrode stimulation within the cat L6 spinal cord: influences of electrode combinations and stimulus interleave time on knee joint extension torque. *IEEE Trans. Rehabil. Eng.* 8, 1–10. doi: 10.1109/86. 830943

Takmakov, P., Zachek, M. K., Keithley, R. B., Walsh, P. L., Donley, C., McCarty, G. S., et al. (2010). Carbon microelectrodes with a renewable surface. *Anal. Chem.* 82, 2020–2028. doi: 10.1021/ ac902753x

Tan, W., Zou, Q., Kim, E. S., and Loeb, G. E. (2004). "Sensing human arm posture with implantable sensors," in *IEEE* (San Francisco, CA), 4290–4293.

Tanae, H., Holcomb, W. G., Yasuda, R., Hogan, J. F., and Glenn, W. W. (1973). Electrical nerve fatigue: advantages of an alternating bidirectional waveform. *J. Surg. Res.* 15, 14–21. doi: 10.1016/0022-4804(73)90158-3

Taylor, D. M., Tillery, S. I. H., and Schwartz, A. B. (2002). Direct cortical control of 3D neuroprosthetic devices. *Science* 296, 1829–1832. doi: 10.1126/science.1070291

Teixeira, E., Jayaraman, G., Shue, G., Crago, P. E., Loparo, K., and Chizek, H. J. (1991). "Feedback control of nonlinear multiplicative system using neural networks: an application to electrically stimulated Muscle," in *IEEE* (Dayton, OH), 1–3.

Tresch, M. C., and Bizzi, E. (1999). Responses to spinal microstimulation in the chronically spinalized rat and their relationship to spinal systems activated by low threshold cutaneous stimulation. *Exp. Brain Res.* 129, 401–416. doi: 10.1007/s002210050908

Triolo, R. J., Bieri, C., Uhlir, J., Kobetic, R., Scheiner, A., and Marsolais, E. B. (1996). Implanted functional neuromuscular stimulation systems for individuals with cervical spinal cord injuries: clinical case reports. *Arch. Phys. Med. Rehabil.* 77, 1119–1128.

Triolo, R. J., Liu, M. Q., Kobetic, R., and Uhlir, J. P. (2001). Selectivity of intra-muscular stimulating electrodes in the lower limbs. *J. Rehabil. Res. Dev.* 38, 533–544.

van den Brand, R., Heutschi, J., Barraud, Q., DiGiovanna, J., Bartholdi, K., Huerlimann, M., et al. (2012). Restoring voluntary control of locomotion after paralyzing spinal cord injury. *Science* 336, 1182–1185. doi: 10.1126/sci-ence.1217416

Wang, W., Collinger, J. L., Degenhart, A. D., Tyler-Kabara, E. C., Schwartz, A. B., Moran, D. W., et al. (2013). An electrocorticographic brain interface in an individual with Tetraplegia. *PLoS ONE* 8:e55344. doi: 10.1371/jour-nal.pone.0055344

Wang, W., Degenhart, A. D., Collinger, J. L., Vinjamuri, R., Sudre, G. P., Adelson, P. D., et al. (2009). Human motor cortical activity recorded with Micro-ECoG electrodes, during individual finger movements. *Conf. Proc. IEEE Eng. Med. Biol. Soc.* 2009, 586–589. doi: 10.1109/IEMBS.2009. 5333704

Wang, W., Sudre, G. P., Xu, Y., Kass, R. E., Collinger, J. L., Degenhart, A. D., et al. (2010). Decoding and cortical source localization for intended movement direc-tion with MEG. *J. Neurophysiol.* 104, 2451–2461. doi: 10.1152/ jn.00239.2010

Watson, C., Paxinos, G., and Kayalioglu, G. (2009). *The Spinal Cord.* London: Academic Press. Wessberg, J., Stambaugh, C. R., Kralik, J. D., Beck, P. D., Laubach, M., Chapin, J. K., et al. (2000). Real-time prediction of hand trajectory by ensembles of cortical neurons in primates. *Nature* 408, 361–365. doi: 10.1038/35042582

Wilson, J. A., Felton, E. A., Garell, P. C., Schalk, G., and Williams, J. C. (2006). ECoG factors underlying multimodal control of a brain-computer interface. *IEEE Trans. Neural Syst. Rehabil. Eng.* 14, 246–250. doi: 10.1109/ TNSRE.2006. 875570

Yakovenko, S., Kowalczewski, J., and Prochazka, A. (2007). Intraspinal stimulation caudal to spinal cord transections in rats. Testing the propriospinal hypothesis. *J. Neurophysiol.* 97, 2570–2574. doi: 10.1152/jn.00814.2006

Yanagisawa, T., Hirata, M., Saitoh, Y., Goto, T., Kishima, H., Fukuma, R., et al. (2011). Real-time control of a prosthetic hand using human electrocorticog-raphy signals. *J. Neurosurg.* 114, 1715–1722. doi: 10.3171/2011.1.JNS101421

Yang, L., Wilke, C., Brinkmann, B., Worrell, G. A., and He, B. (2011). Dynamic imaging of ictal oscillations using non-invasive high-resolution EEG. *Neuroimage* 56, 1908–1917. doi: 10.1016/j. neuroimage.2011.03.043

Yoshida, N., Tomita, Y., Honda, S., and Saitoh, E. (2002). Functional neuromus-cular stimulation for articular angle control with an inverse dynamics model tuned by a neural network. *Ergonomics* 45, 649–662. doi: 10.1080/00140130210 142074

Zhang, Q., Hayashibe, M., and Azevedo-Coste, C. (2013). Evoked electromyography-based closed-loop torque control in functional electrical stimulation. *IEEE Trans. Biomed. Eng.* 60, 2299–2307. doi: 10.1109/TBME.2013.2253777

Modular neuronal assemblies embodied in a closed-loop environment: toward future integration of brains and machines

Jacopo Tessadori[1], Marta Bisio[1], Sergio Martinoia[1,2] and Michela Chiappalone[1]*

[1] Department of Neuroscience and Brain Technologies, Istituto Italiano di Tecnologia, Genova, Italy
[2] Department of Informatics, Bioengineering, Robotics and System Engineering, University of Genova, Genova, Italy

Edited by:
Ahmed El Hady, Max Planck Institute for Dynamics and Self Organization, Germany

Reviewed by:
Guo-Qiang Bi, University of Pittsburgh, USA
Wolfgang Stein, Illinois State University, USA

*Correspondence:
Michela Chiappalone, NeuroTech Unit, Department of Neuroscience and Brain Technologies, Istituto Italiano di Tecnologia, Via Morego 30, 16163 Genova, Italy.
e-mail: michela.chiappalone@iit.it

Behaviors, from simple to most complex, require a two-way interaction with the environment and the contribution of different brain areas depending on the orchestrated activation of neuronal assemblies. In this work we present a new hybrid neuro-robotic architecture based on a neural controller bi-directionally connected to a virtual robot implementing a Braitenberg vehicle aimed at avoiding obstacles. The robot is characterized by proximity sensors and wheels, allowing it to navigate into a circular arena with obstacles of different sizes. As neural controller, we used hippocampal cultures dissociated from embryonic rats and kept alive over Micro Electrode Arrays (MEAs) for 3–8 weeks. The developed software architecture guarantees a bi-directional exchange of information between the natural and the artificial part by means of simple linear coding/decoding schemes. We used two different kinds of experimental preparation: "random" and "modular" populations. In the second case, the confinement was assured by a polydimethylsiloxane (PDMS) mask placed over the surface of the MEA device, thus defining two populations interconnected via specific microchannels. The main results of our study are: (i) neuronal cultures can be successfully interfaced to an artificial agent; (ii) modular networks show a different dynamics with respect to random culture, both in terms of spontaneous and evoked electrophysiological patterns; (iii) the robot performs better if a reinforcement learning paradigm (i.e., a tetanic stimulation delivered to the network following each collision) is activated, regardless of the modularity of the culture; (iv) the robot controlled by the modular network further enhances its capabilities in avoiding obstacles during the short-term plasticity trial. The developed paradigm offers a new framework for studying, in simplified model systems, neuro-artificial bi-directional interfaces for the development of new strategies for brain-machine interaction.

Keywords: bi-directional, *in vitro*, hippocampal cultures, confinement, micro electrode array, robot

INTRODUCTION

Algorithms based on classical models of computation cannot compare with living beings capabilities in terms of dealing with unexpected situations. Different fields of study, such as developmental biology (West-Eberhard, 2003; Gilbert, 2009), embodied cognition (Clark, 1997), evolutionary robotics (Bongard, 2011), seem to indicate as a likely cause for this shortcoming the lack of a developmental phase in traditional silicon-based technology. This process is especially evident in the Central Nervous System (CNS), where morphological changes, both reversible and permanent, occur on a wide range of different time scales. One possible way to deal with this issue is the realization of hybrid systems, where biological components could be exploited for their plastic properties.

In the recent past, several different hybrid model systems have been developed (DeMarse et al., 2001; Martinoia et al., 2004; Mussa-Ivaldi et al., 2010; Warwick et al., 2010; Kudoh et al., 2011), consisting of living neurons coupled to a robotic system.

This solution allows the use of an artificial body whose dynamics can be easily and completely modeled, as opposed to the case of even the simplest animals. Furthermore, the exchange of information in a hybrid system can be limited to the desired level of complexity.

Following this "embodied neurophysiology" approach, we built a closed-loop electrophysiological system by interfacing a virtual mobile robot with a population of neurons, extracted from rat embryos and cultured over Micro Electrode Arrays (MEA; Novellino et al., 2007). The proposed paradigm represents an innovative, simplified, and controllable closed-loop system where it is possible to investigate the dynamic and adaptive properties of a neural population interacting with an external environment by means of an artificial body (i.e., the mobile robot). The main innovations of this experimental setup are: (i) the flexible software architecture at the base of the closed-loop experiments, here described in detail; (ii) the introduction of a modular network design. Starting from the observation of the high degree of modularity in the brain, different studies point out how such a property is likely to have a profound impact on neural activity (Hubel et al., 1977; Sporns et al., 2000; Derdikman et al., 2003; Kumar et al., 2010; Pan et al., 2010; Boucsein et al., 2011). In this work, we took advantage of the modular structure of the network to obtain a better separation between interacting cell assemblies. A significant improvement to previous works would be the added capability of inducing plastic changes in a controlled fashion. A step in this direction is taken in this setup by the use of a tetanic stimulation to enhance interconnected pathways to improve robot behavior (Jimbo et al., 1999; Chiappalone et al., 2008), following a collision with an obstacle. It is worth pointing out that the final objective of this work is not to achieve the best possible control of the robot: excluding any biological component would, at this stage, easily provide better performance and more reliable results. What is being developed here is groundwork for the integration of electronic systems and neural networks, with the twofold long-term objectives of taking advantage of neural plasticity in more complex control systems and performing closed-loops experiment to gage the computational and learning properties of relatively simple neural preparations.

MATERIALS AND METHODS

The setup developed for experiments of embodied electrophysiology is characterized by several different software, hardware and wetware components (**Figure 1**). The wetware part consists of hippocampal neurons cultured onto a standard 60-electrode MEA. The front-end electronics are constituted by a MEA1060-Inv-BC amplification system (Multichannel Systems, MCS, Reutlingen, Germany) and the computer used is a desktop machine (Dell Precision T5500, 2.66 GHz, 3.43 GB RAM) equipped with a DAQ E NI6255 (National Instruments, Austin, TX, USA) data acquisition board. An *ad hoc* adaptor was realized to interface the DAQ board with the amplification system. The software used for the

management and acquisition is HyBrain2, a specifically developed software based on what is described in a previous work (Mulas et al., 2010): it allows control of all the parameters of the neurorobotics experiments and performs the required data processing, such as the implementation of the coding, decoding and short-term plasticity schemes. Information is sent to the culture as a series of electrical stimulations through a Stimulus Generator 4002 (Multichannel Systems). Three different robots can be used for the experiments: two physical ones (Khepera II and its successor Khepera III, from K-Team, Zi les Plains-Praz, Switzerland) and a virtual implementation within the HyBrain2 architecture. The relevant elements of the robot are a set of distance sensors and two independently controlled wheels. Both the physical and the virtual ones have a circular arena with obstacles to move in. In all of the experiments, the task the robot is trying to perform is obstacle avoidance. While both physical robots have been tested and are properly working within the setup, in the following, only experiments with the virtual one are reported. The main problems with the physical robot are the fact that it requires actual tracking from an image to compute its position (which is both machine-time consuming and occasionally fails) and the non-idealities of its sensors: among the other, ambient lighting conditions have an impact on the performance of the infrared distance sensor and it has been reputed unwise to add such a factor of unpredictability at this stage of the development.

NETWORK MODULE
Neuronal preparation: random and modular cultures
Dissociated neuronal cultures were prepared from hippocampi of 18-day-old embryonic rats (pregnant female rats were obtained from Charles River Laboratories). Culture preparation was performed as previously described (Frega et al., 2012). Briefly, the hippocampi of 4–5 embryos were dissected out from the brain and dissociated first by enzymatic digestion in trypsin solution

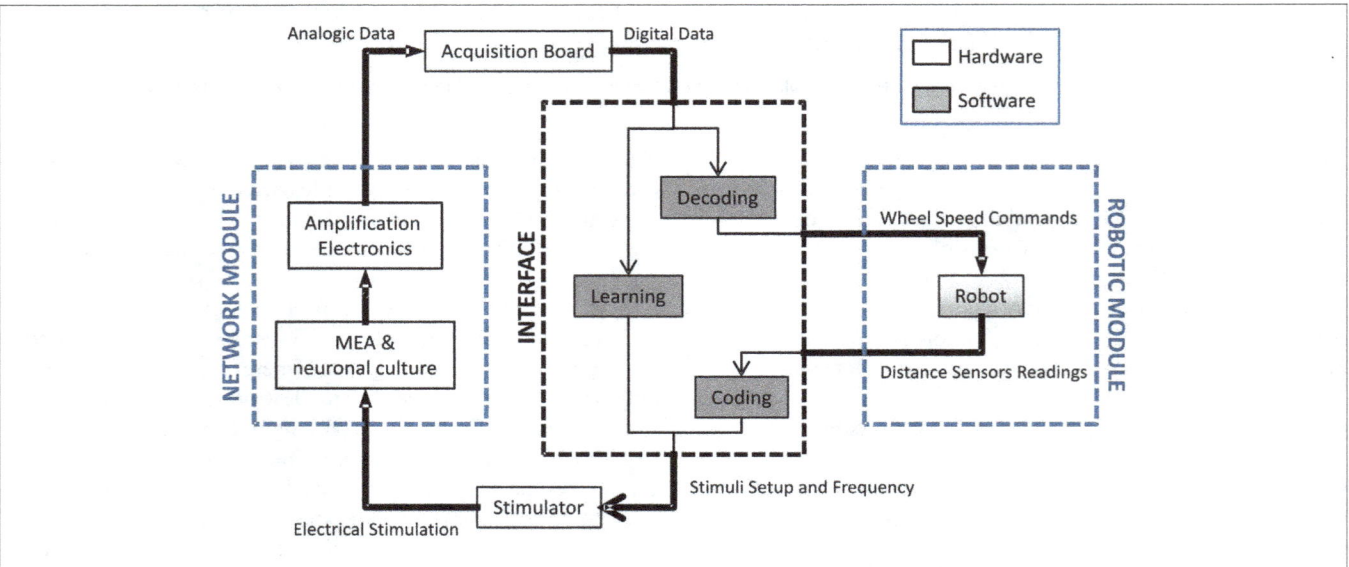

FIGURE 1 | Block diagram of the neuro-robotic architecture. From left to right: (i) the network module, constituted by a network of living neurons coupled to a micro electrode array; (ii) a computer which hosts the developed software tool (i.e., HyBrain2) which manages the communication between the biological and the artificial part; (iii) the robotic module composed by a robot, either real or virtual, with sensors and actuators navigating into a circular arena with obstacles.

0.125% (30 min at 37°C) and subsequently by mechanical disso-ciation with a fine-tipped Pasteur pipette. The resulting tissue was re-suspended in Neurobasal medium supplemented with 2% B-27, 1% Glutamax-I, 1% Pen-Strep solution, and 10% Fetal Bovine Serum (Invitrogen, Carlsbad, CA, USA), at the final concentration of 60 k cells/ml.

Cells were afterward plated onto standard 60-channel MEAs previously coated with poly-D-lysine and laminin to promote cell adhesion (final density around 1200 cells/mm^2) and maintained with 1 ml of nutrient medium (**Figures 2A,B**). They were then placed in a humidified incubator having an atmosphere of 5% CO_2 and 95% air at 37°C. Half of the medium was changed weekly. Recordings were performed on cultures between 20 and 60 days *in vitro* (DIVs).

Considering the multitude of connections that usually forms in a random culture, a way to better control the network complex-ity consists of imposing a constraint to the neuronal cells growth along specific pathways (Chang et al., 2001; Boehler et al., 2012). To do this, a dual-compartment chamber with two interconnecting microchannels has been realized in polydimethylsiloxane (PDMS), a biocompatible, inert, and non-toxic polymer often used to this extent (Raichman and Ben-Jacob, 2008; Levy et al., 2012). The realization of the modular structures has been realized by replica molding using specific master with a previously developed tech-nique (Berdondini et al., 2006). The obtained structures have been then placed on MEA substrates, in order to confine the growth of the neuronal cells that will be plated on it, as shown in **Figure 2B**.

Micro electrode arrays

Micro electrode arrays (Multichannel Systems, MCS, Reutlingen, Germany) consist of 60 TiN/SiN planar round electrodes (30 μm diameter; 200 μm center-to-center inter-electrode distance, see

Figure 2A) arranged in an 8 × 8 square grid excluding corners. In some devices, one recording electrode is replaced by a larger ground electrode. Each electrode provides information on the activity of the neural network in its immediate area. A microwire connects each micro electrode of the MEA to a different channel of a dedicated amplifying system with a gain of 1100. The ampli-fied 60-channel data is then conveyed to the data acquisition card which samples them at 10 kHz per channel and converts them into digital, 12 bit data (**Figures 2C,D**).

HYBRAIN2 SOFTWARE

The need for real-time access to data led to the adoption of a general-purpose acquisition card (NI6255, National Instruments, Austin, TX, USA) and required the development of a specific soft-ware: Hybrain2. The core of the program handles incoming data from the acquisition card and graphically displays them in a panel such as the one shown in **Figure 3A**. Spike detection options can be selected from this panel, such as threshold amplitudes or update times, as well as software blanking of stimulus arti-facts. While a rather sophisticated algorithm (i.e., SALPA filtering; Wagenaar and Potter, 2002) for blanking has been included and validated, it has not been used in the described experiments, as it tends to compete for CPU-time with the rest of the system, leading to occasional resource starvation. In its current version, Hybrain2 does not make use of raw data other than for displaying. Instead, incoming data is processed by a spike detection algo-rithm (Maccione et al., 2009) whose output is a series of time stamps.

As explained later in more detail, both the coding and decoding algorithms for the closed-loop control of the robot are rate-based, therefore spike time stamps are a lossless representation of incom-ing data. **Figure 3B** shows the panels used for configuration of

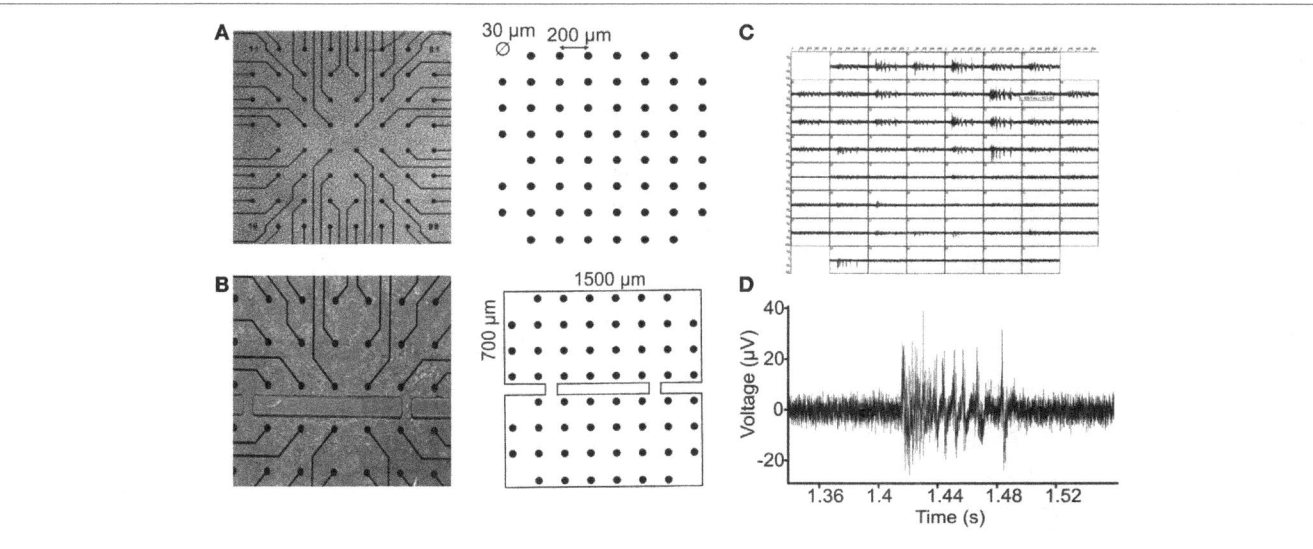

FIGURE 2 | Random and modular neuronal assemblies over micro electrode arrays. (A) On the left, a random culture grown on a standard MEA device. On the right, the MEA layout is shown: a squared matrix of 59 micro electrodes (the missing one is the reference electrode), in which the inter-electrode distance is 200 μm and the micro electrode diameter is 30 μm. **(B)** On the left, a confined culture on a MEA substrate. On the right, the bi-compartmental system realized in PDMS with two interconnection microchannels. Compartments height is 700 μm, and width is 1500 μm. Microchannels height is 100 μm, and width is 50 μm. **(C)** Spontaneous electrophysiological activity of a confined culture of hippocampal neurons, registered from all the micro electrodes. **(D)** A typical hippocampal burst waveform recorded from a single channel.

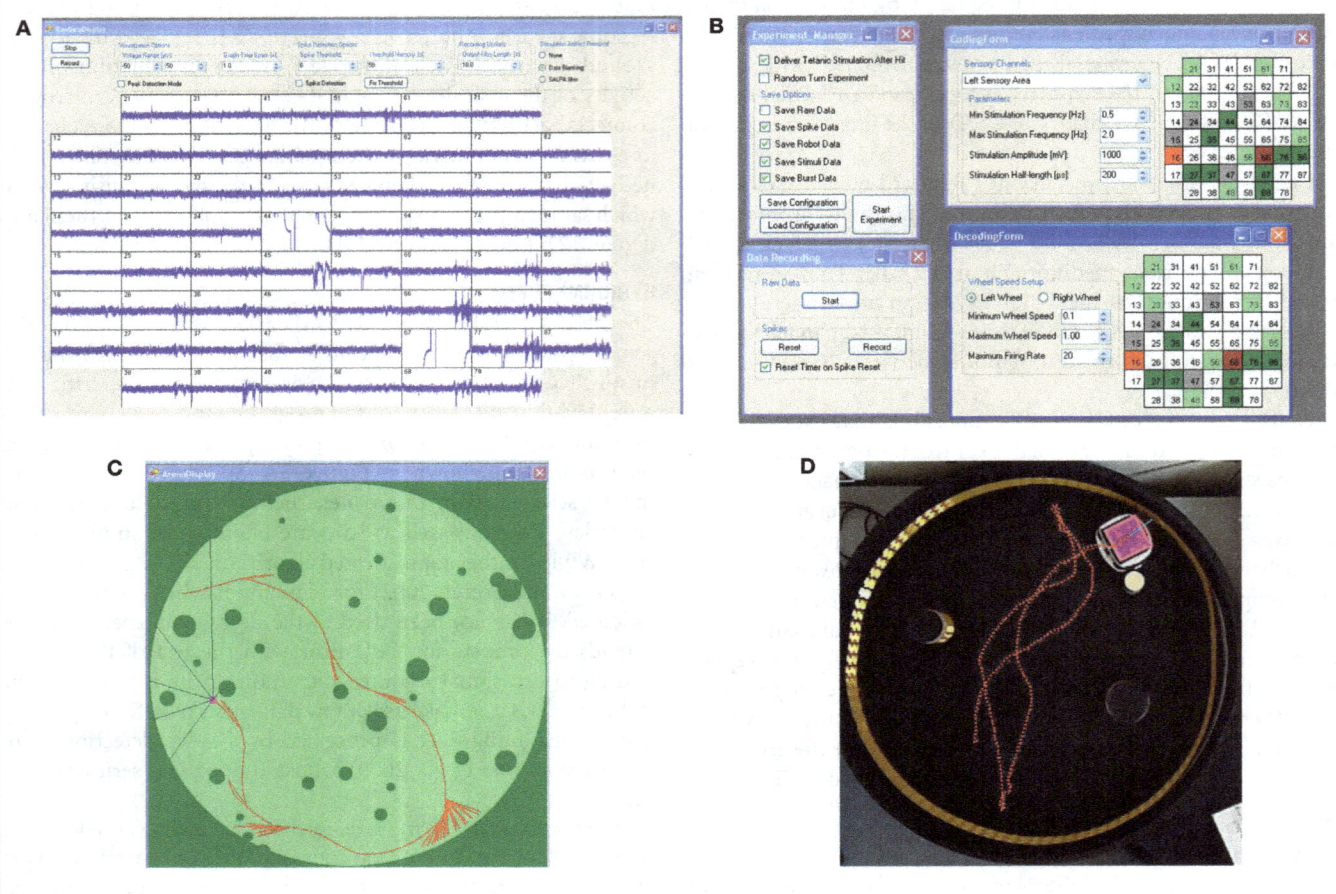

FIGURE 3 | Hybrain2 panels and robotic module. (A) Raw electrodes data display panel, including options for data visualization, artifact filtering, and spike detection. **(B)** Several panels allow the configuration of coding and decoding algorithms and saving of data during experiments. **(C)** The robot arena panel shows the environment of the arena. In the case of a virtual robot, this can also be used to draw the arena itself. **(D)** The physical robot inside the arena where two obstacles are placed. The dotted red line represents the trajectory of the robot inside the arena.

the parameters of these algorithms, such as selection of recording and stimulation electrodes, pulses amplitudes and lengths, and maximum and minimum allowed wheel speeds for the robot.

A module of the software is dedicated to managing the robot itself: in **Figure 3C**, a sample experiment with a virtual robot is shown. Here, the software is generating the robot environment as well as controlling all the relevant parameters of the robot itself, while, in the case of a physical robot (such as that in **Figure 3D**), the software provides a simple tracking feature on images provided by a webcam positioned over the arena and the required communication with the robot itself. All the data produced during experiments, including electrode readings, time stamps, and robot navigation data can be stored for later analysis both in text and/or binary format, while common parameters configurations can be saved and loaded in order to minimize experiment setup times and human errors.

ROBOTIC MODULE

The robot, either virtual or physical, is basically a two-wheeled sensor platform: six infrared sensors are mounted on the robot at different angles, providing information about the distance of surrounding objects in different directions, whereas the speed profile of each wheel determine the direction and velocity of the robot itself.

The arena consists of an enclosed space containing several different round obstacles in random positions and the robot. A typical experiment with the virtual robot is shown in **Figure 3C**: the robot is moving in a 400 × 400 pixels circular arena, where dark green pixels represent obstacles or arena walls, whereas light green pixels are free for the robot to move in. The robot (small pink circle) is collecting information about its environment through its six sensors: each black line departing from the robot represents the line of sight of a different sensor; their angles are fixed with respect to the robot heading (in this case, 30°, 45°, and 90° on both sides of the robot direction), while the length of each line is equal to the distance from the robot center to the closest obstacle in the sensor direction. This distance defines the reading of the sensor: the output is 0 if the robot is in direct contact with an obstacle, 1 if the closest obstacle is at the maximum distance possible (the diameter of the arena, in this case). The three sensor readings on each side are averaged to provide the neuronal network with a single value per side.

In the case shown in **Figure 3C**, the robot is performing an obstacle avoidance task, as can be inferred by the red trajectory. The speed of a wheel is inversely proportional to the average of the sensor readings on the same-side, therefore the robot turns away from close obstacles. The ideal behavior of the robot is that of a Braitenberg vehicle (Braitenberg, 1984) in the case of no loss of information and no significant delays between sensor data collection and motor command execution. Obtaining a behavior as close as possible to this one is the goal of the coding-decoding-short-term plasticity process implemented here.

During experiments, collisions with obstacles or walls are unavoidable: following such an event, the robot moves back to a previous position in its path, at a fixed distance from any obstacle.

INTERFACING THE NETWORK AND THE ROBOTIC MODULE
Decoding scheme
Although many different decoding schemes are possible, so far the only one implemented has been a frequency rate-based algorithm (Adrian, 1928; Rieke et al., 1997; Martinoia et al., 2004). For this scheme, only a feature of the recorded signals is useful: the frequency of spikes at each location. A group of electrodes (i.e., a sub-population of neurons) on the MEA is selected and defined as the "output area" through the procedure described in the Section "Experimental protocol." The number of spikes occurring over that area in 100 ms, non-overlapping windows constitutes the basis for calculating the motor signal for the corresponding wheel. In the current architecture, a linear relation is implemented between wheel speed and motor signal: if no spikes are detected in a time window, the corresponding wheel turns at a set minimum speed, increasing linearly with the number of detected spikes, up to a defined maximum rate. A low-pass filtering effect is added by taking into account previous samples, in order to smooth robot movements.

Dissociated neural networks are especially prone to bursting (Chiappalone et al., 2006) and this pattern of activity has been shown to code different information than just the sum of its spikes (Cozzi et al., 2006). A module for the detection of bursts has been already added to the Hybrain2 software, but its output is not yet part of the control loop of the robot.

For each wheel, the speed is therefore defined as:

$$\omega_i = \begin{cases} \frac{f_{i,t} + f_{i,t-1}}{2 f_i^{MAX}} \left(\omega_i^{MAX} - \omega_i^{min} \right) + \omega_i^{min} & \text{for } f_i < f_i^{MAX} \\ \omega_i^{MAX} & \text{for } f_i \geq f_i^{MAX} \end{cases}$$

where subscript i denotes wheel side, ω is the wheel speed, and f_i,t is the averaged firing rate over all the electrodes corresponding to the i-th recording area at time sample t. ω^{MAX}, ω^{min}, and f^{MAX} are parameters set by the experimenter before the start of the experiment.

Coding scheme
Likewise, the coding scheme is linear and rate-based: two groups of electrodes are defined as "input areas" and assigned to the sensors on the left and right side of the robot body. The details for area selection are fully explained in the Section "Experimental Protocol." Each sensor provides a reading, normalized to 1 for an object in direct contact with the robot and 0 for an object at the far end of the designed arena (while this behavior is nearly ideal for the virtual robot, it is far from so in the case of the physical robot, as already mentioned in the Section "Materials and Methods." The readings from the sensors on the same-side of the robot are then averaged and coded back to the corresponding sensory area. As mentioned before, the coding is linear and frequency based: a fixed stimulus is delivered at the sensory area at a frequency directly proportional to the averaged, same-side sensors readings. The stimulation rate for each input region is determined as:

$$s_i = \left(s_i^{MAX} - s_i^{min} \right) r_i + s_i^{min}$$

where s_i is the stimulation rate of the i-th input area and r_i the normalized average of all the sensor readings on the corresponding side of the robots, whereas s_i^{MAX} s_i^{min} are user-set parameters fixing the maximum and minimum stimulation rate.

Short-term plasticity protocol
In order to progress toward the desired behavior, it is necessary to define a learning rule that allows a modification of connectivity between input and output areas by rewarding "good behavior," while discouraging "bad behavior." The effect of tetanic stimulation in these networks was already demonstrated by our group and by others in the past, showing that a 20 Hz stimulation should strengthen the synaptic connections of receiving neurons (Jimbo et al., 1999; Tateno and Jimbo, 1999; Madhavan et al., 2007; Chiappalone et al., 2008; le Feber et al., 2010). In all these papers the effect of the tetanus on the change of firing rate was studied in a time frame comparable to that of our experiments (30 min to 1 h). Additionally, in a previous paper from our group (Chiappalone et al., 2008), we were able to demonstrate that a single tetanic shock to a neuronal network had an immediate effect in terms of increase in the Post Stimulus Time Histograms (PSTH) area (i.e., increase in the number of spikes evoked by a stimulus), a medium-term effect (i.e., few hours after the tetanus delivery), and a long-term effect (i.e., 1 day after the tetanus delivery).

The above observations have been used to define the learning rule in the current implementation of the software: following each robot collision, a 2-s-long, 20 Hz stimulation is delivered to the same-side input area. The rationale for this choice is that collisions are usually caused by poor correlation between stimulation in an input area and detected activity in the corresponding output area, thus making the network responses to stimulation insufficient to steer the robot in the correct direction. Our hypothesis is that tetanic stimulation strengthens all participating connections, thus correcting the problem, as demonstrated in the studies cited above. A tetanic stimulation induces short-term plasticity effects which allow the groups of neurons involved in the obstacle avoidance tasks to fire at a higher frequency, thus inducing the corresponding wheel to increase the angular velocity. Since input-output regions were selected according to connection strength (see Experimental Protocol below), this should increase responses detected from the desired electrodes upon delivery of a stimulus from the input electrodes. This bring to a generalized strengthening of connections in the network and to an improvement in the driving of the robot.

ON-LINE PROCESSING OF ELECTROPHYSIOLOGICAL SIGNALS
Spike detection
The electrophysiological signals acquired from MEA electrodes must be preprocessed in order to remove the stimulus artifact and to isolate spikes from noise. The spike detection algorithm uses a differential peak-to-peak threshold to follow the variability of the signal and a set of controls are performed in order to make the algorithm as reliable as possible (Maccione et al., 2009). The threshold is proportional to noise SD and is calculated separately for each individual channel (typically as six or seven times SD) before the beginning of the actual experiment (i.e., during phase 1 of the protocol described below).

Blanking of stimulus artifact
Stimulus artifacts are detected when the recorded signal exceeds a defined threshold much higher than the one used for spike detection. The artifact is then suppressed by canceling the first samples in the spike train occurring immediately after it, corresponding to a signal blanking of 4 ms after stimulus delivery.

EXPERIMENTAL PROTOCOL
The typical experimental protocol followed in this work consists of a five-step procedure:

1. Monitoring of the spontaneous activity of the culture;
2. Test stimulus from a set of electrodes in order to choose the I/O of the network, necessary for the connection with the robot;
3. 20-min run without short-term plasticity protocol
4. 20-min run with short-term plasticity protocol
5. Evaluation of the robot's performances on the basis of specific navigation's parameters.

During the first step of the experimental session, spontaneous activity of the network is subject to observation, in order to determine, empirically, which electrodes are the most likely candidate as "input" sites (i.e., sites from which stimulation must be delivered). Typical features to look for in this phase are a sustained mean firing rate (i.e., sufficient number of spikes per second, usually higher than 0.1 spikes/s) and patterns of activity not synchronous with other regions. The best candidates (usually a set of 8–10 sites) are then selected for the second step of the experiment. From each of the candidate "input" channel, in turn, a 500-μs, 1.5 V peak-to-peak, bipolar square wave is delivered every 5 s, until a total of 40 stimuli per channels have been delivered, while spiking activity is detected from other electrodes.

At the end of this phase, for every stimulation electrode involved, 59 PSTH are generated (Chiappalone et al., 2007): these graphs report the average number of spikes detected from each electrode in the 600 ms following each stimulation and therefore provide information on the strength of the connections in the culture. Through a custom-made script developed in the Matlab environment (The Matworks, Natick, MA, USA), the generated PSTHs are then compared in order to look for areas that present a significant degree of specificity, i.e., where responses are not elicited by stimulation delivered from all the electrodes, but from some of them. In this way, it is possible to define an output (recording) area that will respond mostly to stimulation from the corresponding input area, while remaining silent during stimulation from the opposite input area (cf., see "Input and Output Sites of a Neuronal Population" of the Results).

During steps 3 and 4, the robot is left free to roam the arena with the rules described above, with a tetanic stimulus following each collision with an obstacle delivered during step 4. If the starting hypotheses hold true, this will progressively drive the network toward the desired condition of reliable and specific evoked responses.

Finally, we collect the data on the robot performances. In order to verify the neural-based behavior of the robot, we compared the results obtained (i) in a neuron-controlled experiment (a MEA with living neurons grown on, bi-directionally connected to the robot), (ii) in a open-loop experiment (a MEA with living neurons grown on, but without sensory feedback), and (iii) in an "empty" MEA experiment (a MEA with culturing medium only). In case (ii), the robot performs in a way imposed by the spontaneous firing rate of the neural network, usually in a random pattern, while in the case of the "empty" MEA (iii) the robot basically drives in a straight line (see the Supplementary Videos and Closed-Loop Robot Navigation of the Results).

DATABASE OF EXPERIMENTS, DATA ANALYSIS, AND STATISTICS
Experiments on a total of $N = 17$ different cultures, ranging from 20 to 60 DIV, have been conducted: 11 of those were random hippocampal cultures, while the other six experiments were conducted on hippocampal cultures, divided into sub-populations by a confinement mask, as described above. Those six cultures were also compared for spontaneous activity evaluation with a subset of six random cultures (age range of the subset: 21–42 DIV).

In order to highlight differences in term of synchronization between the two populations, a cross-correlation algorithm was applied to spike trains, a technique already introduced previously (Frega et al., 2012). Briefly, the cross-correlation function (i.e., cross-correlogram) is defined by the incidence of a spike at electrode y after that a spike was fired at electrode x. More specifically, given two spike trains (i.e., x and y) from two electrodes of a MEA, we count the number of spikes in the y train within a time frame around the spikes of the x train of $\pm T$ (in the order of tens of milliseconds), using bins of amplitude $\Delta \tau$ (usually set at multiple of the sampling frequency). The correct $C_{xy}(\tau)$ is obtained by means of a normalization procedure, by dividing each element of the array by the square root of the product between the number of peaks in the x and the y train. If the obtained $C_{xy}(\tau)$ shows a distribution that clearly deviated from flat, electrodes x and y are considered correlated. For each cross-correlogram $C_{xy}(\tau)$ we then estimated the coefficient C_{peak}. C_{peak} represents the value of the cross-correlogram in an area around the maximum detected peak and it is usually evaluated in order to quantify the *correlation level* among two recording channels. The statistical distribution of all C_{peak} values was computed for the two experimental groups during spontaneous activity (i.e., random vs. modular cultures). For each robot run, two different parameters have been computed in order to evaluate the performance of the robot, namely the average distance traveled by the robot between hits (measured in pixels) and the average number of hits per second. The virtual robot is implemented so that following a collision against an obstacle, it is immediately moved to the last location where its center was at least 20 pixels away from any other object. Since the robot radius is 5 pixels, the lower limit for the average distance traveled by the robot during each robot run is that of 15 pixels.

Statistical tests were employed to assess the significant difference among diverse experimental conditions. The normal distribution of experimental data was assessed using the Kolmogorov-Smirnov normality test. According to the distribution of the data, we performed either parametric (e.g., ANOVA, **Figure 7**) or non-parametric (e.g., Mann–Whitney U test, **Figures 4–6** and **8**) tests and p values < 0.05 were considered significant. Statistical analysis was carried out by using OriginPro (OriginLab Corporation, Northampton, MA, USA).

RESULTS

NETWORK DYNAMICS: SPONTANEOUS ACTIVITY IN RANDOM AND MODULAR NETWORKS

Hippocampal cultures grown *in vitro* over MEAs show a spontaneous (i.e., ongoing) activity, similar to that exhibited by *in vivo* systems during their development (Ben-Ari, 2001) or during deep sleep (Corner, 2008). Their electrophysiological behavior is characterized by spontaneous spiking which becomes synchronized with the maturation of the network, giving rise to phenomena called "bursts," network bursts (Pasquale et al., 2010) or network spikes (Eytan and Marom, 2006). These network bursts are the fingerprints of a steady-state in which the network dynamic found a

balance between excitation and inhibition (on average 70–80% of neurons are excitatory ones and the remaining 20–30% is constituted by inhibitory interneurons). Such state can be easily pharmacologically disrupted by acting on the glutamatergic as well as on the gabaergic receptors or by adding neuromodulators (Keefer et al., 2001; Eytan et al., 2004; Frega et al., 2012). Another possibility to alter such stereotyped behavior is to introduce modularity (i.e., interconnected populations) instead of having a single uniform and random culture (Raichman and Ben-Jacob, 2008; Shein Idelson et al., 2010; Kanagasabapathi et al., 2012).

Figure 4 shows the spontaneous activity from a representative random (**Figure 4A**, top) and a modular culture (**Figure 4A**, bottom) during the fourth week of development. While in the random culture the activity is highly synchronized and packed in the form of "network bursts" (van Pelt et al., 2004; Pasquale et al., 2010), in the modular culture we can identify two different temporal patterns of activity with moments of synchronized bursts interleaved with sparse spiking periods. Synchronized network bursts spread to the whole culture also in the modular networks, even if, globally, modular cultures are much less correlated than the random ones (**Figure 4B**).

NETWORK DYNAMICS: EVOKED ACTIVITY IN RANDOM AND MODULAR NETWORKS

It is possible to electrically modulate the activity of the network by means of electrical stimulation. The typical response of a

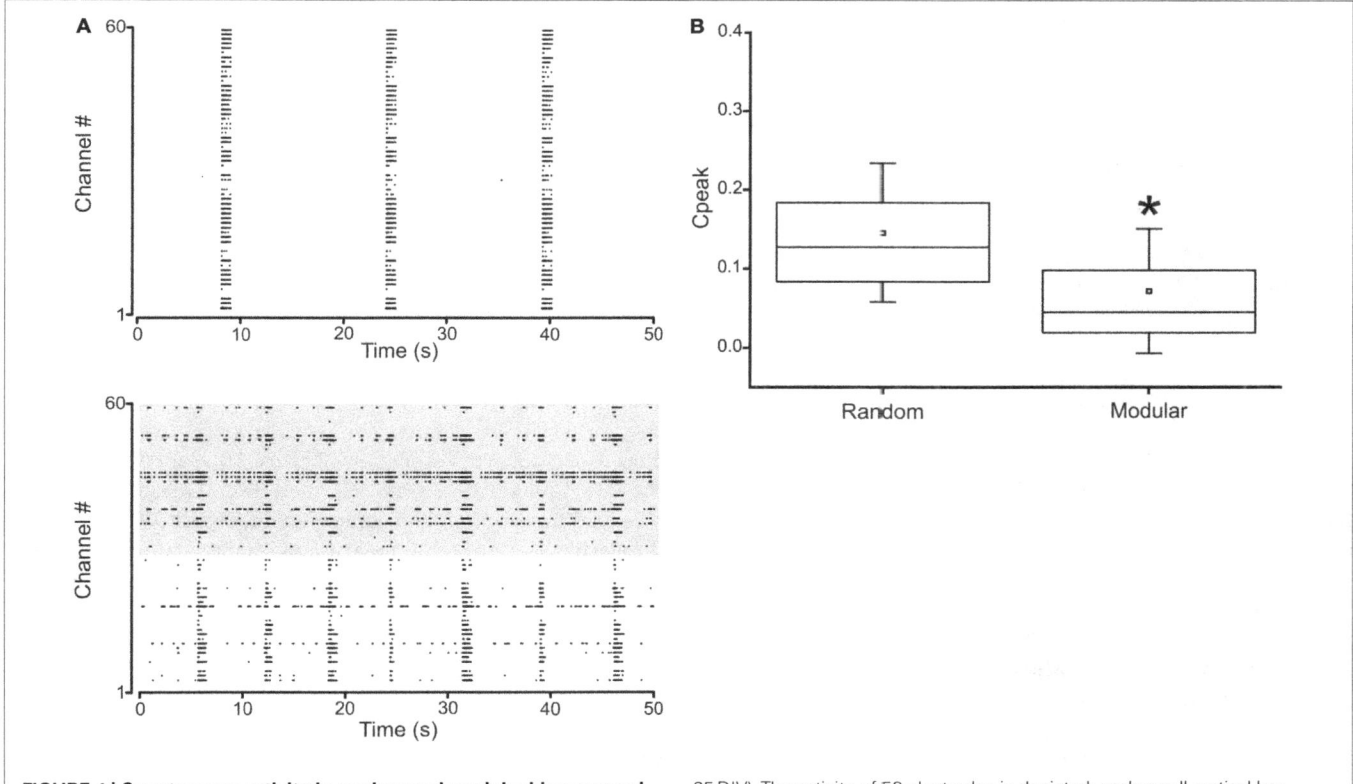

FIGURE 4 | Spontaneous activity in random and modular hippocampal networks. (A) Top. Raster plot of the activity exhibited by a random hippocampal culture (50 s of activity acquired from a representative culture of 28 DIV). Bottom. Raster plot of the activity exhibited by a modular hippocampal culture (50 s of activity acquired from a representative culture of 25 DIV). The activity of 59 electrodes is depicted: each small vertical bar represents a spike, each line an electrode. **(B)** Box-plot of the cross-correlation peaks in $N = 6$ random and $N = 6$ modular cultures. Box range: percentile 25–75; box whiskers: percentile 5–95; line: median; square: mean. Mann–Whitney test for not-normal data, significance level = *$p < 0.05$.

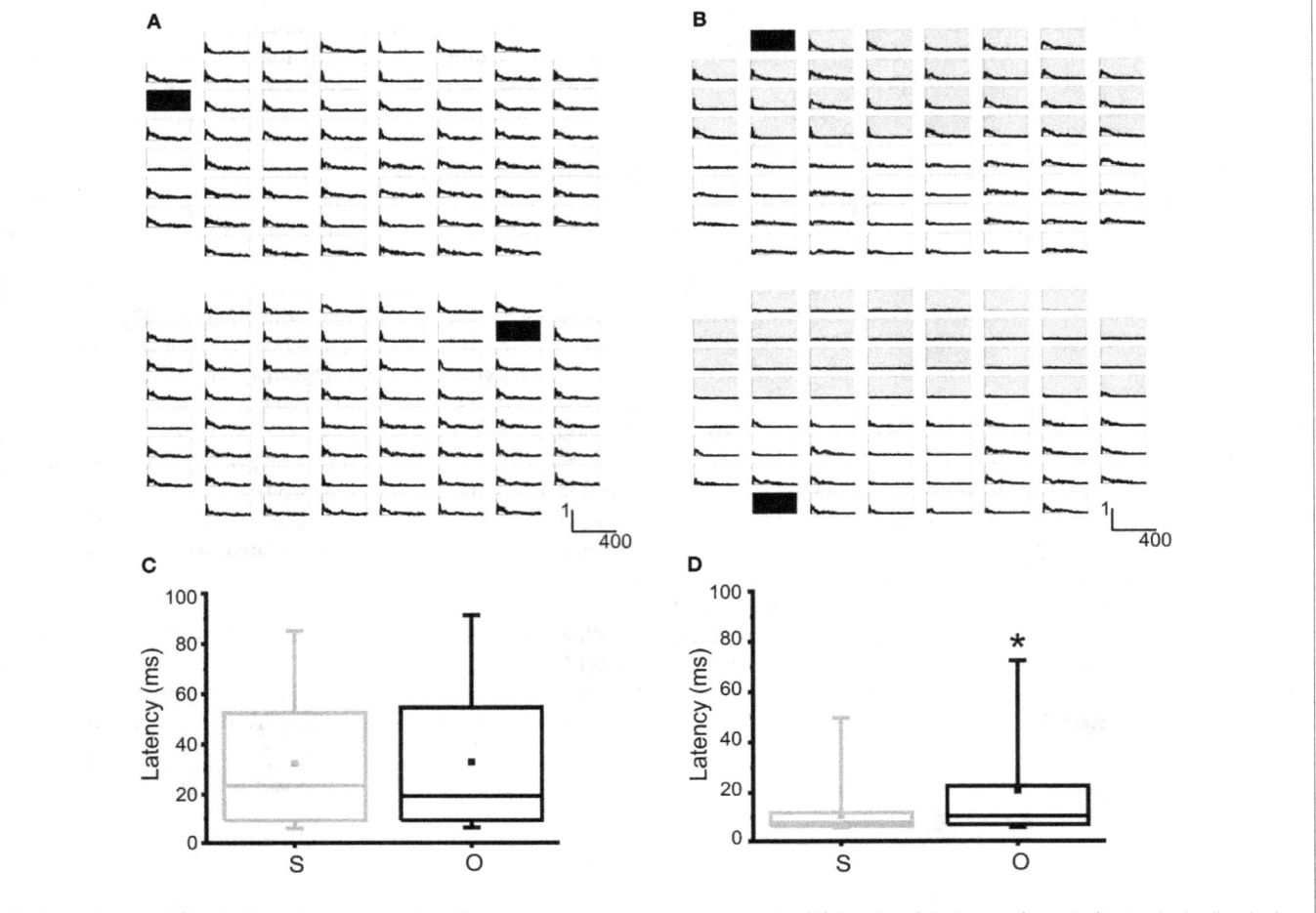

FIGURE 5 | Evoked activity in random and modular hippocampal networks. (A) *Top.* PSTH map obtained from 59 channels as a consequence of the stimulation from electrode 13 (black square). *Bottom.* PSTHs obtained by stimulating electrode 72 (black square) in the same network. *X*-axis: time (0, 400) ms, bin 4 ms; *Y*-axis: probability of evoking a spike. **(B)** *Top.* PSTH map obtained from 59 channels as a consequence of the stimulation from electrode 21 (black square) in the top compartment of a confined network. *Bottom.* PSTHs obtained by stimulating electrode 28 (black square) in the bottom compartment of the same confined network. Shaded area indicates the top compartment. *X*-axis: time (0, 400) ms, bin 4 ms; *Y*-axis: probability of evoking a spike. **(C)** Box-plot of the latency from the first evoked spikes in the same (S) or other (O) compartment with respect to stimulating electrodes. No statistical differences can be noted in a random culture. $N = 11$ random cultures. **(D)** Box-plot of the latency from the first evoked spikes in the same (S) or other (O) compartment with respect to stimulating electrodes. In a modular network, the latency between the stimulus and the first evoked spike is statistically lower for the electrodes belonging to the same cluster of the stimulating electrodes. $N = 6$ modular cultures. Box range: percentile 25–75; Box whiskers: percentile 5–95; line: median; square: mean. Mann–Whitney test for not-normal data, significance level = $*p < 0.05$.

network can be evaluated through the Post Stimulus Time Histogram (PSTH, cf., see Materials and Methods). In **Figure 5A** the maps of the PSTH obtained as a consequence of the stimulation from site 13 (top) and site 72 (bottom) are reported in a non-confined culture. Typically, the PSTH is characterized by an "early response," lasting 20–40 ms, and by a late response, lasting more than 100–200 ms, usually due to the generation of an evoked burst synchronized over the whole network (Gal et al., 2010). The integral calculated over the PSTH profile represents the average number of evoked spikes at a specific site and it is used for quantifying the strength of the connection between a specific stimulation site and all the recording ones (Chiappalone et al., 2008). This parameter is at the base of the choice of the input-output connections for our neuro-robotic studies (cf., see Input and Output

Sites of a Neuronal Population). **Figure 5B** reports the maps of the PSTH obtained in a modular network. When stimulation is delivered from site 21 (top compartment, **Figure 5B** top), mainly the electrodes of the top compartment respond to the stimulation. Few activations can be observed also in the bottom compartment, but with a dominant late response and an almost absent early one. In the same network, when stimulation comes from one electrode of the bottom compartment (electrode 28, **Figure 5B** bottom) practically only that compartment responds to the stimulus.

To further test the actual confinement of the evoked responses, we also analyzed the distribution of the mean latencies (i.e., the distance between the stimulus and the first evoked spike) obtained for each couple of stimulation-recording electrodes (Mainen and Sejnowski, 1995; Tateno and Jimbo, 1999): simply by eye, it is

Modular neuronal assemblies embodied in a closed-loop environment: toward future integration of brains...

21

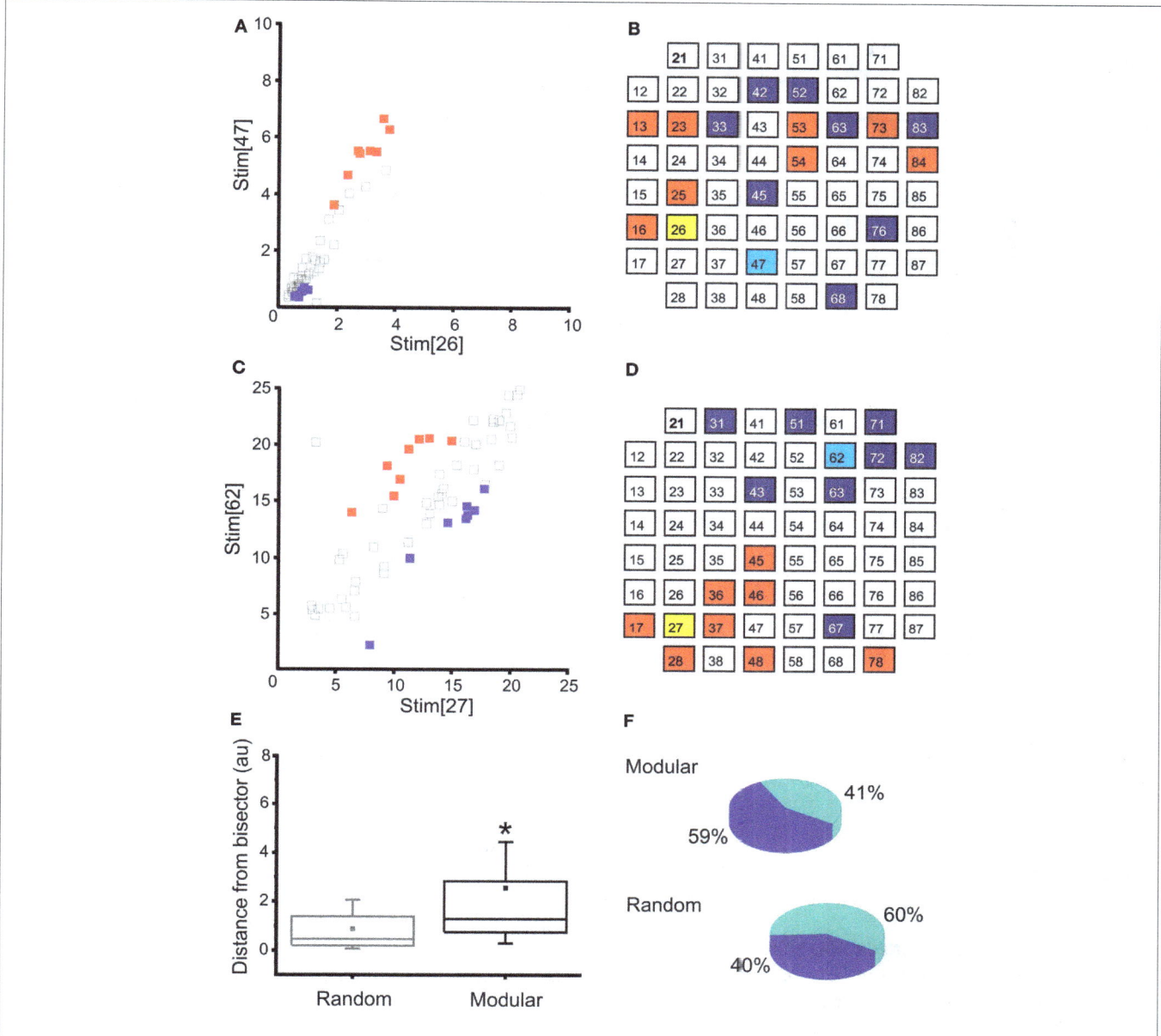

FIGURE 6 | Input-output selection. (A) Map obtained in a representative "random" culture for the selection of the output sites, given two inputs sites (e.g., 26 and 47): red, left recording area; blue, right recording area. **(B)** Schematic representation of the input (yellow and light blue) and respective recording (red and blue) areas for the same experiment reported in A ("random" culture): note that the selected electrodes are quite spread over the entire recording area. **(C)** Map obtained in a representative "confined" culture for the selection of the output sites, given two inputs sites (e.g., 27 and 62): red, left recording area; blue, right recording area. **(D)** Schematic representation of the input (yellow and light blue) and respective recording (red and blue) areas for the same experiment reported in **(B)** ("confined" culture): note that the selected recording electrodes are close to the stimulating electrode and they follow the structure of the underlying network. **(E)** A box-plot representing the distances from bisector of the selected recording electrodes in the set of random and confined cultures used within this study ($N = 11$ random and $N = 6$ modular cultures). The distribution of the distances in the modular case is significantly higher than in the random case. Box range: percentile 25–75; box whiskers: percentile 5–95; line: median; square: mean. Mann–Whitney test for not-normal data, significance level = *$p < 0.05$. **(F)** Pie chart representing the percentage of networks in which at least 50% of the recording electrodes were selected in the same compartment of the stimulating electrode. The percentage is higher for the modular networks ($N = 11$ random and $N = 6$ modular cultures).

clear that the evoked response is (mostly) limited to the compartment hosting the stimulation electrode. **Figures 5C,D** reports the distribution of the latencies from the electrodes in the same compartment (i.e., top or bottom) of the stimulating electrode (S) compared to those from the electrodes in the other compartment (O). Only in the case of confined networks (**Figure 5D**) the two distributions are statistically different, being the latencies evaluated in the electrodes belonging to the same compartment of the

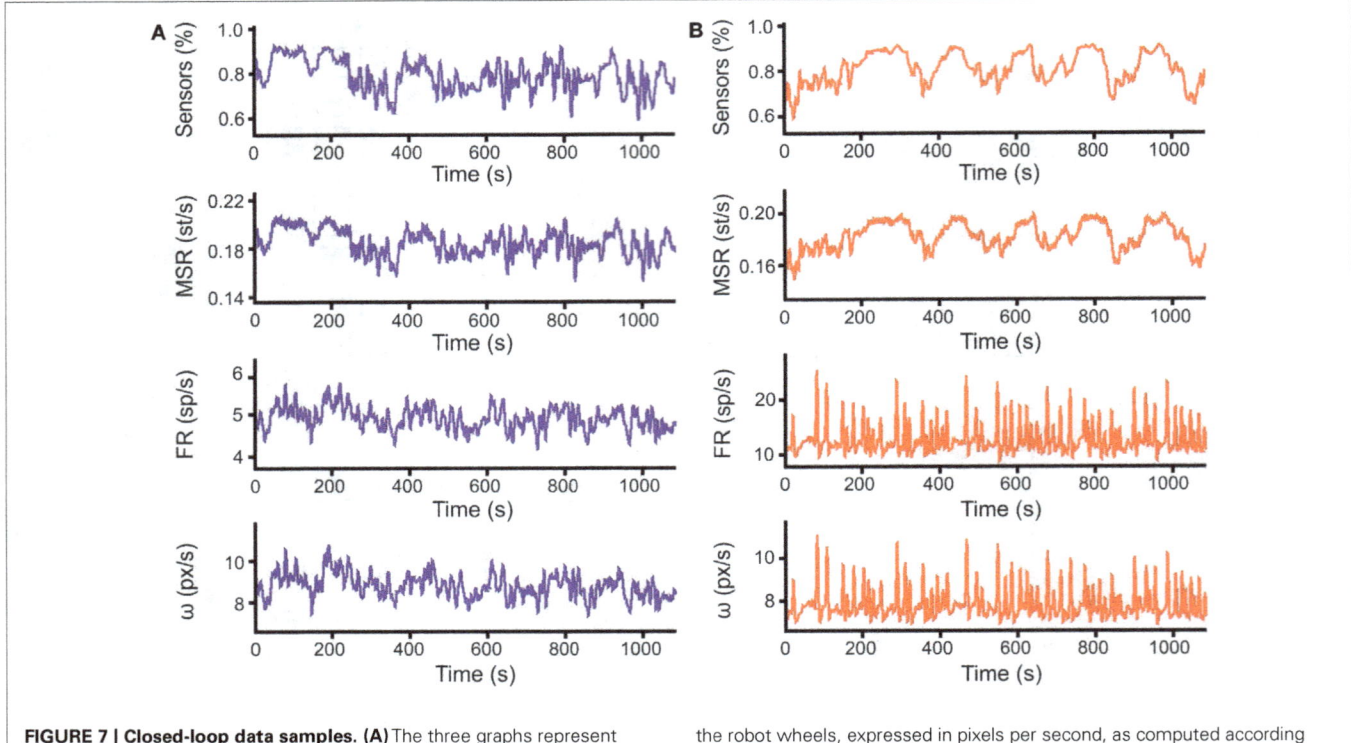

FIGURE 7 | Closed-loop data samples. (A) The three graphs represent 1100 s of data recorded during a robot run under close-loop control. From top to bottom, the graphs represent: (i) the average readings of the three proximity sensors on the left side of the robot, ranging from 1 (obstacle in contact with the robot) to 0 (obstacle at the distance of the arena diameter); (ii) mean rates of delivery of stimulation (i.e., Mean Stimulation Rate, MSR); (iii) mean firing rates by averaging over all the electrodes belonging to the same recording area (i.e., Firing Rate, FR); (iv) speed of the robot wheels, expressed in pixels per second, as computed according to Eq. 1 from firing rates. Data for stimulation and firing rate are point events at times of delivery (for stimulations) or detection (for spikes), while sensor data and wheel speeds are sampled at 10 Hz. The graphs reported above are obtained after low-pass filtering of actual data (sliding Gaussian window over 100 samples – 10s, with an alpha value of 2.5). **(B)** Same set of graphs as **(A)**, displaying information for sensors and wheel of the right side.

stimulation significantly lower than those of the electrodes in the other compartment. This proves that dividing the neural network in two sub-populations has indeed an effect on stimulus response.

INPUT AND OUTPUT SITES OF A NEURONAL POPULATION

The simplest architecture that can be adopted for the proposed task includes two electrodes to deliver coded sensory information, one for each set of sensors. While the same could be said for output sites, the point of interest in this work was the response of the network, therefore a set of 8–10 electrodes is chosen to act as output sites for each wheel.

The main disadvantage in dealing with dissociated cultures instead of experimental models with a preserved neural structure is the lack of predefined architecture. For this reason, before starting an experiment, a procedure has been performed to define the stimulation (sensory input) and recording (motor output) areas of the network. During this procedure (i.e., phase 2 of our experimental protocol, cf., see Materials and Methods), we stimulated the cultures by delivering trains of 40 electrical stimuli (1.5 V peak-to-peak, biphasic pulses, 500 μs total duration) from 8 to 10 sites in a serial way. Then, the PSTH area (i.e., the number of spikes in the 600 ms following each stimulation) between each pair of stimulation-recording electrodes is computed and the related maps, like the one reported in **Figures 6A,C**, are

produced. The coordinates of each square in that map represent the PSTH areas at a specific recording site relative to stimulation from the two stimulating sites reported on the axis (Stim[26] and Stim[47] in **Figure 6A**, for example). All the possible input-output combinations are explored and only the pathways producing "selective" responses are retained. These "selective" pathways are identified by pool of recording sites with respect to a couple of stimulating sites for which the responses measured fall far away from the bisector (i.e., pool of recording site closer to the axis).

Those specific pathways of sensory-motor activations can be then conveniently utilized for driving the robot and for implementing simple reactive behaviors (e.g., obstacle avoidance). **Figures 6B,D** report the selected inputs (i.e., two electrodes, one for the left and one for the right area) and output regions, characterized by eight electrodes each, corresponding with maps **Figures 6B,D**, respectively for two representative cultures (i.e., random and modular).

The presence of a confinement structure tends to generate networks showing a higher degree of functional separation (i.e., selectivity), as well as a physical one, when compared to totally random networks: as can be seen in **Figure 6E**, the average distance from the bisector of the evoked response pair is significantly increased in the case of the modular network. The geometry of the stimulation-recording pairs is also affected, as they are more likely to be clustered together on the same half of the culture (**Figure 6F**).

CLOSED-LOOP ROBOT NAVIGATION

All the parameters relevant to the movement of the robot are recorded during the experiment. In **Figures 7A,B**, more than 1000 s of signal recordings are plotted (**Figure 7A** for the left side and **Figure 7B** for the right side). The top panels are showing sensory information, with the blue trace representing the average value of proximity sensors on the left side of the robot and the red one the average value of those on the right. In the second graph, a measure of stimulation is shown, expressed as the mean stimulation rate. The third line of graphs reports the firing rates, measured in spikes per second; wheel speeds (shown in the lower graph, expressed in pixels per seconds), closely follow neural activity.

The results of the behavior described so far can be observed in **Figures 8A–C**, where a virtual arena is shown along with the path drawn by the robot (in red) in a 20-min long robot run, respectively in an "empty" experiment (**Figure 8A**), an open-loop experiment

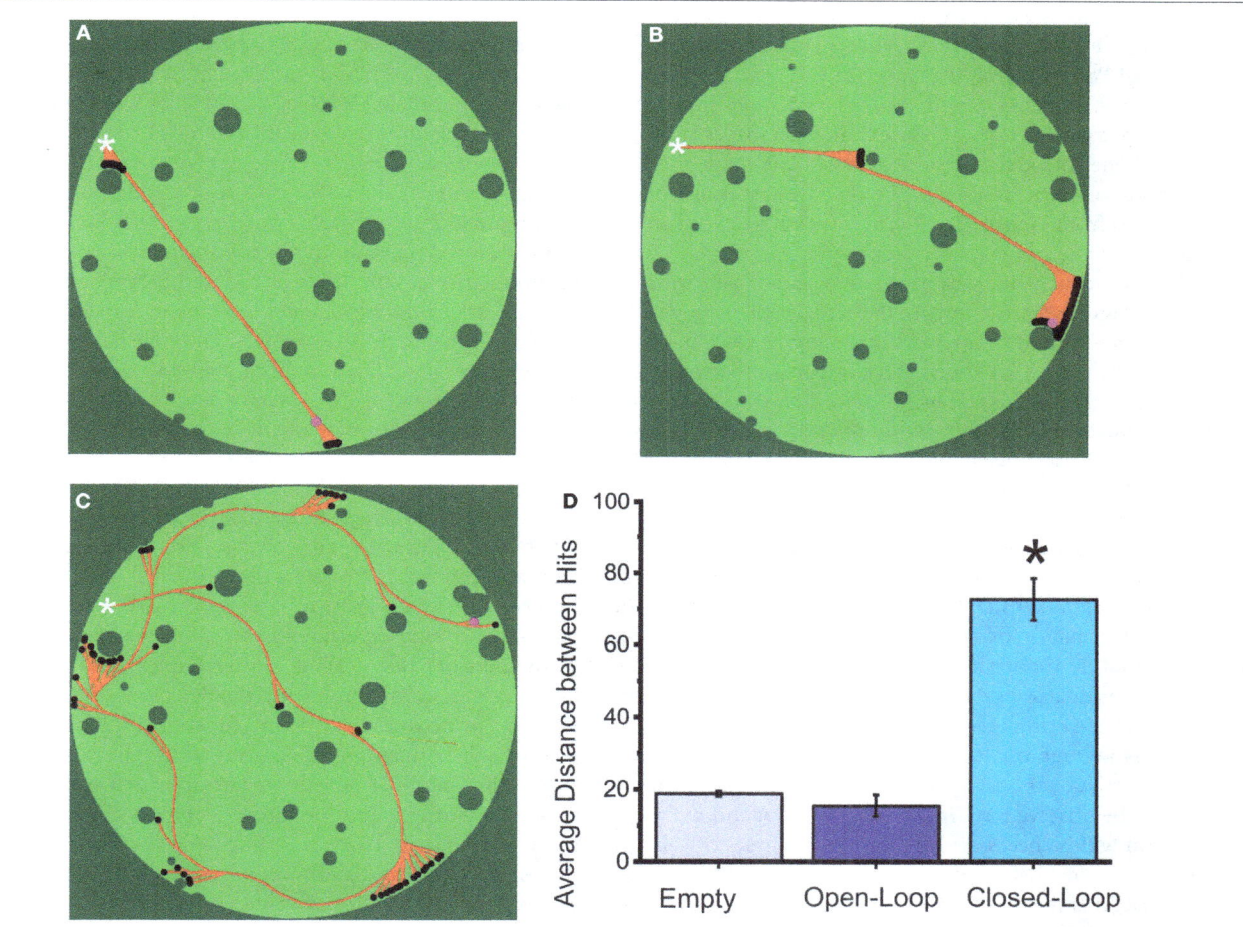

FIGURE 8 | Robot navigation and evaluation of the closed-loop system. (A) Reconstruction of a 20-min long robot trajectory, in an empty MEA configuration. The white cross marks the starting position of the robot and the red path its movement during the observation period, up to its final position (pink circle, in the upper right corner). Dark green pixels are either arena walls or obstacles, while light ones are free for the robot movement. Black dots represent robot impacts with the environment. Total lack of biological material on the MEA prevents a closing of the sensory-motor loop. As a consequence, the robot shows a total inability to navigate its environment. The small changes in robot heading are likely false positives in the spike detection algorithm on background noise or stimulation artifacts. As can be inferred from the image, though, their total impact is almost null and the robot moves almost precisely in a straight line. **(B)** Reconstruction of a 20-min long robot trajectory in open-loop. During this robot run the control loop has been opened by stopping stimulation to the neural culture. As a result, the robot is, similarly to the previous case, lacking any capability of navigating its environment. Changes in robot direction are, in this case, provoked by the spontaneous activity of the neural network. **(C)** Reconstruction of a 20-min long robot trajectory in closed-loop. While the amount of obstacles hit by the robot shows that control is not perfect, the robot is able to take advantage of sensory information to extricate itself from all the situations encountered in a limited amount of time and hits. **(D)** Performance of the neuro-controlled robot during an obstacle avoidance task in terms of the mean distance between two consecutive collisions, calculated in pixels. The values are obtained in $N = 5$ experiments for the empty and the open-loop case and in the $N = 17$ experiments reported in the text (light blue = empty MEA; blue = open-loop MEA; cyan = closed-loop MEA). The closed-loop experiments give the best results. Statistical analysis was carried out by using one-way ANOVA (*$p < 0.05$) for normal distributions (Kolmogorov–Smirnov test of normality), while for mean comparison both the Tukey and the Bonferroni tests were used.

(**Figure 8B**) and finally a closed-loop experiment (**Figure 8C**). While collisions are fairly frequent even in the latter case the behavior of the robot is still much closer to the desired one rather than in an open-loop configuration, or (obviously) in the absence of a biological substrate. As can be observed from the graph in **Figure 8D**, the average path traveled between hits is significantly higher in the case of a close-loop.

IMPACT OF MODULARITY AND TETANIC STIMULATION ON ROBOT NAVIGATION

Despite the improvement in performance of the closed-loop scenario compared to the control cases, robot collisions against obstacles are still a frequent occurrence in random networks. Observation of PSTHs reveals that random networks show a very high degree of connectivity, with evoked responses showing a strong overlap regardless of the stimulating electrodes position (**Figure 5A**). The introduction of a confinement mask shows a marked separation in the responses obtained from stimulation, as can be observed from **Figure 5B**. This, in turn, leads to a reduction in the amount of "cross talk" between input and output channels, with a consequent increase in the navigation performance of the robot. **Figures 9A,C** compare the improvement in performance between the random network structure and the modular one. Specifically, **Figure 9A** shows the comparison between performances evaluated as the average distance between consecutive collisions in different conditions (without and with tetanic stimulation, respectively on the left and right graphs), while **Figure 9C** displays the same performances evaluated through a different parameter, average number of hits per second. The tetanic stimulation leads to a further improvement in the performance, especially when performed on a network with a modular geometry, as can be observed in **Figures 9B,D**: the first couple of graphs show the increase in performance following the introduction of the tetanic stimulation routine (in a random network, left, and in a modular one, right) evaluated as distance between collisions, while the graphs in **Figure 9D** show the performance obtained in the same experiment as average number of hits per second. Examples of changes in effective connectivity obtained in modular and random networks can be observed in **Figure A1** in the Appendix. Even if quantification will be necessary, preliminary analyses of changes in connectivity show that tetanic stimulation does affect the network response, by strengthening the connections on one side and weakening or not affecting the connections on the opposite side.

While all of the described comparisons yield statistically significant results in the case of the average distance parameter, it is not the case for the average number of collisions: the only condition that causes a large enough change to be significant is the introduction of a tetanic stimulation on a modular network.

DISCUSSION AND FUTURE DEVELOPMENT

In this paper we successfully interfaced, in a bi-directional way, a network of neurons coming from the hippocampus of embryonic rats with a virtual robot. The robot, which has sensors and wheels, is forced to move in a static arena with obstacles and its task consists in avoiding collisions. Looking at the spontaneous electrophysiological activity of the network, we first select a set of possible "inputs," then we evaluate the evoked response of the entire culture

by delivering patterns of electrical stimulation. This procedure allows us to select the "outputs" of our network. Then, by applying a linear rate-based decoding strategy, we were able to transform the spike frequency into velocity and the sensory information collected by the robot "eyes" into stimulation frequency for our neurons. The behavior of the robot during the closed-loop experiments resulted significantly better than that in open-loop (i.e., without any sensory feedback) or the "empty" MEA condition, proving that the activity driving the robot is actually neural-based (cf. **Figure 8**). In general, these results prove that an *in vitro* network of biological neurons can control an external agent. While ours is not the first setup to achieve this goal, in our knowledge, no previous work reports an extensive set of experiments like the ones we performed (DeMarse et al., 2001; Martinoia et al., 2004; Novellino et al., 2007; Bakkum et al., 2008; Kudoh et al., 2011), but, rather they focus on a single thesis supported by data obtained from a limited number of analogous preparations. Here, we introduce for the first time statistical comparisons obtained on a sizable number of different preparations with highly different spiking behaviors, such as those observed on random and modular networks. Furthermore, bi-modularity of cultures is introduced here for the first time in the context of closed-loop interfaces and its impact is shown to be relevant for the performance of the embodied agent.

Early experiments on random networks showed the tendency of these cultures to evolve toward a degenerate state where mostly network-wide synchronous activity can be observed. The addition of a confinement mask and the consequent modularity qualitatively changed the behavior of the network, preventing or at least strongly reducing the appearance of synchronized network bursts (cf. **Figure 4**). This change alone was enough to provide a significant increase in the performance of the robot (cf. **Figures 5, 6**, and **9**). These results lead to two possible investigation lines on the same experimental setup: increasing the modularity of the network might allow more complex behavior to emerge, while chronic stimulation since the day of plating might be used in future experiments to define functionally but not physically distinct sub-populations of neurons within the same culture.

Another point of novelty in our approach has been the systematic use of tetanic stimulation on hippocampal cultures over MEA. Previous approaches aiming at demonstrating plasticity in neuronal assemblies by using stimulation protocols from embedded extracellular electrodes were always applied to cortical cultures (Jimbo et al., 1999; Madhavan et al., 2007; Chiappalone et al., 2008; Stegenga et al., 2010). Here we used hippocampal cells and we proved that tetanic stimulation worked successfully, providing an increase in performance both in random and modular networks (cf. **Figure 9**). A further analysis on data is being conducted to determine whether it is possible to define a clear relationship between spontaneous activity of the network and its impact on the observed changes in connectivity strength, since the patterns of induced change proved to be more complex than expected (see **Figure A1** in the Appendix for a preliminary example of effective connection changes induced by tetanic stimulation). This could allow the design of a more successful learning scheme. The exact biological mechanisms linking performance increase and tetanic stimulation are still unclear and further investigations and targeted experiments are needed. Along this direction, the use of

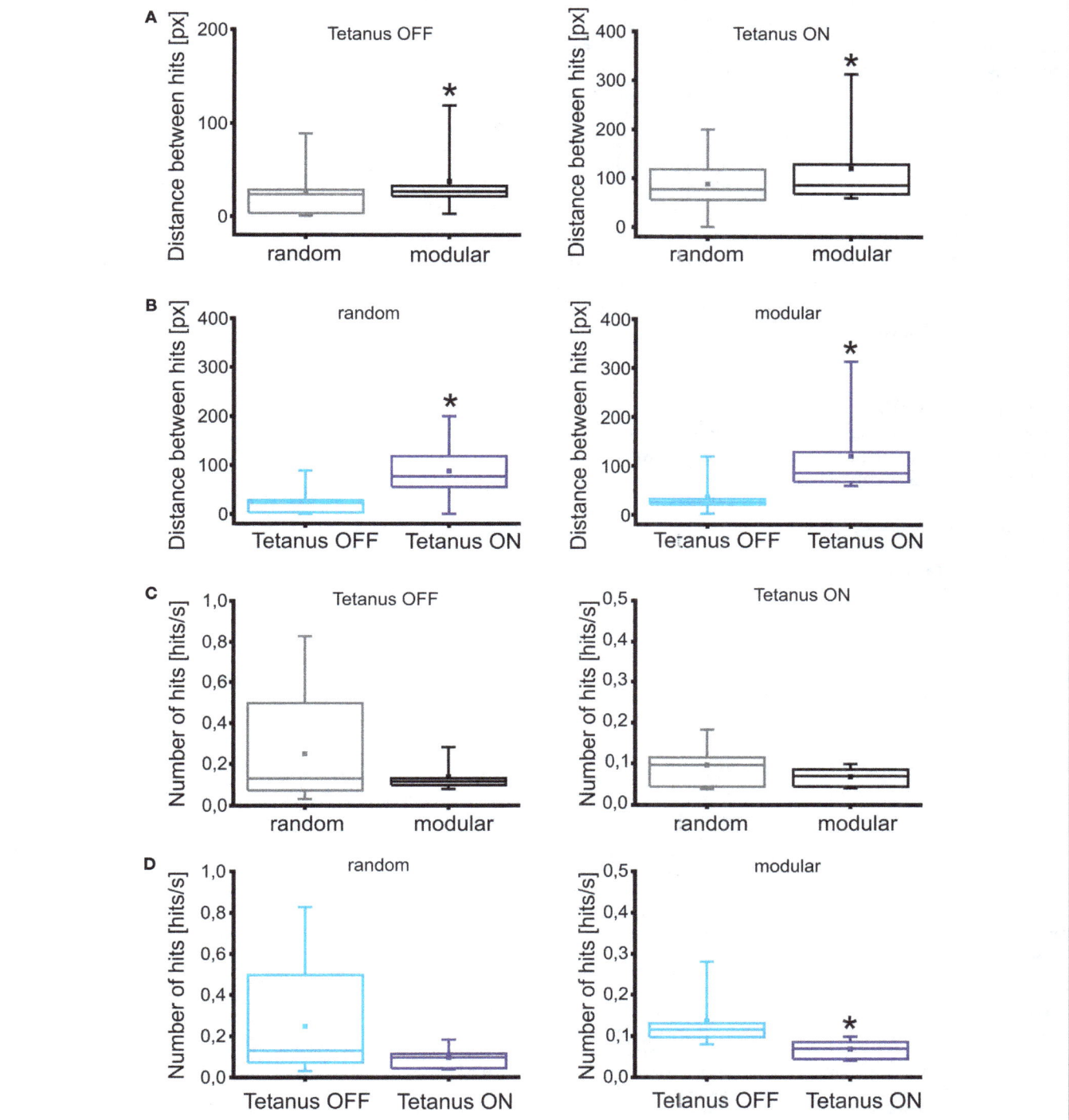

FIGURE 9 | Impact of modularity and tetanic stimulation on robot navigation. (A) Comparison of robot performances in random and modular networks, in the absence or presence of tetanic stimulation (respectively, left and right graph), evaluated as average distance (in pixels) between consecutive hits. **(B)** Comparison of robot performances between different conditions of tetanic stimulation, in random (left graph) and modular networks (right graph), evaluated as average distance between hits. **(C)** Comparison between robot performance in random and modular networks, in the absence or presence of tetanic stimulation (respectively, left and right graph),

evaluated in terms of average number of hits per second. **(D)** Comparison of robot performances in different conditions of tetanic stimulation, in random (left graph) and modular networks (right graph), evaluated in hits per second. All the values are obtained in the experiments described in text ($N = 11$ experiments for the random condition, $N = 6$ for the modular), with a tetanic stimulation session following each standard robot run. Box range: percentile 25–75; box whiskers: percentile 5–95; line: median; square: mean. Statistical analysis was carried out by using Mann–Whitney test for not-normal data, significance level $= *p < 0.05$.

pharmacological manipulation could allow to change the state of the network and thus to investigate roles of synaptic transmission and receptors involved in the process of adaptation and learning depending on specific stimulation protocols.

As expected, the final performance of the robot is worse than what was possible to achieve without including biological components in the closed-loop (data not shown): for the task of obstacle avoidance, it would be possible to program the robot so that it can perform the navigation task with no risk of hitting obstacles. However, our neuro-robotic framework proved to be a valid tool for the study of mechanisms of neural coding and the computational and adaptive properties of neuronal assemblies with the final goal to facilitate progress in understanding neural pathologies, designing neural prosthetics, and creating fundamentally different types of artificial or hybrid intelligence.

ACKNOWLEDGMENTS

The authors wish to thanks Dr. Marina Nanni for the technical assistance in cell culture preparation. The authors would like to thank Alessandro Bosca and Luca Berdondini for their help and technical assistance in the realization of the PDMS masks used for part of the experiments reported in the paper.

Video S1 | Video of a closed-loop robot run. This video of a virtual robot run is running at 40× real speed. The arena is composed of dark green solid obstacles and light green "floor" which the robot can move upon. The magenta circle is the virtual robot itself, the red dots highlight the path followed by the robot center over time, while black circles represent hits against obstacles. While the amount of obstacles hit by the robot shows that control is not perfect, the robot is able to take advantage of sensory information to extricate itself from all the situations encountered in a limited amount of time and hits.

Video S2 | Video of an "empty MEA" robot run. This video of a virtual robot run is running at 40× real speed. The arena is composed of dark green solid obstacles and light green "floor" which the robot can move upon. The magenta circle is the virtual robot itself; the red dots highlight the path followed by the robot center over time, while black circles represent hits against obstacles. The starting direction of the robot in this trial is rotated 90° clockwise with respect to the other two shown videos. Total lack of biological material on the MEA prevents a closing of the sensory-motor loop. As a consequence, the robot shows a total inability to navigate its environment. The small changes in robot heading are likely false positives in the spike detection algorithm on background noise or stimulation artifacts. As can be inferred from the video, though, their total impact is almost null and the robot moves almost precisely in a straight line.

Video S3 | Video of an open-loop robot run. This video of a virtual robot run is running at 40× real speed. The arena is composed of dark green solid obstacles and light green "floor" which the robot can move upon. The magenta circle is the virtual robot itself, the red dots highlight the path followed by the robot center over time, while black circles represent hits against obstacles. During this robot run the control loop has been opened by stopping stimulation to the neural culture. As a result, the robot is, similarly to the previous case, lacking any capability of navigating its environment. Changes in robot direction are, in this case, provoked by the spontaneous activity of the neural network.

REFERENCES

Adrian, E. D. (1928). *The Basis of Sensation: The Action of Sense Organs.* New York: W. W. Norton & Co.

Bakkum, D. J., Chao, Z. C., and Potter, S. M. (2008). Spatio-temporal electrical stimuli shape behavior of an embodied cortical network in a goal-directed learning task. *J. Neural Eng.* 5, 310–323.

Ben-Ari, Y. (2001). Developing networks play a similar melody. *Trends Neurosci.* 24, 353–360.

Berdondini, L., Chiappalone, M., van der Wal, P. D., Imfeld, K., de Rooij, N. F., Koudelka-Hep, M., et al. (2006). A microelectrode array (MEA) integrated with clustering structures for investigating in vitro neurodynamics in confined interconnected subpopulations of neurons. *Sens. Actuators B Chem.* 114, 530–541.

Boehler, M. D., Leondopulos, S. S., Wheeler, B. C., and Brewer, G. J. (2012). Hippocampal networks on reliable patterned substrates. *J. Neurosci. Methods* 203, 344–353.

Bongard, J. C. (2011) "Morphological and environmental scaffolding synergize when evolving robot controllers: artificial life/robotics/evolvable hardware," in *13th Annual Conference on Genetic and Evolutionary Computation (GECCO '11)*, ed. N. Krasnogor (New York: ACM).

Boucsein, C., Nawrot, M. P., Schnepel, P., and Aertsen, A. (2011). Beyond the cortical column: abundance and physiology of horizontal connections imply a strong role for inputs from the surround. *Front. Neurosci.* 5:32. doi:10.3389/fnins.2011.00032

Braitenberg, V. (1984). *Vehicles – Experiments in Synthetic Psychology.* Cambridge, MA: The MIT Press.

Chang, J. C., Brewer, G. J., and Wheeler, B. C. (2001). Modulation of neural network activity by patterning. *Biosens. Bioelectron.* 16, 527–533.

Chiappalone, M., Bove, M., Vato, A., Tedesco, M., and Martinoia, S. (2006). Dissociated cortical networks show spontaneously correlated activity patterns during in vitro development. *Brain Res.* 1093, 41–53.

Chiappalone, M., Massobrio, P., and Martinoia, S. (2008). Network plasticity in cortical assemblies. *Eur. J. Neurosci.* 28, 221–237.

Chiappalone, M., Vato, A., Berdondini, L., Koudelka, M., and Martinoia, S. (2007). Network dynamics and synchronous activity in cultured cortical neurons. *Int. J. Neural Syst.* 17, 87–103.

Clark, A. (1997). *Being There.* Cambridge, MA: MIT Press.

Corner, M. A. (2008). Spontaneous neuronal burst discharges as dependent and independent variables in the maturation of cerebral cortex tissue cultured in vitro: a review of activity-dependent studies in live 'model' systems for the development of intrinsically generated bioelectric slow-wave sleep patterns. *Brain Res. Rev.* 59, 221–244.

Cozzi, L., D'Angelo, P., and Sanguineti, V. (2006). Encoding of time-varying stimuli in population of cultured neurons. *Biol. Cybern.* 94, 335–349.

DeMarse, T. B., Wagenaar, D. A., Blau, A. W., and Potter, S. M. (2001). The neurally controlled animat: biological brains acting with simulated bodies. *Auton. Robots* 11, 305–310.

Derdikman, D., Hildesheim, R., Ahissar, E., Arieli, A., and Grinvald, A. (2003). Imaging spatiotemporal dynamics of surround inhibition in the barrels somatosensory cortex. *J. Neurosci.* 23, 3100–3105.

Eytan, D., and Marom, S. (2006). Dynamics and effective topology underlying synchronization in networks of cortical neurons. *J. Neurosci.* 26, 8465–8476.

Eytan, D., Minerbi, A., Ziv, N., and Marom, S. (2004). Dopamine-induced dispersion of correlations between action potentials in networks of cortical neurons. *J. Neurophysiol.* 92, 1817–1824.

Frega, M., Pasquale, V., Tedesco, M., Marcoli, M., Contestabile, A., Nanni, M., et al. (2012). Cortical cultures coupled to micro-electrode arrays: a novel approach to perform in vitro excitotoxicity testing. *Neurotoxicol. Teratol.* 34, 116–127.

Gal, A., Eytan, D., Wallach, A., Sandler, M., Schiller, J., and Marom, S. (2010). Dynamics of excitability over extended timescales in cultured cortical neurons. *J. Neurosci.* 30, 16332–16342.

Gilbert, S. F. (2009). *Ecological Development Biology.* Sunderland: John Wiley & Sons, Ltd.

Hubel, D. H., Wiesel, T. N., and LeVay, S. (1977). Plasticity of ocular dominance columns in monkey striate cortex. *Philos. Trans. R. Soc. Lond. B Biol. Sci.* 278, 377–409.

Jimbo, Y., Tateno, Y., and Robinson, H. P. C. (1999). Simultaneous induction of pathway-specific potentiation and depression in networks of cortical neurons. *Biophys. J.* 76, 670–678.

Modular neuronal assemblies embodied in a closed-loop environment: toward future integration of brains...

27

Kanagasabapathi, T. T., Massobrio, P., Barone, R. A., Tedesco, M., Martinoia, S., Wadman, W. J., et al. (2012). Functional connectivity and dynamics of cortical-thalamic networks co-cultured in a dual compartment device. *J. Neural Eng.* 9, 036010.

Keefer, E. W., Gramowski, A., and Gross, G. W. (2001). NMDA receptor-dependent periodic oscillations in cultured spinal cord networks. *J. Neurophysiol.* 86, 3030–3042.

Kudoh, S. N., Tokuda, M., Kiyohara, A., Hosokawa, C., Taguchi, T., and Hayashi, I. (2011). Vitroid – the robot system with an interface between a living neuronal network and outer world. *Int. J. Mech. Manuf. Syst.* 4, 135–149.

Kumar, A., Rotter, S., and Aertsen, A. (2010). Spiking activity propagation in neuronal networks: reconciling different perspectives on neural coding. *Nat. Rev. Neurosci.* 11, 615–627.

le Feber, J., Stegenga, J., and Rutten, W. L. (2010). The effect of slow electrical stimuli to achieve learning in cultured networks of rat cortical neurons. *PLoS ONE* 5:e8871. doi:10.1371/journal.pone.0008871

Levy, O., Ziv, N. E., and Marom, S. (2012). Enhancement of neural representation capacity by modular architecture in networks of cortical neurons. *Eur. J. Neurosci.* 35, 1753–1760.

Maccione, A., Gandolfo, M., Massobrio, P., Novellino, A., Martinoia, S., and Chiappalone, M. (2009). A novel algorithm for precise identification of spikes in extracellularly recorded neuronal signals. *J. Neurosci. Methods* 177, 241–249.

Madhavan, R., Chao, Z. C., and Potter, S. M. (2007). Plasticity of recurring spatiotemporal activity patterns in cortical networks. *Phys. Biol.* 4, 181–193.

Mainen, Z. F., and Sejnowski, T. J. (1995). Reliability of spike timing in neocortical neurons. *Science* 268, 1503–1506.

Martinoia, S., Sanguineti, V., Cozzi, L., Berdondini, L., Tomas, J., Le Masson, G., et al. (2004). Towards an embodied in-vitro electrophysiology: the NeuroBIT project. *Neurocomputing* 58–60, 1065–1072.

Mulas, M., Massobrio, P., Martinoia, S., and Chiappalone, M. (2010). A simulated neuro-robotic environment for bi-directional closed-loop experiments. *Paladyn J. Behav. Robot.* 1, 179–186.

Mussa-Ivaldi, F. A., Alford, S. T., Chiappalone, M., Fadiga, L., Karniel, A., Kositsky, M., et al. (2010). New perspectives on the dialogue between brains and machines. *Front. Neurosci.* 4:44. doi:10.3389/neuro.01.008.2010

Novellino, A., D'Angelo, P., Cozzi, L., Chiappalone, M., Sanguineti, V., and Martinoia, S. (2007). Connecting neurons to a mobile Robot: an in vitro bidirectional neural interface. *Comput. Intell. Neurosci.* 2007, 13.

Pan, R. K., Chatterjee, N., and Sinha, S. (2010). Mesoscopic organization reveals the constraints governing Caenorhabditis elegans nervous system. *PLoS ONE* 5:e9240. doi:10.1371/journal.pone.0009240

Pasquale, V., Martinoia, S., and Chiappalone, M. (2010). A self-adapting approach for the detection of bursts and network bursts in neuronal cultures. *J. Comput. Neurosci.* 29, 213–229.

Raichman, N., and Ben-Jacob, E. (2008). Identifying repeating motifs in the activation of synchronized bursts in cultured neuronal networks. *J. Neurosci. Methods* 170, 96–110.

Rieke, F., Warland, D., de Ruyter van Steveninck, R., and Bialek, W. (1997). *Spikes: Exploring the Neural Code.* Cambridge, MA: The MIT Press.

Shein Idelson, M., Ben-Jacob, E., and Hanein, Y. (2010). Innate synchronous oscillations in freely-organized small neuronal circuits. *PLoS ONE* 5:e14443. doi:10.1371/journal.pone.0014443

Sporns, O., Tononi, G., and Edelman, G. M. (2000). Theoretical neuroanatomy: relating anatomical and functional connectivity in graphs and cortical connection matrices. *Cereb. Cortex* 10, 127–141.

Stegenga, J., Le Feber, J., Marani, E., and Rutten, W. L. (2010). Phase-dependent effects of stimuli locked to oscillatory activity in cultured cortical networks. *Biophys. J.* 98, 2452–2458.

Tateno, T., and Jimbo, Y. (1999). Activity-dependent enhancement in the reliability of correlated spike timings in cultured cortical neurons. *Biol. Cybern.* 80, 45–55.

van Pelt, J., Corner, M. A., Wolters, P. S., Rutten, W. L. C., and Ramakers, G. J. A. (2004). Long-term stability and developmental changes in spontaneous network burst firing patterns

in dissociated rat cerebral cortex cell cultures on multi-electrode arrays. *Neurosci. Lett.* 361, 86–89.

Wagenaar, D. A., and Potter, S. M. (2002). Real-time multi-channel stimulus artifact suppression by local curve fitting. *J. Neurosci. Methods* 120, 113–120.

Warwick, K., Xydas, D., Nasuto, S. J., Becerra, V. M., Hammond, M. W., Downes, J. H., et al. (2010). Controlling a mobile robot with a biological brain. *Def. Sci. J.* 60, 5–14.

West-Eberhard, M. J. (2003). *Developmental Plasticity and Evolution.* New York: Oxford University Press.

APPENDIX

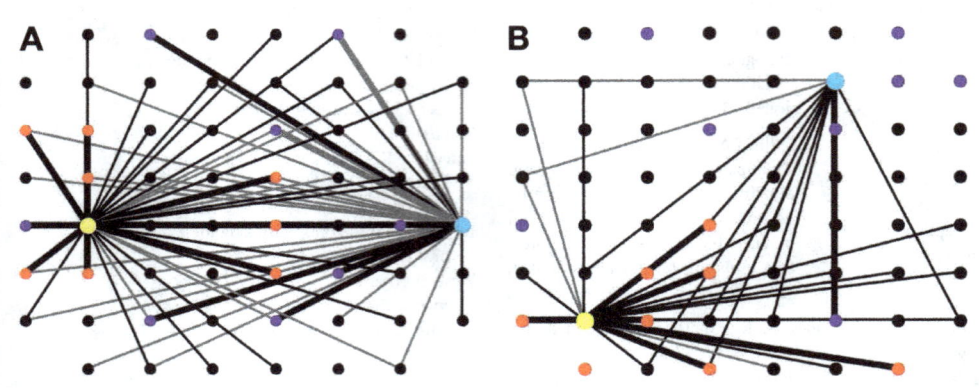

FIGURE A1 | Maps of changes in effective connectivity. (A) Changes in effective connectivity occurring during a tetanic stimulation experiment. The large dots, in yellow and light blue, represent electrodes used for delivery of both tetanic stimulation and sensory information for the left and right inputs. The smaller dots in blue and red indicate the position of electrodes used for recording from the two "motor" areas. Change in effective connectivity is defined as the difference in the area of PSTHs measured after and before the short-term plasticity experiment, divided by the average of these two values. Variations greater than 20% are represented as lines on the maps, with gray and black lines indicating, respectively, a decrease and an increase in functional connectivity. Only connections involving either stimulating electrode have been represented for clarity, with thicker lines highlighting the connections used in the closed-loop control of the robot (left input-left output and right input-right output areas). This map, in particular, is displaying the change in connectivity observed on a random culture during a 30-min short-term plasticity experiment. In this culture, tetanic stimulation led to a widespread increase of connection strengths involving the electrode represented in yellow, while those involving the one in light blue underwent a mixed change, with about half of them resulting strengthened and half of them weakened. **(B)** Same map as **(A)** obtained from recordings on a modular culture before and after a 30-min short-term plasticity experiment. While tetanic stimulation was delivered to both the yellow and light blue electrodes (respectively in the "lower" and "upper" halves of the culture), only one of the sub-populations was significantly affected, with a diffuse increase in connectivity.

3

Virtual sensory feedback for gait improvement in neurological patients

*Yoram Baram**

Computer Science Department, Technion – Israel Institute of Technology, Haifa, Israel

Edited by:
Alberto J. Espay, University of Cincinnati, USA

Reviewed by:
Mariana Moscovich, Universidade Federal do Paraná, Brazil
Fredy J. Revilla, University of Cincinnati College of Medicine, USA
Rahul Gupta, Medtronic Neuromodulation, USA

*Correspondence:
Yoram Baram, Computer Science Department, Technion – Israel Institute of Technology, Haifa 32000, Israel
e-mail: baram@cs.technion.ac.il

We review a treatment modality for movement disorders by sensory feedback. The natural closed-loop sensory-motor feedback system is imitated by a wearable virtual reality apparatus, employing body-mounted inertial sensors and responding dynamically to the patient's own motion. Clinical trials have shown a significant gait improvement in patients with Parkinson's disease using the apparatus. In contrast to open-loop devices, which impose constant-velocity visual cues in a "treadmill" fashion, or rhythmic auditory cues in a "metronome" fashion, requiring constant vigilance and attention strategies, and, in some cases, instigating freezing in Parkinsons patients, the closed-loop device improved gait parameters and eliminated freezing in most patients, without side effects. Patients with multiple sclerosis, previous stroke, senile gait, and cerebral palsy using the device also improved their balance and gait substantially. Training with the device has produced a residual improvement, suggesting virtual sensory feedback for the treatment of neurological movement disorders.

Keywords: sensory feedback, gait improvement, virtual reality, closed-loop gait regulation, sensory-motor control

INTRODUCTION

Neurological disorders, such as Parkinson's disease (PD), multiple sclerosis (MS), previous stroke (PS), senile gait (SG), and cerebral palsy (CP), often entail mobility impairment. Traditionally, gait rehabilitation, whether by means of physiotherapy or pharmacological treatment, has focused on improvement of muscle strength and reduction of spasticity (1–3). However, the main causes of motor impairment in such cases appear to lie in dysfunctional brain structures and neural information pathways. In particular, it has been suggested that PD patients suffer from deficient internal cue production (4–6). Visual feedback cues in the form of transverse lines marking on the ground have been found to improve the walking abilities of patients with PD (7, 8). Moreover, deficits in the functional neuroanatomy underlying gait in PD patients were found to be compensated by visual cues (9). Specifically, the right lateral pre-motor cortex, which is mainly regulated by cerebellar inputs, was activated to a greater extent in PD patients than in age-matched healthy individuals by visual transverse lines. On the other hand, healthy individuals activated mainly the supplementary motor area (SMA), which was under-activated in PD patients. It appears, then, that visually enhanced gait employs different brain pathways in PD patients compared to healthy individuals. It has been suggested that external sensory cues help patients with PD switch from one movement component of a sequence to the next, bypassing the defective internal trigger of the SMA (10, 11). It seems plausible that the concept of sensory bypass of deficient brain structures can apply to other categories of neurological disorders.

Early attempts to improve gait by artificially generated auditory and visual signals have produced open-loop systems which impose sensory signals, generated by an external source, not affected by the patient's own motion, such as fixed-velocity (treadmill-like) visual cues or rhythmic (metronome-like) auditory cues. While such strategies have been found to produce gait improvement in several studies (12–18), others have reported a need for constant vigilance and attention strategies to prevent reversion to impaired gait patterns caused by repetitive stimuli (11), confirming the role of predictive novelty and saliency in dopamine reward (19). Moreover, open-loop systems are known to be inherently inaccurate and unstable (20), which, in the present context, would be manifested by the patient "falling out of sync" with the repetitive sensory stimulus. A comparison of open-loop visual cuing by technological means to transverse lines marking on the ground (21) has found the first to have a marginal effect and the second to have a significant positive effect on walking parameters in PD patients. The advantage of closed-loop over open-loop control of arm motion has been noted (10). More recently, closed-loop sensory feedback strategies have been implemented in such specific motor control functions, related to locomotion, as stationary balance (22), planar pelvis and trunk movement (23), step symmetry (24), knee hyperextension (25), and partial weight-bearing (26). Yet, closed-loop virtual sensory feedback of whole-body forward movement in locomotion, as presently reviewed, does not appear to have been implemented, tested, or analyzed in other works.

CLOSED-LOOP SENSORY FEEDBACK GAIT CONTROL

An examination of the natural sensory-motor control system underlying human locomotion with respect to a visual scenery (27) reveals that it is the physical motion of the body which generates the visual cue and not the other way around. This seemingly obvious observation is crucial to understanding the difference between open-loop and closed-loop sensory control of locomotion. The two control paradigms are illustrated in **Figure 1**. In the open-loop system, a visual cue is generated artificially and fed

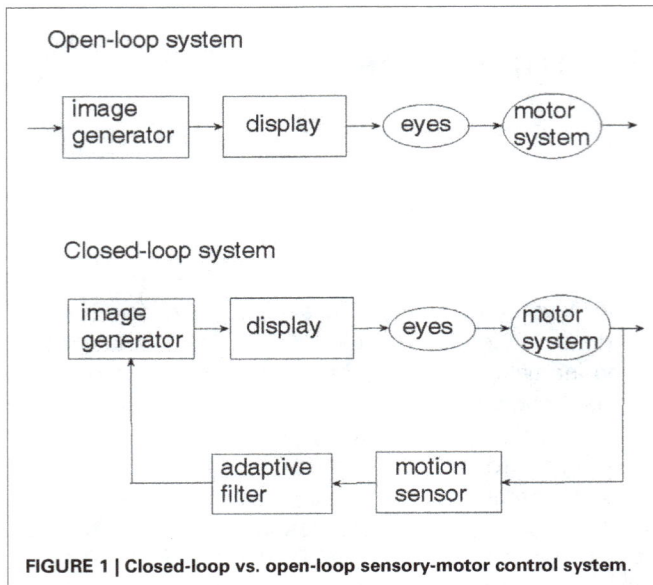

FIGURE 1 | Closed-loop vs. open-loop sensory-motor control system.

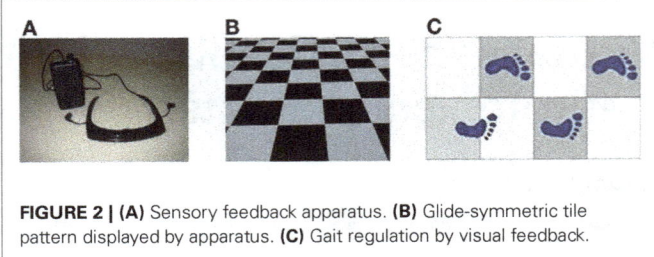

FIGURE 2 | (A) Sensory feedback apparatus. **(B)** Glide-symmetric tile pattern displayed by apparatus. **(C)** Gait regulation by visual feedback.

through the eyes to the brain, which may or may not activate the limbs so as to respond to the visual cue. On the other hand, an artificial realization of the natural sensory-motor control system is the closed-loop feedback system, where the generation of the visual cue is controlled and regulated by the body movement caused by locomotion. The motion of the visual cue is matched to that of the body. When there is no motion of the body, there is no visual cue.

Depicted in **Figure 2A**, a sensory device, employing body-mounted inertial sensors, generates earth-stationary visual cues (28). The checkerboard tiles geometry of the visual display, **Figure 2B**, matched to the glide-reflection symmetry of human locomotion (29), regulates the motor task, producing an even (glide-reflection symmetric) gait pattern, better balance, and safer, more efficient mobility. Even if the resulting gait pattern is not perfectly matched to the visual tile pattern, improvement in that direction translates into improvement in gait. **Figure 2C** illustrates the transition from uneven to even gait resulting from such visual feedback regulation (a short first step is followed by longer, more even steps). In addition to the visual feedback cue delivered by the display, the device also produces an auditory feedback cue in the form of a clicking sound delivered through earphones in response to every step taken by the patient. In contrast to open-loop, metronome-like devices, which attempt to impose a walking pace on the patient by a constant auditory cue, the feedback device produces an auditory cue matched to the walking pattern. A balanced steady walk will generate a rhythmic auditory cue. Any deviation from such a gait pattern will result in a deviation from the auditory rhythm and will be corrected by a change of gait in a feedback fashion. The head-mounted display and earphones bring the sensory feedback signals closer to the sensors – the eyes and the ears, making the sensory effect more pronounced, easier to follow and to learn. An open-loop capability, producing constant movement of the visual cue and a constant rhythmic auditory cue, was also added to an early version of the device for experimental comparison purposes.

MEDICAL STUDIES

Medical studies, described below and summarized in **Table 1**, were performed during different stages in the development of the concept, the apparatus, and the medical assessment methods. Consequently, these studies varied not only in the different research groups and their focus on different neurological disorders, but also in the test parameters. Some of the studies tested visual feedback only, some auditory feedback only, and some both visual and auditory feedback. Some of the tests examined on-line (device on) performance only, some extended to examination of short-term (a few minutes) residual effects, and some examined long-term (a few weeks) residual effects as well. The results of the different studies also differed in their methods of statistical representation. Yet, most of the studies shared some common features, particularly the following three steps:

Step 1: baseline performance. The patient was verbally instructed to walk "normally" without the device along a straight track of 10 m. The time to complete the track and the number of steps were recorded for calculation of baseline walking speed (BWS) and stride length.

Step 2: on-line training and performance. The device was placed on the patient and turned on. The patient was instructed to walk along the 10-m track for the purpose of training. Patients training with visual feedback were asked to imagine, while walking, stepping on the tiles. They were told that stepping on tile boundaries was allowed, and that there was no particular order of black or white tiles that needed to be kept with respect to the stepping sequence. Patients training with auditory feedback were asked to maintain, by controlling their gait pattern, a rhythmic auditory cue. The track walking was repeated twice for training and four more times for measurement and recording of on-line walking speed and stride length.

Step 3: residual effect. The device was taken off the patient, who was given a 20-min break. After the break, the patient was instructed to walk the 10-m track without the device. Walking speed and stride length were recorded four times and averaged. The purpose of this stage was to measure the residual short-term effect of training with the sensory feedback cue.

The results were then averaged across all patients and the average change due to device use was calculated along with the significance parameter p.

While there are several on-going studies on the effects of the GaitAid virtual sensory feedback device, performed by different research groups concerning different disorders and different issues

Table 1 | Clinical test settings.

Study	Disease	Number of patients	Patient condition	Feedback channel	Feedback modality	Training location	Effect measured	Typical change
In-clinic comparison of open and closed-loop strategies	PD	14	Off	V	O	C	OL	13.8%
In-clinic comparison of open and closed-loop strategies	PD	14	Off	V	C	C	OL	25.6%
At-home training with joint visual and auditory feedback	PD	13	On	VA	C	H	OL	17.9%
At-home training with joint visual and auditory feedback	PD	13	On	VA	C	H	LTR	17.1%
Gait initiation and the significance of prior instructions and training	PD	47	On	V	C	C	GI	6.2%
Long-term effects on PD patients with "on"-predominant freezing of gait	PD	13	On	VA	C	H	UPDRS	35.4%
Visual feedback	SG	20	On	V	C	C	OL	6.3%
Level of education effect	SG	20	On	V	C	C	EL	6.7%
Visual feedback	PS	6	On	V	C	C	OL	13.2%
Visual feedback	MS	16	On	V	C	C	OL	13.4%
Visual feedback	MS	16	On	V	C	C	STR	24.4%
Auditory feedback	MS	16	On	A	C	C	OL	12.8%
Auditory feedback	MS	16	On	A	C	C	STR	18.7%
Visual cue geometry effect	MS	16	On	V	C	C	VCG	21.0%
Visual feedback	CP	10	On	V	C	C	STR	21.7%
Auditory feedback	CP	10	On	A	C	C	STR	25.4%

Patient condition: Off, without medication for 12 h; On, on regular medication schedule. Feedback channel: V, visual channel; A, auditory channel; VA, combined visual and auditory channels. Feedback modality: O, open-loop; C, closed-loop. Training location: C, clinic; H, home. Effect measured: OL, on-line; STR, short-term residual; LTR, long-term residual; GI, gait initiation; UPRDS, unified Parkinson's disease rating scale; EL, education level; VCG, visual cue geometry. Typical change: percentage improvement in walking speed compared to baseline, except where corresponding to GI, UPDRS.

of interests, we provide an account of earlier studies, detailed in previous publications.

PARKINSON'S DISEASE

In-clinic comparison of open and closed-loop strategies

A clinical study comparing the on-line effects of visual cues in open-loop and closed-loop configurations on PD patients off their regular medication (30) has found that patients who used the open-loop system improved their gait on average by 13.8% ($p = 0.230$) in walking speed and by 15.0% ($p = 0.056$) in stride length. Two of the patients went into freezing midway when using the open-loop system. The high p values indicate low likelihood of the improvement results being attributable to a specific cause. Patients who used the closed-loop system improved their gait on average by 25.7% ($p = 0.001$) in walking speed and by 30.8% ($p = 0.0085$) in stride length. None of the patients experienced freezing when using the closed-loop system. This study revealed that the gait parameters which are most sensitive to anti-Parkinson medication (31), namely, walking speed and stride length, can also be manipulated, to a similar extent and without some adverse effects, by a closed-loop display of virtual visual cues. These parameters have also been reported to be

improved by pallidotomy [brain surgery (32)], however, a more recent study has shown adverse effects of deep brain stimulation (DBS) of the globus pallidus internus (GPi) in PD patients with dystonia (33).

At-home training with joint visual and auditory feedback

Clinical testing before and after 2-week at-home training with joint visual and auditory feedback (34) found that average improvement with device on was 17.9% ($p = 0.006$) in walking speed and 13.1% ($p = 0.004$) in stride length. Residual improvement in walking without the device was 17.1% ($p = 0.0004$) in walking speed and 12.4% ($p = 0.003$) in stride length. Residual improvement of two thirds of the patients was at least 20% ($p < 0.03$) in either walking speed or stride length or both. Improvement in FOGQ (35) was 14.5% ($p = 0.02$). This shows that although the immediate improvement with device use, or immediately following such use, was somewhat higher (30), residual improvement was sustained at least for a few days following training.

Gait initiation and the significance of prior instructions and training

A study of visual feedback without prior instructions or prior training (36) has shown a decrease in the average time of first-step initiation (−6.2%), with smaller changes in subsequent average walking speed (−0.8%) and cadence (−1.8%). The improvement in step initiation by device use suggests a role for predictive salience and dopamine reward in movement (19). A comparison of the present study to previous studies, in which patients were given prior instructions and training, resulting in the sustainment of an improved gait pattern, suggests that predictive salience and dopamine reward are enhanced by prior instructions and training.

Long-term effects on PD patients with "on"-predominant freezing of gait

A study on the long-term effects of training with sensory feedback has examined PD patients with "on"-predominant freezing of gait (37). Of the 13 initial patients only 2 completed the study, which was attributed to severe burden of the disability and the fragility of these patients, limiting the opportunities to fulfill the required daily training sessions and preventing their return for the scheduled study visits. The single patient who was documented showed a sustained improvement in the UPDRS-III (38) and the FOGQ (35) measures, following 4 weeks of at-home training (UPDRS-III: 24 at baseline, 15.5 at 12 weeks; FOGQ: 16 at baseline, 13 at 12 weeks). Benefits were renewed after a "booster" training once the residual gait improvement weaned at about 16 weeks post-training. Yet, the high dropout rate did not support generalization of these results.

SENILE GAIT
Gait improvement

A study of randomly selected old-age home residents suffering from lower-body Parkinsonism, or SG, but without PD (39) showed that, in patients with baseline performance above the median, the average on-line improvement when using visual feedback was considerably higher ($6.31 \pm 12.59\%$ in walking speed and $6.41 \pm 11.11\%$ in stride length) than in patients with baseline performance below the median ($-0.72 \pm 22.75\%$ in walking speed and $3.39 \pm 11.26\%$ in stride length). This stands in sharp contrast to the results obtained for patients with PD, whose gait improvement was inversely correlated with baseline performance.

Level of education effect on SG improvement

The same study (39) found that, for patients with a maximum of 8 years of study, average improvement in walking speed was -8.83 ± 23.81 and $-4.67 \pm 15.30\%$ in stride length. For patients with 12 years of study, average improvement was $-1.85 \pm 26.83\%$ in walking speed and $3.82 \pm 9.75\%$ in stride length. For patients with 20 years of study, average improvement was $6.75 \pm 0.49\%$ in walking speed and $14.55 \pm 12.66\%$ in stride length. As might have been expected, the ability to make use of sensory feedback information appeared to be positively correlated with cognitive abilities. Conversely, improved performance by sensory feedback may be regarded as a relevant measure of cognitive function in the present context.

PREVIOUS STROKES

Two thirds of the patients with SG also suffering from PS (39), using on-line visual feedback as specified in steps 1 and 2, improved their walking speed or stride length or both by more than 10%. While patients with left-hemisphere vascular accident improved their gait, patients with right-hemisphere vascular accident did not improve. In patients with baseline performance above the median, improvement was considerably higher ($13.2 \pm 6.0\%$ in walking speed and $16.6 \pm 4.7\%$ in stride length) than in patients with baseline performance below the median ($-9.9 \pm 27\%$ in walking speed and $-7.7 \pm 12.3\%$ in stride length). The visual feedback cues did not improve gait in patients with vascular risk factors but without history of PS. As the gait improvement in patients with PS was more pronounced than in patients with SG but without PS, so was the contrast between these patients and patients with PD in the correlation between the level of improvement and baseline performance.

MULTIPLE SCLEROSIS

In contrast to patients with PD, SG, or PS, who are predominantly of advanced age, patients with MS range from teen-agers to mid-agers.

Visual feedback

A study of the effects of visual feedback on patients with MS (40) found that patients whose BWS was below the median showed an average on-line improvement of 13.46% in their walking speed when using the visual feedback channel of the GaitAid device, while patients whose BWS was above the median improved their walking speed by 1.47%. The average short-term residual improvement in walking speed was 24.49% in patients with BWS below the median and 9.09% in patients with BWS above the median. Similar results were obtained for improvement in stride length. These trends are consistent with those found in patients with PD. No gait improvement was found in age-matched controls using visual feedback.

Auditory feedback

A study of the effects of auditory feedback on patients with MS (41) showed an average improvement of $12.84 \pm 18.74\%$ on-line and $18.75 \pm 18.53\%$ residually in walking speed. Average improvement in stride length was $8.30 \pm 11.87\%$ on-line and $9.93 \pm 9.46\%$ residually. No gait improvement was found in age-matched controls using auditory feedback.

Visual cue geometry

A study aimed at comparing the effects of gait training with distinct glide-reflection symmetry (checkerboard tiles) visual feedback cues, to the effects of training with visual cues with no distinct symmetry [earth-stationary transverse lines, as used in early studies (7, 8)] was performed on subjects with gait disorders due to MS (42). It found that the average improvement in the group using the transverse lines was $7.79 \pm 4.24\%$ in walking speed and $7.20 \pm 3.92\%$ in stride length. The average improvement in the group using the visual cue of checkerboard tiles was $21.09 \pm 18.39\%$ in walking speed and $12.99 \pm 1.72\%$ in stride length. This shows that matching the visual cue pattern to the glide-reflection symmetric pattern of human locomotion results in significant additional improvement.

CEREBRAL PALSY

Cerebral palsy has predominantly pre-natal causes and is symptomatically addressed at a young age. A study of patients with gait disorders due to CP (43) found that, for patients training with visual feedback, the short-term residual improvement was $21.70 \pm 36.06\%$ in the walking speed and $8.72 \pm 9.47\%$ in the stride length. For patients training with auditory feedback, the short-term residual improvement was $25.43 \pm 28.65\%$ in the walking speed and $13.58 \pm 13.10\%$ in the stride length. Age-matched controls who trained with either visual or auditory feedback showed no improvement in gait. The relatively large standard deviations in the results may be attributed to the very diverse nature of the disorder and the subsequent disabilities.

MEDICAL STUDIES SUMMARY

The reviewed medical studies are summarized in **Table 1**.

It can be seen that, as indicated by the last column of **Table 1**, all these medical studies show positive effects of sensory feedback on gait in patients with the neurological disorders under consideration. Yet, any comparison between these results must take into account the differences between the disorders, the testing conditions and the measures used, as indicated in the specific subsections, and, in further detail, in the cited references. For instance, the percentage improvements in gait initiation time (GI) and in UPDRS bring into light different aspects of gait improvement in PD patients, but cannot be used to compare the benefits for MS patients to those for PD patients. It should also be noted that while these studies employed various versions of monocular and binocular displays, on the one hand, and either or both visual and auditory feedback channels, the results do not necessarily generalize to all forms of sensory feedback, which may present additional benefits or drawbacks.

DISCUSSION

We have reviewed the use of sensory feedback for improving gait in movement disorders patients. While certain studies have found open-loop sensory stimulation to result in balance and gait improvement, others have raised questions as to the effectiveness of monotone sensory cues, which, lacking the predictive novelty and saliency associated with dopamine reward, require constant vigilance and attention strategies, and instigate freezing in Parkinson's patients who fall out of sync with the sensory stimuli. Realizing that the natural sensory-motor stabilization effect is produced by the sensory cues generated by motion in a stationary environment, we created a closed-loop augmented reality device which produces earth-stationary visual and auditory cues in response to the patient's own motion. The device has been found to improve gait in patients with a variety of neurological disorders, maintaining patient's safety and well-being, without the adverse effects associated with medication and deep brain surgery. Neurological patients are often subject to high levels of fragility and fatigue, which may affect their ability to sustain long periods of physical training in general, and training with sensory feedback in particular. We did not encounter, however, significant levels of such effects in our studies, where particularly disabled patients were excluded. With the exclusion of patients with very low or very high level of impairment, the level of improvement is normally related to the level of impairment. Training with the device has been found to have short-term and long-term residual improvement effects, suggesting virtual sensory feedback as a treatment modality for neurological movement disorders. While, due to conceptual and technological developments, the device took different forms, the concepts tested were quite general (e.g., visual feedback, auditory feedback, and combined visual and auditory feedback). Moreover, for the same concept (e.g., on-line visual feedback in PD patients), the results were quite consistent. It is therefore believed that if other devices, based on the same concepts, become available, they will produce similar results.

As the clinical studies performed on a variety of patient populations with different neurological impairments were of a preliminary nature, future studies, involving larger patient cohorts under streamlined controlled conditions, should investigate the same and other aspects of such treatment in greater detail. The possibility of fitting the sensory feedback device to individual patient limitations and needs should be explored. Long-term treatment programs should be developed and tested in clinic, home and, possibly, a variety of natural environments. The integration of sensory feedback components of specific motor tasks associated with gait and balance, such as head, pelvis, trunk, and knee movement, in a comprehensive motor rehabilitation program, should also be investigated. Mobile technology advancement, improving vision, hearing and sensing, should be adopted to improve device utility and effectiveness.

REFERENCES

1. Gibberd FB, Page NGR, Spencer KM, Kinnear E, Hawksworth JB. Controlled trial of physiotherapy and occupational therapy for Parkinson's disease. *BMJ* (1981) **282**: 1196. doi:10.1136/bmj.282.6280.1970-a

2. Palmer SS, Mortimer JA, Webster DD, Bistevins R, Dickinson GL. Exercise therapy for Parkinson's disease. *Arch Phys Med Rehabil* (1986) **67**:741–745. doi:10.1016/0003-9993(86)90007-9

3. Armutlu K, Karabudak R, Nurlu G. Physiotherapy approaches in the treatment of ataxic multiple sclerosis: a pilot study. *Neurorehabil Neural Repair* (2001) **15**:203–11. doi:10.1177/154596830101500308

4. Georgiou N, Iansek R, Bradshaw JL, Phillips JG, Mattingley JB, Bradshaw JA. An evaluation of the role of internal cues in the pathogenesis of parkinsonian hypokinesia. *Brain* (1993) **116**: 1575–87. doi:10.1093/brain/116.6.1575

5. Morris ME, Iansek R, Matyas TA, Summers JJ. The pathogenesis of gait hypokinesia in Parkinson's disease. *Brain* (1994) **117**: 1169–81. doi:10.1093/brain/117.5.1169

6. Cunnington R, Iansek R, Bradshaw JL, Phillips J. Movement-related potentials in Parkinson's disease: presence and predictability of temporal and spatial cues. *Brain* (1995) **118**:935–50. doi:10.1093/brain/118.4.935

7. Martin JP. Locomotion and the basal ganglia. In: Martin JP, editor. *The Basal Ganglia and Posture*. London: Pitman Medical (1967). p. 20–35.

8. Azulay JP, Mesure S, Amblard B, Blin O, Sangla I, Pouget J. Visual control of locomotion in Parkinson's disease. *Brain* (1999) **122**(Pt 1):111–20. doi:10.1093/brain/122.1.111

9. Hanakawa T, Fukuyama H, Katsumi Y, Honda M, Shibasaki H. Enhanced lateral premotor activity during paradoxical gait in patients with Parkinson's disease. *Ann Neurol* (1999) **45**:329–36. doi:10.1002/1531-8249(199903)45:3<329::AID-ANA8>3.0.CO;2-S

10. Flowers KA. Visual 'closed loop' and 'open loop' characteristics of voluntary movement in patients with parkinsonism and intension tremor. *Brain* (1976) **99**:269–310. doi:10.1093/brain/99.2.269

11. Morris ME, Iansek R, Matyas TA, Summers JJ. Sride length regulation in Parkinson's disease: normalizations strategies and underlying mechanisms. *Brain* (1996) **119**:551–68. doi:10.1093/brain/119. 2.551

12. Prothero J. *The Treatment of Akinesia Using Virtual Images [M. Sc. Thesis]*. Seattle: University of Washington, College of Engineering (1993).

13. Behrman AL, Teielbaum P, Cauraugh JH. Verbal instructional sets to normalize the temporal and spatial gait variables in Pakinson's disease. *J Neurol Neurosurg Psychiatry* (1998) **65**:580–2. doi:10.1136/jnnp. 65.4.580

14. Lewis GN, Byblow WD, Walt SE. Stride length regulation in Parkinson's disease: the use of extrinsic, visual cues. *Brain* (2000) **123**:2077–90. doi:10.1093/brain/123.10.2077

15. Rubinstein TC, Giladi N, Hausdorff JM. The power of cueing to circumvent dopamine deficits: a review of physical therapy treatment of gait disturbances in Parkinson's disease. *Mov Disord* (2002) **17**:1148–60. doi:10.1002/mds.10259

16. Mak MKY, Hui-Chan CWY. Audiovisual cues can enhance sit-to-stand in patients with Parkinson's disease. *Mov Disord* (2004) **19**:1012–9. doi:10.1002/mds.20196

17. Nieuwboer A, Kwakkel G, Rochester L, Jones D, van Wegen E, Willems AM, et al. Cueing training in the home improves gait-related mobility in Parkinson's disease. The RESCUE trial. *J Neurol Neurosurg Psychiatry* (2007) **78**:134–40. doi:10.1136/jnnp.200X.097923

18. Kaminsky TA, Dudgeon BJ, Billingsley FF, Mitchell PH, Weghorst SJ. Virtual cues and functional mobility of people with Parkinson's disease: a single-subject pilot study. *J Rehabil Res Dev* (2007) **44**(3):437–48.

19. Schultz W. Predictive reward signal of dopamine neurons. *J Physiol* (1998) **80**(1):1–27.

20. Kuo BC. *Automatic Control Systems*. Englewood Cliffs, NJ: Prentice-Hall (1962).

21. Griffin HJ, Greenlaw R, Limousin P, Bhatia K, Quinn NP, Jahanshahi M. The effect of real and virtual visual cues on walking in Parkinson's disease. *J Neurol* (2011) **258**(6):991–1000. doi:10.1007/s00415-010-5866-z

22. Esculier JF, Vaudrin J, Bériault P, Gagnon K, Tremblay LE. Home-based balance training programme using Wii Fit with balance board for Parkinsons's disease: a pilot study. *J Rehabil Med* (2012) **44**(2):144–50. doi:10.2340/16501977-0922

23. Hamacher D, Bertram D, Fölsch C, Schega L. Evaluation of a visual feedback system in gait retraining: a pilot study. *Gait Posture* (2012) **36**(2):182–6. doi:10.1016/j.gaitpost.2012.02.012

24. Kim SJ, Krebs HI. Effects of implicit visual feedback distortion on human gait. *Exp Brain Res* (2012) **218**(3):495–502. doi:10.1007/s00221-012-3044-5

25. Teran-Yengle P, Birkhofer R, Weber MA, Patton K, Thatcher E, Yack HJ. Efficacy of gait training with real-time biofeedback in correcting knee hyperextension patterns in young women. *J Orthop Sports Phys Ther* (2011) **41**(12):948–52. doi:10.2519/jospt.2011.3660

26. Hurkmans HL, Bussmann JB, Benda E, Verhaar JA, Stam HJ. Effectiveness of audio feedback for partial weight-bearing in and outside the hospital: a randomized controlled trial. *Arch Phys Med Rehabil* (2012) **93**(4):565–70. doi:10.1016/j.apmr.2011.11.019

27. Baram Y. Walking on tiles. *Neural Proc Lett* (1999) **10**:81–7. doi:10.1023/A:1018713516431

28. Baram Y. *Closed-Loop Augmented Reality Apparatus*. US Patent No. 6,734,834-B1 (2004).

29. Livio M. *The Equation that Couldn't be Solved*. New York: Simon & Schuster (2005).

30. Baram Y, Aharon-Peretz J, Simionotici Y, Ron L. Walking on virtual tiles. *Neural Proc Lett* (2002) **16**:227–33. doi:10.1023/A:1021778608344

31. Pedersen SW, Eriksson T, Oberg B. Effects of withdrawal of antiparkinson medication on gait and clinical score in the Parkinson patient. *Acta Neurol Scand* (1991) **84**(1):7–13. doi:10.1111/j.1600-0404.1991.tb04894.x

32. Siegel KL, Metman LV. Effects of bilateral posteroventral pallidotomy on gait in subjects with Parkinson's disease. *Arch Neurol* (2000) **57**:198. doi:10.1001/archneur.57.2.198

33. Schrader C, Capelle HH, Kinfe TM, Blahak C, Bäzner H, Lütjens G, et al. GPi-DBS may induce a hypokinetic gait disorder with freezing of gait in patients with dystonia. *Neurology* (2011) **77**(5):483–8. doi:10.1212/WNL.0b013e318227b19e

34. Espay J, Baram Y, Dwivedi AK, Shukla R, Gartner M, Gaines L, et al. At-home training with closed-loop augmented-reality cueing device for improvement of gait in patients with Parkinson's disease. *J Rehabil Res Dev* (2010) **47**(6):573–82.

35. Giladi N, Shabtai H, Simon ES, Biran S, Tal J, Korczyn AD. Construction of freezing of gait questionnaire for patients with Parkinsonism. *Parkinsonism Relat Disord* (2000) **6**:165–70. doi:10.1016/S1353-8020(99)00062-0

36. Chong R, Lee KH, Morgan J, Mehta S, Griffin J, Marchant J, et al. Closed-loop VR-based interaction to improve walking in Parkinson's disease. *J Nov Physiother* (2011) **1**:1–7. doi:10.4172/2165-7025.1000101

37. Espay AJ, Gaines L, Gupta R. Sensory feedback in Parkinson's disease patients with "on"-predominant freezing of gait. *Front Neurol* (2013) **4**:14. doi:10.3389/fneur.2013.00014

38. Fahn S, Elton RL, The UPDRS Development Committee. Unified Parkinson's disease rating scale. In: Fahn S, Marsden CD, Calne D, Goldstein M, editors. *Recent Developments in Parkinson's Disease*. Florham Park, NJ: Macmillan Health Care Information (1987). p. 153–64.

39. Baram Y, Aharon-Peretz J, Lenger R. Virtual reality feedback for gait improvement in patients with idiopathic senile gait disorders and in patient with history of strokes. *J Am Geriatr Soc* (2010) **58**(1):191–2. doi:10.1111/j.1532-5415.2009.02654.x

40. Baram Y, Miller A. Effects of virtual reality cues on gait in multiple sclerosis patients. *Neurology* (2006) **66**:178–81. doi:10.1212/01.wnl.0000194255.82542.6b

41. Baram Y, Miller A. Auditory feedback for improvement of gait in multiple sclerosis patients. *J Neurol Sci* (2007) **254**:90–4. doi:10.1016/j.jns.2007.01.003

42. Baram Y, Miller A. Glide-symmetric locomotion reinforcement in patients with multiple sclerosis by visual feedback. *Disabil Rehabil Assist Technol* (2010) **5**(5):323–6. doi:10.3109/17483101003671717

43. Baram Y, Lenger R. Gait improvement in patients with cerebral palsy by visual and auditory feedback. *Neuromodulation* (2012) **15**(1):48–52. doi:10.1111/j.1525-1403.2011.00412.x

4

Spatial vision in insects is facilitated by shaping the dynamics of visual input through behavioral action

Martin Egelhaaf*, Norbert Boeddeker, Roland Kern, Rafael Kurtz and Jens P. Lindemann

Neurobiology and Centre of Excellence "Cognitive Interaction Technology", Bielefeld University, Germany

Edited by:
Eberhard E. Fetz, University of Washington, USA

Reviewed by:
Vladimir Brezina, Mount Sinai School of Medicine, USA
Alexander Borst, Max Planck Institute of Neurobiology, Germany

*Correspondence:
Martin Egelhaaf, Neurobiology and Centre of Excellence "Cognitive Interaction Technology", Bielefeld University, Germany.
e-mail: martin.egelhaaf@ uni-bielefeld.de

Insects such as flies or bees, with their miniature brains, are able to control highly aerobatic flight maneuvres and to solve spatial vision tasks, such as avoiding collisions with obstacles, landing on objects, or even localizing a previously learnt inconspicuous goal on the basis of environmental cues. With regard to solving such spatial tasks, these insects still outperform man-made autonomous flying systems. To accomplish their extraordinary performance, flies and bees have been shown by their characteristic behavioral actions to actively shape the dynamics of the image flow on their eyes ("optic flow"). The neural processing of information about the spatial layout of the environment is greatly facilitated by segregating the rotational from the translational optic flow component through a saccadic flight and gaze strategy. This active vision strategy thus enables the nervous system to solve apparently complex spatial vision tasks in a particularly efficient and parsimonious way. The key idea of this review is that biological agents, such as flies or bees, acquire at least part of their strength as autonomous systems through active interactions with their environment and not by simply processing passively gained information about the world. These agent-environment interactions lead to adaptive behavior in surroundings of a wide range of complexity. Animals with even tiny brains, such as insects, are capable of performing extraordinarily well in their behavioral contexts by making optimal use of the closed action–perception loop. Model simulations and robotic implementations show that the smart biological mechanisms of motion computation and visually-guided flight control might be helpful to find technical solutions, for example, when designing micro air vehicles carrying a miniaturized, low-weight on-board processor.

Keywords: spatial behavior, optic flow, saccades, flying insects, obstacle avoidance, navigation behavior

OPTIC FLOW AS AN IMPORTANT SPATIAL CUE FOR FAST MOVING ANIMALS

Behavior is a phenomenon that takes place in space and is intricately entangled with it. The organism is required to interact with its surroundings in a way appropriate to the respective situational context. It should be able to respond appropriately to objects, for instance, by avoiding collisions with obstacles or by detecting and fixating inanimate objects of interest or other organisms, such as a predator, prey, or mate. On a larger spatial scale, organisms should be able to navigate from one place to another and to localize a goal on the basis of environmental spatial cues.

Insects are obviously well able to cope with these behavioral challenges in a highly virtuosic and efficient way. Think of a blowfly, for example, landing on the rim of a cup, or two flies chasing each other; without technical assistance, our visual system is incapable of resolving the complexity of such flight maneuvres, and the speed at which they are executed exceeds by far the capacities of our own motor system. During their virtuosic flight maneuvres, blowflies can make up to ten sudden ("saccadic") turns per second, during which they may reach angular velocities of up to 4000°/s. The extraordinary navigational skills of bees are another awe inspiring example of insect spatial behavior: spatial cues enable bees to localize previously learnt, barely visible goals, such as a food source or the entrance to their nest, over large distances even in cluttered environments. All these feats are accomplished with visual systems of comparatively poor spatial resolution and extremely small brains that consist of no more than a million neurons, underlining the resource efficiency of the underlying mechanisms.

We will argue in this review that biological agents, such as flying insects, are such efficient and adaptive autonomous systems because they rely, to a large extent, on strategies by which they shape their sensory input through the specific way they move and change their gaze direction. In this way, they actively reduce the complexity of their sensory input and, thus, the computational load for the underlying brain mechanisms. Therefore, by exploiting the consequences of the action–perception cycle, animals with even tiny brains, such as insects, are enabled to perform extraordinarily well in solving spatial vision tasks in a wide range of behavioral contexts. This view somehow contrasts with common conceptions of how spatial vision is accomplished.

If laypeople are asked for the requirements of spatial vision, they are likely to reply that most animals, including humans, are equipped with two eyes which allow them to view the world from slightly different vantage points, and that the nervous system makes use of the resulting disparity information for depth vision. However, the spatial range that can be resolved in this way is critically restricted by the distance between the eyes, the overlap of their visual fields and their spatial resolution (Collett and Harkness, 1982). Hence, stereoscopic vision—if it is available at all to a particular animal species—is functional only in the near range. This poses a problem, especially for fast moving animals, such as many flying insects (as well as for human car drivers), because, in order to control appropriate reactions, such as avoiding collisions with obstacles, spatial information is required at much greater distances than may be available through stereoscopic mechanisms. Amongst the depth cues that are available in addition to binocular information, for example, contrast differences between near and distant objects (Collett and Harkness, 1982), the retinal image motion induced by self-movements of the animal ("optic flow") is particularly relevant (Koenderink, 1986; Rogers, 1993; Poteser and Kral, 1995; Lappe, 2000; Redlick et al., 2001; Vaina et al., 2004).

Whenever an animal moves in its environment, the retinal images are continually displaced. During translatory movements, these displacements depend on the distance of environmental objects to the eyes, their angular location relative to the direction of motion and the velocity of locomotion. Only translational optic flow is distance dependent and, thus, contains spatial information, whereas rotational optic flow is useless for spatial vision, because all objects during rotations are displaced at the same angular velocity irrespective of their distance (**Figure 1**; Koenderink, 1986). Hence, the translatory optic flow component contains information about the relative distance of environmental objects from the animal: objects nearby pass quickly, while objects far-off appear virtually stationary. This motion-induced spatial information is based on behavioral action, because it is only available during self-motion, but not when the animal is stationary. Many animals, ranging from insects to humans, were concluded to exploit optic flow information for depth cueing.

We will focus in this review on the spatial behavior of insects that is based on depth information derived from optic flow. Since optic flow is particularly relevant during fast locomotion in three dimensions, we will mainly cover spatial vision in flight and address four major issues: (1) Components of insect behavior that are thought to be involved in solving basic spatial tasks and how they may depend on motion-based information; (2) the processing of motion-dependent spatial information and how it is facilitated by active gaze movements; (3) the representation of behaviorally relevant spatial information in the visual system; and (4) the behavioral significance of neurons extracting information about self-motion of the animal, as well as the environment, from the image flow generated on the eyes as a consequence of the action–perception loop being closed. Obviously, solving any spatial vision task—especially by flying insects that lack passive stability—requires, as a precondition, the animal's flight attitude to be somehow stabilized by appropriate feedback control systems. This issue, though very important for spatial orientation behavior and widely analysed for decades, will be touched on only briefly, because it has already been thoroughly reviewed (Hengstenberg, 1993; Taylor and Krapp, 2008).

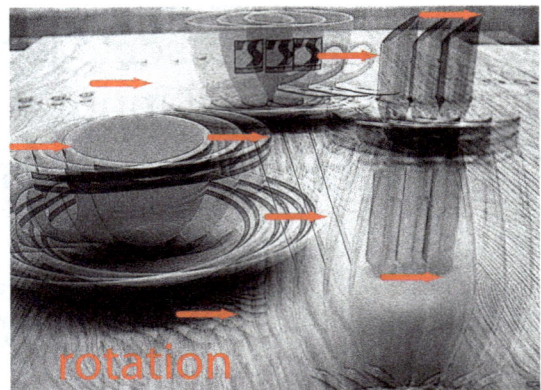
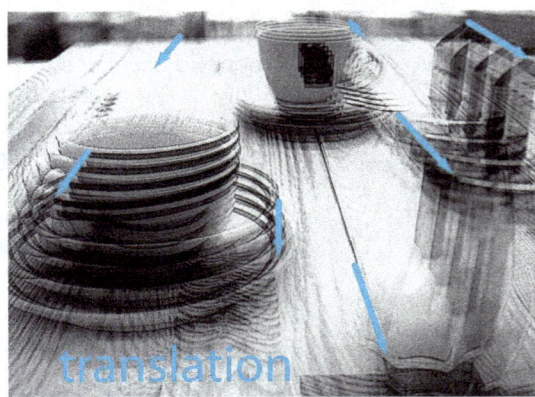

FIGURE 1 | Schematic illustration of the consequences of rotational (upper diagram) or translational self-motion (bottom diagram) for the resulting optic flow. Superimposed images were either generated by rotating a camera around its vertical axis or by translating it forward. Rotational self-motion leads to image movements (red arrows) of the same velocity (reflected in the arrow length) irrespective of the distance of environmental objects from the observer. In contrast, the optic flow elicited by translational self-motion (blue arrows) depends on the distance between objects from the observer. Hence, translational optic flow contains spatial information.

BEHAVIOR INVOLVED IN SPATIAL TASKS AND ITS CONTROL BY VISUAL MOTION CUES

Many animals, including humans, use optic flow for the control of spatial behavior. Since spatial information can most easily be extracted from the retinal image flow during translatory self-motion, some animals execute translatory movements of their body and/or head that appear to be dedicated to generate optic flow suitable for depth cueing. Locusts, mantids, and dragonflies, for instance, sitting in ambush perform lateral body and head movements in preparation for a jump or for catching prey, respectively (Collett, 1978; Sobel, 1990; Collett and Paterson, 1991; Kral and Poteser, 1997; Olberg et al., 2005). Some bird species bob their heads back and forth, most likely to acquire depth information (Davies and Green, 1988; Necker, 2007). Moreover, flying insects, such as flies and bees (Schilstra and van Hateren, 1999; Boeddeker et al., 2010; Braun et al., 2010, 2012; Geurten et al., 2010), but also birds (Eckmeier et al., 2008), perform a saccadic flight and gaze strategy in which short and rapid head and body saccades are separated by largely translatory locomotion. This strategy facilitates access to spatial information from the resulting optic flow.

The use of optic flow to gain spatial information has been shown most convincingly in behavioral experiments in which animals responded to objects that were camouflaged by covering them with the same texture as their background. Thus, these objects could be discriminated only on the basis of optic flow cues

elicited during self-motion. *Drosophila*, for instance, is well able to discriminate the distance of different objects on the basis of slight differences in their retinal velocities (Schuster et al., 2002). Bees (Srinivasan et al., 1987; Lehrer et al., 1988) and blowflies (Kimmerle et al., 1996) use relative motion cues mainly at the edges of objects to discriminate between their height and to land on them (**Figure 2A**; Srinivasan et al., 1990; Kimmerle et al., 1996; Kern et al., 1997). Bees also use motion contrast in discrimination

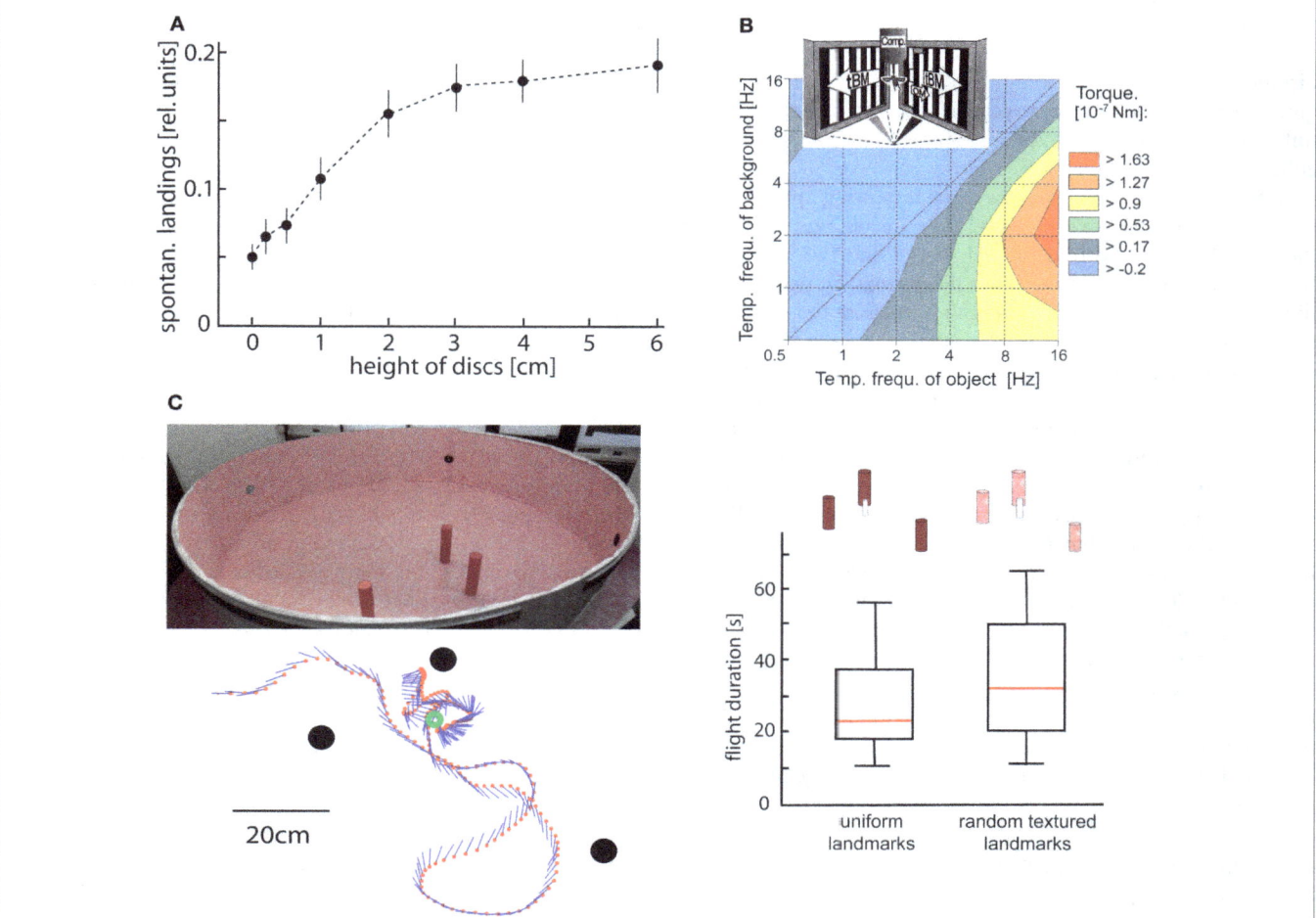

FIGURE 2 | Object detection by relative motion cues. **(A)** Relative number of spontaneous landings of free-flying flies on discs covered with a random texture of different heights. The floor and walls of the flight arena were covered with the same texture. Hence, the discs could only be discriminated by relative motion cues induced on the eyes by the self-motion of the animal. Flies landed on discs raised at least 1 cm above the floor significantly more often than on a reference disc on the floor (data from Kimmerle et al., 1996). **(B)** Contour plot of the turning responses of tethered flying flies measured with a yaw torque compensator (comp) for different combinations of temporal frequencies of object motion (OM) and translatory background motion (tBM). The motion stimuli were striped patterns (spatial period 6.3°) presented on two monitor screens placed at an angle of 90° symmetrically in front of the fly. OM was displayed within a vertical 6.3° wide window in front of the right eye. Object-induced responses are given in a color coded way with warmer colors indicating larger responses. Flies show strong turning responses when OM is faster than tBM. The strongest

responses are induced when the background is not stationary, but moves slowly (data from Kimmerle et al., 1997). **(C)** Landmark navigation of honeybees in a cylindrical flight arena with three cylindrical landmarks (upper left diagram) The landmarks were either homogeneously red or were covered by the same random pattern as the background. Bees were trained to find a barely visible feeder placed between the homogeneous landmarks. The trajectory of one search flight maneuvre is shown in the top view (bottom left diagram). The feeder (green circle) and the landmarks (black dots) are indicated. The position of the bee is indicated by red dots at each 32 ms interval; straight lines represent the orientation of the long axis of the bee. The duration of search flights until landing on the feeder was not significantly increased when the pattern of the landmarks was changed from homogeneous red to the random dot texture that also covered the background (right diagram). Red lines indicate median values, the upper and lower margins of the boxes, the 75th and 25th percentiles; the whiskers indicate the data range (Data from Dittmar et al., 2010).

tasks (Lehrer and Campan, 2005) and for navigating back to the previously learnt location of a barely visible goal (**Figure 2C**; see below; Dittmar et al., 2010). Moreover, hawk-moths hovering in front of a flower use motion cues to control their distance to the nectar donating blossom (Pfaff and Varjú, 1991; Farina et al., 1994; Kern and Varjú, 1998). However, motion information is also used for spatial tasks that are not related to objects. Bees, for instance, exploit optic flow information to estimate distances traveled during navigation flights. The dependence of optic flow information on the depth structure of the environment is also relevant in this context: experimental manipulation of the environment between flights can induce characteristic errors in distance estimation because estimates of distances traveled in a given environment cannot be generalized to environments with different depth structures (Srinivasan et al., 2000; Esch et al., 2001; review: Wolf, 2011).

What are the mechanisms involved in solving spatial behavioral tasks? Insects play a pivotal role in systems analyses of these mechanisms, both at the behavioral and the neural level. Behavioral systems analyses have been mainly performed in flight simulators on tethered flying flies, because the visual input can be perfectly controlled by the experimenter while, in most experimental paradigms, turning responses are recorded. Here, the visual consequences of locomotion are emulated by motion stimuli to which the tethered animal is exposed. However, the degrees of freedom of movement that can be executed by the animal and monitored by the experimenter in these behavioral paradigms are constrained, thus providing only limited access to the rich behavioral repertoire of the animal. Apart from a few exceptions (e.g., Land and Collett, 1974; Collett and Land, 1975; Wagner, 1982; Zeil, 1986), it has only recently become possible to investigate spatial behavior systematically under free-flight conditions with high spatial and temporal resolution and to also reconstruct what an animal has seen during largely unconstrained behavior (Lindemann et al., 2003). In the following, we restrict the review to only a few components of spatial behavior that have been experimentally investigated in detail.

OBJECT DETECTION AND OBJECT-DIRECTED RESPONSES

It has been known for a long time from experiments in tethered flight that flies can discriminate objects from their background on the basis of motion cues and attempt to fixate them in the frontal visual field (Virsik and Reichardt, 1976; Reichardt and Poggio, 1979; Reichardt et al., 1983; Egelhaaf, 1985a; Egelhaaf and Borst, 1993a; Kimmerle et al., 1997, 2000; Maimon et al., 2008; Aptekar et al., 2012). In these experiments, the tethered animal could not move, and only its yaw torque was measured. Relative motion was generated by specifically controlling object and background displacements. In real life, this situation usually occurs as a consequence of the action–perception cycle being closed while the animal moves in a three-dimensional environment and actively generates relative motion cues on its eyes through its behavior (see above).

Only three features of the control system mediating object detection in flies will be mentioned here. (1) The detectability of objects depends to a large extent on the dynamical

properties of object and background motion. Object detection is facilitated if the background moves at a moderate velocity, such as during translation in an environment where the background is at a medium distance from the animal (**Figure 2B**) (Kimmerle et al., 1997). (2) The visual pathways extracting motion-dependent object information and those processing other types of motion information (e.g., those controlling compensatory optomotor responses or translation velocity) are commonly assumed to segregate at the level of the fly's third visual neuropile. The object system appears to be distinguished by its dynamical and other properties. In particular, the object system responds to high-frequency changes of the retinal position and velocity of the object, whereas strong compensatory optomotor responses are evoked by low-frequency velocity changes (Egelhaaf, 1987; Aptekar et al., 2012). The object pathway appears to be kept separate from the other pathways up to the level of the steering muscles that mediate object-induced turns (Egelhaaf, 1989). (3) Even when the object moves exactly in the same way in subsequent stimulus presentations, it may either be fixated by the fly or no fixation responses may be elicited at all. Such a bimodal distribution of responses in the behavioral context of object detection—a full response or no response—suggests a gating mechanism in the neural pathway mediating motion-induced object fixation (Kimmerle et al., 2000).

Currently we can only speculate about the functional significance under real-life conditions of a control system that induces turning responses in tethered flight toward an object moving in front of its background. Potentially, an object may initiate landing behavior under free-flight conditions. This is plausible in blowflies as well as in bees, because (1) an object is most effective in eliciting fixation responses when the ventral part of the visual field is stimulated (Virsik and Reichardt, 1976), and (2) when detecting and approaching a landing site in free-flight, relative motion cues are exploited mainly in the ventral visual field (Wagner, 1982; Lehrer et al., 1988; Kimmerle et al., 1996; Kern et al., 1997; van Breugel and Dickinson, 2012). Similar object-detection systems could play an important role in bees during local navigation when landmarks based on contrast, texture, and relative motion cues need to be detected to guide the animal to its goal (see below).

COLLISION AVOIDANCE

In many situations, objects or other structures in the environment (e.g., extended surfaces, such as walls) are not goals the animal may aim for, but may interfere with the animal's trajectory as obstacles that need to be avoided. Thus, collision avoidance represents a basic, but highly relevant spatial task. Again, optic flow has been shown in a variety of animals, including humans, to be one of the most relevant cues that may signal an impending collision (e.g., Lappe, 2000; Vaina et al., 2004).

Optic flow has been shown to be relevant in collision avoidance behavior for both tethered and free-flying flies. There is consensus amongst studies that asymmetries in the optic flow across the two eyes, for instance, when approaching environmental structures on one side, are decisive for eliciting collision avoidance responses: (1) Flies tend to turn away from the eye experiencing image expansion (Tammero and Dickinson, 2002a,b; Tammero et al., 2004; Bender and Dickinson, 2006b; Budick et al., 2007; Reiser and Dickinson, 2010). (2) The probability of eliciting an evasive turn has been concluded to be highest if the focus of image expansion is located in the lateral rather than in the frontal part of the visual field (Tammero and Dickinson, 2002a; Tammero et al., 2004; Bender and Dickinson, 2006b). Such optic flow might occur during flights with a strong sideways component. These results do not imply that the focus of expansion in the retinal motion pattern during object approach is explicitly extracted by the neuronal circuits that mediate collision avoidance. Based on experiments done in free-flight in different types of flight arenas that allow for more complex behavior than in tethered flight, mechanisms that rely on asymmetries in the optic flow field across the two eyes other than explicitly extracting the focus of expansion are well able to account for relevant aspects of collision avoidance (see below; Lindemann et al., 2008; Mronz and Lehmann, 2008; Kern et al., 2012).

INTERACTION BETWEEN OBJECT FIXATION AND COLLISION AVOIDANCE

Expanding visual flow fields are encountered by flying insects not only when they encounter an obstacle, but also when flying straight toward an object that may serve as a landing site or as a landmark in the context of navigation behavior. As sketched above, tethered flying *Drosophilae* turn away from an expanding retinal image. Given the strength of this evasive response, it is difficult to explain how flies can fly straight in natural surroundings with ample objects surrounding them. This apparent paradox is partially resolved by the finding that *Drosophila*, when flying toward a conspicuous object, tolerates a level of expansion that would otherwise induce avoidance (Reiser and Dickinson, 2010). This suggests that the gain of the control system mediating evasive turns is reduced if prominent visual features are attractive and represent a behavioral goal. Therefore, flies appear to require a goal to keep an overall flight direction, either toward a salient object (Heisenberg and Wolf, 1979; Götz, 1987; Maimon et al., 2008; Reiser and Dickinson, 2010), toward an attractive odorant (Budick and Dickinson, 2006), when flying upwind (Budick et al., 2007), or while pursuing a moving target such as a potential mate (Trischler et al., 2010).

SPATIAL INFORMATION RELEVANT FOR LOCAL NAVIGATION

Whereas collision avoidance and landing are spatial tasks that must be solved by any flying insect, local navigation is relevant especially for particular insects, such as bees, some wasps and ants, which care for their brood and, thus, have to return to their nest after foraging. Consequently, the full complexity of spatial navigation has been analysed mainly in bees, wasps, and ants both in artificial and natural environments. Nonetheless, basic elements of local navigation could be found also in *Drosophila* (Foucaud et al., 2010; Ofstad et al., 2011). Since various aspects of insect navigation and the underlying mechanisms have been reviewed recently (Collett and Collett, 2002; Collett et al., 2006; Zeil et al., 2009; Zeil, 2012), only selected issues will be addressed here, and spatial information processing during flight will be the major focus.

Visual landmarks represent crucial spatial cues and are employed to localize a goal, especially if it is barely visible itself. Information about the landmark constellation around the goal is memorized during elaborate learning flights: the animal flies characteristic sequences of ever increasing arcs while facing the area around the goal. During these learning flights, the animal somehow gathers relevant information that is subsequently used to relocate the goal when returning to it after an excursion. A variety of visual cues, such as contrast, texture and color, are suitable to define landmarks and are employed to find the goal (reviews: Collett and Collett, 2002; Collett et al., 2006; Zeil et al., 2009; Zeil, 2012). Recently, landmarks that are defined by motion cues alone were shown to be sufficient for bees to locate the goal (Dittmar et al., 2010). In this study, several landmarks that were camouflaged by their texture and, thus, could not be discriminated from the background by stationary cues were placed in particular locations surrounding the goal (**Figure 2C**). The mechanisms by which the landmark constellation is learnt and how the memorized information is eventually used to locate the goal are not yet fully understood. However, it is clear that optic flow information generated actively during the bees' typical learning and searching flights is essential for the acquisition of a spatial memory of the goal environment. Moreover, in the vicinity of the landmarks, the animals were found to adjust their flight movements according to specific textural properties of the landmarks (Dittmar et al., 2010; Braun et al., 2012).

Landmarks close to the goal are, for geometrical reasons, most suitable to define the goal location, because the retinal locations of close landmarks are displaced more than distant ones during the translational movements of the animal (Stürzl and Zeil, 2007). Emerging as a direct consequence of the closed action–perception cycle, this property "weighs" the relevance of environmental objects to serve as landmarks for local navigation in the vicinity of the goal.

SPATIAL INFORMATION BASED ON SACCADIC GAZE AND FLIGHT STRATEGY

Saccadic gaze changes have a rather uniform time course and are shorter than 100 ms. Angular velocities of up to several thousand °/s can occur during saccades (**Figure 3**). Since roll movements of the body that are performed for steering purposes during saccades, and also during sideways translations, are compensated by counter-directed head movements, the animals' gaze direction is kept virtually constant during intersaccades (Schilstra and van Hateren, 1999; Boeddeker and Hemmi, 2010; Boeddeker et al., 2010; Braun et al., 2010, 2012; Geurten et al., 2010, 2012). Saccade dynamics in flies have been shown to be fine-tuned by mechanosensory feedback from the halteres, the gyroscopic sense organs of dipteran flies, evolutionarily developed from the hind wings. Haltere feedback may thus contribute to increasing the duration of intersaccadic intervals (Sherman, 2003; Bender and Dickinson, 2006a). Nevertheless, halteres are no prerequisite for a saccadic gaze strategy, given that bees and wasps show similar flight dynamics as flies without halteres (**Figure 3**) (Boeddeker et al., 2010). By squeezing body and head rotations into the brief saccades, translational gaze displacements last for more than 80% of the entire flight time (van Hateren and Schilstra, 1999;

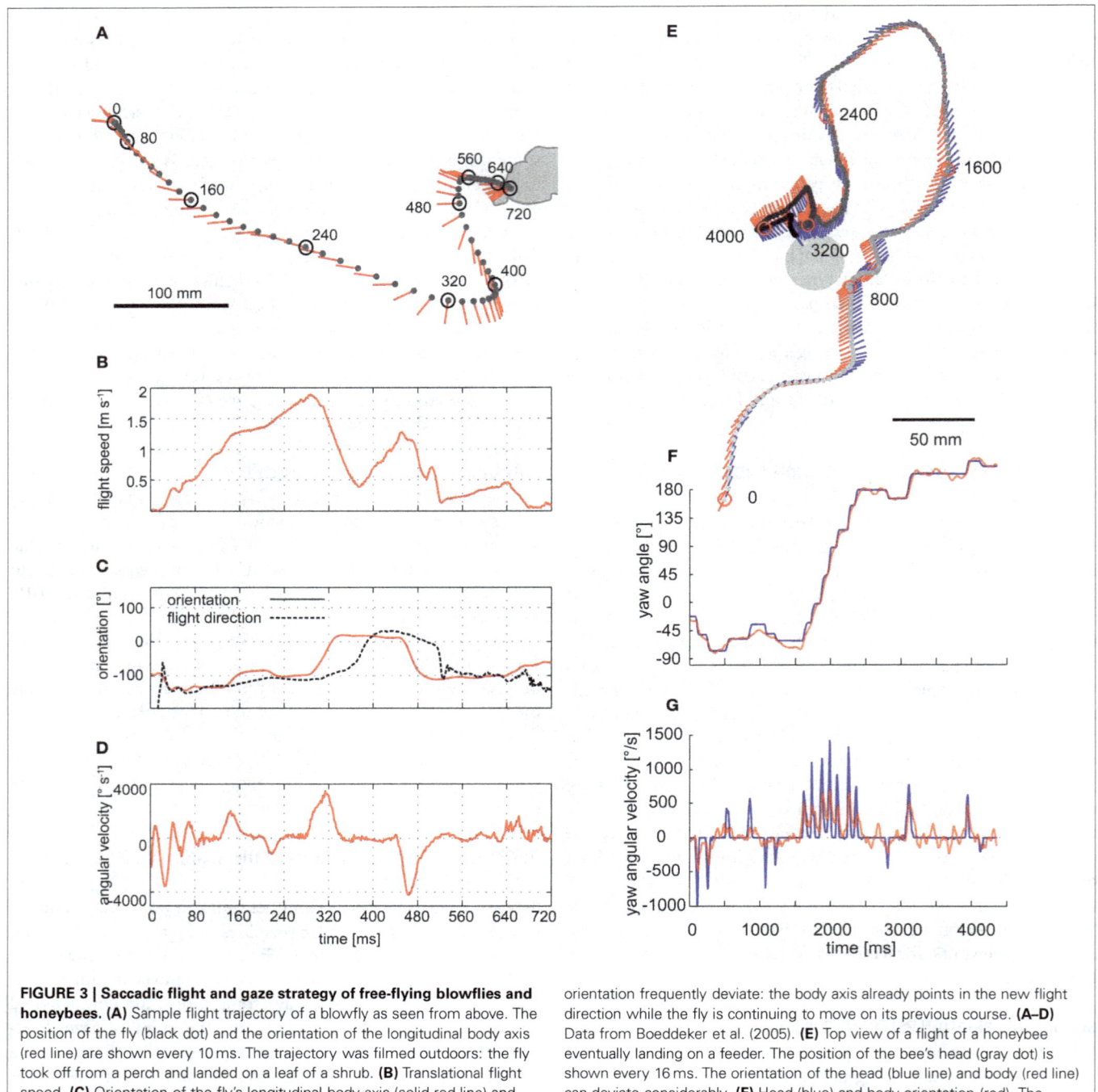

FIGURE 3 | Saccadic flight and gaze strategy of free-flying blowflies and honeybees. (A) Sample flight trajectory of a blowfly as seen from above. The position of the fly (black dot) and the orientation of the longitudinal body axis (red line) are shown every 10 ms. The trajectory was filmed outdoors: the fly took off from a perch and landed on a leaf of a shrub. **(B)** Translational flight speed. **(C)** Orientation of the fly's longitudinal body axis (solid red line) and flight direction (broken black line) in the external coordinate system. **(D)** Angular velocity of the fly. The fly changed its gaze and heading direction through a series of short and fast body turns. Flight direction and body axis orientation frequently deviate: the body axis already points in the new flight direction while the fly is continuing to move on its previous course. **(A–D)** Data from Boeddeker et al. (2005). **(E)** Top view of a flight of a honeybee eventually landing on a feeder. The position of the bee's head (gray dot) is shown every 16 ms. The orientation of the head (blue line) and body (red line) can deviate considerably. **(F)** Head (blue) and body orientation (red). The head usually turns with the thorax but at a higher angular speed, starting, and finishing slightly earlier. **(G)** Head (blue) and body (red) angular velocity. **(E–G)** Data from Boeddeker et al. (2010).

Boeddeker and Hemmi, 2010; Boeddeker et al., 2010; Braun et al., 2010, 2012; van Breugel and Dickinson, 2012).

It should be noted that flying insects may appear to meander smoothly when their overall flight trajectory is inspected (Boeddeker et al., 2005; Kern et al., 2012). Having frequently been an issue of misunderstandings, this smoothness does not contradict a saccadic flight style. As a consequence of inertial forces, flying insects, in particular large ones, may move for some time after a saccadic change in body orientation in their previous direction. Thus, the saccadic gaze strategy is reflected only to some extent in the overall flight trajectories. (**Figure 3**). This may be different in the much smaller *Drosophila* where at least some rapid large-amplitude turns can be seen in the overall flight trajectories (Tammero and Dickinson, 2002b).

Blowflies do not fly exactly straight even in straight flight tunnels without any obstacles. Rather they perform sequences of saccades, alternating their direction and the saccade amplitude depending on the clearance of the animal with respect to the walls of the flight tunnel (Kern et al., 2012). A saccadic flight style may be functionally relevant, even if the overall flight course pursued by the animal is straight. This is because the animal normally has no prior knowledge about the spatial structure of the environment. Thus, the uncertainty about whether it can fly on a straight course or not needs to be resolved on the basis of optic flow information. Regular changes of flight and gaze direction might, therefore, be a useful flight strategy, because it would allow the animal to check (during intersaccadic intervals) the translational optic flow for environmental information (Kern et al., 2012).

Since the saccadic flight and gaze strategy leads to either primarily rotational or primarily translational optic flow on the eyes, it can be interpreted as a behavioral adaptation to facilitate spatial vision. This is because only translational optic flow depends on the distance of the animal to environmental objects and, thus, contains spatial information (see above). A segregation of optic flow fields into their rotational and translational components can, at least in principle, be accomplished computationally for most realistic situations (Longuet-Higgins and Prazdny, 1980; Prazdny, 1980; Dahmen et al., 2000). However, such a computational strategy for the nervous system appears to be a lot more demanding than preventing the formation of composite rotational and translational optic flow by behavioral means. Thus, a saccadic gaze and flight strategy can be regarded as an efficient way to provide the nervous system with input from which spatial information can be extracted with relatively little computational effort.

CONTROL OF SACCADES AS THE MAIN ROTATIONAL COMPONENTS OF FLIGHT BEHAVIOR

The saccadic gaze strategy of insects has been characterized in various functional contexts: flies exhibit a saccadic flight pattern during spontaneous behavior, for instance, when cruising around without any obvious goal. This was shown in a wide range of environments including outdoors conditions (**Figure 3A**). Saccade frequencies of up to 10 per second were observed (Schilstra and van Hateren, 1999; van Hateren and Schilstra, 1999; Tammero and Dickinson, 2002b; Boeddeker et al., 2005, 2010; Braun et al., 2010, 2012; Dittmar et al., 2010; Geurten et al., 2010). The direction, amplitude and frequency of saccades depend not only on the spatial outline, but also on the texture of the environment. Thus, saccades are, at least to some extent, under visual control and serve purposes in spatial behavior, such as in collision avoidance behavior (Frye and Dickinson, 2007; Geurten et al., 2010; Braun et al., 2012; Kern et al., 2012).

There is consensus that intersaccadic optic flow during collision avoidance behavior plays a decisive role in controlling the direction and amplitude of saccades. However, which optic flow parameters may be most relevant is still inconclusive.

Notwithstanding, all proposed mechanisms of evoking saccades rely on some sort of asymmetry in the optic flow pattern in front of the two eyes. The asymmetry may be due to the location of the expansion focus in front of one eye or to a difference between the overall optic flow in the visual fields of the two eyes (Tammero and Dickinson, 2002b; Lindemann et al., 2008; Mronz and Lehmann, 2008; Kern et al., 2012).

Not all of the visual field has been concluded to be involved in saccade control, at least for blowflies. The optic flow in the lateral parts of the visual field does not play a role in determining saccade direction (Kern et al., 2012). This feature might be related to the way in which blowflies fly: during intersaccades, they predominantly fly forwards with some sideways component after saccades that shifts the pole of expansion of the flow field slightly toward frontolateral locations (Kern et al., 2012). In contrast, in *Drosophila*—which are able to hover and fly sideways (Ristroph et al., 2009)—lateral and even rear parts of the visual field have also been shown to be involved in saccade control. Therefore, in *Drosophila*, a mechanism that also takes lateral retinal areas into account for saccade control is plausible from a functional point of view (Tammero and Dickinson, 2002b).

CONTROL OF INTERSACCADIC TRANSLATIONAL MOTION

Whereas saccades are fairly stereotyped across different behavioral contexts, the intersaccadic translational movements may vary to a much larger extent, depending on the behavioral context as well as the spatial layout of the environment (Braun et al., 2010, 2012). This aspect has been addressed systematically in two different behavioral contexts: (1) The dependence of translation velocity on the spatial layout of the environment, and (2) the control of translational movements during visual landmark navigation in the vicinity of an invisible goal.

Insects tend to decelerate when their flight path is obstructed. Flight speed is thought to be controlled by optic flow generated during translational flight (David, 1979, 1982; Farina et al., 1995; Kern and Varjú, 1998; Baird et al., 2005, 2006, 2010; Frye and Dickinson, 2007; Fry et al., 2009; Dyhr and Higgins, 2010; Straw et al., 2010; Kern et al., 2012). Flies, bees, and moths were concluded to keep the optic flow on their eyes at a "preset" total strength by adjusting their flight speed. Accordingly, they decelerate when the translational optic flow increases, for instance, while passing a narrow gap or flying in a narrow tunnel (**Figures 4A,B**) (Srinivasan et al., 1991, 1996; Verspui and Gray, 2009; Baird et al., 2010; Portelli et al., 2011; Kern et al., 2012). However, not all parts of the visual field contribute equally to the input of the velocity controller. Whereas the intersaccadic optic flow generated in eye regions looking well in front of the insect has a strong impact on flight speed, the lateral visual field plays only a minor role (Baird et al., 2010; Portelli et al., 2011; Kern et al., 2012).

Translational flight maneuvres during the spatial navigation of bees have a particularly elaborate fine structure and can be described by a distinct set of prototypical movements (**Figure 4C**). The optic flow generated during flight sequences close to visual landmarks appears to be systematically employed to localize a virtually invisible goal. Not only the overall velocity, but also the relative distribution of sideways and forward

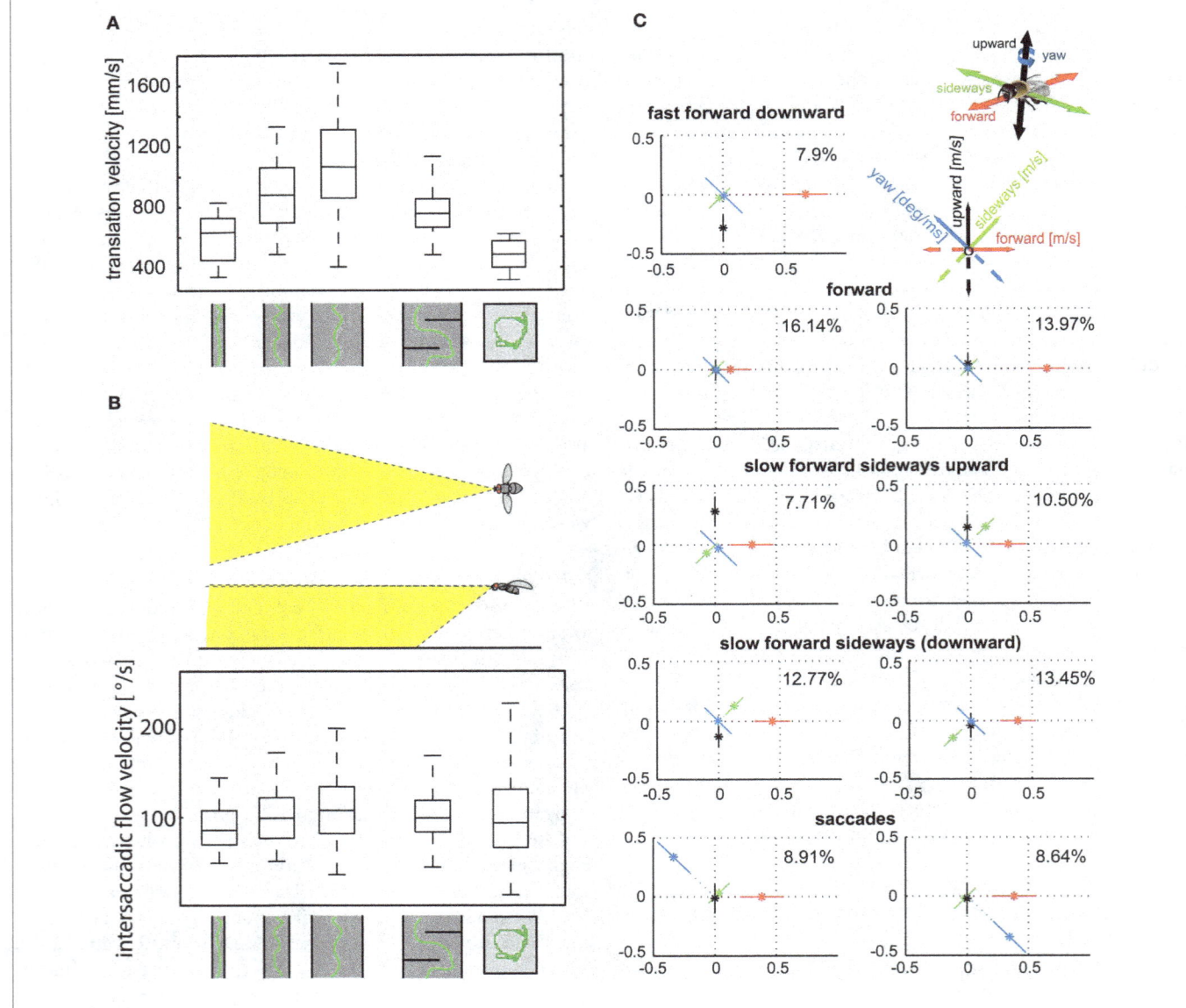

FIGURE 4 | (A) Control of translational velocity in blowflies. Boxplot of the translational velocity in flight tunnels of different widths, in a flight arena with two obstacles and in a cubic flight arena (sketched below data). Translation velocity strongly depends on the geometry of the flight arena. **(B)** Boxplot of the retinal image velocities within intersaccadic intervals experienced in the fronto-ventral visual field (see inset) in the different flight arenas. In this area of the visual field, the intersaccadic retinal velocities are kept roughly constant by regulating the translation velocity according to clearance with respect to environmental structures. The upper and lower margins of the boxes in **(A)** and **(B)** indicate the 75th and 25th percentiles, and the whiskers the data range (Data from Kern et al., 2012). **(C)** Translational and rotational prototypical movements of honeybees during local landmark navigation (see example in **Figure 2C**). Homing flight sequences can be decomposed into nine prototypical movements using clustering algorithms in order to reduce the behavioral complexity. Each prototype is depicted as a star plot containing the four velocity components drawn onto color-coded lines equally dividing the drawing plane (see inset). For each line, the distance of the dot from the center determines the value of the corresponding velocity component, and the error bars give the standard deviation of this value. Percentage values provide the relative occurrence of each prototype. More than 80% of flight-time corresponds to a varied set of translational prototypical movements and less than 20% has significantly non-zero rotational velocity corresponding to the saccades (Data from Braun et al., 2012).

translational movements depend on the insect's distance and orientation relative to the landmarks and the goal (Zeil et al., 2009; Dittmar et al., 2010, 2011; Braun et al., 2012; Zeil, 2012). Bees, for example, frequently tend to perform translational movements with a strong sideways component close to landmarks, as if they wanted to scrutinize them in detail. These sideways movements are more pronounced if the landmarks are camouflaged by the same texture as their background and, thus, can be detected only by relative motion cues in the optic flow fields (Dittmar et al., 2010; Braun et al., 2012).

PROCESSING OF OPTIC FLOW IN THE INSECT NERVOUS SYSTEM

Separating the rotational and translational optic flow components behaviorally can be viewed as an efficient strategy to reduce the computational load for the nervous system when extracting information about the environment and, especially, about its spatial layout. Nonetheless, the retinal image flow resulting from the closed action–perception cycle still has complex spatiotemporal properties, and its processing represents a demanding challenge for the nervous system. In particular, there is not much time for gathering environmental information between saccades. With up to 10 saccades per second being generated, intersaccadic intervals may be as short as only a few ms and rarely longer than 100–200 ms. Time is a critical issue for at least three reasons: (1) All neural processing is time-consuming, beginning with the biophysical mechanisms of signal transduction in the photoreceptors, and ending with transmitter signaling at neuromuscular junctions. (2) Sensory input is encoded by nerve cells with only limited reliability. Repeated presentation of the same input may lead to variable neural responses, which constrain the information which can be transmitted within a given time interval. (3) Neural computations are not necessarily rigid, but may flexibly adjust to the prevailing stimulus conditions. To be functionally beneficial, the time constants of such adaptive processes need to match the behaviorally relevant timescale of changes of the various visual stimulus parameters.

These three issues become particularly challenging if information is to be processed and represented with sufficient reliability on the very short timescales that are behaviorally relevant for fast flying insects. The virtuosity of the spatial behavior of many insects is proof that their sensory and nervous systems somehow cope successfully with this challenge. Since insects accomplish all this with very small brains comprising only a million or less neurons, they seem to be champions of resource efficient information processing and behavioral control.

So far, we only have vague conceptions of how all this is accomplished. In the following, we briefly sketch the available knowledge about the processing of retinal image flow. Particular focus is placed on how the spatiotemporal properties of image flow are shaped by the closed action–perception cycle.

SPATIOTEMPORAL VISUAL INPUT OF INSECTS IS SHAPED BY ACTIVE GAZE STRATEGIES

From what has been sketched above, it may be obvious that the spatiotemporal characteristics of the input to the visual system will depend strongly not only on the features of the behavioral surroundings, but also on the specific dynamical characteristics of locomotion. These movements, resulting from the closed-loop nature of the behavior, may, in turn, depend on the environmental properties. The statistical properties of a wide variety of natural scenes have been characterized in many studies. The scenes analysed were usually stationary, or they resulted from movements either at constant velocities or with dynamics that differ a lot from that of unrestrained gaze changes during natural locomotion (e.g., Eckert and Buchsbaum, 1993; Dong and Attick, 1995; van Hateren, 1997; Simoncelli and Olshausen,

2001; Betsch et al., 2004; Geisler, 2008). In a recent study, we simulated the natural dynamics of the saccadic gaze strategy of insects and registered the resulting image sequences in a large variety of natural environments (Schwegmann et al., in preparation).

Given the characteristic temporal structure of behavioral dynamics, the parameters within these image sequences also change in a temporally structured way. Two aspects of such changes may be particularly relevant for extracting behaviorally relevant environmental information from the retinal image flow: (1) Relevant image parameters, such as brightness, contrast, and spatial frequency composition, vary according to image region and viewing direction, and fluctuate more rapidly during saccadic turns than during intersaccades. (2) During translatory intersaccadic movements, image parameters resulting from close structures fluctuate in general much more than those resulting from distant structures (**Figure 5**).

The dynamical properties imposed by the saccadic gaze change and the image statistics of natural environments constrain the time constants of information processing. Furthermore, the adaptive mechanisms that are thought to adjust the sensitivity of the visual system to the prevailing stimulus conditions have to operate on a suitable timescale. In particular, to optimize the encoding of the fluctuations of environmental image features during the intersaccadic intervals, adaptation in the visual system should essentially take place on a timescale shorter than the duration of these intervals (i.e., within some tens of milliseconds) and may be driven by the high-frequency changes of the respective image parameters. Several physiological components of motion adaptation have been described at the different levels of the fly visual system (e.g., Maddess and Laughlin, 1985; Brenner et al., 2000a; Harris et al., 2000; Fairhall et al., 2001; Kurtz, 2007; Kalb et al., 2008; Liang et al., 2008). To what extent the time constants of these processes, which have been identified with experimenter designed motion stimuli, match the dynamics of parameter changes in the natural visual input, and how these adaptive processes are controlled, is still not clear.

PERIPHERAL PROCESSING OF MOTION INFORMATION

How is the environmental and, in particular, the spatial information extracted from the retinal image flow and represented in the visual motion pathway? The retinal input is transformed at the level of photoreceptors in basically two ways: (1) The retinal input is sampled by the array of photoreceptors. Compared with technical imaging systems, the number of image points and, thus, the spatial resolution is very low, with only approximately 750 image points per eye in *Drosophila* (Hardie, 1985), 5000 in the blowfly *Calliphora* (Beersma et al., 1977) and 5400 in honeybees (Seidl and Kaiser, 1981). The visual angle between photoreceptors is matched by their acceptance angle resulting in a blurred retinal image (Götz, 1965; van Hateren, 1993). Despite the low spatial resolution of the eyes of insects, they are obviously able to accomplish even intricate spatial vision tasks (see above). The low number of retinal input channels reduces the computational load for subsequent information processing tremendously and, thus, may be one reason why insects are so efficient with respect to computational expenditure. (2) As a consequence of

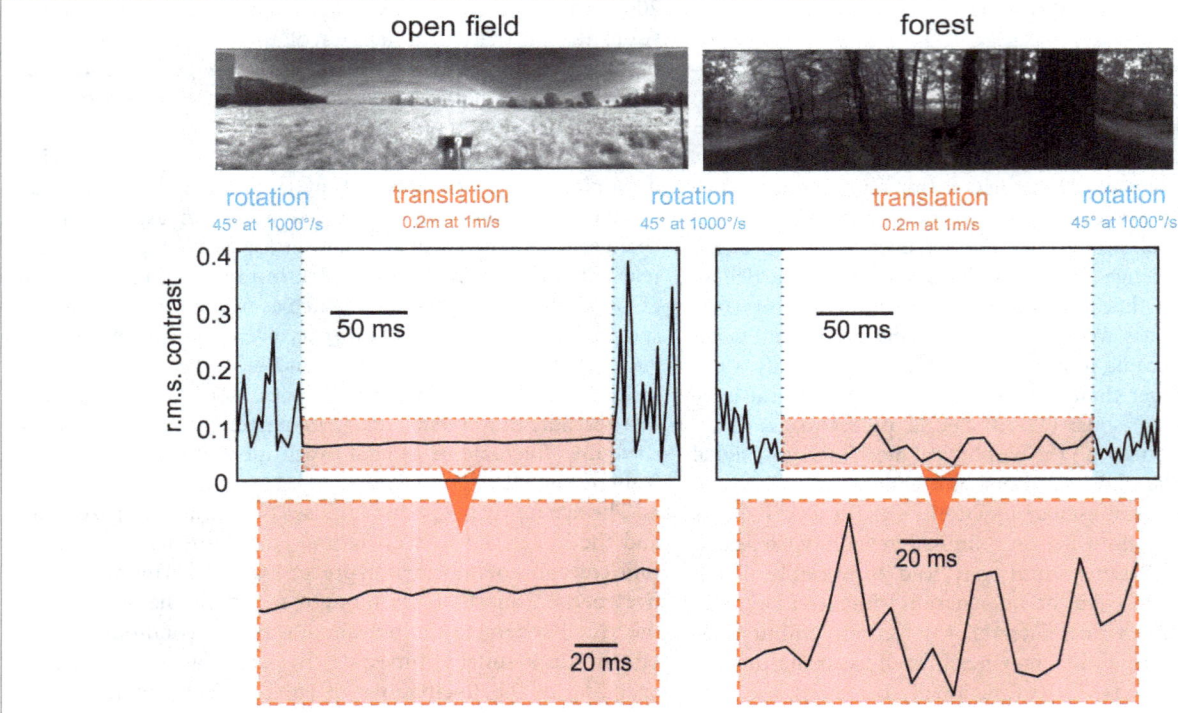

FIGURE 5 | Consequences of flight dynamics for contrast fluctuations in a small patch (2 × 2°, corresponding to approximately the aperture of a local movement detector) of the visual field at the equator and 90° relative to the direction of motion in two typical environments: an open field (left column) and a forest (right column). The movement sequence of the panoramic camera system corresponds to an initial 45° rightward rotation at a saccade-like angular velocity (1000°/s), followed by a translation for 20 cm at a velocity of 1 ms and then another 45° rightward turn. In general, contrast fluctuations are much larger during saccade-like turns than during translational phases. If environmental objects are relatively close (as in the forest environment), translations may also lead to considerable contrast fluctuations, though on a slower timescale. The data are based on high dynamic range image sequences, which are rescaled to the printable contrast range. (Data from Schwegmann et al., in preparation).

the biophysical transduction machinery, the photoreceptors represent a kind of temporal low-pass filter. Owing to adaptive mechanisms, the strength of this temporal blurring depends on the ambient brightness, with the time-constants of blurring reflecting a trade-off between fast transmission and the reliability of the retinal output signals given the stochastic nature of the photons impinging on the photoreceptors (Juusola et al., 1994, 1996; Juusola, 2003).

The photoreceptor output is fed into the neural network of the first visual neuropile, the lamina (**Figure 6A**). Here, those photoreceptors looking at the same point in visual space converge on common second order neurons (Kirschfeld, 1972), thereby increasing the reliability of signal transmission, especially at low-light intensities (Laughlin, 1994). The photoreceptor signals are further processed in the lamina. (1) They are temporally band-pass filtered, thereby enhancing the representation of contrast changes in the retinal images (Laughlin, 1994; van Hateren, 1997). Owing to the special properties of the synapses between photoreceptors and second order neurons, the signal time course becomes faster and more transient with increasing background intensity (Juusola et al., 1995). Given the noisiness of the input signals and the limited dynamic range of nerve cells, the overall brightness-dependent spatiotemporal filter properties of the peripheral visual system are thought to

maximize the flow of information about natural moving images (van Hateren, 1992). It should be noted that these conclusions are based so far on image sequences resulting from smoothly superimposed rotational and translational movements, without taking the different dynamical properties of image changes during saccades and intersaccades into account. During translational intersaccadic movements, the image dynamics can be expected to depend on the depth structure of the scenery, because the retinal images of distant objects move at lower velocities than those of near objects (**Figure 5**). (2) Recent evidence based on targeted genetic manipulations of individual cell types in the peripheral visual system of *Drosophila* indicate, though there are differences in details between studies, that the lamina output is segregated into parallel ON and OFF pathways, signaling either brightness increases or decreases (Joesch et al., 2010; Reiff et al., 2010; Clark et al., 2011). One functional consequence of splitting the visual input into ON and OFF components is to facilitate the biophysical implementation of the mechanism of motion detection at subsequent stages of the visual system. The core of this mechanism is a multiplication-like interaction between neighboring retinal input channels (see below), which gives a positive output for two positive as well as for two negative inputs (Egelhaaf and Borst, 1992, 1993b; Eichner et al., 2011).

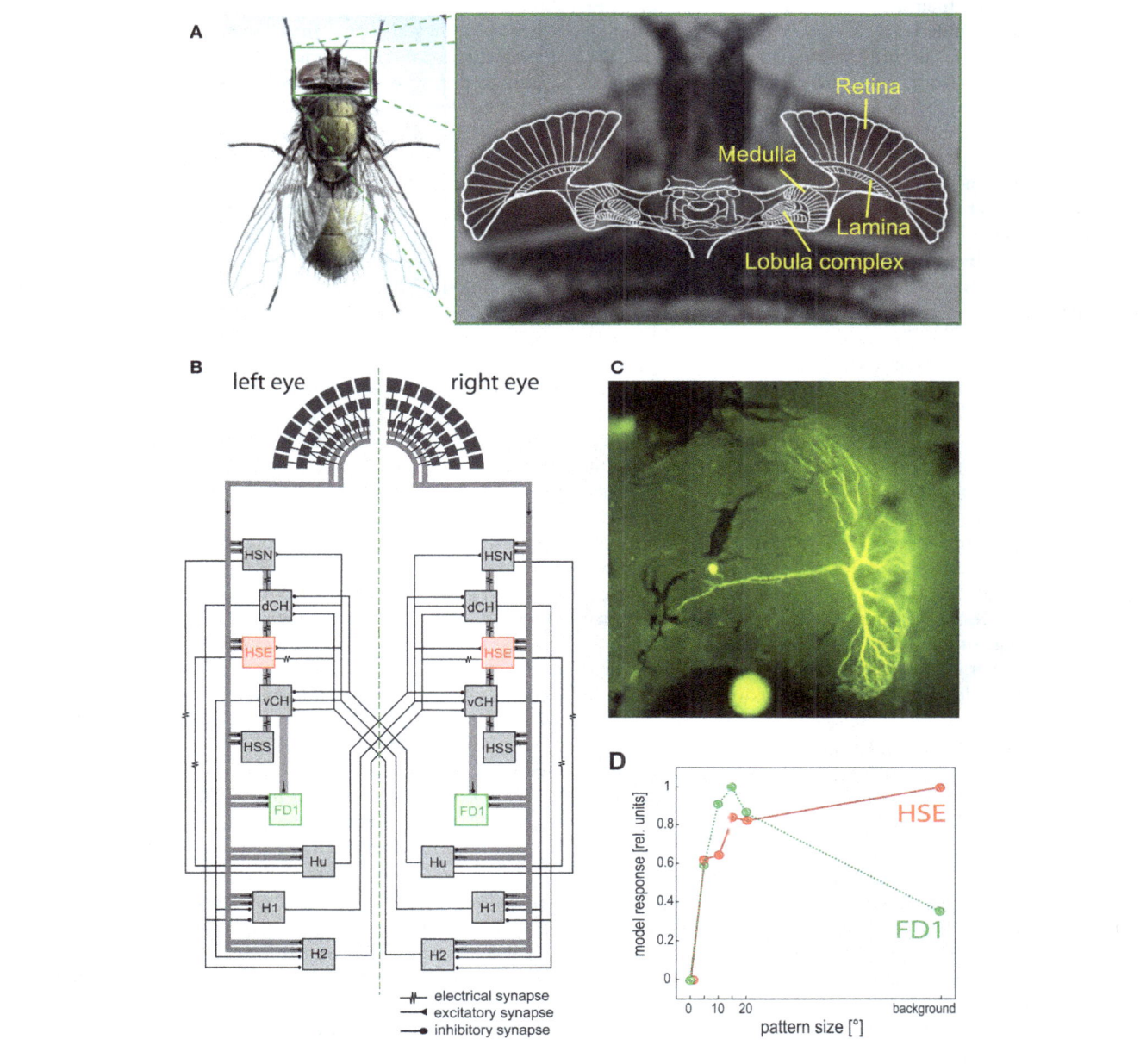

FIGURE 6 | Visual system of the blowfly and neural circuits extracting optic flow information from the retinal image sequences. (A) Schematic of a horizontal section of the fly's brain projected onto a photograph of its head, with the retina and the three main visual neuropiles labeled. **(B)** Wiring sketch of some LWCs sensitive to different types of horizontal motion in the lobula plate of the blowfly. The HSE cells, one type of HS cells, which respond best to coherent wide-field motion, and the FD1 cells, a special type of FD cells, which are most sensitive to the motion of objects, are highlighted. **(C)** Structure of an FD1 cell with its dendritic tree residing in the lobula plate. The cell is shown in a whole-mount preparation after it has been injected with the fluorescent dye Lucifer Yellow. **(D)** Dependence of the normalized response amplitude of an HSE and a FD1 cell on the angular horizontal extent of a moving pattern. The responses are based on computer simulations of a circuit model [as shown in **(B)**]; the model responses mimic the physiologically determined responses (Data from Hennig and Egelhaaf, 2012).

LOCAL MOTION COMPUTATION

A lot is known, especially in flies, about the computations underlying motion vision. The available evidence on bees suggests that motion information is processed in their visual system according to similar principles. Local motion detection is assumed to be accomplished in the second visual neuropile, the medulla (**Figure 6A**). Motion-specific responses have been found in the two most proximal layers of the medulla. Most motion sensitive medulla neurons that could be functionally characterized have small receptive fields, as is expected from neurons involved in local motion detection (review: Strausfeld et al., 2006). As a consequence of the small size of the neurons in this brain area and the difficulty of recording their activity, conclusions concerning the cellular mechanisms underlying motion detection are still tentative. A lot of progress is currently being made by combining the sophisticated repertoire of genetic and molecular approaches in *Drosophila* with electrophysiological and imaging techniques to identify the different components of the neural circuits underlying motion detection (Rister et al., 2007; Joesch et al., 2008, 2010; Katsov and Clandinin, 2008; Borst, 2009; Reiff et al., 2010; Clark et al., 2011; Schnell et al., 2012).

A large number of features of motion detection can be accounted for by a computational model, the so-called correlation-type motion detector. In its simplest form, a local motion detector is composed of two mirror-symmetrical subunits. In each subunit, the signals of adjacent light-sensitive cells receiving the filtered brightness signals from neighboring points in visual space are multiplied after one of them has been delayed. The final detector response is obtained by subtracting the outputs of two such subunits with opposite preferred directions, thereby considerably enhancing the direction selectivity of the motion detection circuit. Each motion detector reacts with a positive signal to motion in a given direction and with a negative signal to motion in the opposite direction (reviews: Reichardt, 1961; Borst and Egelhaaf, 1989; Egelhaaf and Borst, 1993b). Various elaborations of this basic motion detection scheme have been proposed to account for the responses of insect motion-sensitive neurons under a wide range of stimulus conditions including even natural optic flow as experienced under free-flight conditions (see e.g., Borst et al., 2003; Lindemann et al., 2005; Brinkworth et al., 2009).

EXTRACTION OF OPTIC FLOW INFORMATION

Since the optic flow as induced during locomotion has a global structure, it cannot be represented in any specific way by local mechanisms alone. Rather, local motion measurements from large parts of the visual field need to be combined. This is accomplished in the third visual neuropile, the lobula complex, by directionally selective wide-field neurons (**Figure 6**) in all insect species analysed so far. Independent of the species under investigation, these neurons will here be collectively referred to as LWCs (lobula complex wide-field cells). LWCs have been investigated in particular detail in flies, where they reside in the distinct posterior part of the lobula complex; they are, therefore, often termed lobula plate tangential cells (LPTCs). In bees, the lobula complex is undivided; however, bees have very similar motion-sensitive wide-field neurons to those characterized in the lobula plate of flies (DeVoe et al., 1982; Ibbotson, 1991). Most LWCs spatially pool the outputs of many retinotopically arranged local motion-sensitive neurons on their large dendrites and, accordingly, have large receptive fields. These local motion-sensitive neurons are thought to correspond to the local motion detectors, as described above. LWCs are excited by motion in their preferred direction and are inhibited by motion in the opposite direction (reviews: Hausen and Egelhaaf, 1989; Krapp, 2000; Borst and Haag, 2002; Egelhaaf et al., 2002; Egelhaaf, 2006; Taylor and Krapp, 2008; Borst et al., 2010).

For fly LWCs, the local motion-sensitive elements that synapse onto their dendrites have been concluded to differ in their preferred direction of motion. As a consequence, local preferred

directions of LWCs change gradually over their receptive field and it has been suggested that they coincide with the directions of the velocity vectors characterizing the flow fields that are induced during certain types of self-motion (Hausen, 1982; Krapp et al., 1998, 2001; Petrowitz et al., 2000; Taylor and Krapp, 2008).

Despite the characteristic patterns of preferred directions in the receptive fields of LWCs, dendritic pooling of motion input is not sufficient to obtain specific responses during particular types of self-motion. Network interactions, mediated by both electrical and chemical synapses, between LWCs within one brain hemisphere and between both halves of the visual system are important for shaping their specific sensitivities for optic flow (**Figure 6B**; reviews: Borst and Haag, 2002; Egelhaaf et al., 2002; Egelhaaf, 2006; Borst et al., 2010). To enhance the specificity of LWCs for particular global optic flow patterns, interactions between both visual hemispheres are particularly relevant. The optic flow, for instance, across both eyes during forward translation is directed backwards. In contrast, during a pure rotation about the animal's vertical axis, optic flow is directed backwards across one eye, but forwards across the other eye. Thus, translational and rotational optic flow can, at least in principle, be distinguished if motion from both eyes is taken into account (Hausen, 1982; Egelhaaf et al., 1993; Horstmann et al., 2000; Farrow et al., 2003, 2006; Karmeier et al., 2003; Borst and Weber, 2011; Hennig et al., 2011). Other LWCs of blowflies, the figure detection (FD) cells, respond best to the motion of objects rather than to global optic flow patterns. This object sensitivity could be shown for one prominent element of this group of cells to be a consequence of inhibitory synaptic interactions with other LWCs (**Figures 6B–D**) (Egelhaaf, 1985b; Warzecha et al., 1993; Kimmerle and Egelhaaf, 2000a,b; Hennig et al., 2008, 2011; Hennig and Egelhaaf, 2012; Liang et al., 2012). FD cells are thought to play a prominent role in detecting stationary objects in the environment, such as landing sites that are distinguished from their background by motion, and also other visual cues. Other LWCs found in various fly species respond to much smaller objects than do FD cells. These cells were interpreted as being involved in detecting and pursuing prey and/or mates (Olberg, 1981, 1986; Gilbert and Strausfeld, 1991; Nordström et al., 2006; Nordström and O'Carroll, 2006; Barnett et al., 2007; Geurten et al., 2007; Trischler et al., 2007) and it is suggested they owe their exquisite sensitivity for extremely small targets to a variety of local and global synaptic interactions (Nordström, 2012).

Although the synaptic interactions between LWCs may increase their specificity for particular types of optic flow and stimulus sizes, this specificity is usually far from being perfect, and most neurons still respond to a wide range of "non-optimal" stimuli indicating that behaviorally relevant motion information is encoded by the activity profile of populations of LWCs rather than by the responses of individual cells.

Despite their specific differences, LWCs have general properties which may be functionally relevant in the context of spatial vision.

- *Velocity dependence*: LWCs do not operate like odometers: their mean responses increase with increasing velocity, reach a maximum, and then decrease again. Hence, their response does not reflect pattern velocity unambiguously. This ambiguity is even more complex, since the location of the velocity maximum depends on the textural properties of the moving stimulus pattern. If the spatial frequency of a drifting sine-wave grating is shifted to lower values, the velocity optimum shifts to higher values. In terms of the correlation model of motion detection, the location of the temporal frequency optimum is determined by the time constant of the delay filters in the local motion detectors (review: Egelhaaf and Borst, 1993b). The pattern dependence of velocity tuning is reduced if the stimulus pattern consists of a broad range of spatial frequencies, as is characteristic of natural scenes (Dror et al., 2001; Straw et al., 2008). Despite these ambiguities, flies and bees appear to regulate their intersaccadic translation velocity during free-flight to keep the retinal velocities in that part of the operating range of the motion detection system in which responses increase monotonically with retinal velocities (Baird et al., 2010; Portelli et al., 2011; Kern et al., 2012).

- *Time course of motion responses*: The representation of image velocity becomes even more complex if we take time-varying pattern velocities into account, as are characteristic of behavioral situations. The time course of LWC responses is roughly proportional to pattern velocity only as long as the velocity changes are small (Egelhaaf and Reichardt, 1987; Haag and Borst, 1997, 1998). However, as a consequence of the computational structure of local motion detectors, LWC responses do not only depend on pattern velocity, but also on higher-order temporal derivatives (Egelhaaf and Reichardt, 1987). This is reflected, for instance, in the response transients to sudden changes in pattern velocity (Egelhaaf and Borst, 1989; Egelhaaf and Warzecha, 1998; Warzecha et al., 1998). The rapid saccadic turns characterizing insect free-flight probably lead to the most transient retinal image displacements that occur under natural conditions. The retinal peak velocities attained during saccades of up to several thousands of degrees per second are far beyond the velocity optima determined even for transient conditions (Maddess and Laughlin, 1985; Warzecha et al., 1999). Nonetheless, saccade direction can be encoded by LWCs by transient responses with corresponding signs. However, this is the case only as long as the cell is not excited by translational optic flow during intersaccades, for example, when the animal flies close to environmental structures. In this case, the cell may be depolarized more strongly by the translational optic flow than by a preferred-direction saccade, even though the translational velocities are much smaller than the velocities evoked by the saccades (Kern et al., 2005; van Hateren et al., 2005).

- *Motion adaptation*: Motion vision systems operate under a variety of dynamical conditions. Accordingly, several response features of LWCs have been shown to depend on stimulus history in a characteristic way. A number of mechanisms are involved in the corresponding changes in the visual motion pathway. Some of them operate locally and, thus, presynaptic to the LWCs; they are, to some extent, independent of the direction of motion. Other mechanisms originate after spatial pooling of local motion signals at the level of LWCs, making them dependent on the direction of motion (reviews: Clifford and Ibbotson, 2003; Egelhaaf, 2006; Kurtz, 2009). All these processes are usually regarded as adaptive, although their functional significance is still not entirely clear. Several non-exclusive possibilities have been proposed, such as adjusting the dynamic range of motion sensitivity to the prevailing stimulus dynamics (Brenner et al., 2000a; Fairhall et al., 2001), saving energy by adjusting the neural response amplitudes without affecting the overall information that is conveyed (Heitwerth et al., 2005), and increasing the sensitivity to changes in stimulus parameters resulting from environmental discontinuities (Maddess and Laughlin, 1985; Liang et al., 2008, 2011; Kurtz et al., 2009).

- *Gain control by dendritic integration of antagonistic motion input*: Dendritic integration of signals from local motion-sensitive elements by LWCs is a highly non-linear process. When the signals of an increasing number of input elements are pooled, saturation non-linearities make the response largely independent of pattern size. However, the response saturates at different levels for different velocities. Hence, LWC responses are almost invariant against changes in pattern size, while they still depend on velocity. This gain control can be explained on the basis of the passive membrane properties of LWCs and the antagonistic nature of their motion input. Even motion in the preferred direction activates both types of the two mirror-symmetrical subunits of the motion detector, for instance, excitatory and inhibitory inputs of LWCs, though to a different extent, depending on the velocity of motion. As a consequence, the saturation levels reached by the membrane potential of an LWC with increasing numbers of activated input elements are different for different velocities (Hausen, 1982; Egelhaaf, 1985a; Borst et al., 1995; Single et al., 1997).

- *Pattern dependence*: The responses of the local input elements of LWCs are temporally modulated even during pattern motion at a constant velocity owing to their small receptive fields. These modulations are the consequence of the texture of the environment. Since the signals of neighboring input elements are phase-shifted with respect to each other, their pooling by the dendrites of LWCs reduces mainly those pattern-dependent response modulations that originate from the high spatial frequencies of the stimulus pattern. The pattern-dependent response modulations decrease with the increasing size of the receptive field (**Figure 7**) depending, to some extent, on its aspect ratio (Egelhaaf et al., 1989; Single and Borst, 1998; Dror et al., 2001; Meyer et al., 2011; O'Carroll et al., 2011; Hennig and Egelhaaf, 2012; Kurtz, 2012). From the perspective of velocity coding, the pattern-dependent response modulations have been viewed as "pattern noise" because they deteriorate the quality of the neural representation of pattern velocity (Dror et al., 2001; O'Carroll et al., 2011). Alternatively, these pattern-dependent modulations may be functionally relevant, as they reflect the textural properties of the surroundings (Meyer et al., 2011; Hennig and Egelhaaf, 2012). We will argue below that the latter interpretation might be relevant especially during translatory locomotion during intersaccadic intervals.

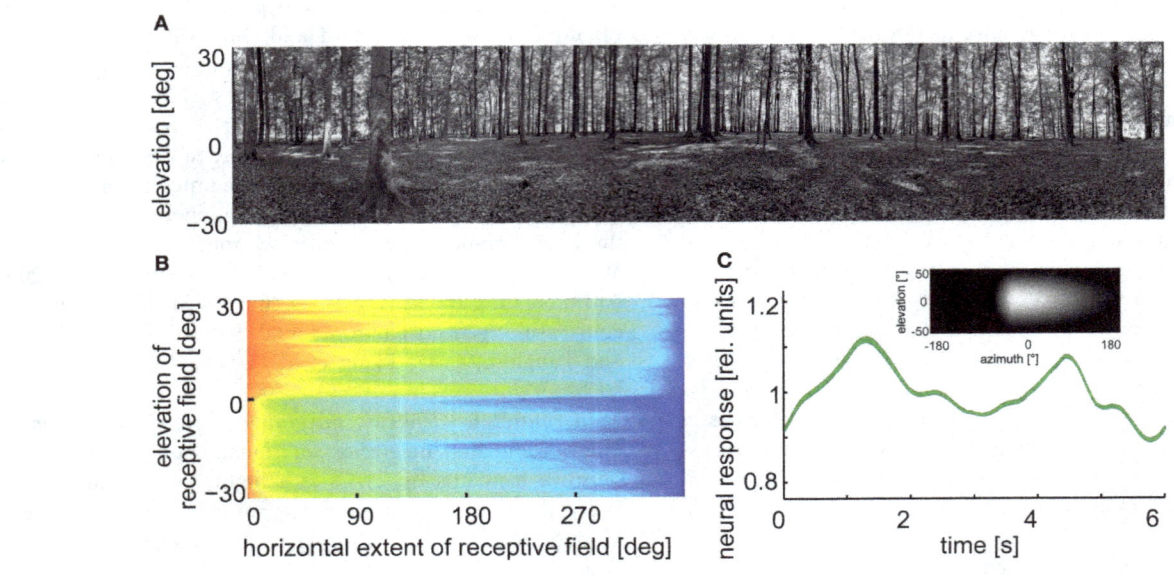

FIGURE 7 | Pattern-dependent response modulations of modeled arrays of movement detectors. (A) Panoramic high dynamic range image of a forest scene (rescaled in contrast for printing purposes). **(B)** Logarithmic color-coded standard deviation describing the mean pattern-dependent modulations for one-dimensional receptive fields differing in the elevation of receptor position and azimuthal receptive field size. Pattern-dependent modulations decrease with horizontal receptive field extent. Modulation amplitude depends on the contrast distribution of the input image, as can be seen when comparing pattern-dependent modulation amplitudes corresponding to the upper (trees) and lower part (ground) of the input image. **(C)** Time-dependent response of an array of movement detectors with an estimated HSE cell receptive field. Inset: Weight field of the spatial sensitivity distribution of a HSE cell. The brighter the gray level, the larger the local sensitivity. The frontal equatorial viewing direction is at 0° azimuth and 0° elevation. Image motion was performed for 12 s in the preferred direction of the model cell at an angular velocity of 60°/s (Data from Meyer et al., 2011).

BEHAVIORAL SIGNIFICANCE OF OPTIC FLOW NEURONS

What is the functional significance of the response characteristics of the motion sensitive and directionally selective LWCs described above? Two related and, to some extent, interdependent views are prevalent in the literature: (1) LWCs are conventionally conceived as self-motion sensors and, in particular, rotation detectors, in other words, neural elements sensing deviations of the animal from its normal attitude and/or flight course. (2) It is often implicitly assumed that the motion detection system should produce responses that come close to a veridical representation of the retinal velocities. Deviation from this velocity representation, such as the ambiguities in the responses resulting from the pattern properties of the stimulus and the fact that the response first increases with increasing velocity, but then decreases again beyond some velocity level (see above), are then regarded as deficiencies of an imperfect biological mechanism. However, it is becoming increasingly obvious from recent research that both views need to be qualified given the peculiar spatiotemporal characteristics of the retinal image flow resulting from the active vision strategies of insects. Moreover, constraints imposed by the timescale of behavior need to be taken into account when interpreting the functional significance of LWCs.

A ROLE OF LWCs IN MEDIATING COMPENSATORY OPTOMOTOR TURNING RESPONSES

LWCs are commonly thought to mediate compensatory optomotor turning responses of the entire body as well as the head. The strongest, though not very specific, evidence is based on the fact

that many characteristics of the behavioral responses correlate well with the response characteristics of LWCs: they show similar velocity sensitivity, and the local preferred directions of various LWCs appear to match with rotational optic flow fields and, thus, were interpreted as an adaption to detect rotational self-motion of the animal around different axes (Krapp and Hengstenberg, 1996; Krapp et al., 1998, 2001; Krapp, 2000; Elyada et al., 2009).

Optomotor following of the entire animal is often analysed in tethered flight both under open- and closed-loop conditions: Here, the fly generates turning responses of the head and the body and follows the moving pattern. This response is usually interpreted to reflexively stabilize the retinal images by minimizing the retinal velocities, for instance, resulting from external and/or internal disturbances (Hausen and Egelhaaf, 1989; Krapp, 2000; Borst and Haag, 2002; Egelhaaf, 2006; Taylor and Krapp, 2008; Borst et al., 2010). However, only rotational optic flow can be eliminated in this way, and the retinal images cannot be stabilized entirely during flight, because the animal needs to translate if it wants to move from one place to another.

A general feature of compensatory optomotor responses is that they are relatively slow. Their response dynamics differ considerably from the much faster object-induced fixation responses (Egelhaaf, 1987, 1989; Warzecha and Egelhaaf, 1996; Duistermars et al., 2007; Rosner et al., 2009). What is the functional significance of such slow compensatory optomotor responses under natural behavioral conditions? Since intersaccadic gaze stabilization is very fast, it is hardly conceivable that it could be controlled by optomotor feedback. Optomotor feedback can play a role only at a much slower timescale, for instance, to compensate for steady asymmetries at the level of the sensory input (e.g., dirt on one eye or internal gain differences) or the motor output (e.g., worn-out wings). Evidence for this comes from experiments where asymmetries were introduced to the visual system by occluding one of the eyes (Kern et al., 2000, in preparation). These behavioral results indicate that LWCs may play a role in mediating compensatory responses of the animal to slow unintended deviations from course, after their output signals are considerably low-pass filtered. So far, it is not clear where in the nervous system downstream of the lobula complex and by what mechanisms this filtering is accomplished.

In addition to the body, the head of flies and bees also performs compensatory optomotor responses in both tethered and free-flight. Compensatory head movements are most prominent during roll rotations of the body as are generated during banked saccadic turns and during sideways translations (Hengstenberg, 1993; van Hateren and Schilstra, 1999; Boeddeker and Hemmi, 2010; Boeddeker et al., 2010; Geurten et al., 2010). Fast gaze stabilization in flies is mainly achieved by mechanosensory input from halteres that act as gyroscopes (Sandeman and Markl, 1980). However, some LWCs have a rather direct impact on head muscles and, thus, on mediating head rotations (Milde et al., 1987, 1995; Gronenberg and Strausfeld, 1990; Gronenberg et al., 1995; Huston and Krapp, 2008, 2009). Bees, like most other insects, lack specialized inertial sensors like halteres. Nonetheless, they also show an optomotor reflex that uses visual motion to stabilize the head with respect to the visual environment under free-flight conditions at retinal velocities of up to 300°/s (Boeddeker and Hemmi, 2010). Experiments on fruit flies provide a similar picture: whereas the visual system is tuned to relatively slow rotation, the haltere-mediated response to mechanical oscillation increases with rising angular velocity (Hengstenberg, 1993; Sherman and Dickinson, 2003, 2004).

In conclusion, LWCs are likely to mediate optomotor responses on a relatively slow timescale, and might thus help compensating rotational optic flow arising from internal asymmetries of the animal. Given the extremely rapid timescale on which gaze direction is stabilized during saccadic flight maneuvres and the response latencies of visually mediated head responses, the functional role of LWCs for compensatory head rotations under free-flight conditions is still not entirely clear.

A ROLE OF LWCs IN GATHERING INFORMATION ABOUT THE ENVIRONMENT DURING INTERSACCADIC INTERVALS

The time that flies and bees keep their gaze straight amounts to more than 80% of the overall flight-time (Schilstra and van Hateren, 1999; van Hateren and Schilstra, 1999; Boeddeker et al., 2005, 2010; Braun et al., 2010, 2012; Geurten et al., 2010; van Breugel and Dickinson, 2012). Hence, rotations are squeezed into relatively short and rapid saccadic turns. This flight and gaze strategy has been interpreted as a way to facilitate gathering environmental information that is contained in the retinal image flow during translatory self-motion (see above). Therefore, motion-sensitive neurons appear to be predestined to provide environmental information during intersaccadic intervals.

This suggestion is plausible, because the specificity of most LWCs for rotational optic flow is not exclusive and they also respond strongly to translational optic flow (Hausen, 1982; Horstmann et al., 2000; Karmeier et al., 2003, 2006; Taylor and Krapp, 2008). Moreover, the most prominent rotations performed by insects in free-flight, the saccadic turns, lead to angular velocities that are much beyond the monotonic operating range of the motion detection system (see above); rather the monotonic operating range roughly matches the intersaccadic translational velocities in those retinal regions that are probably involved in controlling the translation velocity of the animal (Kern et al., 2012).

As has been stressed above, LWCs are not veridical sensors of velocity and, thus, do not provide unambiguous information about self-motion. This is particularly obvious for the translatory movements during intersaccadic intervals, because here, retinal velocities do not only depend on the velocity of locomotion, but also on the three-dimensional layout of the environment. This dependency is reflected in the responses of HS cells; a group of three fly LWCs with a main preferred direction from the front to the back in the visual field of one eye. These neurons depolarize if environmental structures are sufficiently close, especially during translatory self-motion with a strong sideways component (**Figure 8**) (Boeddeker et al., 2005; Kern et al., 2005; Lindemann et al., 2005; Liang et al., 2012). Similar results were obtained in further LWCs during translatory movements in other directions (Karmeier et al., 2006). However, spatial information is only provided by LWCs if rotational movements are largely eliminated during the intersaccadic intervals, emphasizing the importance of the active saccadic flight and gaze strategy in the context of spatial vision (Kern et al., 2006). The responses to objects nearby are even more augmented by adaptation mechanisms, which depend on stimulus history, and, thus, on the properties of previous flight sequences (Liang et al., 2008, 2011).

What is the range within which spatial information is encoded in this way? Under spatially constrained conditions where the flies flew at translational velocities of only slightly more than 0.5 metres per second, the spatial range within which significant distance dependent intersaccadic responses are evoked amounts to approximately two metres (Kern et al., 2005; Liang et al., 2012). Since a given retinal velocity is determined in a reciprocal way by distance and velocity of self-motion, respectively, the spatial range that is represented by LWCs can be expected to increase with increasing translational velocity. In other words, the behaviorally relevant spatial range can be assumed to scale with locomotion velocity. From an ecological point of view, this consequence of the closed-loop nature of vision is economical and efficient, since the behaviorally relevant spatial depth range increases during fast self-motion. A fast moving animal can thus initiate an avoidance maneuver earlier and at a greater distance from an obstacle than when moving slowly.

Recently, we found that the responses of bee LWCs to visual stimuli as experienced during navigation flights in the vicinity of an invisible goal also strongly depend on the spatial layout of the environment. The spatial landmark constellation that guides the bees to their goal leads to a characteristic time-dependent

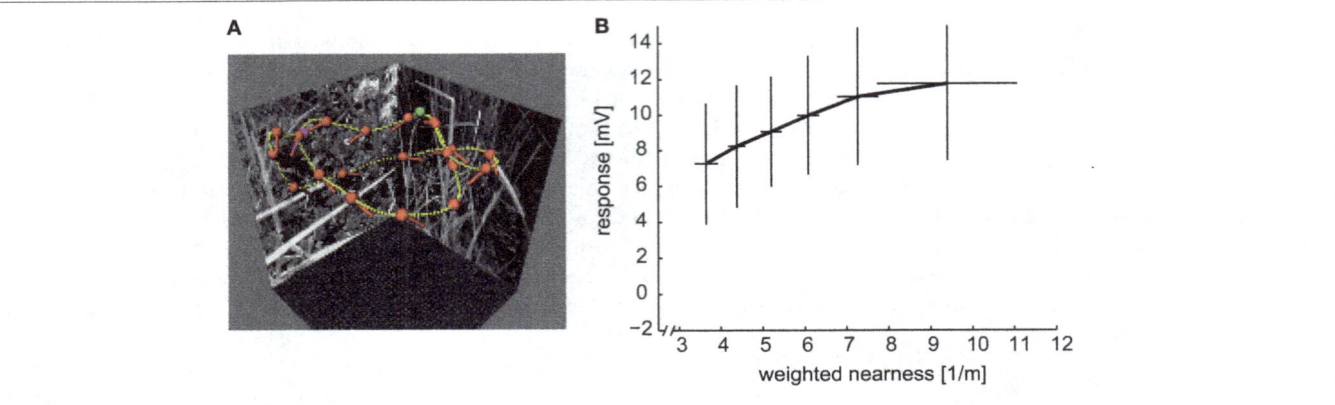

FIGURE 8 | Distance dependence of intersaccadic responses in the HSE cell, a prominent LWC in the blowfly lobula plate. (A) Sample flight trajectory of a blowfly in a cubic arena used for the reconstruction of optic flow. The track of the fly is indicated by the yellow lines; red dots and short dashes indicate the position of the fly's head and its orientation, respectively; green and violet dots indicate the start and end of the trajectory, respectively. **(B)** Average intersaccadic responses of HSE cell recordings from three different flight trajectories plotted versus the corresponding average weighted nearness. The responses were sorted by increasing nearness and then attributed to six groups. The vertical and horizontal lines show the standard deviations of responses and nearness, respectively, across the data values within one group. The intersaccadic responses were related to the nearness of the fly to the respective arena walls (nearness = 1/distance), weighted by the HSE cell's spatial sensitivity distribution (see inset of **Figure 7C**). The intersaccadic responses increase with increasing nearness to the walls of the flight arena (Data from Liang et al., 2012).

response profile in LWCs during the intersaccadic intervals of navigation flights (Mertes et al. in preparation).

The responses of LWCs of flies and bees do not only depend on the retinal velocities, but are also sensitive to pattern properties (**Figure 7**; see above). Although the pattern-dependent modulations in the neural responses have been conventionally viewed as detrimental to the velocity signal, they may reflect functionally relevant information about the environment (Meyer et al., 2011; Hennig and Egelhaaf, 2012). This may be the case especially during intersaccadic translatory movements: since the retinal velocity scales with distance, an object nearby will lead to larger intersaccadic depolarization than a more distant one. Assuming that objects nearby are especially functionally relevant, object detection via optic flow automatically weighs objects according to their distance and, thus, their functional relevance. In other words, cluttered spatial scenery is segmented in this way, without much computational expenditure, into nearby and distant objects.

The amplitude of pattern-induced neural responses depends to a large extent on the size of the neuron's receptive field. Large receptive fields blur pattern-dependent response fluctuations and, thus, improve the quality of velocity signals (**Figure 7**). However, they do this at the expense of how well the signals can be localized. Hence, if motion signals originating from an object need to be localized by a neuron in the visual field, its receptive field should be sufficiently small; then, however, velocity coding is only poor and the signal provides local pattern information (Meyer et al., 2011). Hence, a neuron that is to encode spatial information on the basis of optic flow elicited during translatory self-motion should possess a receptive field that matches the size of the behaviorally relevant objects or textures. Sensitivity to objects may be further augmented by inhibitory spatial interactions, as is characteristic of blowfly FD cells (Hennig and Egelhaaf, 2012), and also by adaptive mechanisms (Liang et al., 2008, 2011). The enhanced sensitivity to objects in FD cells results from

non-linearities in the synaptic interactions between an inhibitory neuron and the FD cell, on the one hand (Egelhaaf, 1985c; Hennig et al., 2008), and from the excitatory receptive field of the FD cell being smaller than that of its inhibitory input, on the other hand (**Figures 6B–D**) (Egelhaaf, 1985b; Egelhaaf et al., 1993; Krapp et al., 2001). In addition, the larger receptive field of the inhibitory LWC enhances the pattern-dependent response fluctuations in the FD cell (Hennig and Egelhaaf, 2012). Thus, the same mechanism which accounts for the FD cells being highly sensitive to objects defined by relative motion cues is also responsible for their sensitivity to objects which are defined by discontinuities in the textural properties of the environment.

It became evident in recent studies that the response properties of fly LWCs are affected by the behavioral state of the animal. Most prominently, the response amplitudes of LWCs increase if the animal is behaviorally active during the electrophysiological recording (Chiappe et al., 2010; Maimon et al., 2010; Rosner et al., 2010; Jung et al., 2011). This effect can be mimicked to some extent by application of the octopamine agonist CDM, which may induce an increase in overall spike rate and a slight shift in the velocity tuning (Longden and Krapp, 2009, 2010; Jung et al., 2011; de Haan et al., 2012; Rien et al., 2012). Octopamine has already been shown much earlier to increase the overall spike rate of LWCs in honeybees, although changes in velocity tuning have not been tested (Kloppenburg and Erber, 1995). These changes in LWC properties related to the behavioral state of the animal are unlikely to alter the conclusions about how environmental features are represented during intersaccadic LWC responses. High intersaccadic velocities, for instance, occur close to objects or the walls of the flight arena. A shift in velocity tuning toward higher velocities would reduce the likelihood of retinal velocities beyond the monotonic response range of the motion detection system and, thus, would improve the encoding of distance information.

We can conclude that LWCs of flies and bees provide information about the spatial layout and the pattern properties of the environment. This information is linked to the translational self-motion of the flying animal during intersaccadic intervals. As a consequence of the action–perception cycle and the distance dependence of translational optic flow, this spatial information is confined to the behaviorally relevant range of up to a few metres. Within this range, the animal has to take action, for instance, to avoid collisions with obstacles, to select a landing place or to employ environmental objects as landmarks in order to learn and/or find the location of a barely visible goal.

CONSTRAINTS SET BY A TIMESCALE OF NATURAL BEHAVIOR

In classical behavioral paradigms using tethered flying insects, the experimenter-defined motion sequences usually stay constant on a timescale of several hundreds of milliseconds and even seconds. However, during unrestrained behavior, the retinal motion patterns continually change. As a consequence of the typical saccadic flight and gaze strategy of insects (see above), optic flow dynamics during natural locomotion also deviate considerably from dynamic stimuli (e.g., white-noise velocity fluctuations) that are often employed in characterizing LWCs. In the context of spatial vision, the intersaccadic intervals are of particular interest. Although they take up, on the whole, more than 80% of the entire flight time, they may be as short as 30 ms.

Why is the duration of intersaccadic intervals and, thus, the timescale on which information about the environment needs to be processed an issue at all? On the one hand, neurons are relatively unreliable computing devices and, on the other hand, the spatial behavior of flying insects takes place on a comparatively rapid timescale. The problem of reliability is particularly daunting, as there is not much redundancy at the output level of the insect visual system which would allow for the pooling of information across equivalent neurons.

When the same stimulus is presented repeatedly to a neuron, the responses may vary a lot between trials. Neuronal activity fluctuates continually even during constant velocity motion (reviews: Pelli, 1991; de Ruyter van Steveninck and Bialek, 1995; Warzecha and Egelhaaf, 2001). On the basis of individual response traces, it is not easily possible to discern stimulus-driven activity changes from those that are due to sources not associated with the stimulus ("noise"). The origin of various potential noise sources in the visual motion pathway and the consequences of the unreliable nature of neural signals have been analysed in flies (e.g., de Ruyter van Steveninck and Bialek, 1995; de Ruyter van Steveninck et al., 1997; Warzecha and Egelhaaf, 1999; Warzecha et al., 2000; Egelhaaf et al., 2001; Lewen et al., 2001; Borst, 2003; Grewe et al., 2003, 2007; Nemenman et al., 2008). These aspects, as well as the impact of neuronal noise on the precision with which motion information can be encoded, have been controversially discussed (Haag and Borst, 1997, 1998; Warzecha and Egelhaaf, 1997; Warzecha et al., 1998, 2000, 2003; Brenner et al., 2000b; Fairhall et al., 2001; Kalb, 2006). One aspect appears to be especially relevant in the context of computing spatial information: given that neuronal responses are noisy, it will take some time to infer reliably behaviorally relevant environmental information from neuronal activity. Bayesian analysis of noisy intersaccadic responses of individual fly LWCs and populations of LWCs reveals that sufficiently reliable information about translatory self-motion and, thus, about spatial parameters of the environment can be decoded already on a timescale of little more than 5 ms and, thus, on a time-scale of even the shortest intersaccadic intervals (Karmeier et al., 2005). Since the neural responses in this analysis were integrated over time, the intersaccadic responses decoded on this basis do not allow for resolving temporal response fluctuations that may arise from pattern properties during an intersaccadic interval. How much the neural responses fluctuate in a pattern-dependent way on a timescale of intersaccades needs to be investigated by scrutinizing individual responses to translations in natural surroundings.

CONCLUSIONS

Despite their small brains with less than a million neurons and a spatial resolution of their eyes much smaller than any useful technical camera system, insects such as flies or bees are able to solve complex spatial tasks, such as avoiding collisions with obstacles, landing on objects or even finding hardly visible goals on the basis of spatial landmark information. Insects outperform man-made autonomous flying systems in these tasks especially if resource efficiency with respect to computational expenditure and energy consumption are conceived as a benchmark. Moreover, insects accomplish this at flight velocities that imply rapid time-varying retinal image flow. The processing of rapid retinal image flow represents great challenges for the neuronal machinery, given the limited reliability of neurons as computing devices. Obviously, as a consequence of millions of years of evolution, insect nervous systems have become well adapted to successfully cope with these computational challenges and to solve those computational tasks that are relevant for the success of the species efficiently and parsimoniously.

One means to accomplish their extraordinary performance is that flies and bees actively shape the image flow on their eyes by their characteristic flight behavior. Neural processing of spatial and textural information about the environment is greatly facilitated by largely segregating the rotational from the translational optic flow through a saccadic flight and gaze strategy. It is suggested that tuning the neural networks of motion computation to the specific spatiotemporal properties of the actively shaped optic flow patterns enables the nervous system to solve apparently complex spatial vision tasks more efficiently and parsimoniously than might be possible without such an active vision strategy. Only by taking into account the characteristics of the retinal image flow that is generated under natural closed-loop conditions did it become clear that the classical interpretations of the functional significance of neurons sensitive to optic flow need to be at least modified and extended: these neurons not only reflect information about the animals' self-motion, but also—through the image flow generated during intersaccadic translational movements—about the outside world. Accordingly, these neurons may be regarded as sensors for environmental information that, as a consequence of the distance dependence of translational optic flow, weigh in computationally inexpensive ways environmental information according to its presumptive significance for spatial vision.

Hence, we can conclude from the experimental work on the spatial behavior of insects and the underlying neural mechanisms, in combination with model simulations, that biological systems such as flies or bees derive part of their power as autonomous systems from scrutinizing their environment during the execution of sets of carefully selected motor routines, instead of just passively gathering information about the world. These animal–environment interactions lead to adaptive behavior in environments of a wide range of complexity. Model simulations and robotic implementations reveal that the smart biological mechanisms of motion computation and flight control might be helpful when designing micro air vehicles that may carry an onboard processor of only relatively small size and weight (Floreano et al., 2009).

REFERENCES

Aptekar, J. W., Shoemaker, P. A., and Frye, M. A. (2012). Figure tracking by flies is supported by parallel visual streams. *Curr. Biol.* 22, 482–487.

Baird, E., Kornfeldt, T., and Dacke, M. (2010). Minimum viewing angle for visually guided ground speed control in bumblebees. *J. Exp. Biol.* 213, 1625–1632.

Baird, E., Srinivasan, M. V., Zhang, S., and Cowling, A. (2005). Visual control of flight speed in honeybees. *J. Exp. Biol.* 208, 3895–3905.

Baird, E., Srinivasan, M. V., Zhang, S., Lamont, R., and Cowling, A. (2006). "Visual control of flight speed and height in the honeybee," in *From Animals to Animats 9*, eds S. Nolfi, G. Baldassare, R. Calabretta, J. Hallam, D. Marocco, O. Miglino, et al. (Berlin, Heidelberg: Springer; Lecture Notes in Computer Science), 40–51.

Barnett, P. D., Nordström, K., and O'Carroll, D. C. (2007). Retinotopic organization of small-field-target-detecting neurons in the insect visual system. *Curr. Biol.* 17, 569–578.

Beersma, D. G. M., Stavenga, D. G., and Kuiper, J. W. (1977). Retinal lattice, visual field and binocularities in flies. *J. Comp. Physiol.* 119, 207–220.

Bender, J. A., and Dickinson, M. H. (2006a). A comparison of visual and haltere-mediated feedback in the control of body saccades in *Drosophila melanogaster*. *J. Exp. Biol.* 209, 4597–4606.

Bender, J. A., and Dickinson, M. H. (2006b). Visual stimulation of saccades in magnetically tethered Drosophila. *J. Exp. Biol.* 209, 3170–3182.

Betsch, B. Y., Einhäuser, W., Körding, K. P., and König, P. (2004). The world from a cat's perspective – statistics of natural videos. *Biol. Cybern.* 90, 41–50.

Boeddeker, N., Dittmar, L., Stürzl, W., and Egelhaaf, M. (2010). The fine structure of honeybee head and body yaw movements in a homing task. *Proc. Biol. Sci.* 277, 1899–1906.

Boeddeker, N., and Hemmi, J. M. (2010). Visual gaze control during peering flight manoeuvres in honeybees. *Proc. Biol. Sci.* 277, 1209–1217.

Boeddeker, N., Lindemann, J. P., Egelhaaf, M., and Zeil, J. (2005). Responses of blowfly motion-sensitive neurons to reconstructed optic flow along outdoor flight paths. *J. Comp. Physiol. A* 25, 1143–1155.

Borst, A. (2003). Noise, not stimulus entropy, determines neural information rate. *J. Comput. Neurosci.* 14, 23–31.

Borst, A. (2009). Drosophila's view on insect vision. *Curr. Biol.* 19, R36–R47.

Borst, A., and Egelhaaf, M. (1989). Principles of visual motion detection. *Trends Neurosci.* 12, 297–306.

Borst, A., Egelhaaf, M., and Haag, J. (1995). Mechanisms of dendritic integration underlying gain control in fly motion-sensitive interneurons. *J. Comput. Neurosci.* 2, 5–18.

Borst, A., and Haag, J. (2002). Neural networks in the cockpit of the fly. *J. Comp. Physiol. A Neuroethol. Sens. Neural Behav. Physiol.* 188, 419–437.

Borst, A., Haag, J., and Reiff, D. F. (2010). Fly motion vision. *Annu. Rev. Neurosci.* 33, 49–70.

Borst, A., Reisenman, C., and Haag, J. (2003). Adaptation to response transients in fly motion vision: II. Model studies. *Vision Res.* 43, 1309–1322.

Borst, A., and Weber, F. (2011). Neural action fields for optic flow based navigation: a simulation study of the fly lobula plate network. *PLoS ONE* 6:e16303. doi: 10.1371/journal.pone.0016303

Braun, E., Dittmar, L., Boeddeker, N., and Egelhaaf, M. (2012). Prototypical components of honeybee homing flight behaviour depend on the visual appearance of objects surrounding the goal. *Front. Behav. Neurosci.* 6:1. doi: 10.3389/fnbeh.2012.00001

Braun, E., Geurten, B., and Egelhaaf, M. (2010). Identifying prototypical components in behaviour using clustering algorithms. *PLoS ONE* 5:e9361. doi: 10.1371/journal.pone.0009361

Brenner, N., Bialek, W., and de Ruyter van Steveninck, R. (2000a). Adaptive rescaling maximizes information transmission. *Neuron* 26, 695–702.

Brenner, N., Strong, S. P., Koberle, R., Bialek, W., and de Ruyter van Steveninck, R. (2000b). Synergy in a neural code. *Neural Comput.* 12, 1531–1552.

Brinkworth, R. S. A., O'Carroll, D. C., and Graham, L. J. (2009). Robust models for optic flow coding in natural scenes inspired by insect biology. *PLoS Comput. Biol.* 5:e1000555. doi: 10.1371/journal.pcbi.1000555

Budick, S. A., and Dickinson, M. H. (2006). Free-flight responses of *Drosophila melanogaster* to attractive odors. *J. Exp. Biol.* 209, 3001–3017.

Budick, S. A., Reiser, M. B., and Dickinson, M. H. (2007). The role of visual and mechanosensory cues in structuring forward flight in *Drosophila melanogaster*. *J. Exp. Biol.* 210, 4092–4103.

Chiappe, M. E., Seelig, J. D., Reiser, M. B., and Jayaraman, V. (2010). Walking modulates speed sensitivity in *Drosophila* motion vision. *Curr. Biol.* 20, 1470–1475.

Clark, D. A., Bursztyn, L., Horowitz, M. A., Schnitzer, M. J., and Clandinin, T. R. (2011). Defining the computational structure of the motion detector in Drosophila. *Neuron* 70, 1165–1177.

Clifford, C. W. G., and Ibbotson, M. R. (2003). Fundamental mechanisms of visual motion detection: models, cells and functions. *Prog. Neurobiol.* 68, 409–437.

Collett, T. S. (1978). Peering – a locust behavior pattern for obtaining motion parallax information. *J. Exp. Biol.* 76, 237–241.

Collett, T. S., and Collett, M. (2002). Memory use in insect visual navigation. *Nat. Rev. Neurosci.* 3, 542–552.

Collett, T. S., Graham, P., Harris, R. A., and Hempel-De-Ibarra, N. (2006). Navigational memories in ants and bees: memory retrieval when selecting and following routes. *Adv. Study Behav.* 36, 123–172.

Collett, T. S., and Harkness, L. I. K. (1982). "Depth vision in animals," in *Analysis of Visual Behaviour*, eds D. J. Ingle, M. A. Goodale, and R. J. W. Mansfield (Cambridge, MA; London England: The MIT Press), 111–176.

Collett, T. S., and Land, M. F. (1975). Visual control of flight behaviour in the hoverfly *Syritta pipiens* L. *J. Comp. Physiol.* 99, 1–66.

Collett, T. S., and Paterson, C. J. (1991). Relative motion parallax and target localization in the locust, *Schistocerca gregaria*. *J. Comp. Physiol. A* 169, 615–621.

Dahmen, H. J., Franz, M. O., and Krapp, H. G. (2000). "Extracting ego-motion from optic flow: limits of accuracy and neuronal filters," in *Computational, Neural and Ecological Constraints of Visual Motion Processing*, eds J. M. Zanker and J. Zeil (Berlin, Heidelberg, New York: Springer), 143–168.

David, C. T. (1979). Optomotor control of speed and height by free-flying Drosophila. *J. Exp. Biol.* 82, 389–392.

David, C. T. (1982). Compensation for height in the control of ground-speed by Drosophila in a new, 'barber's pole' wind tunnel. *J. Comp. Physiol.* 147, 485–493.

Davies, M. N. O., and Green, P. R. (1988). Head-bobbing during walking, running and flying: relative motion perception in the pigeon. *J. Exp. Biol.* 138, 71–91.

de Haan, R., Lee, Y.-J., and Nordström, K. (2012). Octopaminergic modulation of contrast sensitivity. *Front. Integr. Neurosci.* 6:55. doi: 10.3389/fnint.2012.00055

de Ruyter van Steveninck, R., and Bialek, W. (1995). Reliability and statistical efficiency of a blowfly movement-sensitive neuron. *Philos. Trans. R. Soc. Lond. B Biol. Sci.* 348, 321–340.

de Ruyter van Steveninck, R., Lewen, G. D., Strong, S. P., Koberle, R., and Bialek, W. (1997). Reproducibility and variability in neural spike trains. *Science* 275, 1805–1808.

DeVoe, R. D., Kaiser, W., Ohm, J., and Stone, L. S. (1982). Horizontal movement detectors of honeybees. Directionally-selective visual neurons in the lobula and brain. *J. Comp. Physiol.* 147, 155–170.

Dittmar, L., Egelhaaf, M., Stürzl, W., and Boeddeker, N. (2011). The behavioural relevance of landmark texture for honeybee homing. *Front. Behav. Neurosci.* 5:20. doi: 10.3389/fnbeh.2011.00020

Dittmar, L., Stürzl, W., Baird, E., Boeddeker, N., and Egelhaaf, M. (2010). Goal seeking in honeybees: matching of optic flow snapshots. *J. Exp. Biol.* 213, 2913–2923.

Dong, D. W., and Attick, J. J. (1995). Statistics of natural time-varying images. *Network* 6, 345–358.

Dror, R. O., O'Carroll, D. C., and Laughlin, S. B. (2001). Accuracy of velocity estimation by Reichardt correlators. *J. Opt. Soc. Am. A Opt. Image Sci. Vis.* 18, 241–252.

Duistermars, B. J., Reiser, M. B., Zhu, Y., and Frye, M. A. (2007). Dynamic properties of large-field and small-field optomotor flight responses in Drosophila. *J. Comp. Physiol. A Neuroethol. Sens. Neural Behav. Physiol.* 193, 787–799.

Dyhr, J. P., and Higgins, C. M. (2010). The spatial frequency tuning of optic-flow-dependent behaviors in the bumblebee *Bombus impatiens. J. Exp. Biol.* 213, 1643–1650.

Eckert, M. P., and Buchsbaum, G. (1993). Efficient coding of natural time varying images in the early visual system. *Philos. Trans. R. Soc. Lond. B Biol. Sci.* 339, 385–395.

Eckmeier, D., Geurten, B. R. H., Kress, D., Mertes, M., Kern, R., Egelhaaf, M., et al. (2008). Gaze strategy in the free flying zebra finch (*Taeniopygia guttata*). *PLoS ONE* 3:e3956. doi: 10.1371/journal.pone.0003956

Egelhaaf, M. (1985a). On the neuronal basis of figure-ground discrimination by relative motion in the visual system of the fly. I. Behavioural constraints imposed on the neuronal network and the role of the optomotor system. *Biol. Cybern.* 52, 123–140.

Egelhaaf, M. (1985b). On the neuronal basis of figure-ground discrimination by relative motion in the visual system of the fly. II. Figure-Detection Cells, a new class of visual interneurones. *Biol. Cybern.* 52, 195–209.

Egelhaaf, M. (1985c). On the neuronal basis of figure-ground discrimination by relative motion in the visual system of the fly. III. Possible input

circuitries and behavioural significance of the FD-Cells. *Biol. Cybern.* 52, 267–280.

Egelhaaf, M. (1987). Dynamic properties of two control systems underlying visually guided turning in house-flies. *J. Comp. Physiol. A* 161, 777–783.

Egelhaaf, M. (1989). Visual afferences to flight steering muscles controlling optomotor response of the fly. *J. Comp. Physiol. A* 165, 719–730.

Egelhaaf, M. (2006). "The neural computation of visual motion," in *Invertebrate Vision*, eds E. Warrant and D.-E. Nilsson (Cambridge, UK: Cambridge University Press), 399–461.

Egelhaaf, M., and Borst, A. (1989). Transient and steady-state response properties of movement detectors. *J. Opt. Soc. Am. A* 6, 116–127.

Egelhaaf, M., and Borst, A. (1992). Are there separate on- and off-channels in fly motion vision? *Vis. Neurosci.* 8, 151–164.

Egelhaaf, M., and Borst, A. (1993a). A look into the cockpit of the fly: visual orientation, algorithms, and identified neurons. *J. Neurosci.* 13, 4563–4574.

Egelhaaf, M., and Borst, A. (1993b). "Movement detection in arthropods," in *Visual Motion and its Role in the Stabilization of Gaze*, eds F. A. Miles and J. Wallman (Amsterdam: Elsevier), 53–77.

Egelhaaf, M., Borst, A., and Reichardt, W. (1989). Computational structure of a biological motion detection system as revealed by local detector analysis in the fly's nervous system. *J. Opt. Soc. Am. A* 6, 1070–1087.

Egelhaaf, M., Borst, A., Warzecha, A.-K., Flecks, S., and Wildemann, A. (1993). Neural circuit tuning fly visual interneurons to motion of small objects. II. Input organization of inhibitory circuit elements by electrophysiological and optical recording techniques. *J. Neurophysiol.* 69, 340–351.

Egelhaaf, M., Grewe, J., Kern, R., and Warzecha, A.-K. (2001). Outdoor performance of a motion-sensitive neuron in the blowfly. *Vision Res.* 41, 3627–3637.

Egelhaaf, M., Kern, R., Kurtz, R., Krapp, H. G., Kretzberg, J., and Warzecha, A.-K. (2002). Neural encoding of behaviourally relevant motion information in the fly. *Trends Neurosci.* 25, 96–102.

Egelhaaf, M., and Reichardt, W. (1987). Dynamic response properties of movement detectors: theoretical

analysis and electrophysiological investigation in the visual system of the fly. *Biol. Cybern.* 56, 69–87.

Egelhaaf, M., and Warzecha, A.-K. (1998). Encoding of motion in real time by the fly visual system. *Curr. Opin. Neurobiol.* 9, 454–460.

Eichner, H., Joesch, M., Schnell, B., Reiff, D. F., and Borst, A. (2011). Internal structure of the fly elementary motion detector. *Neuron* 70, 1155–1164.

Elyada, Y. M., Haag, J., and Borst, A. (2009). Different receptive fields in axons and dendrites underlie robust coding in motion-sensitive neurons. *Nat. Neurosci.* 12, 327–332.

Esch, H. E., Zhang, S., Srinivasan, M. V., and Tautz, J. (2001). Honeybee dances communicate distances measured by optic flow. *Nature* 411, 581–583.

Fairhall, A. L., Lewen, G. D., Bialek, W., and de Ruyter van Steveninck, R. (2001). Efficiency and ambiguity in an adaptive neural code. *Nature* 412, 787–792.

Farina, W. M., Kramer, D., and Varjú, D. (1995). The response of the hovering hawk moth *Macroglossum stellatarum* to translatory pattern motion. *J. Comp. Physiol.* 176, 551–562.

Farina, W. M., Varjú, D., and Zhou, Y. (1994). The regulation of distance to dummy flowers during hovering flight in the hawk moth *Macroglossum stellatarum. J. Comp. Physiol.* 174, 239–247.

Farrow, K., Haag, J., and Borst, A. (2003). Input organization of multifunctional motion-sensitive neurons in the blowfly. *J. Neurosci.* 29, 9805–9811.

Farrow, K., Haag, J., and Borst, A. (2006). Nonlinear, binocular interactions underlying flow field selectivity of a motion-sensitive neuron. *Nat. Neurosci.* 9, 1312–1320.

Floreano, D., Zufferey, J.-C., Srinivasan, M. V., and Ellington, C. (2009). *Flying Insects and Robots.* Heidelberg, Dordrecht, London, New York: Springer.

Foucaud, J., Burns, J. G., Mery, F., and Zars, T. (2010). Use of spatial information and search strategies in a water maze analog in *Drosophila melanogaster. PLoS ONE* 5:e15231. doi: 10.1371/journal.pone.0015231

Fry, S. N., Rohrseitz, N., Straw, A. D., and Dickinson, M. H. (2009). Visual control of flight speed in *Drosophila melanogaster. J. Exp. Biol.* 212, 1120–1130.

Frye, M. A., and Dickinson, M. H. (2007). Visual edge orientation shapes free-flight behavior in Drosophila. *Fly* 1, 153–154.

Geisler, W. S. (2008). Visual perception and the statistical properties of natural scenes. *Annu. Rev. Psychol.* 59, 10.1–10.26.

Geurten, B. R. H., Kern, R., Braun, E., and Egelhaaf, M. (2010). A syntax of hoverfly flight prototypes. *J. Exp. Biol.* 213, 2461–2475.

Geurten, B. R. H., Kern, R., and Egelhaaf, M. (2012). Species-specific flight styles of flies are reflected in the response dynamics of a homolog motion-sensitive neuron. *Front. Integr. Neurosci.* 6:11. doi: 10.3389/fnint.2012.00011

Geurten, B. R. H., Nordström, K., Sprayberry, J. D. H., Bolzon, D. M., and O'Carroll, D. C. (2007). Neural mechanisms underlying target detection in a dragonfly centrifugal neuron. *J. Exp. Biol.* 219, 3277–3284.

Gilbert, C., and Strausfeld, N. J. (1991). The functional organization of male-specific visual neurons in flies. *J. Comp. Physiol. A* 169, 395–411.

Götz, K. G. (1965). Die optischen Übertragungseigenschaften der Komplexaugen von Drosophila. *Kybernetik* 2, 215–221.

Götz, K. G. (1987). Course-control, metabolism and wing interference during ultralong tethered flight in *Drosophila melanogaster. J. Exp. Biol.* 128, 35–46.

Grewe, J., Kretzberg, J., Warzecha, A.-K., and Egelhaaf, M. (2003). Impact of photon-noise on the reliability of a motion-sensitive neuron in the fly's visual system. *J. Neurosci.* 23, 10776–10783.

Grewe, J., Weckström, M., Egelhaaf, M., and Warzecha, A.-K. (2007). Information and discriminability as measures of reliability of sensory coding. *PLoS ONE* 2:e1328. doi: 10.1371/journal.pone.0001328

Gronenberg, W., Milde, J. J., and Strausfeld, N. J. (1995). Oculomotor control in Calliphorid flies: organization of descending neurons to neck motor neurons responding to visual stimuli. *J. Comp. Neurol.* 361, 267–284.

Gronenberg, W., and Strausfeld, N. J. (1990). Descending neurons supplying the neck and flight motor of Diptera: physiological and anatomical characteristics. *J. Comp. Neurol.* 302, 973–991.

Haag, J., and Borst, A. (1997). Encoding of visual motion information and reliability in spiking and graded potential neurons. *J. Neurosci.* 17, 4809–4819.

Haag, J., and Borst, A. (1998). Active membrane properties and signal encoding in graded potential neurons. *J. Neurosci.* 18, 7972–7986.

Hardie, R. C. (1985). "Functional organization of the fly retina," in *Progress in Sensory Physiology 5*, eds H. Autrum, D. Ottoson, E. R. Perl, R. F. Schmidt, H. Shimazu, and W. D. Willis (Berlin, Heidelberg, New York, Tokyo: Springer), 1–79.

Harris, R. A., O'Carroll, D. C., and Laughlin, S. B. (2000). Contrast gain reduction in fly motion adaptation. *Neuron* 28, 595–606.

Hausen, K. (1982). Motion sensitive interneurons in the optomotor system of the fly. II. The horizontal cells: receptive field organization and response characteristics. *Biol. Cybern.* 46, 67–79.

Hausen, K., and Egelhaaf, M. (1989). "Neural mechanisms of visual course control in insects," in *Facets of Vision*, eds D. G. Stavenga and R. C. Hardie (Berlin, Heidelberg: Springer), 391–424.

Heisenberg, M., and Wolf, R. (1979). On the fine structure of yaw torque in visual flight orientation of *Drosophila melanogaster*. *J. Comp. Physiol.* 130, 113–130.

Heitwerth, J., Kern, R., van Hateren, J. H., and Egelhaaf, M. (2005). Motion adaptation leads to parsimonious encoding of natural optic flow by blowfly motion vision system. *J. Neurophysiol.* 94, 1761–1769.

Hengstenberg, R. (1993). "Multisensory control in insect oculomotor systems," in *Visual Motion and its Role in the Stabilization of Gaze, Bd 1*, eds F. A. Miles and J. Wallman (Amsteram, London, New York, Tokyio: Elsevier), 285–298.

Hennig, P., and Egelhaaf, M. (2012). Neuronal encoding of object and distance information: a model simulation study on naturalistic optic flow processing. *Front. Neural Circuits* 6:14. doi: 10.3389/fncir.2012.00014

Hennig, P., Kern, R., and Egelhaaf, M. (2011). Binocular integration of visual information: a model study on naturalistic optic flow processing. *Front. Neural Circuits* 5:4. doi: 10.3389/fncir.2011.00004

Hennig, P., Möller, R., and Egelhaaf, M. (2008). Distributed dendritic processing facilitates object detection: a computational analysis on the visual system of the fly. *PLoS ONE* 3:e3092. doi: 10.1371/journal.pone.0003092

Horstmann, W., Egelhaaf, M., and Warzecha, A.-K. (2000). Synaptic interactions increase optic flow specificity. *Eur. J. Neurosci.* 12, 2157–2165.

Huston, S. J., and Krapp, H. G. (2008). Visuomotor transformation in the fly gaze stabilization system. *PLoS Biol.* 6:e173. doi: 10.1371/journal.pbio.0060173

Huston, S. J., and Krapp, H. G. (2009). Nonlinear integration of visual and haltere inputs in fly neck motor neurons. *J. Neurosci.* 29, 13097–13105.

Ibbotson, M. R. (1991). Wide-field motion-sensitive neurons tuned to horizontal movement in the honeybee, *Apis mellifera*. *J. Comp. Physiol. A* 168, 91–102.

Joesch, M., Plett, J., Borst, A., and Reiff, D. F. (2008). Response properties of motion-sensitive visual interneurons in the lobula plate of *Drosophila melanogaster*. *Curr. Biol.* 18, 368–374.

Joesch, M., Schnell, B., Raghu, S. V., Reiff, D. F., and Borst, A. (2010). ON and OFF pathways in Drosophila motion vision. *Nature* 468, 300–304.

Jung, S. N., Borst, A., and Haag, J. (2011). Flight activity alters velocity tuning of fly motion-sensitive neurons. *J. Neurosci.* 31, 9231–9237.

Juusola, M. (2003). The rate of information transfer of naturalistic stimulation by graded potentials. *J. Gen. Physiol.* 122, 191–206.

Juusola, M., French, A. S., Uusitalo, R. O., and Weckström, M. (1996). Information processing by graded-potential transmission through tonically active synapses. *Trends Neurosci.* 19, 292–297.

Juusola, M., Kouvalainen, E., Järvilehto, M., and Weckström, M. (1994). Contrast gain, signal-to-noise ratio and linearity in light-adapted blowfly photoreceptors. *J. Gen. Physiol.* 104, 593–621.

Juusola, M., Uusitalo, R. O., and Weckström, M. (1995). Transfer of graded potentials at the photoreceptor-interneuron synapse. *J. Gen. Physiol.* 103, 117–148.

Kalb, J. (2006). Robust integration of motion information in the fly visual system revealed by single cell photoablation. *J. Neurosci.* 26, 7898–7906.

Kalb, J., Egelhaaf, M., and Kurtz, R. (2008). Adaptation changes directional sensitivity in a visual motion-sensitive neuron of the fly. *Vision Res.* 48, 1735–1742.

Karmeier, K., Krapp, H. G., and Egelhaaf, M. (2003). Robustness of the tuning of fly visual interneurons to rotatory optic flow. *J. Neurophysiol.* 90, 1626–1634.

Karmeier, K., Krapp, H. G., and Egelhaaf, M. (2005). Population coding of self-motion: applying Bayesian analysis to a population of visual interneurons in the fly. *J. Neurophysiol.* 94, 2182–2194.

Karmeier, K., van Hateren, J. H., Kern, R., and Egelhaaf, M. (2006). Encoding of naturalistic optic flow by a population of blowfly motion sensitive neurons. *J. Neurophysiol.* 96, 1602–1614.

Katsov, A. Y., and Clandinin, T. R. (2008). Motion processing streams in Drosophila are behaviorally specialized. *Neuron* 59, 322–335.

Kern, R., Boeddeker, N., Dittmar, L., and Egelhaaf, M. (2012). Blowfly flight characteristics are shaped by environmental features and controlled by optic flow information. *J. Exp. Biol.* 215, 2501–2514.

Kern, R., Egelhaaf, M., and Srinivasan, M. V. (1997). Edge detection by landing honeybees: behavioural analysis and model simulations of the underlying mechanism. *Vision Res.* 37, 2103–2117.

Kern, R., Lutterklas, M., and Egelhaaf, M. (2000). Neural representation of optic flow experienced by unilaterally blinded flies on their mean walking trajectories. *J. Comp. Physiol. A* 186, 467–479.

Kern, R., van Hateren, J. H., and Egelhaaf, M. (2006). Representation of behaviourally relevant information by blowfly motion-sensitive visual interneurons requires precise compensatory head movements. *J. Exp. Biol.* 209, 1251–1260.

Kern, R., van Hateren, J. H., Michaelis, C., Lindemann, J. P., and Egelhaaf, M. (2005). Function of a fly motion-sensitive neuron matches eye movements during free flight. *PLoS Biol.* 3:e171. doi: 10.1371/journal.pbio.0030171

Kern, R., and Varjú, D. (1998). Visual position stabilization in the hummingbird hawk moth, Macroglossum stellatarum L.: I. Behavioural analysis. *J. Comp. Physiol. A* 182, 225–237.

Kimmerle, B., and Egelhaaf, M. (2000a). Detection of object motion by a fly neuron during simulated translatory flight. *J. Comp. Physiol. A* 186, 21–31.

Kimmerle, B., and Egelhaaf, M. (2000b). Performance of fly visual interneurons during object fixation. *J. Neurosci.* 20, 6256–6266.

Kimmerle, B., Eikermann, J., and Egelhaaf, M. (2000). Object fixation by the blowfly during tethered flight in a simulated three-dimensional environment. *J. Exp. Biol.* 203, 1723–1732.

Kimmerle, B., Srinivasan, M. V., and Egelhaaf, M. (1996). Object detection by relative motion in freely flying flies. *Naturwiss* 83, 380–381.

Kimmerle, B., Warzecha, A.-K., and Egelhaaf, M. (1997). Object detection in the fly during simulated translatory flight. *J. Comp. Physiol. A* 181, 247–255.

Kirschfeld, K. (1972). "The visual system of Musca: studies on optics, structure and function," in *Information Processing in the Visual System of Arthropods*, ed R. Wehner (Berlin, Heidelberg, New York: Springer), 61–74.

Kloppenburg, P., and Erber, J. (1995). The modulatory effects of serotonin and octopamine in the visual-system of the honey-bee (*Apis mellifera* L.).2. Electrophysiological analysis of motion-sensitive neurons in the lobula. *J. Comp. Physiol. A* 176, 119–129.

Koenderink, J. J. (1986). Optic flow. *Vision Res.* 26, 161–180.

Kral, K., and Poteser, M. (1997). Motion parallax as a source of distance information in locusts and mantids. *J. Insect Behav.* 10, 145–163.

Krapp, H. G. (2000). "Neuronal matched filters for optic flow processing in flying insects," in *Neuronal Processing of Optic Flow, International Review of Neurobiology, Vol. 44*, ed M. Lappe (San Diego, CA: Academic Press), 93–120.

Krapp, H. G., Hengstenberg, B., and Hengstenberg, R. (1998). Dendritic structure and receptive-field organization of optic flow processing interneurons in the fly. *J. Neurophysiol.* 79, 1902–1917.

Krapp, H. G., and Hengstenberg, R. (1996). Estimation of self-motion by optic flow processing in single visual interneurons. *Nature* 384, 463–466.

Krapp, H. G., Hengstenberg, R., and Egelhaaf, M. (2001). Binocular contribution to optic flow processing in the fly visual system. *J. Neurophysiol.* 85, 724–734.

Kurtz, R. (2007). Direction-selective adaptation in fly visual motion-sensitive neurons is generated by an intrinsic conductance-based mechanism. *Neuroscience* 146, 573–583.

Kurtz, R. (2009). The many facets of adaptation in fly visual motion processing. *Commun. Integr. Biol.* 2, 1–3.

Kurtz, R. (2012). "Adaptive encoding of motion information in the fly visual system," in *Frontiers in*

Sensing, eds F. Barth, J. Humphrey, and M. Srinivasan (Wien, New York: Springer), 115–128.

Kurtz, R., Egelhaaf, M., Meyer, H. G., and Kern, R. (2009). Adaptation accentuates responses of fly motion-sensitive visual neurons to sudden stimulus changes. *Proc. Biol. Sci.* 276, 3711–3719.

Land, M. F., and Collett, T. S. (1974). Chasing behaviour of houseflies (*Fannia canicularis*). A description and analysis. *J. Comp. Physiol.* 89, 331–357.

Lappe, M. (ed.). (2000). *Neuronal Processing of Optic Flow*. San Diego, CA: Academic Press (International Review of Neurobiology).

Laughlin, S. B. (1994). Matching coding, circuits, cells, and molecules to signals: general principles of retinal design in the fly's eye. *Prog. Ret. Eye Res.* 13, 165–196.

Lehrer, M., and Campan, R. (2005). Generalization of convex shapes by bees: what are shapes made of? *J. Exp. Biol.* 208, 3233–3247.

Lehrer, M., Srinivasan, M. V., Zhang, S. W., and Horridge, G. A. (1988). Motion cues provide the bee's visual world with a third dimension. *Nature* 332, 356–357.

Lewen, G. D., Bialek, W., and de Ruyter van Steveninck, R. (2001). Neural coding of naturalistic motion stimuli. *Network* 12, 317–329.

Liang, P., Heitwerth, J., Kern, R., Kurtz, R., and Egelhaaf, M. (2012). Object representation and distance encoding in three-dimensional environments by a neural circuit in the visual system of the blowfly. *J. Neurophysiol.* 107, 3446–3457.

Liang, P., Kern, R., and Egelhaaf, M. (2008). Motion adaptation enhances object-induced neural activity in three-dimensional virtual environment. *J. Neurosci.* 28, 1–6.

Liang, P., Kern, R., Kurtz, R., and Egelhaaf, M. (2011). Impact of visual motion adaptation on neural responses to objects and its dependence on the temporal characteristics of optic flow. *J. Neurophysiol.* 105, 1825–1834.

Lindemann, J. P., Kern, R., Michaelis, C., Meyer, P., van Hateren, J. H., and Egelhaaf, M. (2003). FliMax, a novel stimulus device for panoramic and highspeed presentation of behaviourally generated optic flow. *Vision Res.* 43, 779–791.

Lindemann, J. P., Kern, R., van Hateren, J. H., Ritter, H., and Egelhaaf, M. (2005). On the computations analysing natural optic flow: quantitative model analysis of the blowfly motion vision pathway. *J. Neurosci.* 25, 6435–6448.

Lindemann, J. P., Weiss, H., Möller, R., and Egelhaaf, M. (2008). Saccadic flight strategy facilitates collision avoidance: closed-loop performance of a cyberfly. *Biol. Cybern.* 98, 213–227.

Longden, K. D., and Krapp, H. G. (2009). State-dependent performance of optic-flow processing interneurons. *J. Neurophysiol.* 102, 3606–3618.

Longden, K. D., and Krapp, H. G. (2010). Octopaminergic modulation of temporal frequency coding in an identified optic flow-processing interneuron. *Front. Syst. Neurosci.* 4:153. doi: 10.3389/fnsys.2010.00153

Longuet-Higgins, H. C., and Prazdny, K. (1980). The interpretation of a moving retinal image. *Proc. R. Soc. Lond. B Biol. Sci.* 208, 385–397.

Maddess, T., and Laughlin, S. B. (1985). Adaptation of the motion-sensitive neuron H1 is generated locally and governed by contrast frequency. *Proc. R. Soc. Lond. B Biol. Sci.* 225, 251–275.

Maimon, G., Straw, A. D., and Dickinson, M. H. (2008). A simple vision-based algorithm for decision making in flying Drosophila. *Curr. Biol.* 18, 464–470.

Maimon, G., Straw, A. D., and Dickinson, M. H. (2010). Active flight increases the gain of visual motion processing in *Drosophila*. *Nat. Neurosci.* 13, 393–399.

Meyer, H. G., Lindemann, J. P., and Egelhaaf, M. (2011). Pattern-dependent response modulations in motion-sensitive visual interneurons – A model study. *PLoS ONE* 6:e21488. doi: 10.1371/journal.pone.0021488

Milde, J. J., Gronenberg, W., and Strausfeld, N. J. (1995). Oculomotor control in calliphorid flies: organization of descending neurons to neck motor neurons responding to visual stimuli. *J. Comp. Neurol.* 361, 267–284.

Milde, J. J., Seyan, H. S., and Strausfeld, N. J. (1987). The neck motor system of the fly, *Calliphora erythrocephala*. II. Sensory organization. *J. Comp. Physiol. A* 160, 225–238.

Mronz, M., and Lehmann, F.-O. (2008). The free-flight response of Drosophila to motion of the visual environment. *J. Exp. Biol.* 211, 2026–2045.

Necker, R. (2007). Head-bobbing of walking birds. *J. Comp. Physiol.*

A Neuroethol. Sens. Neural Behav. Physiol. 193, 1177–1183.

Nemenman, I., Lewen, G. D., Bialek, W., de Ruyter van Steveninck, R. R., and Friston, K. J. (2008). Neural coding of natural stimuli: information at sub-millisecond resolution. *PLoS Comput. Biol.* 4:e1000025. doi: 10.1371/journal.pcoi.1000025

Nordström, K. (2012). Neural specializations for small target detection in insects. *Curr. Opin. Neurobiol.* 22, 272–278.

Nordström, K., Barnett, P. D., and O'Carroll, D. C. (2006). Insect detection of small targets moving in visual clutter. *PLoS Biol.* 4:e54. doi: 10.1371/journal.pbio.0040054

Nordström, K., and O'Carroll, D. C. (2006). Small object detection neurons in female hoverflies. *Proc. Biol. Sci.* 273, 1211–1216.

O'Carroll, D. C., Barnett, P. D., and Nordström, K. (2011). Local and global responses of insect motion detectors to the spatial structure of natural scenes. *J. Vis.* 11, 1–17. Available online at: http://www.journalofvision.org/content/11/14/20

Ofstad, T. A., Zuker, C. S., and Reiser, M. B. (2011). Visual place learning in *Drosophila melanogaster*. *Nature* 474, 204–207.

Olberg, R. M. (1981). Object- and self-movement detectors in the ventral nerve cord of the dragonfly. *J. Comp. Physiol.* 141, 327–334.

Olberg, R. M. (1986). Identified target-selective visual interneurons descending from the dragonfly brain. *J. Comp. Physiol.* 159, 827–840.

Olberg, R. M., Worthington, A. H., Fox, J. L., Bessette, C. E., and Loosemore, M. P. (2005). Prey size selection and distance estimation in foraging adult dragonflies. *J. Comp. Physiol. A Neuroethol. Sens. Neural Behav. Physiol.* 191, 791–797.

Pelli, D. G. (1991). "Noise in the visual system may be early," in *Computational Models of Visual Processing*, eds M. S. Landy and J. A. Movshon (Cambridge, MA: MIT-Press), 147–151.

Petrowitz, R., Dahmen, H. J., Egelhaaf, M., and Krapp, H. G. (2000). Arrangement of optical axes and the spatial resolution in the compound eye of the female blowfly *Calliphora*. *J. Comp. Physiol. A* 186, 737–746.

Pfaff, M., and Varjú, D. (1991). Mechanisms of visual distance perception in the hawk moth *Macroglossum stellatarum*. *Zool. Jahrb. Physiol.* 95, 315–321.

Portelli, G., Ruffier, F., Roubieu, F. L., Franceschini, N., and Krapp,

H. G. (2011). Honeybees' speed depends on dorsal as well as lateral, ventral and frontal optic flows. *PLoS ONE* 6:e19486. doi: 10.1371/journal.pone.0019486

Poteser, M., and Kral, K. (1995). Visual distance discrimination between stationary targets in praying mantis: an index of the use of motion parallax. *J. Exp. Biol.* 198, 2127–2137.

Prazdny, K. (1980). Ego-motion and relative depth map from optical-flow. *Biol. Cybern.* 36, 87–102.

Redlick, F. P., Jenkin, M., and Harris, L. R. (2001). Humans can use optic flow to estimate distance of travel. *Vision Res.* 41, 213–219.

Reichardt, W. (1961). "Autocorrelation, a principle for the evaluation of sensory information by the central nervous system," in *Sensory Communication*, ed W. A. Rosenblith (New York, London: MIT Press and John Wiley and Sons), 303–317.

Reichardt, W., and Poggio, T. (1979). Figure-ground discrimination by relative movement in the visual system of the fly. Part I: experimental results. *Biol. Cybern.* 35, 81–100.

Reichardt, W., Poggio, T., and Hausen, K. (1983). Figure-ground discrimination by relative movement in the visual system of the fly. Part II: towards the neural circuitry. *Biol. Cybern.* 46, 1–30.

Reiff, D. F., Plett, J., Mank, M., Griesbeck, O., and Borst, A. (2010). Visualizing retinotopic half-wave rectified input to the motion detection circuitry of Drosophila. *Nat. Neurosci.* 13, 973–978.

Reiser, M. B., and Dickinson, M. H. (2010). Drosophila fly straight by fixating objects in the face of expanding optic flow. *J. Exp. Biol.* 213, 1771–1781.

Rien, D., Kern, R., and Kurtz, R. (2012). Octopaminergic modulation of contrast gain adaptation in fly visual motion-sensitive neurons. *Eur. J. Neurosci.* 36, 3030–3039.

Rister, J., Pauls, D., Schnell, B., Ting, C. Y., Lee, C. H., Sinakevitch, I., et al. (2007). Dissection of the peripheral motion channel in the visual system of *Drosophila melanogaster*. *Neuron* 56, 155–170.

Ristroph, L., Berman, G. J., Bergou, A. J., Wang, Z. J., and Cohen, I. (2009). Automated hull reconstruction motion tracking (HRMT) applied to sideways maneuvers of free flying insects. *J. Exp. Biol.* 212, 1324–1335.

Rogers, B. J. (1993). "Motion parallax and other dynamic cues for depth vision," in *Visual motion and its role in the stabilization of gaze*, eds F. A. Miles and J. Wallman (Amsterdam: Elsevier), 119–137.

Rosner, R., Egelhaaf, M., Grewe, J., and Warzecha, A.-K. (2009). Variability of blowfly head optomotor responses. *J. Exp. Biol.* 212, 1170–1184.

Rosner, R., Egelhaaf, M., and Warzecha, A.-K. (2010). Behavioural state affects motion-sensitive neurones in the fly visual system. *J. Exp. Biol.* 213, 331–338.

Sandeman, D. C., and Markl, H. (1980). Head movements in the flies (*Calliphora*) produced by deflexion of the halteres. *J. Exp. Biol.* 85, 43–60.

Schilstra, C., and van Hateren, J. H. (1999). Blowfly flight and optic flow. I. Thorax kinematics and flight dynamics. *J. Exp. Biol.* 202, 1481–1490.

Schnell, B., Raghu, S. V., Nern, A., and Borst, A. (2012). Columnar cells necessary for motion responses of wide-field visual interneurons in *Drosophila*. *J. Comp. Physiol. A Neuroethol. Sens. Neural Behav. Physiol.* 198, 389–395.

Schuster, S., Strauss, R., and Götz, K. G. (2002). Virtual-reality techniques resolve the visual cues used by fruit flies to evaluate object distances. *Curr. Biol.* 12, 1591–1594.

Seidl, R., and Kaiser, W. (1981). Visual field size, binocular domain and the ommatidial array of the compound eyes in worker honey bees. *J. Comp. Physiol.* 143, 17–26.

Sherman, A. (2003). A comparison of visual and haltere-mediated equilibrium reflexes in the fruit fly *Drosophila melanogaster*. *J. Exp. Biol.* 206, 295–302.

Sherman, A., and Dickinson, M. H. (2003). A comparison of visual and haltere-mediated equilibrium reflexes in the fruit fly *Drosophila melanogaster*. *J. Exp. Biol.* 206, 295–302.

Sherman, A., and Dickinson, M. H. (2004). Summation of visual and mechanosensory feedback in Drosophila flight control. *J. Exp. Biol.* 207, 133–142.

Simoncelli, E. P., and Olshausen, B. A. (2001). Natural image statistics and neural representation. *Annu. Rev. Neurosci.* 24, 1193–1225.

Single, S., and Borst, A. (1998). Dendritic integration and its role in computing image velocity. *Science* 281, 1848–1850.

Single, S., Haag, J., and Borst, A. (1997). Dendritic computation of direction selectivity and gain control in visual interneurons. *J. Neurosci.* 17, 6023–6030.

Sobel, E. C. (1990). The locust's use of motion parallax to measure distance. *J. Comp. Physiol. A* 167, 579–588.

Srinivasan, M., Lehrer, M., and Wehner, R. (1987). Bees perceive illusory colours induced by movement. *Vision Res.* 27, 1285–1289.

Srinivasan, M. V., Lehrer, M., and Horridge, G. A. (1990). Visual figure-ground discrimination in the honeybee: the role of motion parallax at boundaries. *Proc. R. Soc. Lond. B* 238, 331–350.

Srinivasan, M. V., Lehrer, M., Kirchner, W. H., and Zhang, S. W. (1991). Range perception through apparent image speed in freely flying honeybees. *Vis. Neurosci.* 6, 519–535.

Srinivasan, M. V., Zhang, S., Altwein, M., and Tautz, J. (2000). Honeybee navigation: nature and calibration of the "odometer". *Science* 287, 851–853.

Srinivasan, M. V., Zhang, S. W., Lehrer, M., and Collett, T. S. (1996). Honeybee navigation en route to the goal: visual flight control and odometry. *J. Exp. Biol.* 199, 237–244.

Strausfeld, N. J., Douglass, J. K., Campbell, H. R., and Higgins, C. M. (2006). "Parallel processing in the optic lobes of flies and the occurrence of motion computing circuits," in *Invertebrate Vision*, eds E. Warrant and D.-E. Nilsson (Cambridge, UK: Cambridge University Press), 349–398.

Straw, A. D., Lee, S., and Dickinson, M. H. (2010). Visual control of altitude in flying drosophila. *Curr. Biol.* 20, 1550–1556.

Straw, A. D., Rainsford, T., and O'Carroll, D. C. (2008). Contrast sensitivity of insect motion detectors to natural images. *J. Vis.* 8, 1–9. Available online at: http://journalofvision.org/8/3/32/

Stürzl, W., and Zeil, J. (2007). Depth, contrast and view-based homing in outdoor scenes. *Biol. Cybern.* 96, 519–531.

Tammero, L. F., and Dickinson, M. H. (2002a). Collision-avoidance and landing responses are mediated by separate pathways in the fruit fly, *Drosophila melanogaster*. *J. Exp. Biol.* 205, 2785–2798.

Tammero, L. F., and Dickinson, M. H. (2002b). The influence of visual landscape on the free flight behavior of the fruit fly *Drosophila melanogaster*. *J. Exp. Biol.* 205, 327–343.

Tammero, L. F., Frye, M. A., and Dickinson, M. H. (2004). Spatial organization of visuomotor reflexes in Drosophila. *J. Exp. Biol.* 207, 113–122.

Taylor, G. K., and Krapp, H. G. (2008). "Sensory systems and flight stability: what do insects measure and why?" in *Advances in Insect Physiology* (Amsterdam: Elsevier), 231–316.

Trischler, C., Boeddeker, N., and Egelhaaf, M. (2007). Characterisation of a blowfly male-specific neuron using behaviourally generated visual stimuli. *J. Comp. Physiol. A Neuroethol. Sens. Neural. Behav. Physiol.* 193, 559–572.

Trischler, C., Kern, R., and Egelhaaf, M. (2010). Chasing behavior and optomotor following in free-flying male blowflies: flight performance and interactions of the underlying control systems. *Front. Behav. Neurosci.* 4:20. doi: 10.3389/fnbeh.2010.00020

Vaina, L. M., Beardsley, S. A., and Rushton, S. K. (2004). *Optic Flow and Beyond*. Dordrecht, Boston, London: Kluwer Academic Publishers.

van Breugel, F., and Dickinson, M. H. (2012). The visual control of landing and obstacle avoidance in the fruit fly *Drosophila melanogaster*. *J. Exp. Biol.* 215, 1783–1798.

van Hateren, J. H. (1992). Theoretical predictions of spatiotemporal receptive fields of fly LMCs, and experimental validation. *J. Comp. Physiol. A* 171, 157–170.

van Hateren, J. H. (1993). Three modes of spatiotemporal preprocessing by eyes. *J. Comp. Physiol. A* 172, 583–591.

van Hateren, J. H. (1997). Processing of natural time series of intensities by the visual system of the blowfly. *Vision Res.* 37, 3407–3416.

van Hateren, J. H., Kern, R., Schwerdtfeger, G., and Egelhaaf, M. (2005). Function and coding in the blowfly H1 neuron during naturalistic optic flow. *J. Neurosci.* 25, 4343–4352.

van Hateren, J. H., and Schilstra, C. (1999). Blowfly flight and optic flow. II. Head movements during flight. *J. Exp. Biol.* 202, 1491–1500.

Verspui, R., and Gray, J. R. (2009). Visual stimuli induced by self-motion and object-motion modify odour-guided flight of male moths (*Manduca sexta* L.). *Exp. Biol.* 212, 3272–3282.

Virsik, R., and Reichardt, W. (1976). Detection and tracking of moving objects by the fly *Musca domestica*. *Biol. Cybern.* 23, 83–98.

Wagner, H. (1982). Flow-field variables trigger landing in flies. *Nature* 297, 147–148.

Warzecha, A.-K., and Egelhaaf, M. (1996). Intrinsic properties of biological motion detectors prevent the optomotor control system from getting unstable. *Philos. Trans. R. Soc. B* 351, 1579–1591.

Warzecha, A.-K., and Egelhaaf, M. (1997). How reliably does a neuron in the visual motion pathway of the fly encode behaviourally relevant information? *Eur. J. Neurosci.* 9, 1365–1374.

Warzecha, A.-K., and Egelhaaf, M. (1999). Variability in spike trains during constant and dynamic stimulation. *Science* 283, 1927–1930.

Warzecha, A.-K., and Egelhaaf, M. (2001). "Neuronal encoding of visual motion in real-time," in *Processing Visual Motion in the Real World: A Survey of Computational, Neural, and Ecological Constraints*, eds J. M. Zanker and J. Zeil (Berlin, Heidelberg, New York: Springer), 239–277.

Warzecha, A.-K., Egelhaaf, M., and Borst, A. (1993). Neural circuit tuning fly visual interneurons to motion of small objects. I. Dissection of the circuit by pharmacological and photoinactivation techniques. *J. Neurophysiol.* 69, 329–339.

Warzecha, A.-K., Horstmann, W., and Egelhaaf, M. (1999). Temperature dependence of neuronal performance in the motion pathway of the blowfly *Calliphora erythrocephala*. *J. Exp. Biol.* 202, 3161–3170.

Warzecha, A.-K., Kretzberg, J., and Egelhaaf, M. (1998). Temporal precision of the encoding of motion information by visual interneurons. *Curr. Biol.* 8, 359–368.

Warzecha, A.-K., Kretzberg, J., and Egelhaaf, M. (2000). Reliability of a fly motion-sensitive neuron depends on stimulus parameters. *J. Neurosci.* 20, 8886–8896.

Warzecha, A.-K., Kurtz, R., and Egelhaaf, M. (2003). Synaptic transfer of dynamical motion information between identified neurons in the visual system of the blowfly. *Neuroscience* 119, 1103–1112.

Wolf, H. (2011). Odometry and insect navigation. *J. Exp. Biol.* 214, 1629–1641.

Zeil, J. (1986). The territorial flight of male houseflies (*Fannia canicularis*). *Behav. Ecol. Sociobiol.* 19, 213–219.

Zeil, J. (2012). Visual homing: an insect perspective. *Curr. Opin. Neurobiol.* 22, 285–293.

Zeil, J., Boeddeker, N., and Stürzl, W. (2009). "Visual homing in insects and robots," in *Flying Insects and Robots*, eds D. Floreano, J. C. Zufferey, M. V. Srinivasan, and C. P. Ellington (Heidelberg, Dordtrecht, London, New York: Springer), 87–99.

5

Neural control and adaptive neural forward models for insect-like, energy-efficient, and adaptable locomotion of walking machines

Poramate Manoonpong[1]***, Ulrich Parlitz**[2,3] **and Florentin Wörgötter**[1]

[1] *Bernstein Center for Computational Neuroscience, The Third Institute of Physics, Georg-August-Universität Göttingen, Göttingen, Germany*
[2] *Max Planck Research Group Biomedical Physics, Max Planck Institute for Dynamics and Self-Organization, Göttingen, Germany*
[3] *Institute for Nonlinear Dynamics, Georg-August-Universität Göttingen, Göttingen, Germany*

Edited by:
Ahmed El Hady, Max Planck Institute for Dynamics and Self Organization, Germany

Reviewed by:
Ralf Der, Max Planck Institute for Mathematics, Germany
Georg Martius, Max Planck Institute for Mathematics in the Sciences, Germany
William Lewinger, University of Surrey, UK

*Correspondence:
Poramate Manoonpong, Bernstein Center for Computational Neuroscience, III Physikalisches Institut - Biophysik, Georg-August-Universität Göttingen, Friedrich-Hund Platz 1, D-37077 Göttingen, Germany.
e-mail: poramate@physik3.gwdg.de; poramate@manoonpong.com

Living creatures, like walking animals, have found fascinating solutions for the problem of locomotion control. Their movements show the impression of elegance including versatile, energy-efficient, and adaptable locomotion. During the last few decades, roboticists have tried to imitate such natural properties with artificial legged locomotion systems by using different approaches including machine learning algorithms, classical engineering control techniques, and biologically-inspired control mechanisms. However, their levels of performance are still far from the natural ones. By contrast, animal locomotion mechanisms seem to largely depend not only on central mechanisms (central pattern generators, CPGs) and sensory feedback (afferent-based control) but also on internal forward models (efference copies). They are used to a different degree in different animals. Generally, CPGs organize basic rhythmic motions which are shaped by sensory feedback while internal models are used for sensory prediction and state estimations. According to this concept, we present here adaptive neural locomotion control consisting of a CPG mechanism with neuromodulation and local leg control mechanisms based on sensory feedback and adaptive neural forward models with efference copies. This neural closed-loop controller enables a walking machine to perform a multitude of different walking patterns including insect-like leg movements and gaits as well as energy-efficient locomotion. In addition, the forward models allow the machine to autonomously adapt its locomotion to deal with a change of terrain, losing of ground contact during stance phase, stepping on or hitting an obstacle during swing phase, leg damage, and even to promote cockroach-like climbing behavior. Thus, the results presented here show that the employed embodied neural closed-loop system can be a powerful way for developing robust and adaptable machines.

Keywords: efference copy, central pattern generators, sensory feedback, recurrent neural networks, local leg control, walking gait, autonomous robots

1. INTRODUCTION

Walking animals, like locusts, stick insects, and cockroaches, can traverse diverse terrains in an energy-efficient way. During traversing, their locomotion can also adapt to deal with terrain changes. Furthermore, their movements are elegant and versatile. These capabilities are the result of the coupling of biomechanics (Dickinson et al., 2000) and neural control. For instance, the appropriate biomechanical structures of body and legs of a cockroach (Ritzmann et al., 2004) allows it to walk naturally, deal with minor disturbances during traversing rough terrain, and even climb over relatively high obstacles as compared to its size. While biomechanics allows for such capabilities, neural control, on the other hand, combines information from different sensor modalities and provides coordinated outputs to many motor joints (Büschges, 2005; Grillner, 2006; Cruse et al., 2009; Mulloney and Smarandache, 2010; Fuchs et al., 2011). This process is fast and adaptive which leads to the generation of locomotion and adaptation.

During the last few decades, roboticists have tried to imitate such natural properties with artificial legged locomotion systems. Several of them have paid attention on the biomechanical design of such systems to have animal-like properties (Cham et al., 2002; Iida and Pfeifer, 2004; Lewinger et al., 2005; Kingsley et al., 2006; Schneider et al., 2012). Others have focused on sensorimotor coordination and control for locomotion and adaptation by using different approaches including machine learning algorithms (Lee et al., 2006; Erden and Leblebicioglu, 2008), classical engineering control techniques (Brooks, 1986; Shkolnik and Tedrake, 2007), and biologically inspired control mechanisms (Beer et al., 1997; Kuo, 2002; Lewis and Bekey, 2002; Dürr et al., 2003; Ekeberg et al., 2004; Cruse et al., 2007; Kimura et al., 2007; Spenneberg and Kirchner, 2007; Amrollah and Henaff, 2010; Daun-Gruhn and Büschges, 2011; Harischandra et al., 2011; Lewinger and Quinn, 2011; von Twickel et al., 2012). With increasing machine complexity, integrating more behaviors, and obtaining adaptability, the control problems become more challenging.

Artificial neural networks (ANNs) appear appropriate for such control problems due to their intrinsically distributed architecture, their capability to integrate new behaviors, as well as synaptic learning (Beer et al., 1997; Dürr et al., 2003; Ekeberg et al., 2004; Cruse et al., 2007; Kimura et al., 2007; Amrollah and Henaff, 2010; Daun-Gruhn and Büschges, 2011; Lewinger and Quinn, 2011; Harischandra et al., 2011; von Twickel et al., 2012). In addition they have a number of excellent properties as follows. They are able to build a controller as a composition of different neural modules to produce desired motor behaviors (von Twickel et al., 2012). And, they are conceptually close to biological systems compared to other solutions. In particular recurrent neural networks (RNNs) exhibit dynamical behavior (oscillatory, hysteresis, chaotic patterns, etc.) for generating basic rhythmic locomotion behavior (Beer et al., 1997; Kimura et al., 2007; Amrollah and Henaff, 2010; Daun-Gruhn and Büschges, 2011; von Twickel et al., 2012). Considering this, here we exploit the features of ANNs to develop locomotion control for walking machines. This is based on a modular structure consisting of different neural modules having main functions that follow three key mechanisms found in animal locomotion (Holst and Mittelstaedt, 1950; Meyrand et al., 1991; Cruse et al., 1998; Katz, 1998; Bläsing and Cruse, 2004; Cruse et al., 2009; Harris-Warrick, 2011): (1) central mechanisms [i.e., central pattern generators (CPGs)] for generating basic rhythmic motions, (2) sensory feedback (i.e., afferent-based control) for shaping the motions, and (3) internal forward models (i.e., efferent-based control) for sensory prediction and walking state estimations. While these three key mechanisms are essential for locomotion control as found in biological legged systems, only individual instances of them had been successfully applied to artificial ones (Beer et al., 1997; Ishiguro et al., 2003; Cruse et al., 2007; Kimura et al., 2007; Spenneberg and Kirchner, 2007; Amrollah and Henaff, 2010; Schroeder-Schetelig et al., 2010; Harischandra et al., 2011; Lewinger and Quinn, 2011; Owaki et al., 2012; von Twickel et al., 2012), thereby providing partial solutions. A few studies have applied all these mechanisms to animal-like legged robots to achieve complex behavior and adaptability (Lewis and Bekey, 2002). However, the mechanisms have been often used for active two-legged walking (Lewis and Simo, 2001).

Taking all these mechanisms into account for the design of our adaptive neural locomotion control leads to robust walking behavior in many situations. Furthermore, the controller can generate a multitude of walking patterns (e.g., 20 patterns), insect-like leg movements, and energy-efficient and adaptable locomotion for a biomechanical six-legged walking machine, like the AMOS II[1] robot used here. It also allows AMOS II to cope with leg damage and even promote cockroach-like climbing behavior. Besides the complex behavior generation, the rationales behind this study are also: (1) to give a better understanding of how a CPG mechanism with neuromodulation, sensory feedback, and adaptive internal forward models with efference copies can be combined in artificial legged locomotion systems and (2) to emphasize that the generated behaviors require the coupling of biomechanics (i.e., physical structure) and neural mechanisms

with sensory feedback embedded in an embodied neural-closed loop system. The work presented here extends our previous works (Manoonpong et al., 2007, 2008b; Steingrube et al., 2010) by modifying a chaotic CPG (Steingrube et al., 2010) into a CPG with neuromodulaiton leading to more gaits and smoother and faster switching between them compared with the chaotic CPG. It also introduces for the first time local leg feedback and adaptive forward models as well as their combination with the CPG in robust walking behaviors.

The following section describes the technical specification of the six-legged walking machine AMOS II used for the experiments, followed by adaptive neural locomotion control. The controller is developed to generate versatile and adaptable locomotion of walking machines. The experimental results are shown in section 3. Discussion is given in section 4.

2. MATERIALS AND METHODS

All the experiments of this work were carried out with the physical six-legged walking machine AMOS II. Thus, the first section describes its biomechanical setup, followed by details of the adaptive neural locomotion controller and its components which are the main contribution of this work. Here, some results are described alongside the introduced components from which they mainly derive because this provides a better understanding of their functionalities.

2.1. THE WALKING MACHINE PLATFORM AMOS II (BIOMECHANICS)

In order to explore and test the performance of the proposed adaptive neural locomotion control in a physical system, the six-legged walking machine AMOS II is employed (**Figure 1A**). It is an improved version of our previous six-legged walking machine AMOS (Steingrube et al., 2010).

AMOS II has six identical legs. Each leg has three joints (**Figure 1B**): the thoraco-coxal (TC-) joint enables forward (+) and backward (−) movements, the coxa-trochanteral (CTr-) joint enables elevation (+) and depression (−) of the leg, and the femur-tibia (FTi-) joint enables extension (+) and flexion (−) of the tibia (**Figures 1C,D**). The morphology of these multi-jointed legs is modeled on the basis of a cockroach leg (Zill et al., 2004) but the tarsus segments are ignored. Each tibia contains a spring compliant element to substitute part of the function of the tarsus; i.e., absorbing the impact force during touchdown on the ground. In addition, a passive coupling is installed at each joint (**Figure 1B**) in order to yield passive compliance and to protect the motor shaft. The maximum and minimum ranges of the joint movements of the legs are shown in **Figures 1C,D**. In a normal walking condition (e.g., walking on flat terrain), we set the default joint movements so that its body is very close to the ground (i.e., low center of mass) and its body falls to the ground before taking the next step during normal walking. However, for walking over rough terrains, these ranges will be automatically shifted such that AMOS II lifts its body up for better locomotion. This walking strategy is inspired by insect walking, like that of a cockroach (Alexander, 1982; Ritzmann et al., 2004, 2012) and it also ensures stability when confronting leg damage.

The body of AMOS II consists of two segments: a front segment where two front legs are installed and a central body

---

[1] Advanced MObility Sensor-driven walking device II.

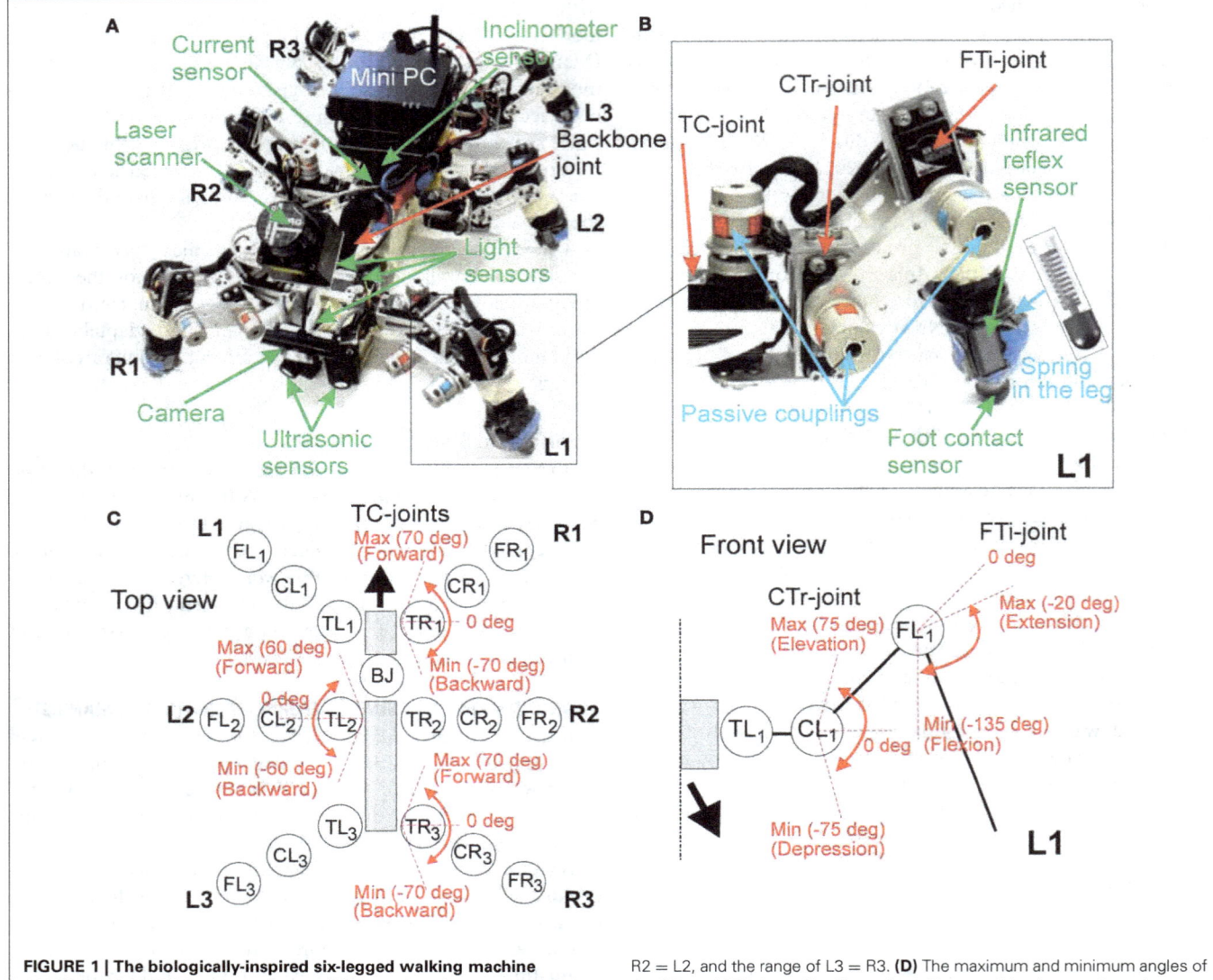

FIGURE 1 | The biologically-inspired six-legged walking machine AMOS II. **(A)** AMOS II with its sensors. **(B)** Examples of components at the left front leg (L1). **(C)** The location of all motor joints on AMOS II and the maximum and minimum angles of the TC-joints of the right front (R1), left middle (L2), and right hind (R3) legs (top view). The remaining legs on the opposite side have the same ranges; i.e., the range of L1 = R1, the range of R2 = L2, and the range of L3 = R3. **(D)** The maximum and minimum angles of the CTr- and FTi-joints of L1 (front view). The remaining legs perform the same joint angle ranges. Abbreviations are: TR1, CR1, FR1 = TC-, CTr-, and FTi-joints of the right front leg (R1); TR2, CR2, FR2 = right middle leg (R2); TR3, CR3, FR3 = right hind leg (R3); TL1, CL1, FL1 = left front leg (L1); TL2, CL2, FL2 = left middle leg (L2); TL3, CL3, FL3 = left hind leg (L3); BJ = a backbone joint.

segment where the two middle and the two hind legs are attached. They are connected by one active backbone joint (BJ) inspired by the invertebrate morphology of the American cockroach's trunk (**Figure A1**). This BJ can rotate around the lateral or transverse axis in a range between −45° (minimum downward position) and +45° (maximum upward position). It stays at zero degree during walking and it leans upwards and bends downwards while climbing. In total, AMOS II has 19 active joints (three at each leg, one BJ). They are driven by digital servomotors (HSR-5990 TG) delivering a stall torque of 2.9 Nm at 5 V. In addition, the body joint torque is tripled by using a gear to achieve a more powerful body joint motion. Besides the motors, AMOS II has 21 sensors: two ultrasonic sensors (US) at the front body part, six foot contact (FC) sensors in its legs, six infrared reflex (IR) sensors at the front

of its legs, one current sensor (CS) and one inclinometer (IM) sensor inside the body, and three light dependent (LD) sensors, one USB camera (CM) and one laser scanner (LS) on the front body part (**Figure 1**). These sensors are used to generate stimulus induced behavior (like, photo tropism and obstacle avoidance) as well as versatile, energy-efficient, and adaptable locomotion. The USB camera is used for terrain classification and the LS is used to measure obstacle height in order to distinguish between a wall and a surmountable obstacle.

We use a Multi-Servo IO Board (MBoard) installed inside the body to digitize all sensory input signals except the CM and LS signals. We also use it to generate a pulse-width-modulated signal to control the position of the servomotor. For experiments here, the MBoard is connected to a personal computer (PC) where the

CM and LS are directly connected and a neural locomotion controller is implemented. The communication between a PC and the MBoard is accomplished via an RS232 interface at 57.6 kb/s. Electrical power supply for all servomotors, the MBoard, and all sensors is given by lithium polymer batteries with a voltage regulator producing a stable 5 V supply.

2.2. ADAPTIVE NEURAL LOCOMOTION CONTROL

The adaptive neural locomotion control (**Figure 2**) has been developed based on a modular structure. It consists of two main components: CPG-based control and local leg control. The CPG-based control basically coordinates all leg joints of AMOS II, thereby generating insect-like leg movements and a multitude of different behavioral patterns. The patterns include forward/backward walking, turning left and right, and insect-like gaits. These gaits allow for energy-efficient locomotion on different terrains. All these patterns can be autonomously controlled by exteroceptive sensors, like a camera, a LS, and US. While the CPG-based control provides versatile autonomous behaviors, the local leg control using proprioceptive sensory feedback (like FC sensors) adapts the movement of an individual leg of AMOS II

to deal with a change of terrain, losing of ground contact during stance phase, or stepping on or hitting an obstacle during swing phase.

Here, the CPG-based control of the entire system has four components: (1) a CPG mechanism with neuromodulation for generating different periodic signals, (2) neural CPG postprocessing for shaping the CPG signals to obtain smooth leg movements, (3) neural motor control consisting of two additional different networks [phase switching network (PSN) and velocity regulating networks (VRNs)] for controlling walking direction (forward/backward and turning), and (4) motor neurons with delay lines for sending final motor commands to all leg joints of AMOS II.

For the local leg control, it has only two components for each leg: (1) an adaptive neural forward model transforming the motor signal (efference copy) generated by the CPG into an expected sensory signal for estimating the walking state and (2) elevation and searching control for adapting leg motion (e.g., extension/flexion and elevation/depression).

All neurons of the control network (**Figures 2, A2**) are modeled as discrete-time non-spiking neurons. They are updated

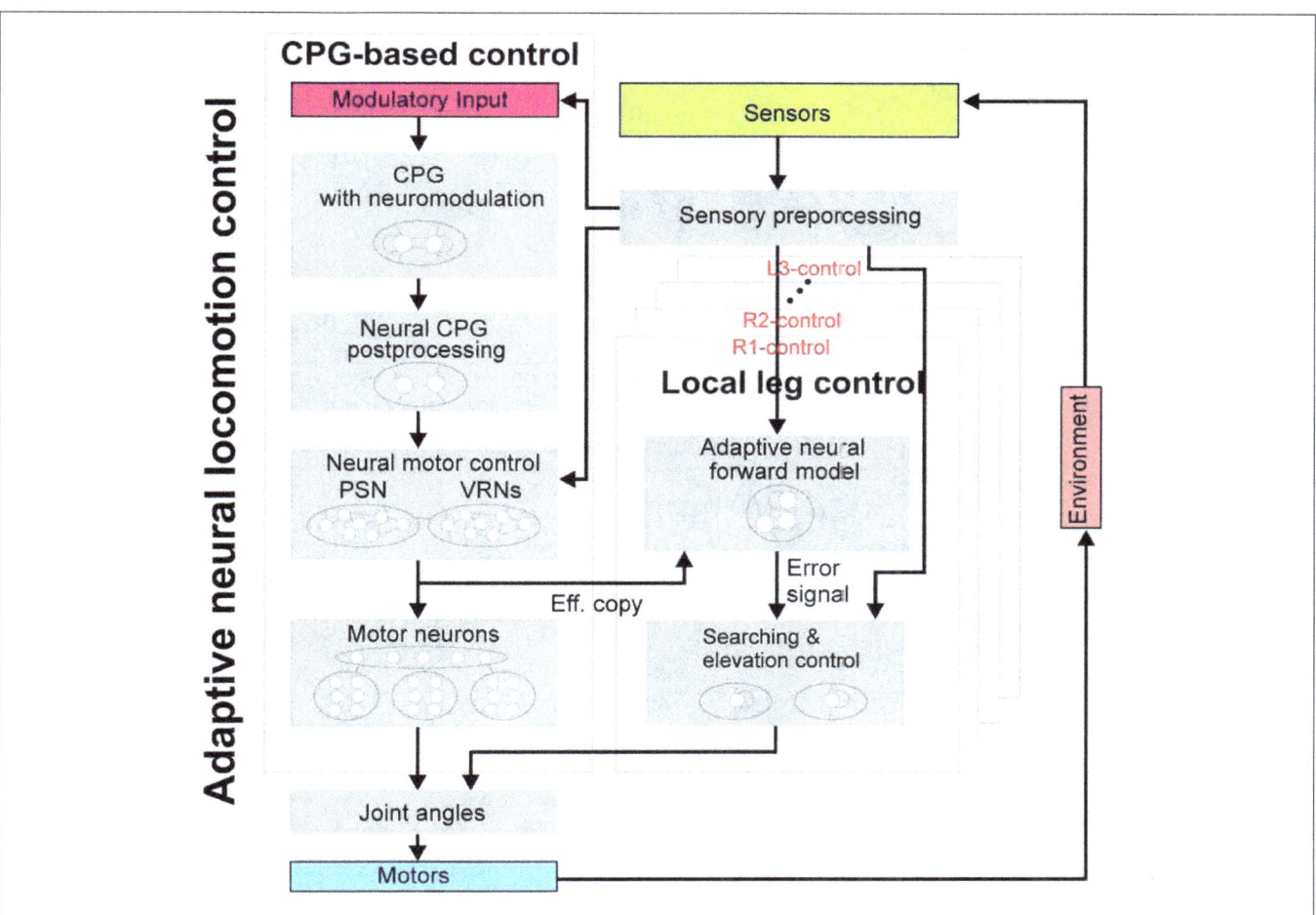

FIGURE 2 | Adaptive neural locomotion control. The controller generates insect-like, energy-efficient, and adaptable locomotion of AMOS II. This adaptive neural closed-loop controller consists of one CPG-based control unit and six local leg control units (R1-, R2-, R3-, L1-, L2-, and L3-control) (see text for functional description and **Figure A2** for the complete circuit). Abbreviations are referred to **Figure 1**.

with a frequency of approximately 27 Hz. The activity a_i of each neuron develops according to:

$$a_i(t) = \sum_{j=1}^{n} W_{ij} o_j(t-1) + B_i, \quad i = 1, \ldots, n, \qquad (1)$$

where n denotes the number of units, B_i an internal bias term or a stationary input to neuron i, W_{ij} the synaptic strength of the connection from neuron j to neuron i. The output o_i of all neurons of the network is calculated by using the hyperbolic tangent (tanh) transfer function, i.e., $o_i = \tanh(a_i), \in [-1, 1]$, except for the CPG postprocessing neurons using a step function, the motor neurons using piecewise linear transfer functions, and neurons in searching and elevation control using a linear transfer function.

2.3. CPG-BASED CONTROL

The structure of this control unit is based on our previous sensor-driven CPG-based controller (Steingrube et al., 2010) in which a chaotic CPG is used as a main component. While the chaotic CPG can produce different periodic output signals including a

chaotic one, only a few number of gaits (e.g., five different gaits) and a chaotic motion have been realized for hexapod locomotion (Steingrube et al., 2010). Furthermore, switching between these gaits cannot be immediately achieved but requires a few steps and the transition is non-smooth. This is because the system has to switch to a chaotic state first before obtaining a new periodic pattern.

Thus to overcome this drawback, in this study we modify the chaotic CPG to a simpler CPG mechanism with neuromodulation. It is inspired by biological findings (Meyrand et al., 1991; Katz, 1998; Harris-Warrick, 2011) (see the section 4 for more details). It provides a large number of periodic output patterns including a chaotic one, resulting in a large number of walking patterns (i.e., more than five stable gaits). It also allows fast and smooth switching between patterns. The circuit consists of two neurons $i \in \{1, 2\}$, fully connected (**Figure 3A**). The discrete-time dynamics of the activity states a_i and the output states o_i of the circuit follows Equation (1) and a tanh transfer function, respectively. Their initial states are set to a small positive value, e.g., 0.1. An extrinsic modulatory input MI is introduced and projected to the synaptic connections of the neurons (**Figure 3A**), thereby

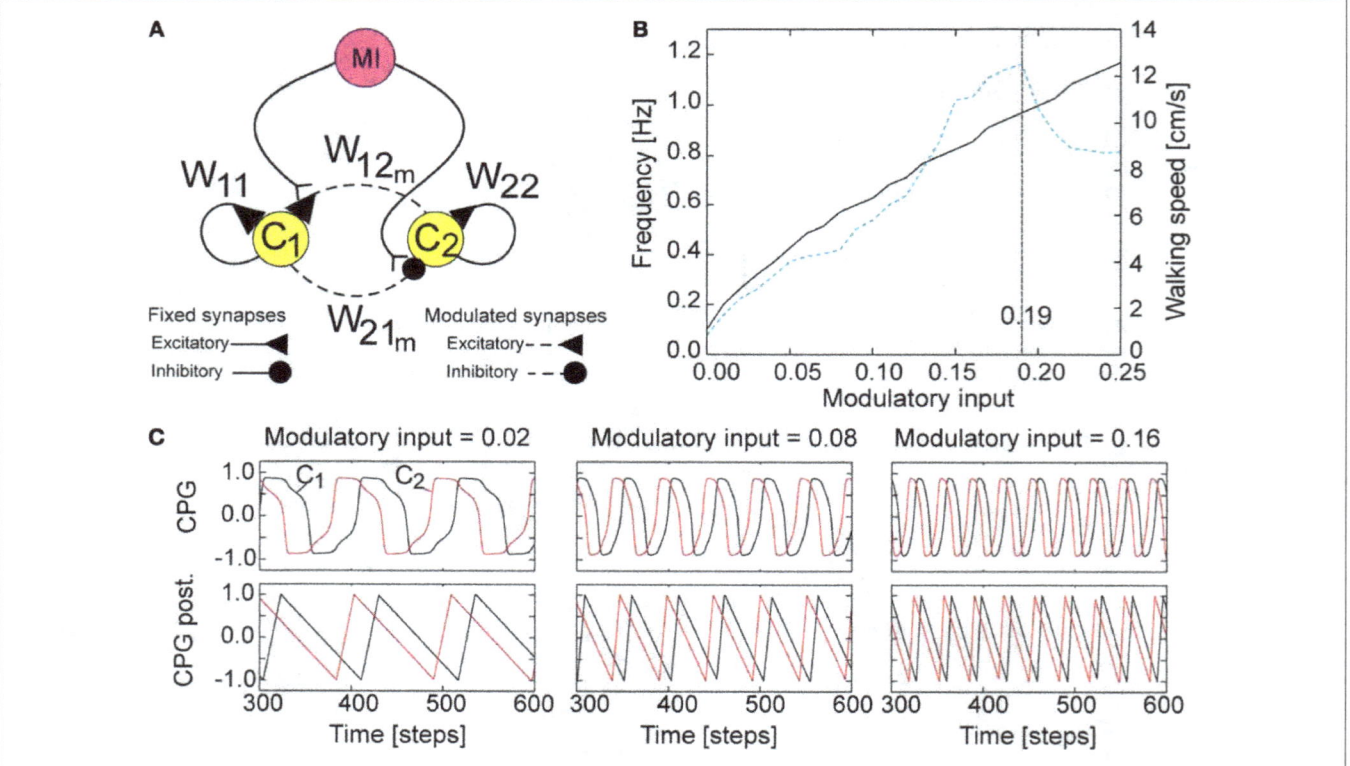

FIGURE 3 | CPG mechanism with neuromodulation. (A) Wiring diagram of the CPG circuit. The extrinsic modulatory input MI alters the synaptic weights of the CPG, thereby modulating the CPG outputs. The synaptic weights are set as $W_{11,22} = 1.4$, $W_{12_m} = 0.18 + MI$, $W_{21_m} = -0.18 - MI$. **(B)** The resulting eigenfrequency of the outputs of the CPG (black solid line, left scale) and the walking speed of AMOS II (blue dashed line, right scale) with respect to MI. Here MI is increased by 0.01. If MI is smaller than 0.0 the network dynamics exhibits only fixed point attractors; i.e., oscillations are switched off. Recall that the

CPG network is updated with a frequency of approximately 27 Hz (i.e., one time step is ≈ 0.037 s). **(C)** Examples of the asymmetrical periodic outputs of the CPG (top) where MI is set to 0.02, 0.08, and 0.16. The signals differ in phase by $\pi/2$ and are shaped by neural CPG postprocessing such that smooth ascending and descending signals are obtained for motor control (bottom). This kind of asymmetrical periodic signals is appropriate for walking found in insects where swing (ascending slope) and stance (descending slope) phases differ in duration, being intrinsically asymmetry (Wilson, 1966).

modulating the outputs of the CPG (**Figures 3B,C**). *MI* will be controlled by a sensory signal (see the section 3). According to this, the synaptic weights are described as:

$$W_{11,22} = W_{d0}, \tag{2}$$

$$W_{12_m} = W_{d1} + MI, \tag{3}$$

$$W_{21_m} = -(W_{d1} + MI), \tag{4}$$

where $W_{11,22}$ are fixed synapses and $W_{12_m,21_m}$ are modulated synapses. W_{d0} and W_{d1} are the default synaptic weights, which are used to create basic periodic signals. They need to be selected in accordance with the dynamics of the system that generates periodic or quasi-periodic attractors (Pasemann et al., 2003).

We empirically adjust and set the parameters to $W_{d0} = 1.4$ and $W_{d1} = 0.18$. This parameter setup with $MI = 0.0$ results in a very low frequency of the periodic outputs. Increasing MI will increase the frequency of the outputs (see black solid line in **Figure 3B**). The investigation of AMOS II walking on a flat floor using this CPG shows that its walking speed is proportional to the value of MI; i.e., increasing MI leads to the increasing of walking speed (see blue dashed line in **Figure 3B**). However, the walking speed will decrease if MI is grater than 0.19. This is because the output frequency is too high such that the motors of AMOS II cannot

follow the driving frequency properly[2]. Interestingly, together with neural motor control and a delay line mechanism embedded in the motor neuron module (described below), AMOS II shows different walking patterns at the different values of *MI* (e.g., 20 patterns) where some of these patterns show similar gaits but differ in stepping frequency in the swing and stance phases. **Figure 4** shows examples of six different patterns or gaits: slow wave gait ($MI = 0.02$), fast wave gait ($MI = 0.04$), tetrapod gait ($MI = 0.06$), caterpillar gait ($MI = 0.09$), intermixed gait ($MI = 0.12$), and fast tripod gait ($MI = 0.19$). Some of them are similar to insect gaits (Wilson, 1966) and allow for energy-efficient locomotion on particular terrains (see the section 3). Here we use visual information to trigger the most energy-efficient gait while AMOS II traverses different terrains. Visual information is obtained from a terrain classification system consisting of the USB camera of AMOS II (**Figure 1A**) and an online feature-based terrain classification algorithm. The camera acquires terrain images while the classification algorithm (i.e., image processing) extracts local features of the images using Scale Invariant Feature Transform (SIFT) (Lowe, 2004), encodes the features

---

[2]Note that this limitation is not because of the CPG but due to the hardware. Applying the CPG to different robots (e.g., light weight robots with fast actuator speed), one might be able to obtain more than 20 different walking speeds on flat terrain.

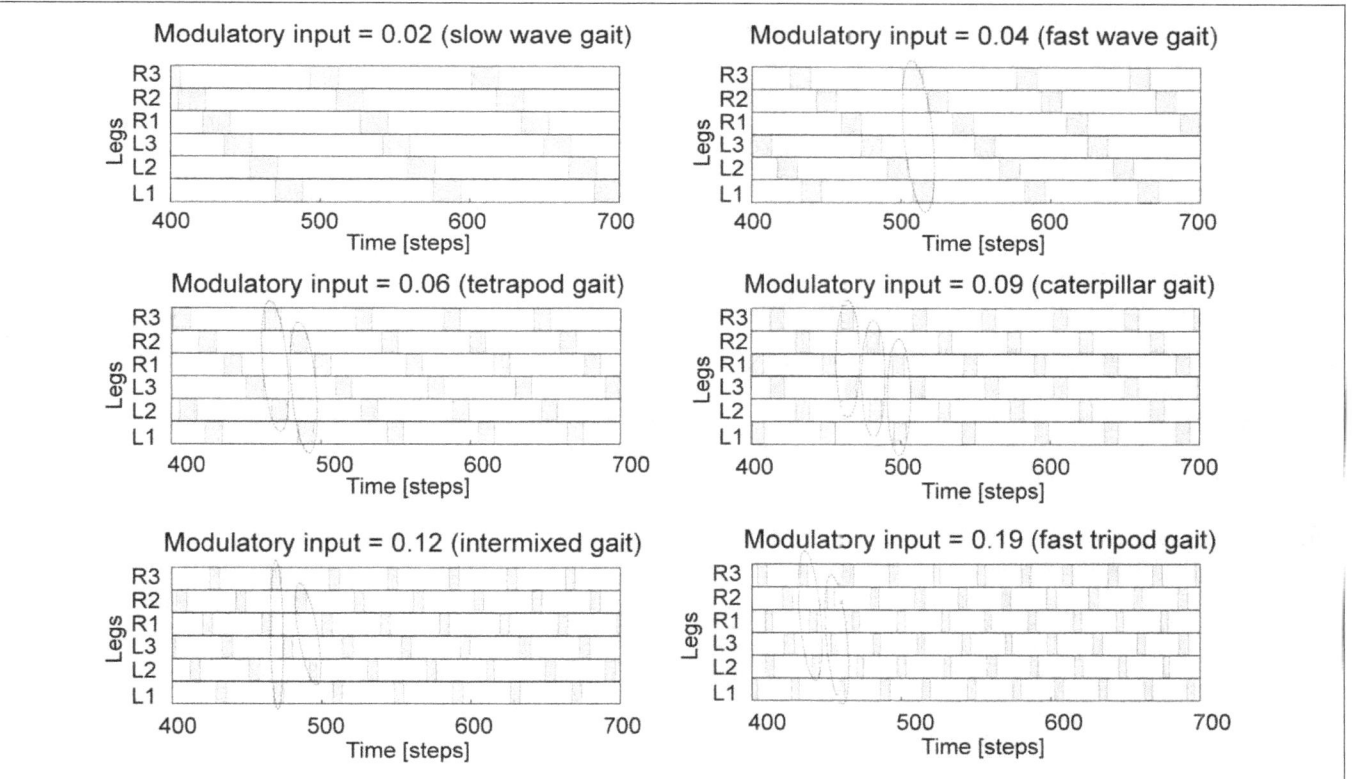

FIGURE 4 | Examples of six different gaits generated by the CPG. They are observed from the motor signals of the CTr-joints (**Figure 1**). White areas indicate ground contact or stance phase and gray areas refer to no ground contact during swing phase. As frequency increases, some legs step in pairs (dashed enclosures). We encourage readers to see also **Figure 3** and **Video S2** for, e.g., 20 walking patterns with respect to $MI = 0.0, 0.01, \ldots, 0.19$. Note that one time step is ≈ 0.037 s.

using the Bag of Words (BoW) technique (Zhang et al., 2010), and then classifies the words using Support Vector Machines (SVMs) with a radial basis function kernel (Cortes and Vapnik, 1995). The output of the algorithm provides terrain information used to set *MI* of the CPG, thereby triggering the corresponding pre-mapped energy-efficient gait (see the section 3).

Fast and smooth switching between gaits in a comparison to our previous chaotic CPG can be seen at **Video S1**. In principle, for the AMOS II system, a transition state from one stable gait to another stable gait using the CPG with neuromodulation requires about 2 s while it needs about 5 s when using the chaotic CPG. This fast switching between gaits is required for situations like escaping from an attack or danger (i.e., fast changing from a slow wave gait to a fast tripod gait). Note that the change of the modulation value occurs instantaneously where the CPG with neuromodulation immediately switches from one frequency to a new frequency. However, the system requires a longer time for a new gait to emerge because of delay lines (described below) transmitting the CPG signals to the motor neurons.

The outputs of the CPG are passed to motor neurons through two hierarchical subcomponents or modules: neural CPG postprocessing and neural motor control. The neural CPG postprocessing (**Figure 2**), which directly receives the CPG outputs, consists of postprocessing neurons with a threshold value of 0.85 and integrator units (**Figure A2**). Specifically, the neurons are for signal shaping while the integrator units are for obtaining continuous signals with asymmetry of ascending and descending slopes (**Figure 3C**). At first the CPG outputs get transformed by the neurons which produce the step function outputs with high (+1) or low (−1) value. Time intervals of the high and low outputs are counted. The high and low outputs are converted to continuous signals with ascending and descending slopes, respectively. The conversion is done by dividing the integrated high and low outputs by the time intervals part. Since the counting of the time intervals is subsequent, each slope is calculated using the time intervals of the previous period. Finally, the integrator outputs are scaled to the range between −1.0 and 1.0. For different frequencies of the CPG, the time intervals are different, thereby generating different ascending and descending slopes (**Figure 3C**).

Note that the CPG with the neural CPG postprocessing presented here has certain advantages over a classical solution (e.g., constructing CPG signals directly by hand or using a simple wavegenerator). This is because the CPG, derived from a RNN with two neurons, in principle exhibits various dynamical behaviors (e.g., periodic patterns, chaotic patterns, and hysteresis effects) which can be exploited for locomotion control (Manoonpong et al., 2008a; Steingrube et al., 2010). While the network can generate various output patterns, the neural CPG postprocessing is used to only translate these output signals into smooth continuous signals (e.g., saw-tooth signals) for motor control and does not change the network dynamics. In fact, the CPG and its postprocessing are independent; therefore, one could also apply different postprocessing mechanisms to shape or transform the CPG outputs into other periodic forms if required. In this neural approach, we can simply change the gaits (flexibility) and obtain

various patterns including chaotic motions[3] (versatility) by only changing the network parameters (i.e., synaptic weights and bias terms). Furthermore, one could also apply learning mechanisms (with an additional neuron) to the CPG such that the CPG can be entrained by sensory feedback in order to adapt to the feedback pattern and memorize it (Nachstedt et al., 2012). This will lead to the adaptivity of the gaits. Implementing this adaptivity on the AMOS II system is one of our major plans for future work. All these features (flexibility, versatility, and adaptivity) would be difficult to be achieved by a classical solution.

The neural motor control, which receives the postprocessed CPG outputs, consists of two different neural networks: one PSN and two VRNs. All neuron outputs of these networks are given by a hyperbolic tangent (tanh) transfer function. The PSN is a generic feedforward network (see **Figure A2** for the network structure). This network is designed by hand and consists of 4 hierarchical layers with 12 neurons. The synaptic weights and bias terms of the network are determined in a way that they do not change the periodic form of input signals (i.e., the postprocessed CPG outputs) and keep the amplitude of the signals as high as possible. Thus, all synaptic weights and bias terms were set to 0.5, which will convert the signals in the linear domain of the transfer function, except the synaptic weights and bias terms of the output neurons. They were set to 3.0 and −1.35, respectively, in order to amplify the signals and to shift the offset of the final output signals such that they have their center at zero. The complete network and parameters (i.e., all synaptic weights and bias terms) are shown in **Figure A2**. As a result, the network can switch the phase of the CPG outputs to lead or lag behind each other by $\pi/2$ in phase with respect to a given input for walking sideways [see Steingrube et al. (2010) and Manoonpong et al. (2008b) for more details]. It also provides additional fine tuning of the phase of the CPG outputs to achieve a proper phase shift between the CTr- and FTi-joints leading to insect-like leg movements (**Figure 5**).

The two VRNs are also simple feed-forward networks (see **Figure A2** for the network structure). The network is derived from a multiplication of two values in the range $x, y \in [-1, 1]$. It was constructed by four hidden neurons, which are connected with an output neuron. The network was trained by using the backpropagation algorithm (Rumelhart et al., 1986). The resulting network parameters (synaptic weights and bias terms) are shown in **Figure A2**. It approximately works as a multiplication operator. Each VRN controls the three ipsilateral TC-joints on one side. Since the VRNs function qualitatively like a multiplication function (Manoonpong et al., 2007), they have capability to increase or decrease the amplitude of the TC-joint signals and even reverse them with respect to their control inputs. Controlling the TC-joint signals in this way results in various walking directions, like forward/backward, turning left/right, turning in different radians, or curve walking in forward and backward directions [see Manoonpong et al. (2008b) for walking experiments].

---

[3]This CPG will show chaotic dynamics if its synaptic weights are set to $W_{11} = -5.5$, $W_{22} = 0.0$, $W_{12_m} = 1.475$, $W_{21_m} = -1.65$ with additional bias terms ($B_1 = -5.725$, $B_2 = 0.25$) projecting to the neurons C_1 and C_2, respectively. The chaotic patterns prove behaviorally useful for self-untrapping from a hole in the ground (Steingrube et al., 2010).

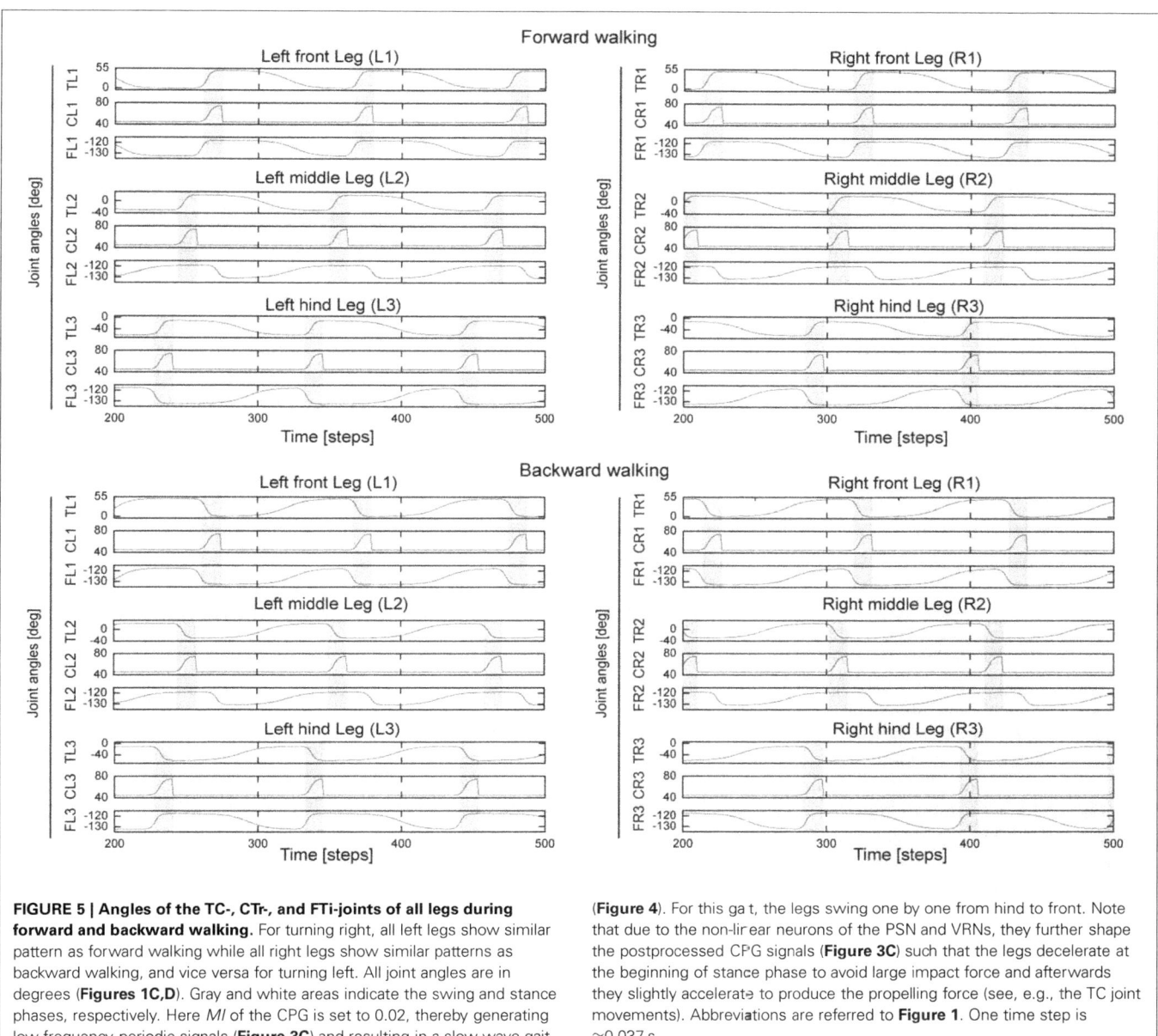

FIGURE 5 | Angles of the TC-, CTr-, and FTi-joints of all legs during forward and backward walking. For turning right, all left legs show similar pattern as forward walking while all right legs show similar patterns as backward walking, and vice versa for turning left. All joint angles are in degrees (**Figures 1C,D**). Gray and white areas indicate the swing and stance phases, respectively. Here *MI* of the CPG is set to 0.02, thereby generating low frequency periodic signals (**Figure 3C**) and resulting in a slow wave gait

(**Figure 4**). For this gait, the legs swing one by one from hind to front. Note that due to the non-linear neurons of the PSN and VRNs, they further shape the postprocessed CPG signals (**Figure 3C**) such that the legs decelerate at the beginning of stance phase to avoid large impact force and afterwards they slightly accelerate to produce the propelling force (see, e.g., the TC joint movements). Abbreviations are referred to **Figure 1**. One time step is ≈0.037 s.

Using exteroceptive sensors, like US (**Figure 1**), together with a neural sensory preprocessing network (see the network $N_{2,3}$ in **Figure A2**) where the network processes the US and provides a final resulting turning signal to the VRNs, allows AMOS II to autonomously avoid obstacles and to escape from a corner and even a deadlock situation (**Video S3**). Currently the network (**Figure A2**) has fixed synaptic weights resulting in a hard-wired anticipatory behavior with a fixed turning angle in front of the obstacles for avoiding them. Instead one could also apply a learning mechanism [e.g., Hebbian learning and synaptic scaling (Tetzlaff et al., 2011)] to adapt the synaptic weights of the network. This would enable AMOS II to learn to anticipate an obstacle and perform different turning behaviors depending on environmental complexity.

Note that the PSN and VRNs have been developed using a neural approach since this allows for adaptation and the use of standard (neural) learning (e.g., backpropagation) to modify the networks' properties and it is also close to biological systems. For example, there is strong evidence for a phase shifting property found in inter-segmental neurons in the connective elements of a cockroach (Pearson and Iles, 1973). Phase relationships between these neurons can change as would be required for emulating the functionality of our PSN. Studies by Akay et al. (2007) show that in stick insect locomotion motorneuron pools are able to not only drive protractor (swing) and retractor (stance) muscle activities but also reverse their activities leading to the change of locomotion directions (e.g., from walking forward to backward and vice versa). The functionality of these motorneuron pools is directly reproduced by our VRN which controls and reverses motor signals. In addition, another specific functionality of the VRN, namely that of regulating the magnitude of the motor signals allowing for different moving speeds, has been already found in another study (Gabriel and Büschges, 2007). This study suggests that in stick insects there are neurons that receive synaptic input, which modifies their activity according to the walking speed of the animal. This input seems specific to only these neurons and it arises via local pre-motor inter-neurons, which could, thus, represent the VRN interneurons as suggested by our network. In addition to this, the PSN and VRNs are generic and transferable. As suggested by their names, the PSN and VRN serve a general purpose (e.g., "phase switching") largely regardless of the robot's specific embodiment. Due to modularity, the PSN and VRN are typically independent of each other in their functioning and do not influence or become influenced by other components. Thus, they can be combined to form controllers of different types of robots (Manoonpong et al., 2007, 2008b; Steingrube et al., 2010; Chadil et al., 2011) where they do not require fine tuning for the specific system in which they are employed.

Finally, the outputs of the PSN and VRNs are sent to the motor neurons through delay lines (**Figure A2**). The ipsilateral lag is determined by a delay τ (i.e., 16 time steps or ≈ 0.6 s) and the phase shift between both left and right sides is given by a delay τ_L (i.e., 48 time steps or ≈ 2 s). These delays are independent of the CPG signals. This setup leads to biologically motivated leg coordination since the legs on each side perform phase shifted waves of the same frequency (Wilson, 1966). The frequency of the waves is defined by MI of the CPG. The connections to the motor neurons are similar to our previous work (Steingrube et al., 2010) except the ones to the FTi-motor neurons. They are modified here (**Figure A2**) to be more similar to insect-like leg movements (Ekeberg et al., 2004; Cruse et al., 2009). **Figure 5** illustrates all leg movements during forward and backward walking. During forward walking, in the swing phase the FTi-joints of the front and middle legs extend while the ones of the hind legs flex. In the stance phase, the FTi-joints of the front legs gradually flex to pull the body forward while the ones of the hind legs gradually extend to also push it forward. For the middle legs, the FTi-joints combine both actions of the FTi-joints of the front and hind legs. They flex rapidly and early during the stance phase in order to pull the body since in this period the legs are at an anterior position [i.e., positive TC-joint angles (**Figure 1C**)]. Afterwards, they stay flexed and then gradually extend in order to push the body since in this period the legs are at a posterior position [i.e., negative TC-joint angles (**Figure 1C**)]. These biologically-inspired leg movements (Ekeberg et al., 2004; Cruse et al., 2009) provide more propelling force, resulting in an increased walking speed of AMOS II by $\approx 15\%$ compared with the fixed FTi-joint version (Steingrube et al., 2010). These movements are reversed for backward walking. We encourage readers to also see the video showing the leg movements of AMOS II at **Video S4**. Since the generated leg movements are independent of other influences, similar movements exist in all gaits. It is important to note that the leg movements shown here, however, are still not completely similar to insect leg movements. This can be further improved by applying additional components, i.e., muscle models (Xiong

et al., 2012), to obtain a smoother foot path and to come closer to insect-like leg movements.

2.4. LOCAL LEG CONTROL

While the CPG-based control in principle can generate a multitude of different behavioral patterns and insect-like locomotion (i.e., leg movements and gaits) without sensory feedback, it cannot adapt an individual leg to deal with a change of terrain, losing of ground contact during stance phase, or stepping on or hitting an obstacle during swing phase. This adaptable locomotion is necessary for traversing rough terrain or climbing over obstacles. To address this issue, we introduce here local leg control consisting of two components: (1) an adaptive neural forward model and (2) elevation and searching control. These two components are applied to each leg of AMOS II (see **Figures 2, A2**).

The adaptive neural forward model serves to estimate the walking state. To do so, it transforms a motor signal (i.e., here the CTr-motor signal[4], efference copy) into an expected sensory signal to be able to compare it to the actual incoming one (i.e., here the FC signal of the leg). The forward model consists of only two neurons (**Figure 6A**). The neuron F transforms the motor signal while the neuron P performs postprocessing. We construct the neuron F as a hysteresis element (Pasemann, 1993) using a single recurrent neuron with synaptic plasticity (described below in details) and the postprocessing neuron P as a standard one (see Equation 1) with a tanh transfer function. Note that this postprocessing neuron P with its large fixed presynaptic weight (i.e., 10.0) basically sharpens a transformed motor signal to perfectly match to a FC signal.

Due to a delay in the relation between FC signal and the CTr-motor signal, a simple thresholding method cannot be applied for signal transformation. Therefore, we use the single recurrent neuron instead since this is a simple neural mechanism providing dynamical properties (e.g., hysteresis effect) that can smooth the motor signal and at the same time provide a delay in the input–output relation required to transform the motor signal into the expected sensory signal. The activation function of this neuron is given by:

$$a_F(t) = W_R(t)o_F(t-1) + W_I(t)I(t) + B(t), \qquad (5)$$

where I is the input of the neuron which is here the CTr-motor signal coming from the CPG-based control. o_F is the output of the neuron given by the tanh transfer function, i.e., $o_F = \tanh(a_F), \in [-1, 1]$. W_R, W_I, and B are the recurrent weight, the presynaptic weight, and the bias term of the neuron, respectively. These parameters need to be adjusted to obtain a proper hysteresis loop for the signal transformation. Therefore, we employ a gradient descent learning rule to adapt them. In principle, the rule attempts to minimize the error E between the target output T and the actual output o_F of the neuron through gradient descent. The error is measured as:

$$E(t) = \frac{1}{2}(T(t) - o_F(t))^2. \qquad (6)$$

---

[4]We use the CTr-motor signal instead of the TC- and FTi-motor signals since its pattern is close to the FC signal.

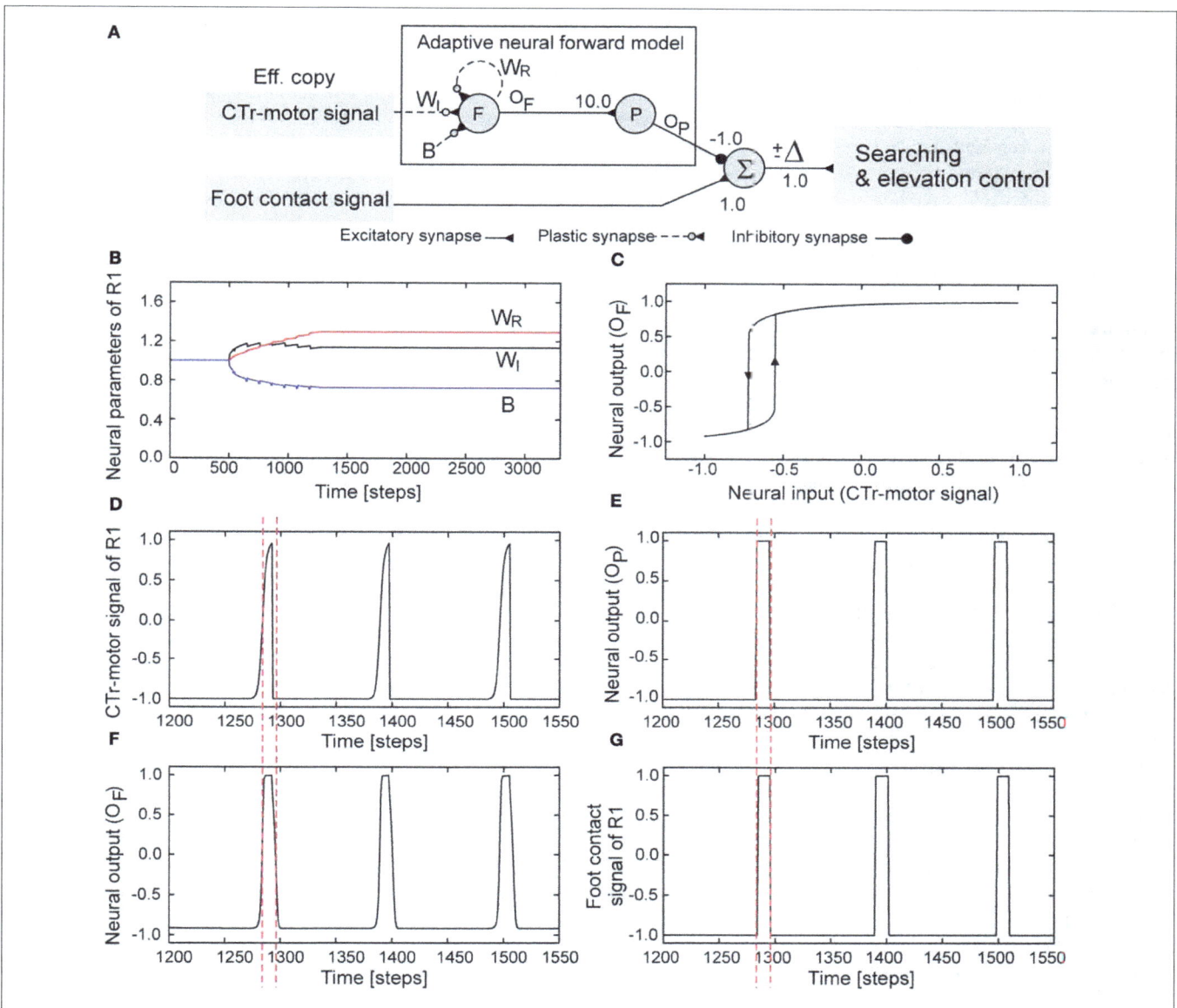

FIGURE 6 | Adaptive neural forward model. (A) The model structure consisting of recurrent and non-recurrent neurons. **(B)** Changes of the parameters of the model of the right front leg (R1). **(C)** The hysteresis effect between the input and output signals of the forward model of R1 where the converged parameters are used (see **B**). In this situation, the input varies between −1.0 and 1.0. Consequently, the output will gradually show high activation (≈ +1.0) when the input increases to value above −0.55. The output will show low activation (≈ −1.0) when the input decreases below −0.715. **(D)** The CTr-motor signal of R1 which is the input of the neuron F. Its high activation drives the leg to swing (i.e., swing phase) while its low activation drives the leg in touching the ground (i.e., stance phase). **(E)** The output of the postprocessing neuron P is used to compare to the foot contact signal for estimating the walking state. **(F)** The output of the neuron F or the transformed motor signal. **(G)** The foot contact signal of R1. It is filtered and mapped onto the interval $[−1, +1]$ where $+1$ is the leg has no ground contact and vice versa. Dashed lines are provided for comparison. Note that the parameter changes of the forward models of the other legs show similar patterns. Their convergence was achieved after about eight to twenty walking steps. The parameters converged at slightly different values, resulting in slightly different hysteresis loops. One time step is ≈0.037 s.

In this study, we use the filtered FC sensor signal, linearly mapped onto the interval $[−1, 1]$, as the target output. According to the learning rule, the parameters (W_R, W_I, and B) are updated every time step ($≈0.037$ s) in proportion to the gradient and given as follows:

$$\Delta W_R = -\mu \frac{\partial E}{\partial W_R} = \mu(T(t) - o_F(t))(1 - o_F(t)^2)o_F(t-1), \quad (7)$$

$$\Delta W_I = -\mu \frac{\partial \bar{E}}{\partial V_I} = \mu(T(t) - o_F(t))(1 - o_F(t)^2)I(t), \quad (8)$$

$$\Delta B = -\mu \frac{\partial E}{\partial B} = \mu(T(t) - o_F(t))(1 - o_F(t)^2), \quad (9)$$

where μ is the learning rate which is set to a small positive value, e.g., 0.01. For the training process, we initialize the neural activity and output states of the forward model to 0.0 and W_R, W_I, and B to 1.0. Due to this simple neural system, the process can perform online. We implemented six forward models on AMOS II where each of them works on one leg. Afterwards, we let AMOS II walk in a normal condition (i.e., walking on floor with a certain gait). The training process will stop as soon as the difference between the filtered FC signal and the postprocessed neural output o_P is smaller than a threshold, e.g., 0.05, over a certain period of times (e.g., 500 time steps). We performed the training process only once and only for the normal walking condition. This walking condition is used as a reference to compare it to other walking conditions in any terrain.

Figure 6B illustrates the parameter changes of the forward model of, e.g., the right front leg (R1, **Figure 1A**) during training. The training process was set to start after 500 time steps (or around four walking steps) and the parameters (W_R, W_I, and B) converged after around 1300 steps (or around seven walking steps). The resulting parameters lead to a proper hysteresis loop (**Figure 6C**). Utilizing this hysteresis property together with the neural postprocessing, the CTr-motor signal is finally transformed into the expected FC signal (**Figures 6D–G**). In this example, AMOS II walked with a slow wave gait (i.e., $MI = 0.02$). It is important to note that the models of all legs that adapted to this gait can be directly applied to other gaits.

After training, the output of each trained forward model (i.e., the expected FC signal, **Figure 6E**) is used to compare it to the actual incoming FC signal of the leg (**Figure 6G**). The difference Δ (**Figure 6A**) between them determines the walking state where a positive value ($+\Delta$) means losing ground contact during the stance phase and a negative one ($-\Delta$) means stepping on or hitting obstacles during the swing phase. Thus, we use the positive value for searching control (**Figure 7A**). The value is accumulated through a recurrent neuron S with a linear transfer function and always reset to 0.0 at the beginning of swing phase. The output of this neuron o_S with significant change (e.g., $o_S > 0.15$) controls vertical shifting of the CTr- and FTi-joints. Consequently, these joints are shifted when the positive difference occurs; thereby, the respective leg searches for a foothold. This searching control only occurs in the stance phase. On the other hand, we use the negative value for elevation control (**Figure 7B**). The value is also accumulated through a recurrent neuron E with a linear transfer function. The output of this neuron with significant change[5] (e.g., $o_E < -15$) shifts the CTr- and FTi-joint movements upwards. At the same time, the TC-joint movement is shortly inhibited. As a consequence, the leg is elevated, thereby avoiding an obstacle or freeing itself from the obstacle. This elevation control only occurs in the swing phase. Note that the IR sensors installed at the legs (**Figure 1B**) can be also used for elevation control. This allows the legs to avoid hitting a large obstacle in the front (**Video S5**).

To illustrate the functionality of the searching control and clearly observe leg motion, we activated one leg [e.g., right middle

leg (R2)] and fixed the other legs to a certain position. Afterwards, we changed ground level during stance phase. Changing it causes different positive errors ($+\Delta$) due to mismatch between the expected FC signal and the actual incoming one. The error is accumulated through the recurrent neuron S. If the accumulated error (**Figure 7C**) is higher than the threshold, the searching controller then controls the CTr- and FTi-joints to depress the leg and at the same time extend the tibia, respectively. This results in searching for a foothold. Note that the TC-joint motion is not influenced. All joint angles of the leg in this experiment are shown in (**Figures 7D–F**). We encourage readers to also see the video of this experiment at **Video S6**.

To illustrate the functionality of the elevation control and clearly observe leg motion, we also activated only one leg [e.g., right middle leg (R2)] and fixed the other legs to a certain position. In addition, we inhibited the searching control such that the leg could not search for a foothold. This is to better see and understand the changes of the joint angles. To force elevation of the leg, we made the foot touch an obstacle during the swing phase. This causes negative errors ($-\Delta$) that are accumulated through the recurrent neuron E. If the accumulated error (**Figure 7G**) is higher than the threshold, the elevation controller then inhibits the TC-joint for the forward motion of the leg and at the same time drives the CTr- and FTi-joints to elevate the leg and fully extend the tibia, respectively. This results in the elevation of the leg, thereby freeing it from the obstacle during the swing phase. After the leg frees from the obstacle, the TC-, CTr-, and FTi-joints immediately return to their unaltered positions. Since the process occurs in a very short time, the gait does not break down (see the section 3). All joint angles of the leg in this experiment are shown in (**Figures 7H–J**). We encourage readers to also see the video of this experiment at **Video S5**.

3. RESULTS

In the previous sections, we showed the individual functionalities and performances of the CPG-based control and the local leg control in part. Here, we present experiments carried out to assess the ability of their combination (i.e., adaptive neural locomotion control, **Figure 2**). The first experiment investigated energy-efficient gaits for different terrains. To do so, we categorized terrains into four different groups: hard terrain (e.g., floor, pavement), loose terrain (e.g., fine gravel), rough terrain (e.g., gravel), and vegetated terrain (e.g., grass).

For each of these terrain groups, we let AMOS II walk from slow to fast gaits by manually increasing MI of the CPG. During locomotion, the local leg control autonomously adapted the legs for a foothold. Thus, in this experiment, the CPG-based control and the local leg control function as open-loop control and closed-loop control, respectively. We calculate the electric energy consumption of each walking pattern as:

$$E = IVt, \tag{10}$$

where I is average electric current in amperes used by the motors during walking 1 m. It is measured using the Zap 25 CS installed inside AMOS II. V is voltage (here 5 V). t is time in seconds for the travel distance (here 1 m). **Figure 8** shows the energy

---

[5]Here, we use a high threshold value for controlling the elevation since a minor disturbance can be handled by passive mechanisms (spring and passive couplings) installed at the leg. Using a small threshold value might lead to an unnecessary elevation of the leg resulting in unstable motion.

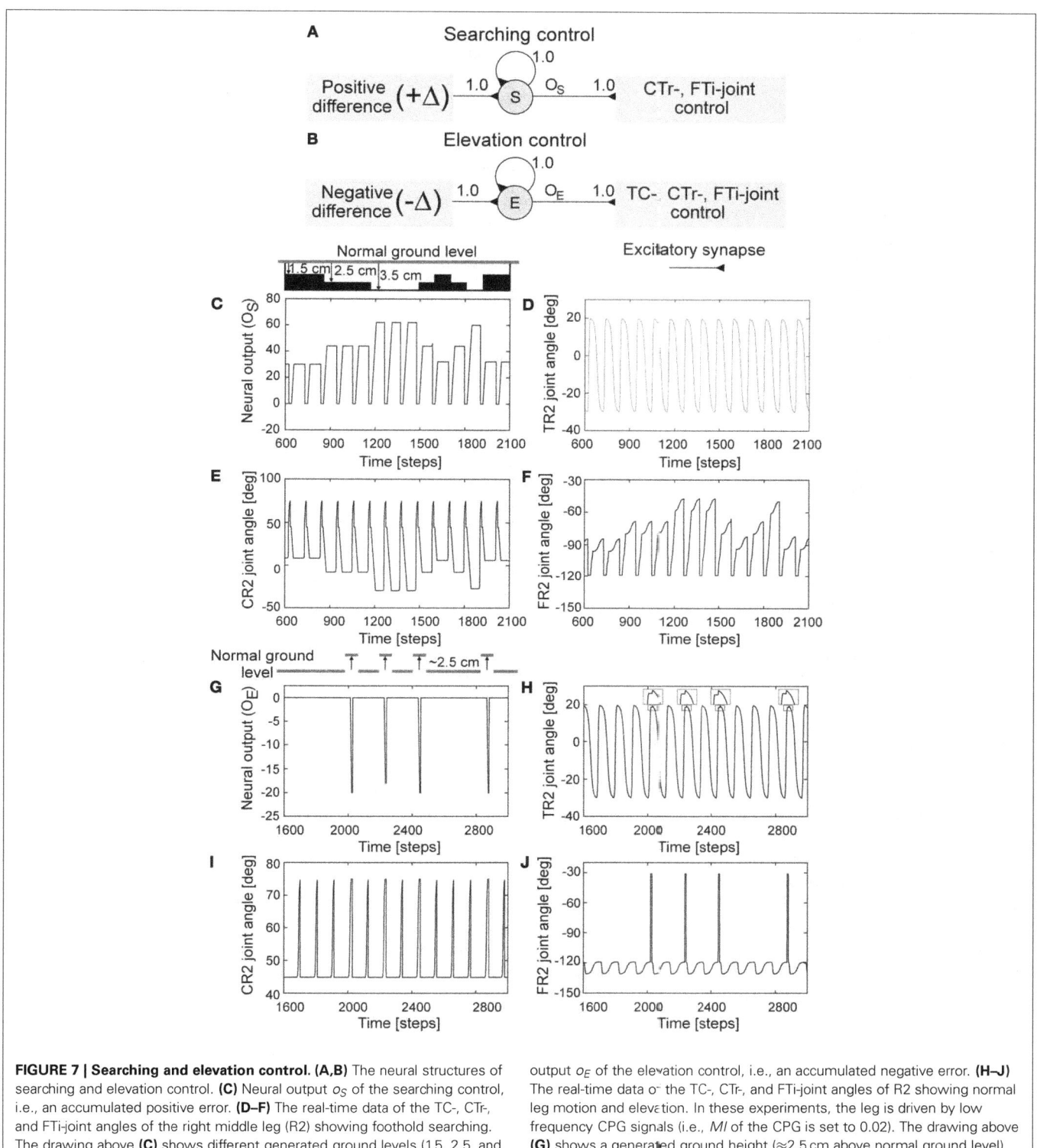

FIGURE 7 | Searching and elevation control. (A,B) The neural structures of searching and elevation control. **(C)** Neural output o_S of the searching control, i.e., an accumulated positive error. **(D–F)** The real-time data of the TC-, CTr-, and FTi-joint angles of the right middle leg (R2) showing foothold searching. The drawing above **(C)** shows different generated ground levels (1.5, 2.5, and 3.5 cm below normal ground level) activating foothold searching. **(G)** Neural

output o_E of the elevation control, i.e., an accumulated negative error. **(H–J)** The real-time data of the TC-, CTr-, and FTi-joint angles of R2 showing normal leg motion and elevation. In these experiments, the leg is driven by low frequency CPG signals (i.e., MI of the CPG is set to 0.02). The drawing above **(G)** shows a generated ground height ($\approx$2.5 cm above normal ground level) activating leg elevation. One time step is $\approx$0.037 s.

consumptions measured in these four terrain groups where the measurement of each group was repeated five times.

Figures 8A,B suggest using the MI values of 0.04 and 0.06 which generate a fast wave gait and a tetrapod gait on loose and

rough terrains, respectively. **Figures 8C,D** suggest using the MI value of 0.19 which produces a fast tripod gait on hard and vegetated terrains. Note that AMOS II started to slip when the value of MI was higher than 0.19 for hard and vegetated terrains and it got

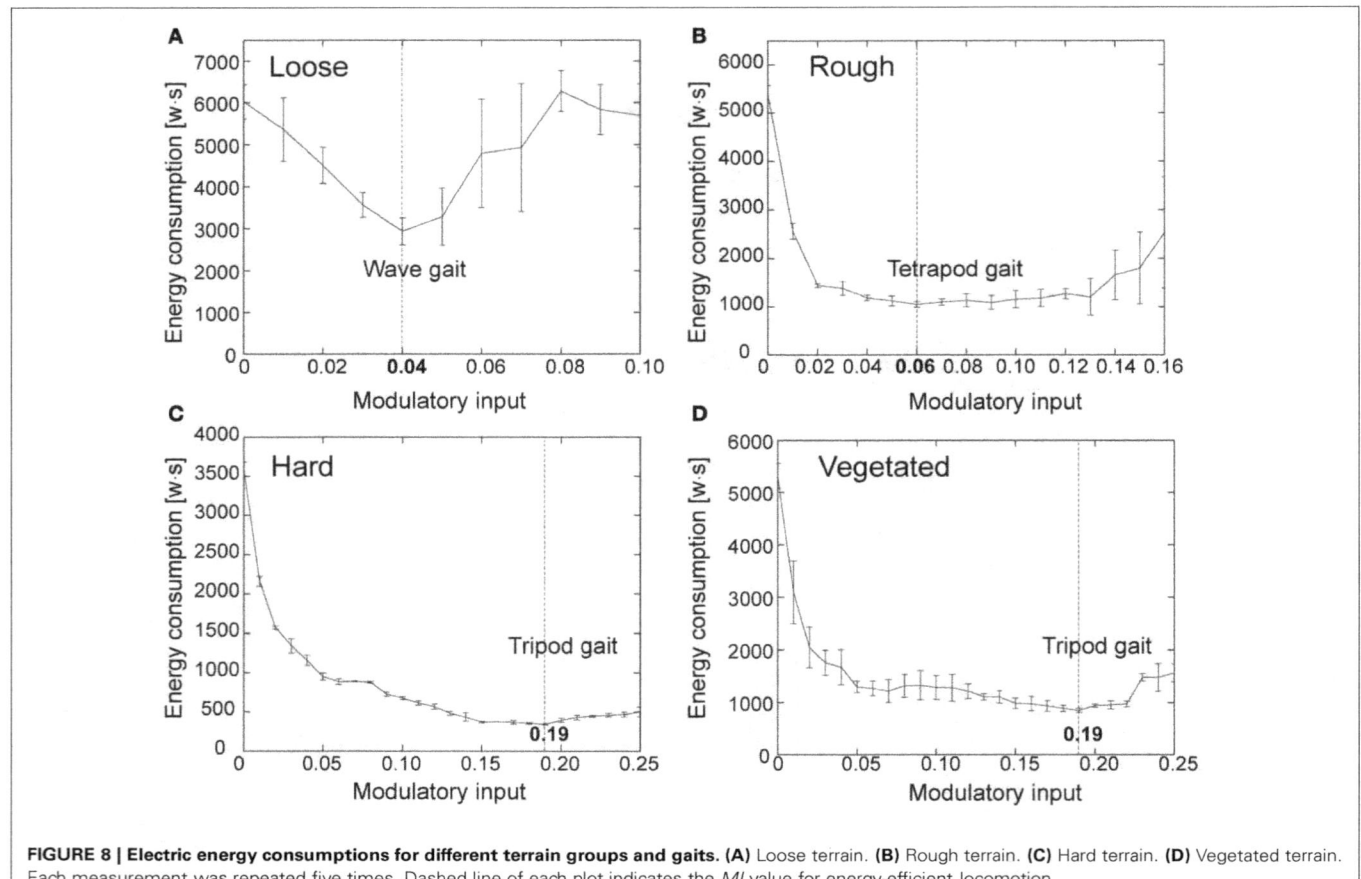

FIGURE 8 | Electric energy consumptions for different terrain groups and gaits. (A) Loose terrain. **(B)** Rough terrain. **(C)** Hard terrain. **(D)** Vegetated terrain. Each measurement was repeated five times. Dashed line of each plot indicates the *MI* value for energy-efficient locomotion.

stuck most of the time when the *MI* values were higher than 0.16 and 0.10 for rough and loose terrains, respectively. This experimental result reveals that each terrain group requires a specific gait which leads to the lowest energy consumption. This allows mapping the four terrain groups to the energy-efficient gaits.

The second experiment employed the investigated energy-efficient gaits together with the visual terrain classification system (described in section 2.3) to allow AMOS II to autonomously perform energy-efficient locomotion while traversing the different terrains. The output of the visual terrain classification system provides terrain information. This information was used as the preprocessed sensory input to set *MI* of the CPG, thereby triggering the corresponding pre-mapped energy-efficient gait. This way, the experiment reflects a complete neural closed-loop system (**Figure 2**). The experimental result is shown in **Figure 9**.

It can be seen that at the beginning AMOS II walked with a fast wave gait (photo 1) since it detected fine gravel (loose terrain) using its visual system. Afterwards, it changed from the wave gait to a tetrapod gait (photo 2) since it detected gravel (rough terrain). Finally, it used a fast tripod gait (photo 3) on the floor (hard terrain). During traversing the different terrains, AMOS II adapted its legs individually to deal with a change of terrain. That is, it depressed its leg and extended its tibia to search for a foothold when losing a ground contact during the stance phase. Losing ground contact information is detected by a significant

change of the positive accumulated error o_S, see black line in **Figure 9C**). However, during the swing phase no leg elevation was observed (i.e., no significant change of the negative accumulated error o_E, see red line in **Figure 9C**) since only minor perturbation occurred, where the perturbation was handled by the passive components of the leg. We encourage readers to see the video of this experiment at **Video S7**. Another test in an outdoor environment where AMOS II walked from gravel to grass can be seen at **Figure A4**. In addition to energy-efficient and adaptable locomotion emphasized in this experiment, the basic leg movements of AMOS II and the used gait follows insect locomotion. Thus, this experiment is an example of the demonstration of insect-like, energy-efficient, and adaptable locomotion of walking machines, like AMOS II.

The third experiment focused on both, leg elevation and foothold searching, of AMOS II to deal with small obstacles. In this scenario, we let AMOS II walk with a certain pattern [e.g., a slow wave gait ($MI = 0.02$)] and placed small obstacles ($\approx$2.5 cm height) on its path. The experimental result is shown in **Figure 10**. It can be seen that, while walking forward, the foot of the right front leg (R1) of AMOS II hit an obstacle during the swing phase (photo 1), thereby preventing the leg from completing the phase. This leads to a significant change of the negative accumulated error o_E (**Figure 10A**). As a consequence, AMOS II elevated the leg to free it from the obstacle (photo 2). Afterwards, it placed the

Neural control and adaptive neural forward models for insect-like, energy-efficient, and adaptable locomotion...

71

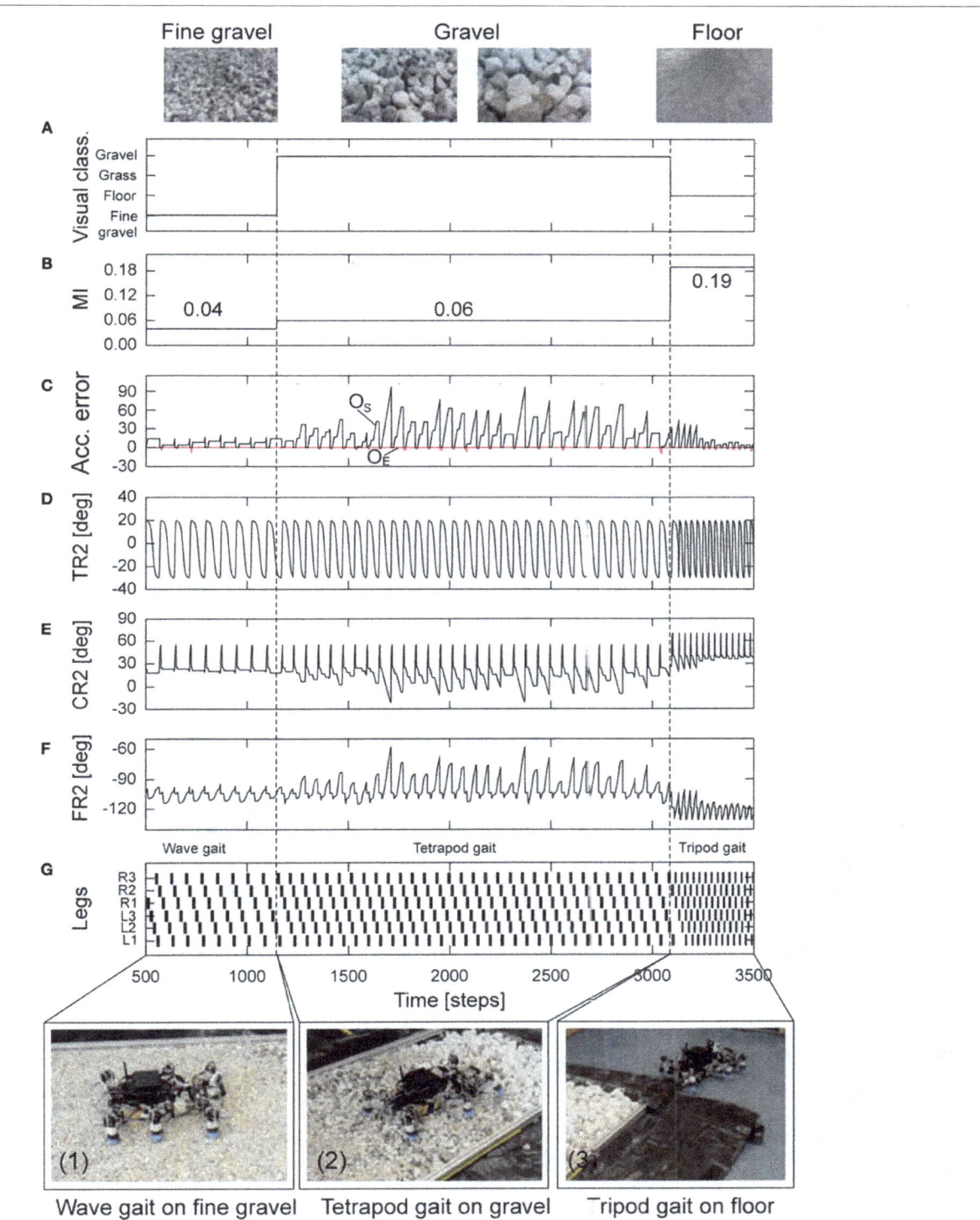

FIGURE 9 | Real-time data of energy-efficient and adaptable locomotion on three different terrains. (A) The output of the online terrain classification system which is a preprocessed visual sensory signal. **(B)** The modulatory input *MI* of the CPG which is directly controlled by the sensory signal. It was set to 0.04 (fast wave gait), then 0.06 (tetrapod gait), and finally 0.19 (fast tripod gait). **(C)** The positive (o_S) and negative (o_E) accumulated errors (**Figures 7A,B**). They control leg adaptation to deal with different terrains. **(D–F)** The TC-, CTr-, and FTi-joint angles of the right middle leg (R2) during walking from fine gravel

(loose terrain) to gravel (rough terrain) to floor (hard terrain). They represent the leg movement including adaptation. **(G)** Gait diagram showing the different energy-efficient gaits of AMOS II while traversing the terrains. Black boxes indicate swing phase while white areas between them indicate stance phase. Abbreviations are referred to **Figure 1**. Above pictures show snap shots from the camera on AMOS II used for the terrain classification while walking. Below pictures show snap shots of locomotion of AMOS II during the experiment. Note that one time step is ≈0.037 s.

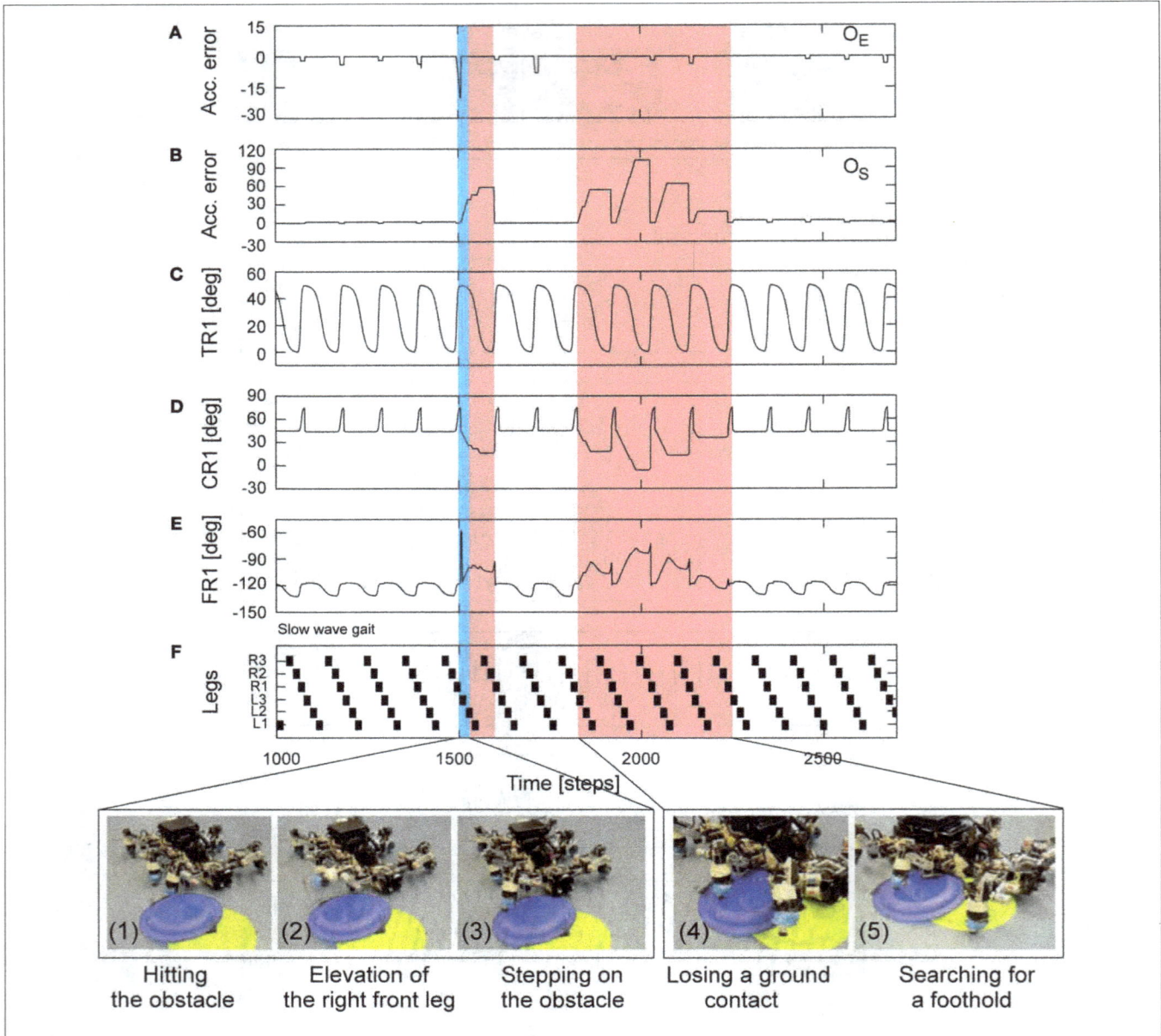

(1) Hitting the obstacle

(2) Elevation of the right front leg

(3) Stepping on the obstacle

(4) Losing a ground contact

(5) Searching for a foothold

FIGURE 10 | Real-time data of adaptable locomotion on terrain with small obstacles. (A,B) The negative (o_E) and positive (o_S) accumulated errors (**Figures 7B,A**). They control leg adaptation to deal with stepping on or hitting obstacles during the swing phase and losing a ground contact during the stance phase. **(C–E)** The TC-, CTr-, and FTi-joint angles of the right front leg (R1) during walking on the floor with small obstacles ($\approx$2.5 cm height). They represent the leg movement including adaptation. **(F)** Gait diagram showing a slow wave gait ($MI = 0.02$) of AMOS II in this experiment. Black boxes indicate swing phase while white areas between them indicate stance phase. Abbreviations are referred to **Figure 1**. Below pictures show snap shots of locomotion of AMOS II during the experiment. Blue and red areas indicate elevation and searching actions, respectively. Note that one time step is $\approx$0.037 s.

leg on top of the obstacle without getting stuck (photo 3). Due to the difference of the ground level, this causes a significant change of the positive accumulated error o_S (**Figure 10B**). AMOS II then lowered the leg more downward to ensure ground contact. After a few steps, the leg again lost a ground contact during the stance phase (photo 4), resulting in searching for a foothold (photo 5). Finally, AMOS II successfully walked away from the obstacles. This experiment reveals that using this leg adaptation mechanism

AMOS II can effectively locomote on terrain with small obstacles without getting stuck. We encourage readers to also see the video of this experiment at **Video S8**.

The fourth experiment was to show that the adaptive neural locomotion control not only generates insect-like, energy-efficient, and adaptable locomotion of AMOS II (as shown above) but also allows it with the help of its BJ to climb over a large obstacle. To do so, we placed AMOS II on rough terrain (i.e., soil with stones) with an 11 cm high obstacle at front. The task of AMOS II was to move forward and climb over the obstacle. For this experiment, the CPG-based control generated a basic walking pattern [e.g., a slow wave gait ($MI = 0.02$)] while the local leg control adapted the legs individually for foothold searching and elevation, thereby enabling effective locomotion and supporting the body of AMOS II during climbing. Note that the slow wave gait was used in this experiment because it is the most effective gait for climbing which allows AMOS II to negotiate the highest climbable obstacle (13 cm height which equals 75% of its leg length) [see Goldschmidt et al. (2012) for details]. In addition to the locomotion control, reactive BJ control was also applied to control the BJ for climbing [see Goldschmidt et al. (2012) for details]. The controller produces an abstraction of body flexion observed in cockroach climbing. It controls the BJ to lean upwards to surmount obstacles and to bend downwards for stable climbing.

This downward motion appears in cockroach climbing while the upward motion does not exist. Instead of leaning the body flexion joint upwards as AMOS II does, a cockroach extends its front and middle legs to raise its reaching height to surmount obstacles, thereby rearing its entire body to a taller pose. Here, we used the US at the front body part of AMOS II (**Figure 1A**) for obstacle detection and BJ control. **Figure 11** presents the experimental result.

At the first period (0–500 time steps), the local leg control was deactivated. Due to the rough terrain, the feet could not perfectly touch the ground during the stance phase; thus, AMOS II could not move forward (photo 1). After 500 time steps, the local leg control was activated. It allows for foothold searching, thereby adapting locomotion to the terrain. As a result, AMOS II moved forward. As AMOS II approached the obstacle, the US detection activated the BJ control such that the BJ

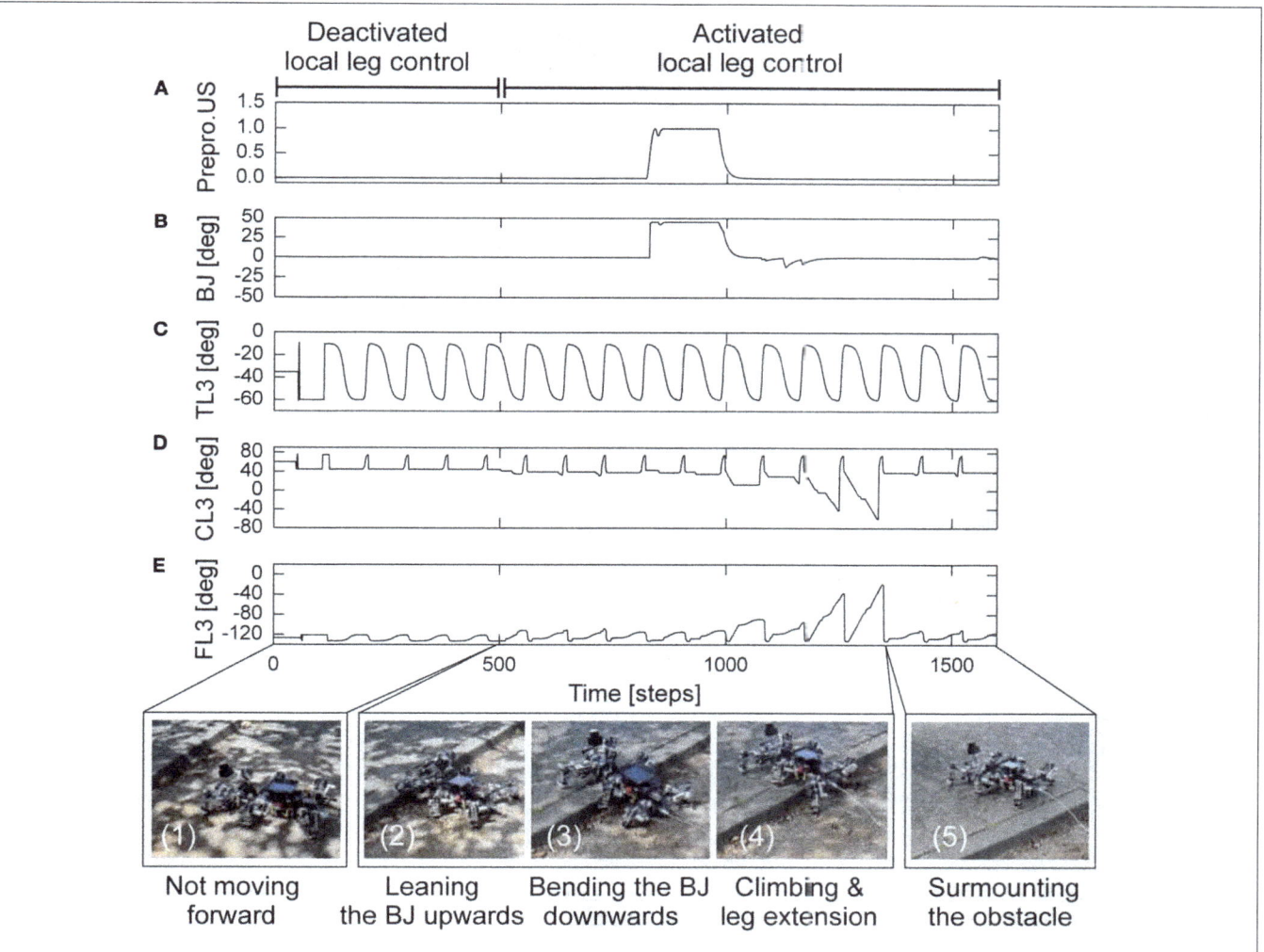

FIGURE 11 | Real-time data of walking and climbing over a large obstacle in an outdoor environment. (A) The preprocessed ultrasonic sensor (US) signal for reactive backbone joint control. **(B)** The backbone joint (BJ) angle during walking and climbing. The BJ stayed at zero angle during walking. It leant upwards and then bent downwards during climbing. **(C–E)** The TC-, CTr-, and FTi-joint angles of the left hind leg (L3)

during walking and climbing. The joint adaptation was controlled by the negative (o_E) and positive (o_S) accumulated errors (**Figures 7B,A**). The changes of the errors have similar patterns as shown in **Figure 9C**. Here AMOS II used a slow wave gait ($MI = 0.02$, **Figure 10F**). Below pictures show snap shots of the locomotion of AMOS II during the experiment. Note that one time step is ≈ 0.037 s.

leant upwards (photo 2). Due to a time-out period after leaning upwards, the BJ moved downwards to ensure stability while climbing (photo 3). During climbing, a hind leg [e.g., left hind leg (L3), photo 4] lowered downwards, showing leg extension, to support the body. Finally, AMOS II successfully locomoted on rough terrain and surmounted the 11 cm high obstacle (photo 5). We encourage readers to also see the video of this experiment at **Video S9**. Besides this experimental result, it is important to note that both adaptive locomotion and reactive BJ controllers have a distributed implementation, but they are indirectly coupled by sensory feedback and the physical components of AMOS II. This way, the combined neural control network driven by the sensor signals synchronizes leg and BJ movements for stable walking and climbing.

The final experiment was to illustrate that the adaptive neural locomotion controller can adapt the remaining legs to deal with a leg damage situation. In this experiment we let AMOS II walk with a slow wave gait ($MI = 0.02$) and then disconnected the power connector of the motor of a leg joint such that the joint became inactive (i.e., uncontrollable). This is to simulate leg damage. After damage, we placed AMOS II on top of an object to observe the adaptation of the remaining legs that allows AMOS II to be able to continue moving forward. **Figure 12** present the experimental result.

As shown in **Figure 12**, AMOS II walked in a normal walking condition at the beginning (photo 1). During walking, we disconnected the motor power connector of the FTi-joint of the left middle leg (photo 2) such that the joint became inactive. Then we

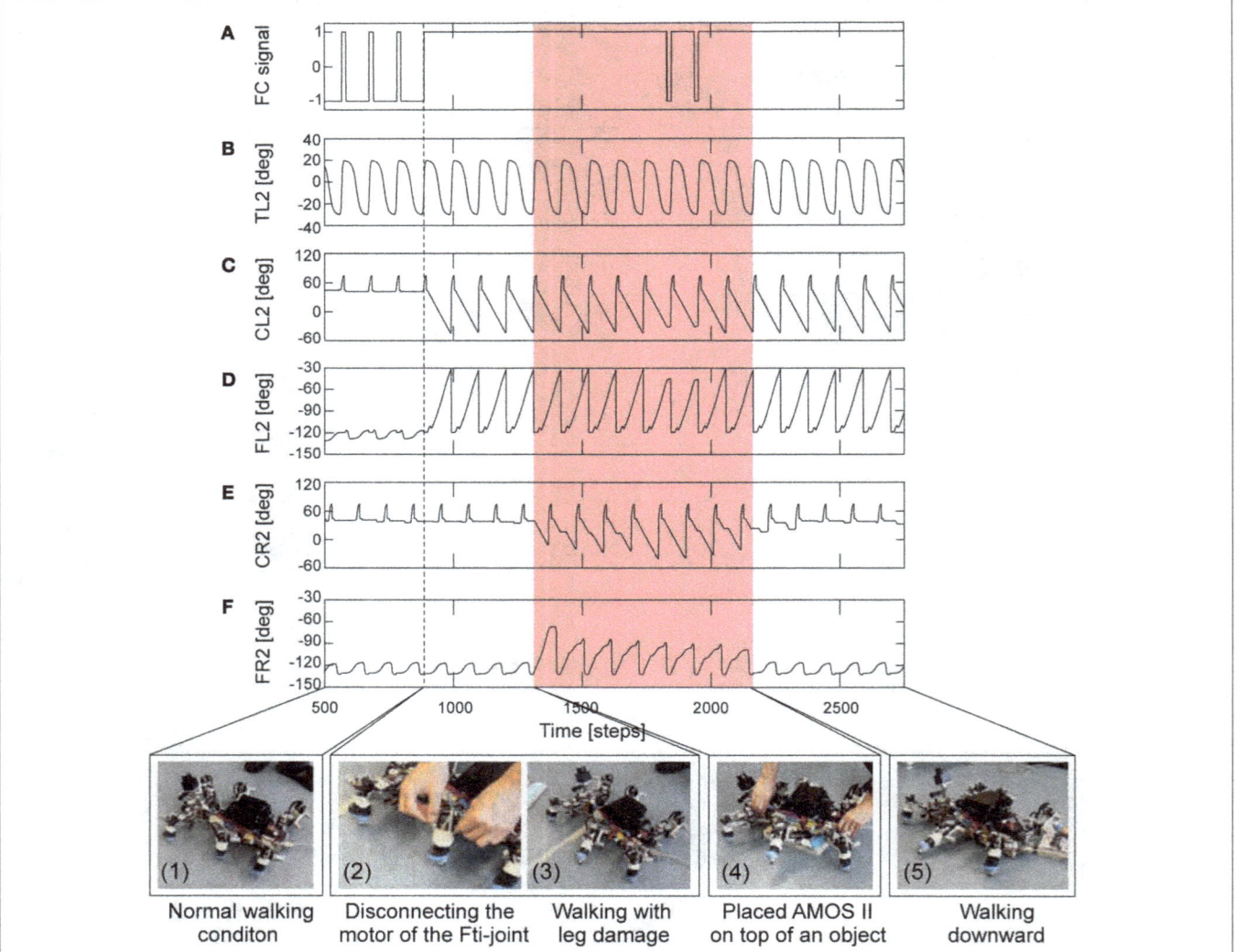

FIGURE 12 | Real-time data of adaptable locomotion during leg damage. **(A)** The filtered foot contact (FC) signal of the left middle leg (L2) where +1 is the leg has no ground contact and −1 is the leg touches the ground. **(B–D)** The TC-, CTr-, and FTi-joint angles of L2. **(E,F)** The CTr- and FTi-joint angles of the right middle leg (R2). The joint adaptation was controlled by the negative (o_E) and positive (o_S) accumulated errors (**Figures 7B,A**). The changes of the

errors have similar patterns as shown in **Figure 9C**. Here AMOS II used a slow wave gait ($MI = 0.02$, **Figure 10F**). Below pictures show snap shots of the locomotion of AMOS II during the experiment. Dashed line indicates the time that the motor power connector of the FTi-joint of L2 was disconnected. Red area indicates the time that AMOS II was on a 3.5 cm high object. Note that one time step is ≈0.037 s.

also tilted the tibia upward; thereby, the foot could not touch the ground properly. This results in the leg adaptation to search for a foothold (photo 3). Afterwards, we placed AMOS II on top of a 3.5 cm high object (photo 4). Since AMOS II was on the object, its legs lost a ground contact. AMOS II adapted its legs to search for a foothold (see, e.g., the FTi- and CTr-joint signals of the right middle leg in **Figures 12E,F**). As a result, it successfully climbed down from the object and continued walking forward (photo 5). The ability of leg adaptation was mainly achieved by the local leg control mechanisms. These mechanisms even allow AMOS II to climb down from the object with a 7 cm height. Without them, AMOS II got stuck on the object. We encourage readers to see the video of this experiment at **Video S10**. This experimental result reveals that the developed adaptive neural locomotion controller can not only generate versatile locomotion behaviors including climbing (shown in the other experiments) but also give robustness to the system by allowing it to cope with damage.

4. DISCUSSION

Here, we briefly discuss some remaining issues concerning the six-legged walking machine AMOS II and its controller, because most of the relevant discussion points have been treated in the above sections.

AMOS II was used as an experimental platform and represents an embodied neural closed-loop system with many degrees of freedom. It was designed with a morphology analogous to a cockroach. It was constructed in a straightforward way as a biomechatronic system consisting of several sensors and actuators. Due to extra rubber coupling elements and springs integrated into the joints and tibiae of AMOS II, this yields passive compliance allowing AMOS II to deal with minor disturbances during locomotion over rough terrain (as described in the second experiment). The joint compliance also enables AMOS II to passively flex its legs to avoid damages when the environment changes (**Video S11**). Besides the physical components of AMOS II that follow biomechanics of walking animals, another special trait of AMOS II is that we configured the ranges of the joint movements of AMOS II such that it has a very low center of mass (i.e., low ground clearance) and its body falls to the ground before taking the next step during normal walking. When negotiating a large obstacle, AMOS II uses its BJ together with additional reactive BJ control (Goldschmidt et al., 2012) to climb over it while its leg movements automatically adapt accordingly (**Video S12**).

In fact, the advantage of low ground clearance is evident in case of leg damage. In this situation, a robot with high ground clearance will tip over or fall down a lot (**Figure A5A**) leading to unstable locomotion and remaining legs need to carry more load. Thus, the motors need to produce high torque to carry the load resulting in high power consumption (**Figure A5B**). Furthermore the legs might have difficulty to swing during swing phase (**Figures A5C,D**); thereby, the robot will not move forwards properly (**Figure A5G** and **Video S10**). In contrast, with low ground clearance the robot will not much fall down (**Figure A5A**) since its body is already close to the ground and the remaining legs need not to carry much more load leading to lower power consumption compared to the high ground clearance case (**Figure A5B**), and they are able to swing during swing phase

(**Figures A5E,F**). As a result, the robot can still move better in a straight way (**Figure A5H** and **Video S10**). However, the drawback of having low ground clearance is that the robot could get stuck often when walking on non-flat terrains. Accordingly, during walking over rough terrains AMOS II will lift its body up to obtain higher ground clearance such that it does not get stuck. Lifting the body up is automatically done by shifting the center of the CTr-joint angles downwards (more depression) and the center of the FTi-joint angles upwards (more extension) and this is the default joint movements for rough terrains. By contrast, most walking machines (Lee et al., 2006; Spenneberg and Kirchner, 2007; Lewinger and Quinn, 2009) always perform locomotion with high ground clearance (**Video S12**). Although such a high ground clearance walking strategy could simplify it for the controller to deal with different terrains, it might lead to instability of the systems (as described above); unless, additional control mechanisms are applied (Spenneberg et al., 2004). In fact, the biologically-inspired locomotion strategy of AMOS II arises not only from biomechanics but is a combination of its biomechanics and adaptive neural locomotion control. While the biomechanics allows for leg and body movements as well as provides some degree of disturbance rejection, the adaptive neural locomotion controller generates versatile motions and adaptation.

The controller consists of two main parts: CPG-based control and local leg control. The CPG-based control is the improved version of our original chaotic CPG-based controller [compare **Figure A2** in Steingrube et al. (2010) with **Figure A2** of this paper]. Two main components of the controller have been modified here while the other parts remain unchanged. We replaced the chaotic CPG by a simpler CPG mechanism with neuromodulation. As a consequence, by exploiting neural dynamics of the new CPG mechanism, we can generate a multitude of walking patterns (e.g., 20 patterns). Some of these patterns are comparable to insect gaits (Wilson, 1966) and allow for energy-efficient locomotion on different terrains, like, fine gravel (loose terrain), gravel (rough terrain), and grass (vegetated terrain). The CPG also provides fast switching between the patterns compared with the chaotic CPG. For motor connections, we modified the connections to the FTi-motor neurons such that the FTi-joints are activated during walking while in the previous work these joints are inhibited; i.e., they stay in a flexed position. The introduced FTi-joint movements are inspired by insect leg movements (Ekeberg et al., 2004; Cruse et al., 2009). During the stance phase of forward walking, the FTi-joints of the front legs flex inward, of the hind legs extend outward, and of the middle legs combine these two movements by first flexion and then extension. As a consequence, the front, hind, and middle legs pull, push, and pull and push the body forward, respectively. This results in faster walking speed compared with the fixed FTi-joint version. This CPG-based control coordinating all joints can be considered as open-loop control since in principle it does not require any sensory feedback for the locomotion generation (i.e., multiple patterns and insect-like leg movements). However, the loop can be simply closed by using, e.g., exteroceptive sensory feedback to generate stimulus induced behavior (like, photo tropism and obstacle avoidance) as well as to select an energy-efficient gait with respect to the terrain in an autonomous manner.

In contrast to the CPG-based control, the local leg control introduced here for the first time employs proprioceptive sensory feedback (i.e., here only FC sensors) for adaptable locomotion. Thus it can be considered as closed-loop control. It has two components applied independently to each leg of AMOS II: an adaptive forward model with efference copy and searching and elevation control. The forward model is constructed by using a simple hysteresis neuron with recurrent connection. It can learn online to transform the CTr-motor signal (efference copy) into the expected FC signal. While the forward model is minimal and sufficient here, one could combine several of them to obtain different forward models for different purposes, e.g., sensory noise cancelation and slope detection (Manoonpong and Wörgötter, 2009) or use them for designing non-linear filters (Manoonpong et al., 2010). Due to our controller being modular, if desired, one could replace this simple hysteresis neuron by more complex neural networks [e.g., reservoir computing networks (Dasgupta et al., 2012)] for transforming motor commands into complex expected sensory signals.

Our forward model presented here can be considered as an adaptive predictor that can learn to predict the sensory consequences (expected sensory feedback) from motor commands (efference copy) (Kawato, 1999). The expected sensory feedback (or transformed motor command) is then used to compare it with the actual FC signal for the walking state estimation. The sensory prediction error enables AMOS II to determine whether its leg loses ground contact during the stance phase or hits or steps on any obstacles during the swing phase. Afterwards, this information is used to adapt the leg accordingly through the searching and elevation control. The adaptive leg motions (i.e., searching and elevation motions) follow the observed locomotion in certain insects, like locusts (Pearson and Franklin, 1984), cockroaches (Tryba and Ritzmann, 2000), and stick insects (Fischer et al., 2001), during walking on rough terrain. As a result, employing closed-loop local leg control mechanisms with the forward models allows AMOS II to not only successfully traverse rough terrains and climb over large obstacles, but to also cope with leg damage.

Besides special features described above, our adaptive neural locomotion controller also combines three key aspects found in animal locomotor control: central mechanism (CPGs) (Meyrand et al., 1991; Katz, 1998; Harris-Warrick, 2011), sensory feedback (afferent-based control) (Cruse et al., 2009), and internal forward models with efference copies (efferent-based control) (Holst and Mittelstaedt, 1950; Cruse et al., 1998; Bläsing and Cruse, 2004). In particular, our CPG-based control or central mechanism for versatile locomotion generation relies on a CPG mechanism with neuronmodulation that is inspired by the function of neural CPG circuits found in lobsters (Selverston et al., 1993; Pulver and Marder, 2002) and the mollusc *Tritonia diomedea* (Katz et al., 1994). These biological findings suggest that extrinsic and intrinsic neuromodulatory inputs to the CPG circuits can alter the cellular changes and synaptic properties of neurons in the circuits. Thereby, these inputs modify the output of the CPG leading to behavioral flexibility and different locomotion modes. This process can be achieved on the fly resulting in the adaptation of behavior to environmental changes in an ongoing fashion. Our local leg control mechanisms based on sensory feedback

(afferent-based control) and adaptive neural forward models with efference copies (efferent-based control) for state estimation and adaptable locomotion follows the evidence of forward model predictions with sensory feedback in the stick insects *Aretaon asperrimus*. It shows that during climbing over very large gaps the stick insects perform an immediate change in the stepping pattern of the legs when losing ground contact at the end of the swing phase (Bläsing and Cruse, 2004). This would reflect an expectation of regular ground contacts. Other results supporting the idea of forward model predictions (Cruse et al., 1998) indicate that, during the swing phase of the stick insects, reactions to obstacles depend on an internal state.

While these three key aspects are essential for locomotion control, some works have taken these aspects into account for developing locomotion control in simulation (Kuo, 2002; Dürr et al., 2003). Only a few have successfully applied it to a real system but with small numbers of inputs and outputs and behavioral restrictions (Lewis and Simo, 2001; Lewis and Bekey, 2002), thereby, reducing the sensor-motor coordination problem substantially. Most studies use a combination of several CPGs and sensory feedback to generate different walking behaviors (Beer et al., 1997; Harischandra et al., 2011) including reflexes (Kimura et al., 2007; Spenneberg and Kirchner, 2007; Lewinger and Quinn, 2011; von Twickel et al., 2012). The reflexes driven by only sensory feedback results in searching and elevation actions when losing ground contact and hitting an obstacle, respectively. However, due to the lack of forward model predictions (internal state) this control approach has difficulties to generate reactions for walking machines to avoid an obstacle when stepping on it during swing phase as the stick insects do. Another interesting approach, like "Walknet" (Cruse et al., 2007), has no central control unit. Instead, it uses a decentralized control architecture with local coordination rules highly depending on different types of proprioceptive sensory feedback, e.g., FC, joint angle, and joint angular velocity signals, to determine an internal state and generate basic locomotion and adaptation. However, this mechanism malfunctions when losing the sensory information, thereby it is less robust.

In contrast to this, our adaptive neural locomotion controller based on a modular structure is robust and has fault tolerance capabilities. Damage to a part of the system can result in a loss of some of the abilities of the system, but, the whole system can still function partially (see the leg damage experiment in **Figure 12**). Its modules (**Figures 2, A2**) generally have a simpler structure as compared to the network as a whole. Thus, their functions and dynamics are analyzable by observing the input/output relationship of an individual module (Manoonpong et al., 2007, 2008b). Its individual modules have been used in earlier studies and successfully provided partial solutions to different walking machines (Manoonpong et al., 2007, 2008b). Furthermore, the controller, using a single CPG, sensory feedback, and forward model predictions providing an internal state, can generate a multitude of walking patterns (e.g., 20 walking patterns), insect-like leg movements, energy-efficient locomotion, and adaptable locomotion (like searching and elevation actions including reactions when stepping on an obstacle during swing phase). It can also handle leg damage and even generate cockroach-like climbing behavior (**Video S12**) when additional reactive BJ control is applied (Goldschmidt et al., 2012). The controller can also be simply transferred to another six-legged walking machine having a different morphology but leg lengths with similar proportion to AMOS II. In this case, the internal network structure and parameters of its CPG-based control (**Figure 2**, left) remain unchanged. We set *MI* of the CPG to 0.15; thereby, the controller generates a tripod gait with a walking frequency of approximately 0.8 Hz for the machine (**Video S13**). Only the maximum and minimum ranges of the joint movements of the legs and the neural parameters of the adaptive forward models (**Figure 2**, right) are different. The neural parameters are adapted to the new system by using the online learning mechanism (Equations 8–9). In principle, applying the controller to other different walking machines might be necessary to also adjust generated walking frequency (i.e., operating range of *MI* of the CPG). The capability of the controller which combines the key aspects of the biological locomotion systems to achieve a very rich behavioral repertoire in an autonomous fashion, to the best of our knowledge, has not been achieved in other walking machine systems so far.

Taken together this work suggests how a CPG mechanism with neuromodulation, sensory feedback, and internal forward models with efference copies can be used for controlling complex robots. It further confirms that this combination plays an important role for locomotion in biological as well as artificial systems. The results presented here show that the employed embodied neural closed-loop system can be an option for developing robust and adaptable machines, thereby bringing the goal of approaching living creatures in their levels of performance a little bit closer. As the controller is modular, it is flexible and offers the future possibility of integrating joint angle and joint CS signals as feedback together with additional entrainment and reflexive mechanisms (Takemura et al., 2005; Cruse et al., 2009; Nachstedt et al., 2012) to avoid leg slipping which currently occurs when the legs work partially against each other. The controller can also be extended to multiple CPGs (Ren et al., 2012) in order to be able to adjust the frequency of each leg individually for some situations like gap crossing (Bläsing, 2006) or damage compensation (Ren et al., 2012). It even can be combined with other neural modules like short term motor memory (Dasgupta et al., 2012) and muscle models (Xiong et al., 2012). This will enable the robotic system to be capable of navigating in complex environments with a certain degree of memory-guided behaviors and at the same time performing more natural movements with active compliances.

ACKNOWLEDGMENTS

This research was supported by the Emmy Noether Program of the Deutsche Forschungsgemeinschaft (DFG, MA4464/3-1), the Federal Ministry of Education and Research (BMBF) by a grant to the Bernstein Center for Computational Neuroscience II Göttingen (01GQ1005A, project D1), and European Communitys Seventh Framework Programme FP7/2007–2013 (Specific Programme Cooperation, Theme 3, Information and Communication Technologies) under grant agreement no. 270273, Xperience. We thank Steffen Zenker, Eren Erdal Aksoy, Xiaofeng Xiong, Eduard Grinke, and Dennis Goldschmidt for technical assistance and Frank Hesse for discussions.

SUPPLEMENTARY MATERIAL

The Supplementary Material for this article can be found online at: http://www.frontiersin.org/Neural_Circuits/10.3389/fncir.2013.00012/abstract

Video S1 | Comparison of gait switching using a CPG with neuromodulation and a chaotic CPG. Using a CPG with neuromodulation, AMOS II shows fast and smooth switching between gaits, while the switching is slower and less smooth when using our previous chaotic CPG. (http://manoonpong.com/Frontiers/SupplementaryVideo1.wmv)

Video S2 | Examples of 20 different walking patterns. AMOS II walks with different patterns from slow to fast speed with respect to $MI = 0.0, 0.01, \ldots, 0.19$. (http://manoonpong.com/Frontiers/SupplementaryVideo2.wmv)

Video S3 | Turning behavior. AMOS II autonomously turns to avoid obstacles and escape from a corner and even a deadlock situation. It detects obstacles and a corner by using its ultrasonic sensors installed at front. (http://manoonpong.com/Frontiers/SupplementaryVideo3.wmv)

Video S4 | Insect-like leg movements. To clearly observe the insect-liked leg movements of AMOS II, we place it on a box and let it perform forward and backward walking. (http://manoonpong.com/Frontiers/SupplementaryVideo4.wmv)

Video S5 | Leg elevation. To clearly observe the leg elevation of AMOS II, we place it on a box and make the foot touch an obstacle during the swing phase. Due to mismatch between the expected foot contact signal, generated by the adaptive forward model, and the actual one, AMOS II can immediately elevate its leg (here right middle leg) to free the leg from the obstacle. In addition, we show that using an IR sensor at the leg also allows AMOS II to elevate its leg in order to avoid hitting the obstacle. The first part of this video corresponds to the result shown in **Figures 7G–J** of the manuscript. (http://manoonpong.com/Frontiers/SupplementaryVideo5.wmv)

Video S6 | Searching for a foothold. To clearly observe searching for a foothold of AMOS II, we place it on a box and change the ground level during the stance phase. Due to mismatch between the expected foot contact signal, generated by the adaptive forward model, and the actual one, AMOS II can immediately lowers its leg (here right middle leg) to search for a foothold. This video corresponds to the result shown in **Figures 7C–F** of the manuscript. (http://manoonpong.com/Frontiers/SupplementaryVideo6.wmv)

Video S7 | Energy-efficient and adaptable locomotion on different terrains. First test shows that AMOS II walks with a fast wave gait since it detects fine gravel (loose terrain) using its visual system. Afterward, it changes from the wave gait to a tetrapod gait since it detects gravel (rough terrain). Finally, it uses a fast tripod gait on the floor (hard terrain). Another test in an outdoor environment shows that AMOS II walks with a tetrapod gait since it detects gravel (rough terrain). Afterward, it changes from the tetrapod gait to a tripod gait since it detects grass (vegetated terrain). Note that during traversing the different terrains, AMOS II adapts its legs individually to the terrains. The first part of this video corresponds to the result shown in **Figure 9** of the manuscript and the second part of this video corresponds to the result shown in **Figure A4**. (http://manoonpong.com/Frontiers/SupplementaryVideo7.wmv)

Video S8 | Adaptable locomotion on terrain with small obstacles. First test shows that AMOS II can free its right front leg after the leg hits an obstacle during the swing phase. Due to the difference of the ground level, AMOS II also adapts its legs by lowering them more downward to ensure ground contact during the stance phase. Other tests also show this kind of adaptable locomotion of AMOS II. The first part of this video corresponds to the result shown in **Figure 10** of the manuscript. (http://manoonpong.com/Frontiers/SupplementaryVideo8.wmv)

Video S9 | Climbing over a large obstacle in an outdoor environment. AMOS II walks on rough terrain and then climbs over an 11 cm high obstacle. This video corresponds to the results shown in **Figure 11** of the manuscript. (http://manoonpong.com/Frontiers/SupplementaryVideo9.wmv)

Video S10 | Adaptable locomotion during leg damage. While AMOS II is walking, we disconnect the motor power connector of the FTi-joint of its left middle leg to simulate leg damage. Local leg control allows AMOS II to adapt its legs to deal with the leg damage. As a result, it could still move forward without problem. This first part of the video corresponds to the results shown in **Figure 12** of the manuscript. Another test is shown in the second part of the video. The third part of the video shows that AMOS II fails to cope with leg damage if local leg control is not activated. The last part of the video shows walking behaviors with low and high ground clearance during leg damage. (http://manoonpong.com/Frontiers/SupplementaryVideo10.wmv)

Video S11 | Passive compliances of the joints and legs of AMOS II. The joint compliance enables AMOS II to passively flex its legs to avoid damages when the environment changes. In addition, its leg compliance allows it to absorb external (ground reaction) forces. (http://manoonpong.com/Frontiers/SupplementaryVideo11.wmv)

Video S12 | Walking and climbing like a cockroach. AMOS II keeps its body very close to the ground during walking. While climbing, it uses its active backbone joint and leg adaptation. The video also compares its locomotion with cockroaches and other walking machines [four legs (Quadruped robot of the Stanford AI Lab, http://ai.stanford.edu), six legs (BILL-Ant-a robot of Case Biorobotics Lab, http://biorobots.cwru.edu/), eight legs (Scorpion robot of DFKI Bremen - Robotics Innovation Center, http://robotik.dfki-bremen.de/)]. Note that cockroach videos are referred to (Ritzmann et al., 2004; Abbott, 2007; Lewinger and Quinn, 2009) while the walking machine videos are referred to (Lee et al., 2006; Spenneberg and Kirchner, 2007; Lewinger and Quinn, 2009). (http://manoonpong.com/Frontiers/SupplementaryVideo12.wmv)

Video S13 | Testing the adaptive neural locomotion controller on another six-legged walking machine. We transfer the adaptive neural locomotion controller to another walking machine. We set MI of the CPG to 0.15; thereby, the controller generates a tripod gait with a walking frequency of approximately 0.8 Hz for the machine. As a result, the controller allows the machine to perform foothold searching when its leg loses ground contact, to adapt its locomotion to deal with irregular terrain or different ground levels, and to climb over a 7 cm high obstacle. For climbing, additional reactive active backbone joint control is also applied. (http://manoonpong.com/Frontiers/SupplementaryVideo13.wmv)

REFERENCES

Akay, T., Ludwar, B., Goritz, M., Schmitz, J., and Büschges, A. (2007). Segment specificity of load signal processing depends on walking direction in the stick insect leg muscle control system. *J. Neurosci.* 27, 3285–3294.

Alexander, R. (1982). *Locomotion of Animals.* Glasgow: Blackie.

Amrollah, E., and Henaff, P. (2010). On the role of sensory feedbacks in rowat-selverston cpg to improve robot legged locomotion. *Front. Neurorobot.* 4:113. doi: 10.3389/fnbot.2010.00113

Beer, R., Quinn, R., Chiel, H., and Ritzmann, R. (1997). Biologically inspired approaches to robotics: what can we learn from insects? *Commun. ACM* 40, 30–38.

Bläsing, B. (2006). Crossing large gaps: a simulation study of stick insect behavior. *Adapt. Behav.* 14, 265–286.

Bläsing, B., and Cruse, H. (2004). Mechanisms of stick insect locomotion in a gap crossing paradigm. *J. Comp. Physiol. A* 190, 173–183.

Brooks, R. A. (1986). A robust layered control systems for a mobile robot. *IEEE J. Robot. Autom.* 2, 14–23.

Büschges, A. (2005). Sensory control and organization of neural networks mediating coordination of multi-segmental organs for locomotion. *J. Neurophysiol.* 93, 1127–1135.

Chadil, N., Phadoognsidhi, M., Suwannasit, K., Manoonpong, P., and Laksanacharoen, P. (2011). "A reconfigurable spherical robot," in *Proceedings of the IEEE International Conference on Robotics and Automation,* (Shanghai), 2380–2385.

Cham, J., Bailey, S., Clark, J., Full, R., and Cutkosky, M. (2002). Fast and robust: hexapedal robots via shape deposition manufacturing. *Int. J. Robot. Res.* 21, 869–883.

Cortes, C., and Vapnik, V. (1995). Support-vector networks. *Mach. Learn.* 20, 273–297.

Cruse, H., Dürr, V., Schilling, M., and Schmitz, J. (2009). "Principles of insect locomotion," in *Spatial Temporal Patterns for Action-Oriented Perception in Roving Robots,* Cognitive Systems Monographs, Vol. 1, eds P. Arena and L. Patanè (Berlin: Springer), 43–96.

Cruse, H., Dürr, V., and Schmitz, J. (2007). Insect walking is based on a decentralized architecture revealing a simple and robust controller. *Philos. Trans. A Math. Phys. Eng. Sci.* 365, 221–250.

Cruse, H., Kindermann, T., Schumm, M., Dean, J., and Schmitz, J. (1998). WALKNET – a biologically inspired network to control six-legged walking. *Neural Netw.* 11, 1435–1447.

Dasgupta, S., Wörgötter, F., and Manoonpong, P. (2012). "Information theoretic self-organised adaptation in reservoirs for temporal memory tasks," in *Proceedings of the International Conference on 13th Engineering Applications of Neural Network Conference (EANN2012), Vol. 311,* (London), 31–40. CCIS.

Daun-Gruhn, S., and Büschges, A. (2011). From neuron to behavior: dynamic equation-based prediction of biological processes in motor control. *Biol. Cybern.* 105, 71–88.

Dickinson, M., Farley, C., Full, R., Koehl, M., Kram, R., and Lehman, S. (2000). How animals move: an integrative view. *Science* 288, 100–106.

Dürr, V., Krause, A., Schmitz, J., and Cruse, H. (2003). Neuroethological concepts and their transfer to walking machines. *Int. J. Robot. Res.* 22, 151–167.

Ekeberg, O., Blümel, M., and Büschges, A. (2004). Dynamic simulation of insect walking. *Arthropod Struct. Dev.* 33, 287–300.

Erden, M., and Leblebicioglu, K. (2008). Free gait generation with reinforcement learning for a six-legged robot. *Robot. Auton. Syst.* 56, 199–212.

Fischer, H., Schmidt, J., Haas, R., and Büschges, A. (2001). Pattern generation for walking and searching movements of a stick insect leg. i. coordination of motor activity. *J. Neurophysiol.* 85, 341–353.

Fuchs, E., Holmes, P., Kiemel, T., and Ayali, A. (2011). Intersegmental coordination of cockroach locomotion: adaptive control of centrally coupled pattern generator circuits. *Front. Neural Circuits* 4:125. doi: 10.3389/fncir.2010.00125

Gabriel, J., and Büschges, A. (2007). Control of stepping velocity in a single insect leg during walking. *Philos. Trans. R. Soc. A* 365, 251–271.

Goldschmidt, D., Wörgötter, F., and Manoonpong, P. (2012). "Biologically inspired reactive climbing behavior of hexapod robots," in *Proceedings of the IEEE International Conference on Intelligent Robots and Systems,* (Vilamoura, Algarve), 4632–4637.

Grillner, S. (2006). Biological pattern generation: the cellular and computational logic of networks in motion. *Neuron* 52, 751–766.

Harischandra, N., Knuesel, J., Kozlov, A., Bicanski, A., Cabelguen, J.-M., Ijspeert, A., et al. (2011). Sensory feedback plays a significant role in generating walking gait and in gait transition in salamanders:a simulation study. *Front. Neurorobot.* 5:3. doi: 10.3389/fnbot.2011.00003

Harris-Warrick, R. M. (2011). Neuromodulation and flexibility in central pattern generator networks. *Curr. Opin. Neurobiol.* 21, 1–8.

Holst, E. V., and Mittelstaedt, H. (1950). Das Reafferenzprinzip. *Naturwissenschaften* 37, 464–476.

Iida, F., and Pfeifer, R. (2004). Cheap rapid locomotion of a quadruped robot: self-stabilization of bounding gait. *Intell. Auton. Syst.* 8, 642–649.

Ishiguro, A., Fujii, A., and Hotz, P. E. (2003). Neuromodulated control of bipedal locomotion using a polymorphic CPG circuit. *Adapt. Behav.* 11, 7–17.

Katz, P., Getting, P., and Frost, W. (1994). Dynamic neuromodulation of synaptic strength intrinsic to a central pattern generator circuit. *Nature* 367, 729–731.

Katz, P. S. (1998). Comparison of extrinsic and intrinsic neuromodulation in two central pattern generator circuits in invertebrates. *Exp. Physiol.* 83, 281–292.

Kawato, M. (1999). Internal models for motor control and trajectory planning. *Curr. Opin. Neurobiol.* 9, 718–727.

Kimura, H., Fukuoka, Y., and Cohen, A. H. (2007). Adaptive dynamic walking of a quadruped robot on natural ground based on biological concepts. *Int. J. Robot. Res.* 26, 475–490.

Kingsley, D., Quinn, R., and Ritzmann, R. (2006). "A cockroach inspired robot with artificial muscles," in *Proceedings of the IEEE International Conference on Intelligent Robots and Systems,* (Beijing), 1837–1842.

Kuo, A. (2002). The relative roles of feedforward and feedback in the control of rhythmic movements. *Motor Control* 6, 129–145.

Lee, H., Shen, Y., Yu, C.-H., Singh, G., and Ng, A. Y. (2006). "Quadruped robot obstacle negotiation via reinforcement learning," in *Proceedings of the IEEE International Conference on Robotics and Automation.* (Orlando, FL).

Lewinger, W., Harley, C., Ritzmann, R., Branicky, M., and Quinn, R. (2005). "Insect-like antennal sensing for climbing and tunneling behavior in a biologically-inspired mobile robot," in *Proceedings of the IEEE International Conference on Robotics and Automation*, (Barcelona), 4176–4181.

Lewinger, W. A., and Quinn, R. D. (2009). "A small autonomous agile robot with an on-board neurologically-based control system," in *Proceedings of the IEEE International Conference on Intelligent Robots and Systems,* (St. Louis, MO), 412–413.

Lewinger, W. A., and Quinn, R. D. (2011). Neurobiologically-based control system for an adaptively walking hexapod. *Ind. Robot.* 38, 258–263.

Lewis, M. A., and Bekey, G. A. (2002). Gait adaptation in a quadruped robot. *Auton. Robot.* 12, 301–312.

Lewis, M. A., and Simo, L. S. (2001). Certain principles of biomorphic robots. *Auton. Robot.* 11, 221–226.

Lowe, D. G. (2004). Distinctive image features from scale-invariant keypoints. *Int. J. Comput. Vis.* 60, 91–110.

Manoonpong, P., Pasemann, F., Kolodziejski, C., and Wörgötter, F. (2010). "Designing simple nonlinear filters using hysteresis of single recurrent neurons for acoustic signal recognition in robots," in *Proceedings of the International Conference on International Conference on Artificial Neural Networks (ICANN2010), Vol. LNCS 6352,* (Thessaloniki), 374–383.

Manoonpong, P., Pasemann, F., and Roth, H. (2007). Modular reactive neurocontrol for biologically-inspired walking machines. *Int. J. Robot. Res.* 26, 301–331.

Manoonpong, P., Pasemann, F., and Wörgötter, F. (2008a). Reactive neural control for phototaxis and obstacle avoidance behavior of walking machines. *Int. J. Mech. Syst. Sci. Eng.* 1, 172–177.

Manoonpong, P., Pasemann, F., and Wörgötter, F. (2008b). Sensor-driven neural control for omnidirectional locomotion and versatile reactive behaviors of walking machines. *Robot. Auton. Syst.* 56, 265–288.

Manoonpong, P., and Wörgötter, F. (2009). Efference copies in neural control of dynamic biped walking. *Robot. Auton. Syst.* 57, 1140–1153.

Meyrand, P., Simmers, J., and Moulins, M. (1991). Construction of a pattern-generating circuit with

neurons of different networks. *Nature* 351, 60–63.

Mulloney, B., and Smarandache, C. (2010). Fifty years of cpgs: two neuroethological papers that shaped the course of neuroscience. *Front. Behav. Neurosci.* 4:45. doi: 10.3389/fnbeh.2010.00045

Nachstedt, T., Wörgötter, F., and Manoonpong, P. (2012). "Adaptive neural oscillator with synaptic plasticity enabling fast resonance tuning," in *Proceedings of the International Conference on Artificial Neural Networks (ICANN2012), Vol. LNCS 7552,* (Lausanne), 451–458.

Owaki, D., Kano, T., Nagasawa, K., Tero, A., and Ishiguro, A. (2012). Simple robot suggests physical interlimb communication is essential for quadruped walking. *J. R. Soc. Interface.* doi: 10.1098/rsif.2012.0669.   [Epub ahead of print].

Pasemann, F. (1993). Dynamics of a single model neuron. *Int. J. Bifurcat. Chaos* 2, 271–278.

Pasemann, F., Hild, M., and Zahedi, K. (2003). "So(2)-networks as neural oscillators," in *Proceedings of the International Work-Conference on Artificial and Natural Networks, 2686,* (Maó, Menorca), 144–151.

Pearson, K., and Franklin, R. (1984). Characteristics of leg movements and patterns of coordination in locusts walking on rough terrain. *Int. J. Robot. Res.* 3, 101–112.

Pearson, K., and Iles, J. (1973). Nervous mechanisms underlying intersegmental coordination of leg movements during walking in the cockroach. *J. Exp. Biol.* 58, 725–744.

Pulver, S., and Marder, E. (2002). Neuromodulatory complement of the pericardial organ in the embryonic lobster, *Homarus americanus*. *J. Comp. Neurol.* 451, 79–90.

Ren, G., Chen, W., Kolodziejski, C., Wörgötter, F., Dasgupta, S., and Manoonpong, P. (2012). "Multiple chaotic central pattern generators for locomotion generation and leg damage compensation in a hexapod robot," in *Proceedings of the IEEE International Conference on Intelligent Robots and Systems*, 2756–2761.

Ritzmann, R., Harley, C., Daltorio, K., Tietz, B., Pollack, A., Bender, J., et al. (2012). Deciding which way to go: how do insects alter movements to negotiate barriers? *Front. Neurosci.* 6:97. doi: 10.3389/fnins.2012.00097

Ritzmann, R., Quinn, R., and Fischer, M. (2004). Convergent evolution and locomotion through complex terrain by insects, vertebrates and

robots. *Arthropod Struct. Dev.* 33, 361–379.

Rumelhart, D. E., Hinton, G. E., and Williams, R. J. (1986). "Parallel distributed processing: explorations in the microstructure of cognition," in *Chap. Learning Internal Representations by Error Propagation, Vol. 1.* eds J. A. Feldman, P. J. Hayes, and D. E. Rumelhart (Cambridge, MA: MIT Press), 318–362.

Schneider, A., Paskarbeit, J., Schaeffersmann, M., and Schmitz, J. (2012). "HECTOR, a new hexapod robot platform with increased mobility – control approach, design and communication," in *Advances in Autonomous Mini Robots*, eds U. Rückert, S. Joaquin, and W. Felix (Bielefeld: Springer), 249–264.

Schroeder-Schetelig, J., Manoonpong, P., and Wörgötter, F. (2010). Using efference copy and a forward internal model for adaptive biped walking. *Auton. Robot.* 29, 357–366.

Selverston, A., Rowat, P., and Boyle, M. (1993). "Modeling a reprogrammable central pattern generating network," in *Locomotion Control in Legged Invertebrates on Biological Neural Networks in Invertebrate Neuroethology and Robotics*, eds R. D. Beer, R. E. Ritzmann, and T. McKenna (San Diego, CA: Academic Press Professional, Inc.), 229–250.

Shkolnik, A., and Tedrake, R. (2007). "Inverse kinematics for a point-foot quadruped robot with dynamic redundancy resolution," in *Proceedings of the IEEE International Conference on Robotics and Automation*, (Rome), 4331–4336.

Spenneberg, D., and Kirchner, F. (2007). "The bio-inspired scorpion robot: design, control & lessons learned," in *Climbing & Walking Robots, Towards New Applications*, eds M. Xie, S. Dubowsky, J.-G. Fontaine, M. O. Tokhi, and G. S. Virk (Singapore: World Scientific), 197–218.

Spenneberg, D., McCullough, K., and Kirchner, F. (2004). "Stability of walking in a multilegged robot suffering leg loss," in *Proceedings of the IEEE International Conference on Robotics and Automation, Vol. 3,* 2159–2164.

Steingrube, S., Timme, M., Wörgötter, F., and Manoonpong, P. (2010). Self-organized adaptation of simple neural circuits enables complex robot behavior. *Nat. Phys.* 6, 224–230.

Takemura, H., Deguchi, M., Ueda, J., Matsumoto, Y., and Ogasawara,

T. (2005). Slip-adaptive walk of quadruped robot. *Robot. Auton. Syst.* 53, 124–141.

Tetzlaff, C., Kolodziejski, C., Timme, M., and Wörgötter, F. (2011). Synaptic scaling in combination with many generic plasticity mechanisms stabilizes circuit connectivity. *Front Comput. Neurosci.* 5:47. doi: 10.3389/fncom.2011.00047

Tryba, A., and Ritzmann, R. (2000). Multi-joint coordination during walking and foothold searching in the Blaberus cockroach. I. Kinematics and electromyograms. *J. Neurophysiol.* 83, 3323–3336.

von Twickel, A., Hild, M., Siedel, T., Patel, V., and Pasemann, F. (2012). Neural control of a modular multilegged walking machine: simulation and hardware. *Robot. Auton. Syst.* 60, 227–241.

Wilson, D. M. (1966). Insect walking. *Annu. Rev. Entomol.* 11, 103–122.

Xiong, X., Wörgötter, F., and Manoonpong, P. (2012). "A virtual musculoskeletal model for variable compliance and joint stabilization of a walking hexapod," in *Front. Comput. Neurosci. Conference Abstract: Bernstein Conference 2012.* (Munich).

Zhang, Y., Jin, R., and Zhou, Z.-H. (2010). Distinctive image features from scale-invariant keypoints. *Int. J. Mach. Learn. and Cyber.* 1, 43–52.

Zill, S., Schmitz, J., and Büschges, A. (2004). Load sensing and control of posture and locomotion. *Arthropod Struct. Dev.* 33, 273–286.

APPENDIX

THE WALKING MACHINE PLATFORM AMOS II (BIOMECHANICS)

The most important specification of AMOS II is presented in the main text of the manuscript. Therefore, we only provide here a clear picture of the active backbone joint (BJ) of AMOS II including its angle range (see **Figure A1**, left). Its minimum downward position ($-45°$) is comparable to the one observed in a cockroach (see **Figure A1**, right). Due to the mechanical design of the BJ, it allows the joint to also lean upwards to a maximum position of $45°$. The leaning upward and downward motions are used for climbing over a large obstacle having a height up to 13 cm or 75% of the leg length of AMOS II.

COMPLETE NEURAL CIRCUIT

Figure A2 shows the complete neural circuit of the adaptive locomotion controller. The controller generates versatile locomotion behavior of AMOS II by means of CPG-based control and local leg control (see main text for details). In total the controller has six neural modules where the modules I–IV belong to the CPG-based control and the modules V, VI belong to the local leg control.

Module I (CPG with neuromodulation): MI = modulatory input; $C_{1,2}$ = output neurons of the CPG. We use a hyperbolic tangent (tanh) transfer function for the CPG neurons.

Module II (neural CPG postprocessing): $CP_{1,2}$ = postprocessing neurons with a step function; $Int_{1,2}$ = integrator units.

Module III (neural motor control): $I_{1,...,4}$ = neural control parameters for generating different walking directions and stopping motion; $H_{1,...,14}$ = interneurons of the phase switching network (PSN); $H_{15,...,28}$ = interneurons of the velocity regulating networks (VRNs). We use a tanh transfer function for the interneurons. Parameters are $A = 1.7246$, $B = -2.48285$, and $C = -1.7246$.

Module IV (motor neurons): $M_{1,...,5}$ = premotor neurons; TR_1, CR_1, FR_1 = TC-, CTr- and FTi-motor neurons of the right front leg (R1); TR_2, CR_2, FR_2 = right middle leg (R2); TR_3, CR_3, FR_3 = right hind leg (R3); TL_1, CL_1, FL_1 = left front leg (L1); TL_2, CL_2, FL_2 = left middle leg (L2); TL_3, CL_3, FL_3 = left hind leg (L3); BJ = a backbone motor neuron which is controlled by reactive BJ control [not shown here but see Goldschmidt et al. (2012)]; τ = ipsilateral lag (i.e., 16 time steps or ≈ 0.6 s); τ_L = the phase shift between both left and right sides (i.e., 48 time steps or ≈ 2 s). We use piecewise linear transfer functions for the premotor and motor neurons.

Module V (adaptive neural forward models): $F_{1,...,6}$ = adaptive hysteresis neurons for motor signal transformation; W_I, W_R, B = learning parameters; $P_{1,...,6}$ = postprocessing neurons; Δ = an error between the expected foot contact (FC) signal and the actual one. We use a tanh transfer function for the hysteresis and postprocessing neurons.

Module VI (searching and elevation control): $PD_{1,...,6}$ = preprocessing neurons which provide only a positive error ($+\Delta$); $ND_{1,...,6}$ = preprocessing neurons which provide only a negative error ($-\Delta$); $E_{1,...,6} = S_{1,...,6}$ = recurrent neurons (i.e., accumulators). We use piecewise linear transfer functions for the preprocessing neurons and use a linear transfer function for the recurrent neurons.

Note that in all modules, all numbers are synaptic weights and the ones marked with subscript "B" refer to fixed bias terms.

Different exteroceptive and proprioceptive sensors are used here as inputs to the adaptive controller to generate stimulus induced behavior, energy-efficient gait, and adaptable locomotion. The sensors are: left and right ultrasonic sensors (US), six FC sensors ($FC_{1,...,6}$), one USB camera (CM), six infrared reflex (IR) sensors ($IR_{1,...,6}$), one current sensor (CS), and left and right light dependent sensors (LD). All raw sensory signals are preprocessed using neural preprocessing except the visual signal which is done by using an online feature-based terrain classification algorithm.

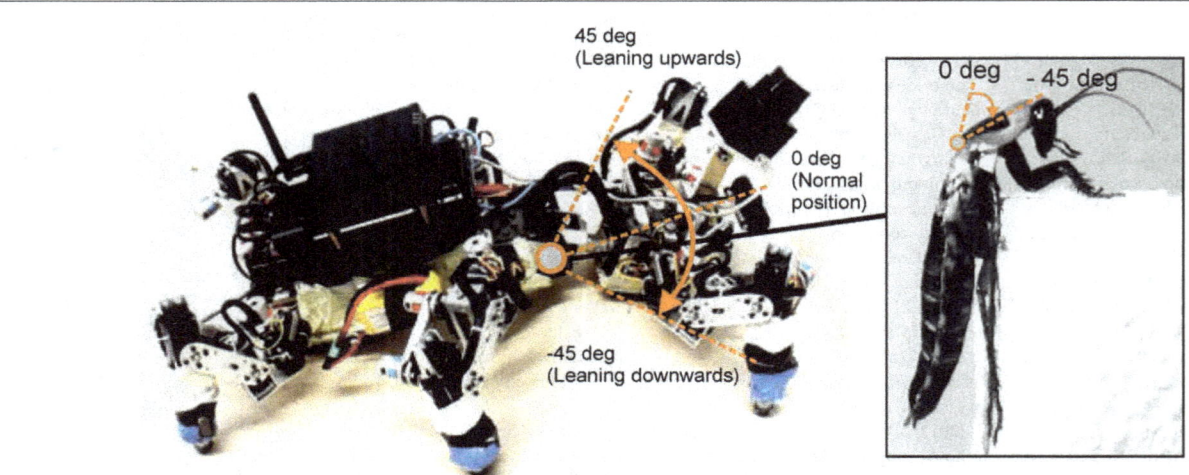

FIGURE A1 | The six-legged walking machine AMOS II inspired by the morphology of a cockroach. Left: Climbing position of AMOS II with a body flexion joint. **Right:** Climbing position of a cockroach. It can bend its front body downwards to keep the legs close to the surface of an object for an optimum climbing position and even to prevent unstable actions (modified from Ritzmann et al., 2004).

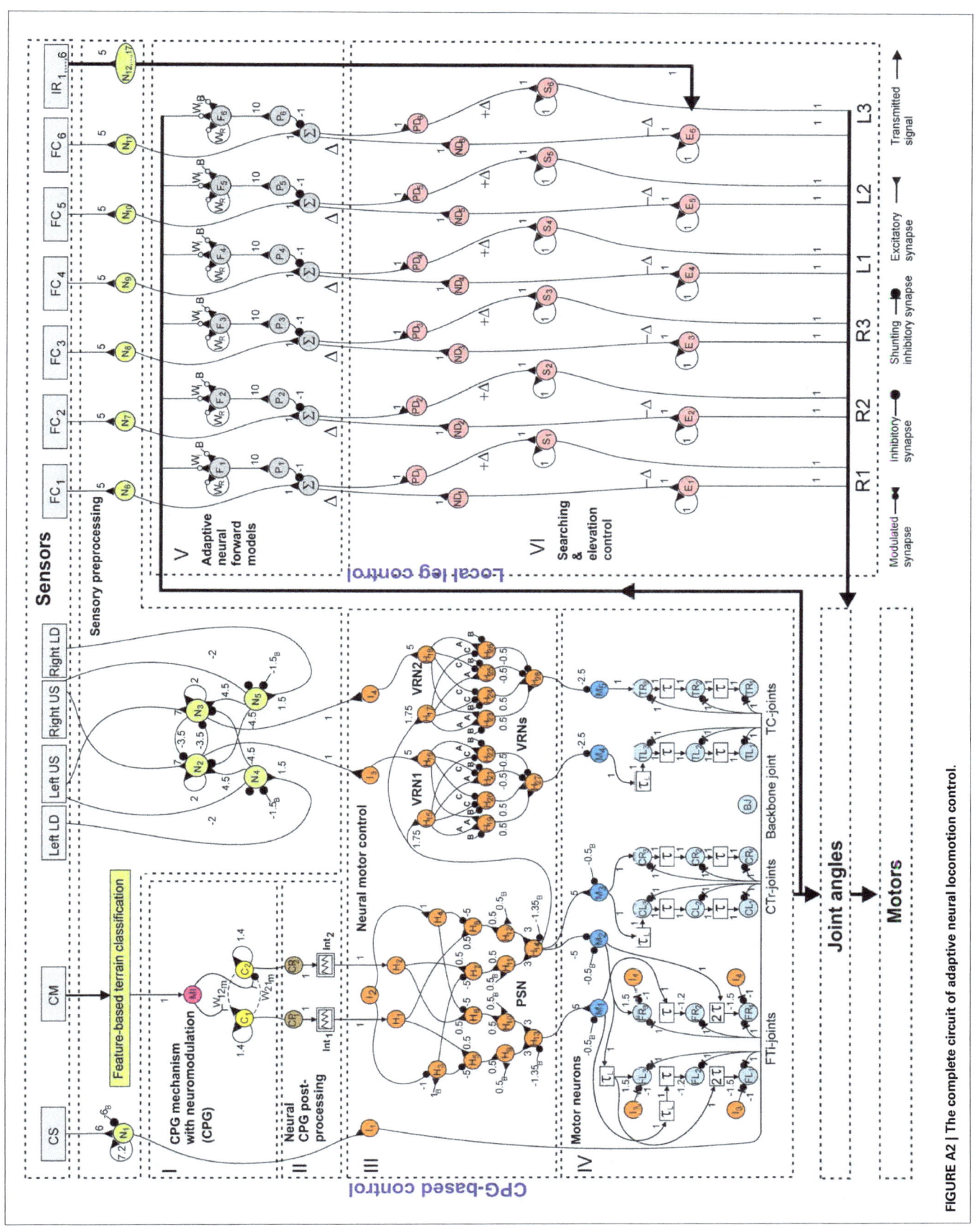

FIGURE A2 | The complete circuit of adaptive neural locomotion control.

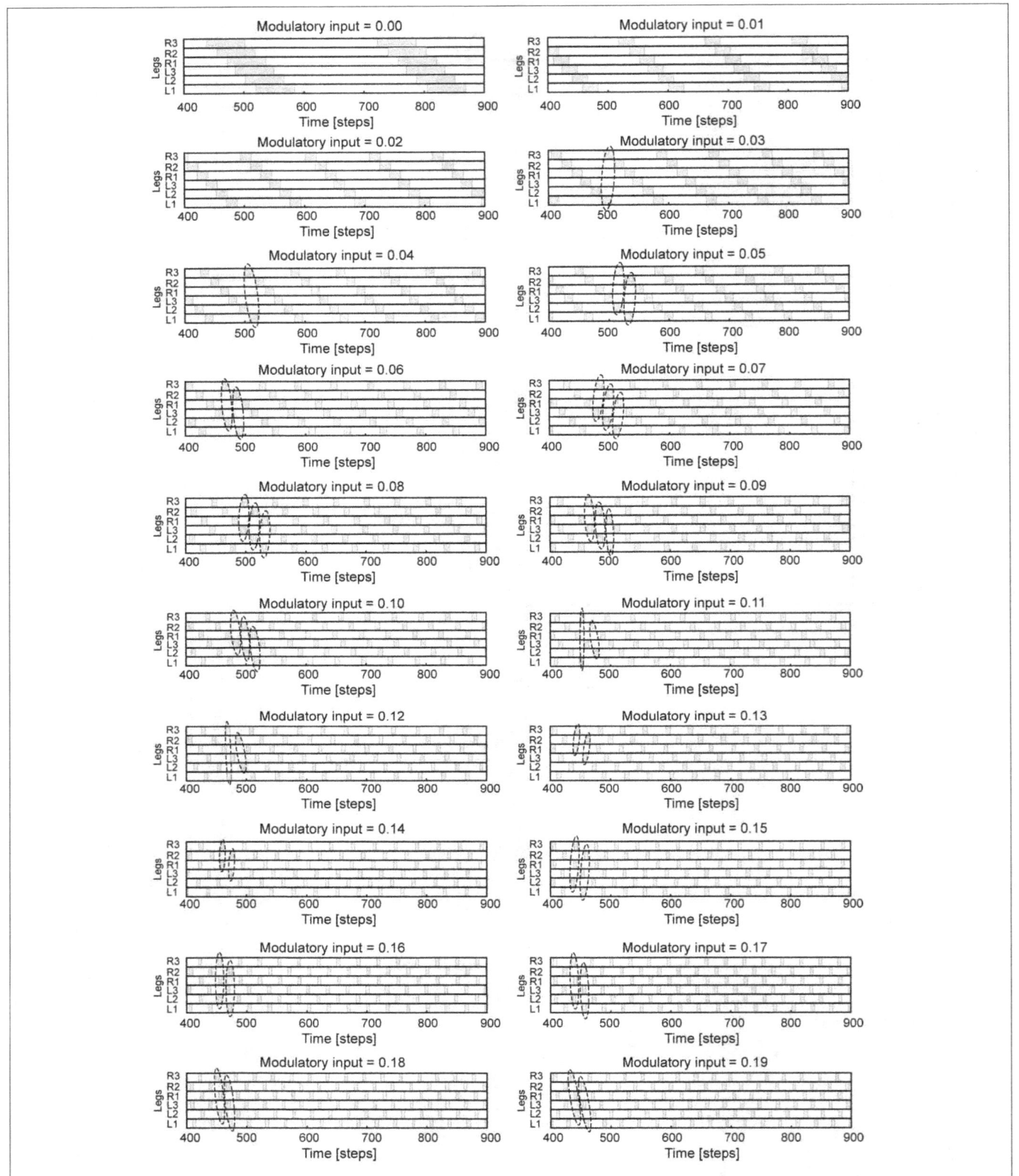

FIGURE A3 | 20 different walking patterns of AMOS II. The patterns are observed from the motor signals of the CTr-joints. White areas indicate ground contact or stance phase and gray areas refer to no ground contact during swing phase. As frequency increases, some legs steps in pairs (dashed enclosures). One time step is ≈0.037 s.

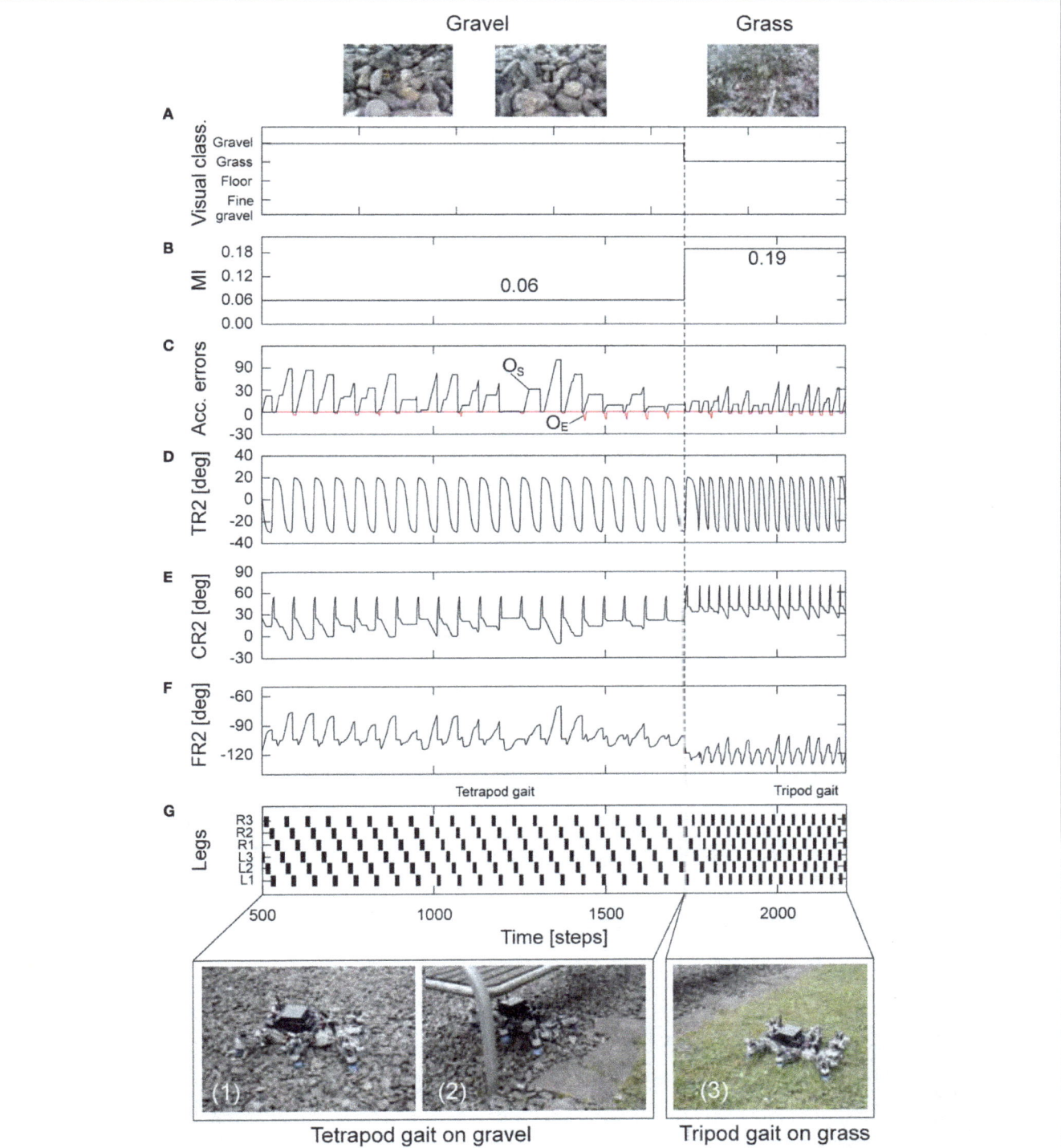

FIGURE A4 | Real-time data for energy-efficient and adaptable locomotion on two different terrains in an outdoor environment. (A) The output of the online terrain classification which is a preprocessed visual sensory signal. **(B)** The modulatory input *MI* of the CPG which is directly controlled by the sensory signal. It was set to 0.06 (tetrapod gait) and then 0.19 (fast tripod gait). **(C)** The positive (o_S) and negative (o_E) accumulated errors of the expected foot contact signal and the actual one (cf. **Figures 7A,B** of the manuscript). They control leg adaptation to deal with different terrains. **(D–F)** The TC-, CTr-, and FTi-joint angles of the right middle leg (R2) during walking from gravel (rough terrain) to grass (vegetated terrain). They represent the leg movement including adaptation. **(G)** Gait diagram showing the different energy-efficient gaits of AMOS II while traversing the terrains. Black boxes indicate swing phase while white areas between them indicate stance phase. Abbreviations are referred to **Figure 1** of the manuscript. Above pictures show snap shots from the camera on AMOS II used for the terrain classification while walking. Below pictures show snap shots of locomotion of AMOS II during the experiment. Note that one time step is ≈ 0.037 s.

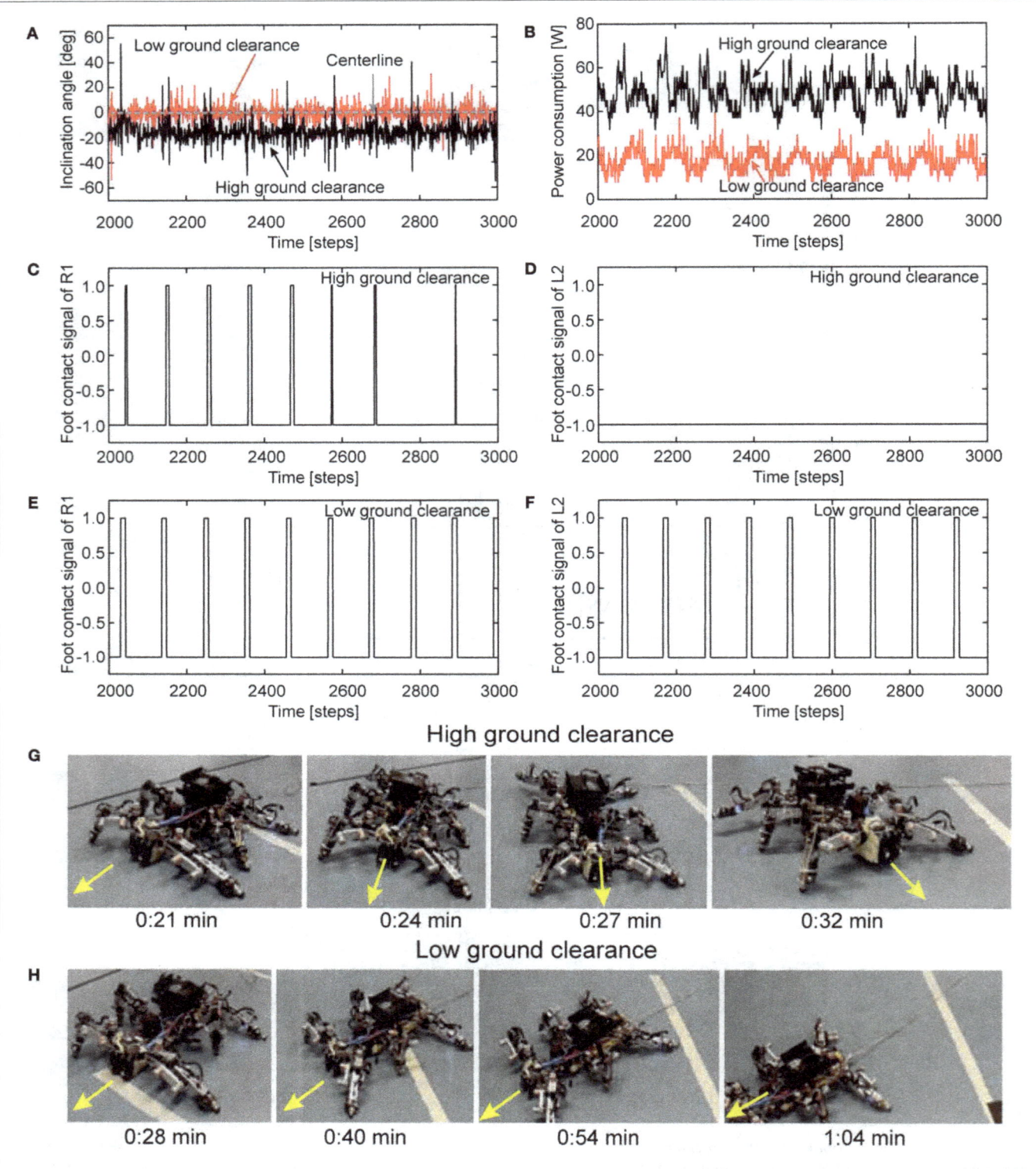

FIGURE A5 | Real-time data for walking with high and low ground clearance during leg damage. (A) The inclination angle of AMOS II obtained from an inclinometer sensor installed inside the body. Negative value means that AMOS II tilts to its left. **(B)** Power consumption. **(C,D)** The foot contact signals of R1 and L2 for the high ground clearance case.

(E,F) The foot contact signals of R1 and L2 for the low ground clearance case. They are filtered and mapped onto the interval [−1, +1] where +1 is the leg has no ground contact and vice versa. **(G,H)** Snap shots of the locomotion of AMOS II during the test with high and low ground clearance, respectively.

Neural control and adaptive neural forward models for insect-like, energy-efficient, and adaptable locomotion...

85

This algorithm is briefly described in the main text of the manuscript.

We use a hysteresis neuron (N_1) with a tanh transfer function for preprocessing the CS signal. The hysteresis principle (Pasemann, 1993) leads to a non-linear transition of two output states (low and high activations). Thus, hysteresis neuron can effectively filter sensory noise (Manoonpong et al., 2008b). The preprocessed CS signal which provides an energy level is used to inhibit all joint movements, thereby stopping robot motion, when the system has low power.

We use four neurons ($N_{2,...,5}$) with a tanh transfer function to form the neural preprocessing network of the left and right LD signals and the left and right US signals. The network is developed based on a minimal recurrent controller (MRC) structure (Pasemann et al., 2003) which allows balancing positive (LD) and negative (US) tropisms. The network outputs (i.e., outputs of $N_{2,3}$) provide orienting control signals which are transmitted to $I_{3,4}$ of the neural motor control module. As a result, AMOS II can effectively perform an appropriate turning angle to avoid obstacles or corners as well as turn toward a light source.

We simply use neurons ($N_{6,...,17}$) with a tanh transfer function for preprocessing the $FC_{1,...,6}$ and $IR_{1,...,6}$ signals. This is because the sensor signals contain small noise which can be eliminated by the non-linearity of the neuron. The preprocessed sensor signals are used for local leg control (described in the main text of the manuscript). All neural preprocessing parameters, e.g., synaptic strengths and bias terms (see **Figure A2**) were obtained by experiments [see Manoonpong et al. (2008a,b) for more details of the neural preprocessing parameters].

ADDITIONAL EXPERIMENTAL RESULTS

Here we present three more experimental results that complement those shown in the main text of the manuscript.

Figure A3 shows 20 walking patterns with different speeds of AMOS II. These patterns are mainly controlled by the CPG-based controller. Setting the modulatory input MI of the CPG to 0.0, each leg steps in a wave on each side of the body with overlap. Increasing MI, stepping frequency increases and some legs steps in pairs (see dashed enclosures). This results in a variety of patterns (or gaits) including insect-like gaits and intermixed gaits. For example, one observes wave gaits with different frequencies ($MI = 0.01–0.04$), tetrapod gaits with different frequencies ($MI = 0.05–0.06$), caterpillar gaits with different frequencies ($MI = 0.07–0.10$), and tripod gaits with different frequencies ($MI = 0.15–0.19$). Legs are labeled from front to back as numbers 1–3 and the left and right sides are L and R, respectively. Note that increasing MI higher than 0.19, we found only two different gaits comparable to tripod gait (e.g., $MI = 0.19$) and caterpillar gait (e.g., $MI = 0.10$).

Figure A4 shows autonomous selection of energy-efficient gaits while traversing from gravel to grass in an outdoor environment. It can be seen that at the beginning AMOS II walked with a tetrapod gait (photos 1,2) since it detected gravel (rough terrain) using its visual system. Afterward, it changed from the tetrapod gait to a tripod gait (photo 3) since it detected grass (vegetated terrain). During traversing the different terrains, AMOS II adapted its legs individually to deal with a change of terrain. That is, it depressed its leg and extended its tibia to search for a foothold when losing a ground contact during the stance phase where this information is detected by a significant change of the positive accumulated error o_S, see black line in **Figure A4C**. However, during the swing phase no leg elevation was observed since only minor perturbation occurred (i.e., no significant change of the negative accumulated error o_E, see red line in **Figure A4C**). We encourage readers to see the video of this experiment at **Video S7**.

Figure A5 shows walking behaviors with high and low ground clearance when legs are damaged. In this test, AMOS II was driven by only the CPG-based control described in the section 2.3 of the manuscript. We let AMOS II walk with a slow wave gait ($MI = 0.02$) and then disconnected the motor power connectors of the CTr- and FTi-joints of the right (R3) and left (L3) hind legs and the left front leg (L1). The joints became inactive (i.e., uncontrollable). This is to simulate leg damage. It can be seen that AMOS II with high ground clearance had large body inclination ($\approx -18°$, **Figure A5A**) leading to unstable locomotion and remaining legs need to carry more load. Thus, the motors need to produce high torque to carry the load resulting in high power consumption (**Figure A5B**). Furthermore the legs could not swing properly during swing phase (**Figures A5C,D**). In this case, the left middle leg (L2) always stayed on the ground; thereby, the robot turned to the left (**Figure A5G** and **Video S10**). In contrast, with low ground clearance the AMOS II fell down a little bit (**Figure A5A**) since its body was already close to the ground and remaining legs need not to carry more load leading to lower power consumption compared to the high ground clearance case (**Figure A5B**). The remaining legs (R1, R2, and L2) were able to swing during swing phase (**Figures A5E,F**). As a result, it could still move more straightforward compared to the high ground clearance case (**Figure A5H** and **Video S10**).

6

Vesicular stomatitis virus with the rabies virus glycoprotein directs retrograde transsynaptic transport among neurons *in vivo*

Kevin T. Beier[1], Arpiar B. Saunders[2], Ian A. Oldenburg[2], Bernardo L. Sabatini[2] and Constance L. Cepko[1]*

[1] Department of Genetics and Department of Ophthalmology, Harvard Medical School, Harvard University and Howard Hughes Medical Institute, Boston, MA, USA
[2] Department of Neurobiology, Harvard Medical School, Harvard University and Howard Hughes Medical Institute, Boston, MA, USA

Edited by:
Eberhard E. Fetz, University of Washington, USA

Reviewed by:
Naoshige Uchida, Harvard University, USA
Jeffrey C. Smith, National Institutes of Health, USA

*Correspondence:
Constance L. Cepko, Department of Genetics, Department of Ophthalmology, Harvard Medical School, Howard Hughes Medical Institute, Boston, MA 02115, USA.
e-mail: cepko@genetics.med.harvard.edu

Defining the connections among neurons is critical to our understanding of the structure and function of the nervous system. Recombinant viruses engineered to transmit across synapses provide a powerful approach for the dissection of neuronal circuitry *in vivo*. We recently demonstrated that recombinant vesicular stomatitis virus (VSV) can be endowed with anterograde or retrograde transsynaptic tracing ability by providing the virus with different glycoproteins. Here we extend the characterization of the transmission and gene expression of recombinant VSV (rVSV) with the rabies virus glycoprotein (RABV-G), and provide examples of its activity relative to the anterograde transsynaptic tracer form of rVSV. rVSV with RABV-G was found to drive strong expression of transgenes and to spread rapidly from neuron to neuron in only a retrograde manner. Depending upon how the RABV-G was delivered, VSV served as a polysynaptic or monosynaptic tracer, or was able to define projections through axonal uptake and retrograde transport. In animals co-infected with rVSV in its anterograde form, rVSV with RABV-G could be used to begin to characterize the similarities and differences in connections to different areas. rVSV with RABV-G provides a flexible, rapid, and versatile tracing tool that complements the previously described VSV-based anterograde transsynaptic tracer.

Keywords: vesicular stomatitis virus, transsynaptic infection, rabies, retrograde transneuronal tracing, *in vivo*, technology, polysynaptic

INTRODUCTION

Mapping neuronal connectivity in the central nervous system (CNS) of even simple organisms is a difficult task. Recombinant viruses engineered to trace synaptic connections and express transgenes promise to enable higher-throughput mapping of connections among neurons than other methods, e.g., serial reconstruction from electron micrographs (Bock et al., 2011; Briggman et al., 2011). The Pseudorabies (PRV) and Rabies viruses (RABV) have been the best characterized and most utilized circuit tracing viruses to date (Ugolini et al., 1989; Kelly and Strick, 2000). RABV was recently modified by Wickersham and colleagues such that it can travel across only one synapse, allowing for a straightforward definition of monosynaptic connections (Wickersham et al., 2007b). This strategy permitted the first unambiguous identification of retrogradely connected cells from an initially infected cell ("starter cell"), without the need for electrophysiology. Moreover, the starter cell could be defined through the expression of a specific viral receptor that limited the initial infection.

Recently, we created an anterograde monosynaptic virus that complements the previously available retrograde viral tracers (Beier et al., 2011). Vesicular stomatitis virus (VSV), a virus related to RABV, with its own glycoprotein (G) gene (VSV-G), or with a G from the unrelated lymphocytic choriomeningitis virus (LCMV-G), spreads in the anterograde direction across synapses.

VSV can be used as a polysynaptic tracer that spreads across many synapses, owing to the fact that the normal, replication-competent form of the virus does not cause serious diseases in humans (Brandly and Hanson, 1957; Johnson et al., 1966; Brody et al., 1967). Whether the virus is a monosynaptic or polysynaptic tracer is determined by the method of delivery of the G gene (**Figure 1A**). Advantages of VSV are that it is well-characterized, is relatively simple in comparison to PRV, and it rapidly grows to high titer in tissue culture cells. It is also being developed as a vaccine vector, often using a G of another virus as the immunogen, as well as being developed as a cytocidal agent that will target tumor cells in humans (Balachandran and Barber, 2000; Stojdl et al., 2000, 2003).

Previous studies of the anatomical patterns of transmission, as well as physiological recordings, have shown that the transmission of VSV and RABV among neurons is via synapses (Kelly and Strick, 2000; Wickersham et al., 2007b; Beier et al., 2011). In addition, it has been shown that RABV, as well as lentiviruses with RABV-G in their envelope, travel retrogradely from an injection site (Mazarakis et al., 2001; Wickersham et al., 2007a). We hypothesized that providing a recombinant VSV (rVSV) with the RABV-G would create a retrograde polysynaptic transsynaptic tracer without the biosafety concerns inherent to RABV. Our initial characterization of rVSV with RABV-G showed that indeed

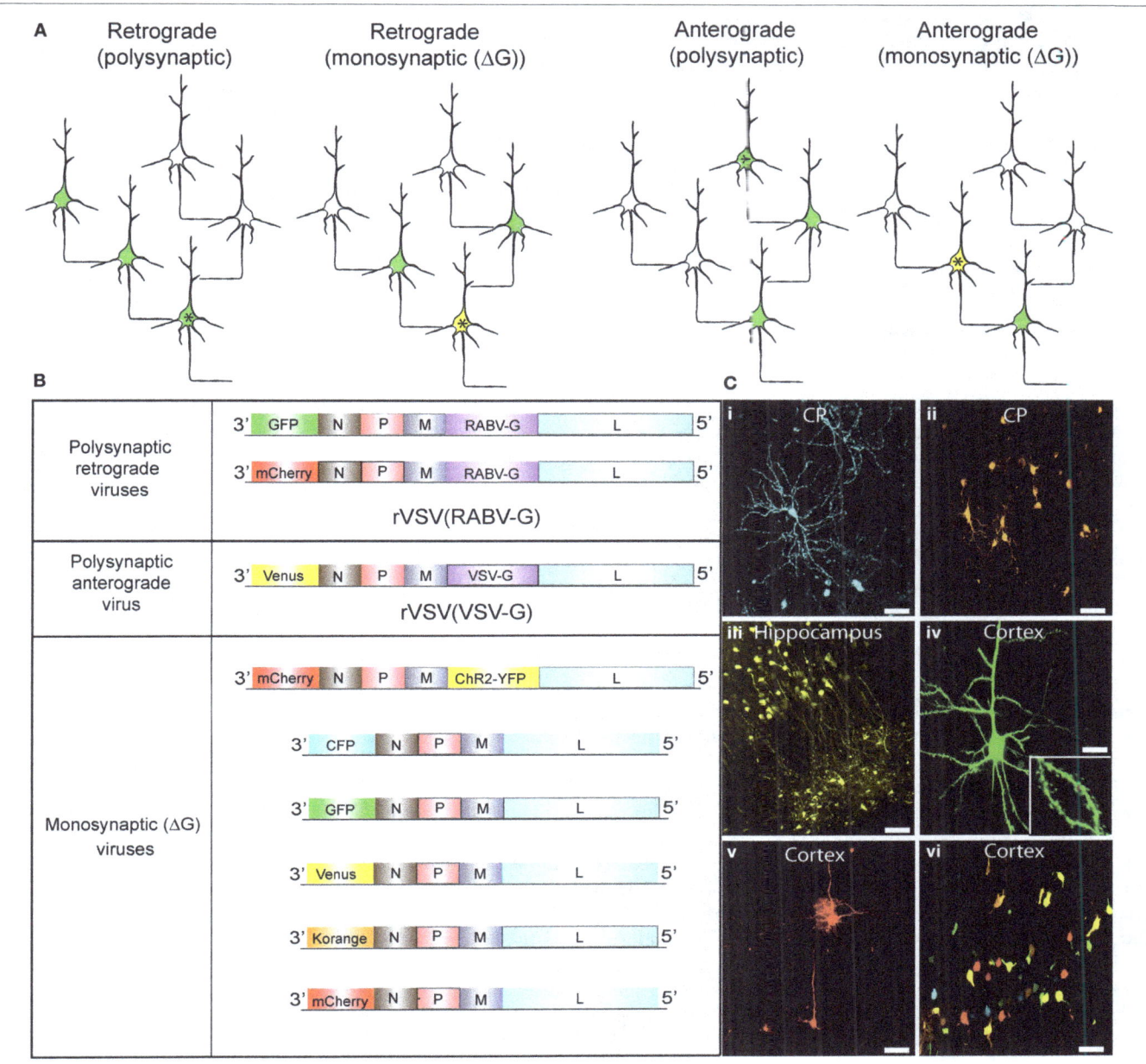

FIGURE 1 | Synaptic tracing strategies using VSV. (A) Schematic illustrating the strategies for polysynaptic or monosynaptic retrograde or anterograde transsynaptic transmission of rVSV encoding GFP. The initially infected cell is indicated by an asterisk. VSV encoding a glycoprotein (G) within its genome can spread polysynaptically. The direction of the spread depends on the identity of the glycoprotein. Infected neurons are shown in green. In some cases, the initially infected starter cell can be defined by the expression of an avian receptor, TVA (tagged with a red fluorescent protein). The TVA-expressing neurons can then be specifically infected by rVSVΔG with the EnvA/RABV-G (A/RG) glycoprotein (Wickersham et al., 2007b) on the virion surface [rVSVΔG(A/RG)]. These starter cells are then yellow, due to viral GFP and mCherry from TVA-mCherry expression. For monosynaptic tracing, the G protein is expressed *in trans* in the TVA-expressing cell, and thus complements rVSVΔG to allow transmission in a specific direction. **(B)** Genomic diagrams of rVSV vectors. All VSVs contain four essential proteins: N, P,

M, and L. Some viruses encode a G gene in their genome, which allows them to spread polysynaptically. rVSV vectors typically encode a transgene in the first position, while others carry an additional transgene in the G position. **(C)** Morphological characterization of rVSV-infected neurons in several locations within the mouse brain. **(i,ii)** Caudate-putamen (CP) neurons at 4 dpi from an injection of the CP with rVSV(VSV-G) viruses encoding **(i)** CFP or **(ii)** Korange. **(iii)** Labeled neurons of the CA1 region of the hippocampus are shown at 5 dpi following injection into the hippocampus of rVSV(VSV-G) encoding Venus. **(iv,v)** Cortical pyramidal neurons are shown following injection into the CP of rVSV(RABV-G) expressing **(iv)** GFP at 24 hpi, or **(v)** mCherry at 48 hpi. Inset in **(iv)** is a high magnification of the neuron in panel **(iv)**, highlighting labeling of dendritic spines. **(vi)** Multiple viruses can be co-injected into the same animal. Here, individual rVSVΔG(VSV-G) viruses encoding CFP, GFP, Venus, Korange, and mCherry were used to infect the cortex. Scale bars = 50 μm.

it could be taken up as a retrograde tracer (Beier et al., 2011). To determine if it could transmit among neurons following its replication in neurons, and to further analyze the transmission patterns of both the monosynaptic and polysynaptic forms of rVSV with RABV-G, we made injections into several CNS and peripheral locations. In addition, we performed co-infections of rVSV with RABV-G and the anterograde form of rVSV in order to exploit the differences in the directionality of transmission of these two viruses in mapping circuits.

RESULTS

VSV CAN ENCODE A VARIETY OF TRANSGENES

Schematics of viruses created and used throughout this study are shown in **Figure 1**. We created rVSV vector plasmids carrying different transgenes in either the first or fifth genomic positions (**Figure 1B**). After rescuing each virus, we tested the ability of each to express transgenes in different brain regions through intracranial injections (**Figure 1C**). All rVSV vectors drove robust fluorophore expression 1 or 2 days post-infection (hpi) (**Figure 1C**) (van den Pol et al., 2009). In fact, by 12 hpi, labeling was sufficiently bright to image fine morphological details, such as dendritic spines (**Figure 1C,iv**).

PHYSIOLOGY OF CELLS INFECTED WITH rVSV ENCODING RABV-G

To characterize the physiological properties of cells infected with rVSV, we tested a replication-competent rVSV encoding GFP, with RABV-G in the genome in place of VSV-G [hereafter designated rVSV(RABV-G)]. van den Pol et al. reported that hippocampal neurons infected with replication-incompetent (G-deleted or "ΔG") rVSV were physiologically healthy at 12–14 hpi, but were less so by 1 day post-infection (dpi) (van den Pol et al., 2009). Given the known toxicity of both VSV and RABV-G (Coulon et al., 1982), we tested the physiology of cortical pyramidal neurons in the motor cortex (M1) infected with rVSV(RABV-G). Between 12 and 18 hpi, the membrane capacitance, input resistance, resting membrane potential, and current-to-action potential firing relationship were indistinguishable between infected and uninfected neurons (**Figure 2**). However, by 2 dpi, electrophysiological properties were so abnormal in the infected cortical pyramidal cells that physiological measurements could not be made.

VSV EXPRESSES TRANSGENES RAPIDLY IN NEURONS

The speed and strength of the expression of transgenes encoded by VSV depends upon the gene's genomic position (van den Pol et al., 2009; Beier et al., 2011). Genes in the first position are expressed the most highly, with a decrease in the level of expression in positions more 3′ within the viral plus strand. When GFP was inserted into the first position of VSV, GFP fluorescence was first detectable at approximately 1 hpi in cultured cells (van den Pol et al., 2009).

In order to quantify the relative expression of a fluorescent protein in the first genomic position in neurons, rat hippocampal slices were infected with a replication-incompetent rVSV that expresses mCherry (rVSVΔG, **Figures 1A,B**). This was a ΔG virus which had the RABV-G supplied in trans during the preparation of the virus stock [referred to as rVSVΔG(RABV-G)].

Average fluorescence intensity of the infected cells was measured every hour over the course of 18 h. By 4 hpi at 37°C, red fluorescence was clearly visible, and reached maximal levels by approximately 14 hpi ($N = 3$, **Figure 3**). Similar results were obtained with a virus encoding GFP in the first genomic position rather than mCherry (i.e., **Figure 1B**) ($N = 3$).

rVSV(RABV-G) SPREADS TRANSSYNAPTICALLY IN THE RETROGRADE DIRECTION

We previously demonstrated that rVSV(RABV-G) could be taken up retrogradely by neurons (Beier et al., 2011), but these experiments did not distinguish between direct axonal uptake of the initial inoculum vs. retrograde transsynaptic transmission following viral replication. To distinguish between these two mechanisms and to extend the previous analyses, we conducted further experiments in the mammalian visual system (**Figures 4A–G**). As visual cortex area 1 (V1) does not receive direct projections from retinal ganglion cells (RGCs), but rather receives secondary input from RGCs via the lateral geniculate nucleus (LGN), infection of RGCs from injection of V1 would demonstrate retrograde transmission from cells which supported at least one round of viral replication. Following a V1 injection with rVSV(RABV-G), GFP-positive RGCs were observed in the retina by 3 dpi ($N = 3$; **Figure 4G**). Importantly, viral labeling in the brain was restricted to primary and secondary projection areas, even at 7 dpi. These included the LGN (**Figure 4D**) and the hypothalamus (**Figure 4E**), two areas known to project directly to V1 (Kandel, 2000). Selective labeling was observed in other areas, such as cortical areas surrounding V1 (**Figure 4C**), which project directly to V1, and also in the superior colliculus (SC) stratum griseum centrale, which projects to the LGN (**Figure 4F**). Labeling was also observed in the nucleus basalis, which projects to the cortex, as well as many components of the basal ganglia circuit, which provide input to the thalamus [such as the caudate-putamen (CP), globus pallidus (GP), and the subthalamic nucleus (STn)]. The amygdala, which projects to the hypothalamus, was also labeled. Consistent with a lack of widespread viral transmission, animals did not exhibit signs of disease at 7 dpi.

These data show that rVSV(RABV-G) can spread in a retrograde direction from the injection site, but do not address whether the virus can spread exclusively in the retrograde direction. Directional transsynaptic specificity can only be definitively addressed using a unidirectional circuit. We therefore turned to the primary motor cortex (M1) to CP connection, in which neurons project from the cortex to the CP, but not in the other direction (**Figure 4H**) (Beier et al., 2011). Injections of rVSV(RABV-G) into M1 should not label neurons in the CP if the virus can only label cells across synapses in the retrograde direction. Indeed, at 2 dpi, areas directly projecting to the injection site, including the contralateral cortex, were labeled (**Figure 4I**). Only axons from cortical cells were observed in the CP, with no GFP-labeled cell bodies present in the CP (**Figure 4J**), consistent with lack of anterograde transsynaptic spread. By 3 dpi, a small number of medium spiny neurons (MSNs) in the CP were observed, likely via secondary spread from initially infected thalamic or GP neurons (data not shown).

Vesicular stomatitis virus with the rabies virus glycoprotein directs retrograde transsynaptic transport...

89

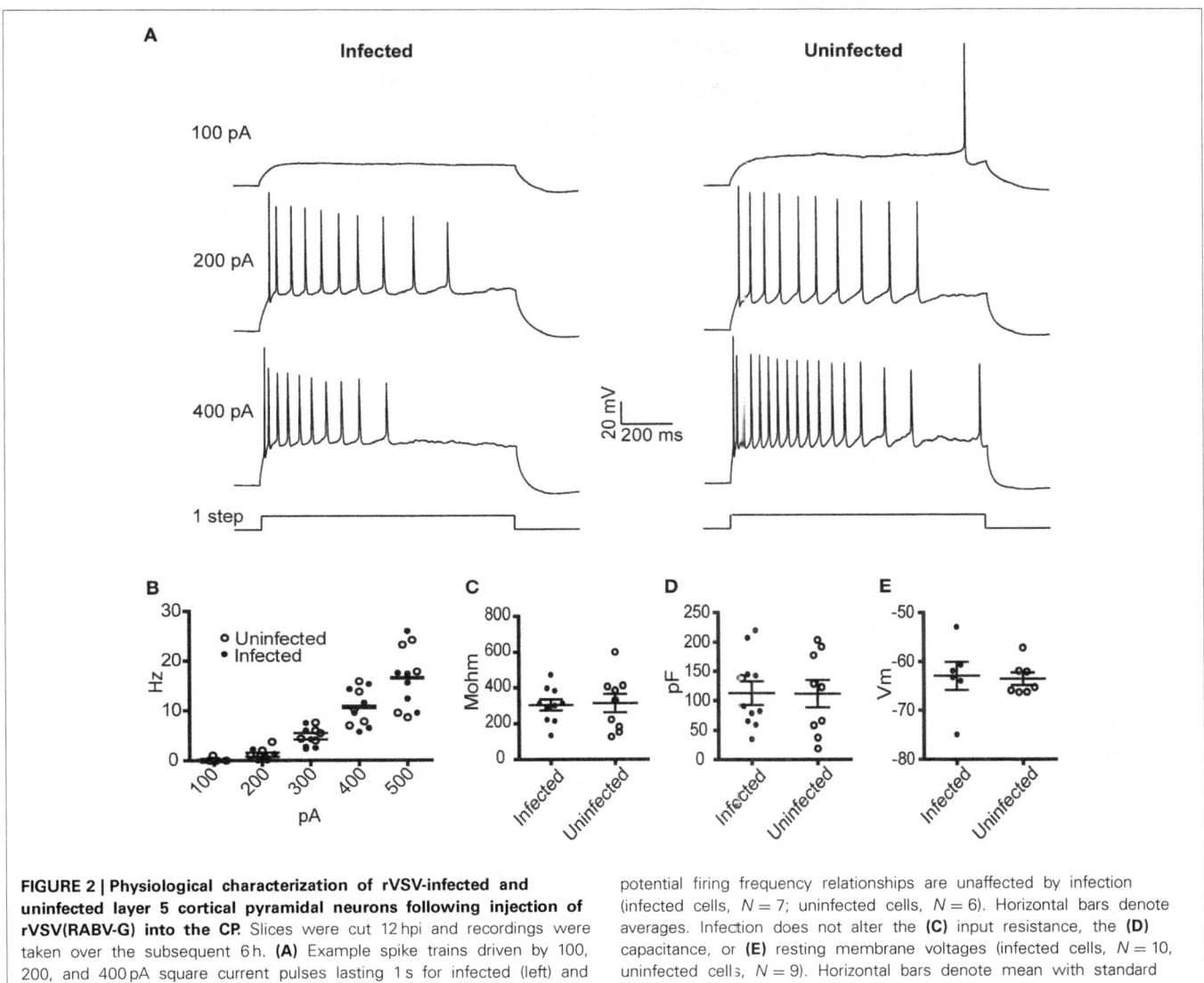

FIGURE 2 | Physiological characterization of rVSV-infected and uninfected layer 5 cortical pyramidal neurons following injection of rVSV(RABV-G) into the CP. Slices were cut 12 hpi and recordings were taken over the subsequent 6 h. **(A)** Example spike trains driven by 100, 200, and 400 pA square current pulses lasting 1 s for infected (left) and uninfected (right) neurons. **(B)** A summary plot showing current/action potential firing frequency relationships are unaffected by infection (infected cells, $N = 7$; uninfected cells, $N = 6$). Horizontal bars denote averages. Infection does not alter the **(C)** input resistance, the **(D)** capacitance, or **(E)** resting membrane voltages (infected cells, $N = 10$, uninfected cells, $N = 9$). Horizontal bars denote mean with standard error of the mean.

PERIPHERAL UPTAKE OF rVSV(RABV-G) AND TRANSMISSION TO THE CNS

A particular advantage of retrograde viral tracers is the ability to label CNS neurons projecting to peripheral sites. This has been a powerful application of both RABV and PRV (Ugolini et al., 1989; Standish et al., 1994). To test if rVSV(RABV-G) could also perform this function, we examined the innervation of the dura surface by neurons of the trigeminal ganglion, a neuronal circuit thought to be involved in migraine headaches (Penfield and McNaughton, 1940; Mayberg et al., 1984). These neurons have axons, but not canonical dendrites, and send projections into the spinal cord and brainstem. Therefore, the only way trigeminal neurons could become labeled from viral application to the dura is through retrograde uptake of the virus.

We applied rVSV(RABV-G) to the intact dura mater and analyzed the dura, trigeminal ganglion, and CNS for labeling (**Figure 4K**). At the earliest time point examined, 3 dpi, we observed axons traveling along the dura, but little other evidence of infection (**Figure 4L**). No labeled neuronal cell bodies on the dura were observed, consistent with the lack of neurons on this surface. In contrast, we did find labeled cell bodies in the trigeminal ganglion (**Figure 4M**). No infection was seen in the CNS, even at 4 dpi, consistent with the lack of inputs from the brain into the trigeminal ganglion ($N = 4$ animals).

THE KINETICS OF RETROGRADE TRANSSYNAPTIC SPREAD

To further characterize patterns and kinetics of viral transmission and directional specificity of transsynaptic spread, injections of rVSV(RABV-G) were made into the CP (**Figure 5A**). In order to determine which cells were labeled by direct uptake of virus in the inoculum, a separate set of animals were injected into the CP with the replication-incompetent rVSVΔG(RABV-G) ($N = 3$ animals, analyzed 3 dpi). Cells labeled by rVSVΔG(RABV-G) were observed in the CP, GP, substantia nigra (SN), thalamus, and

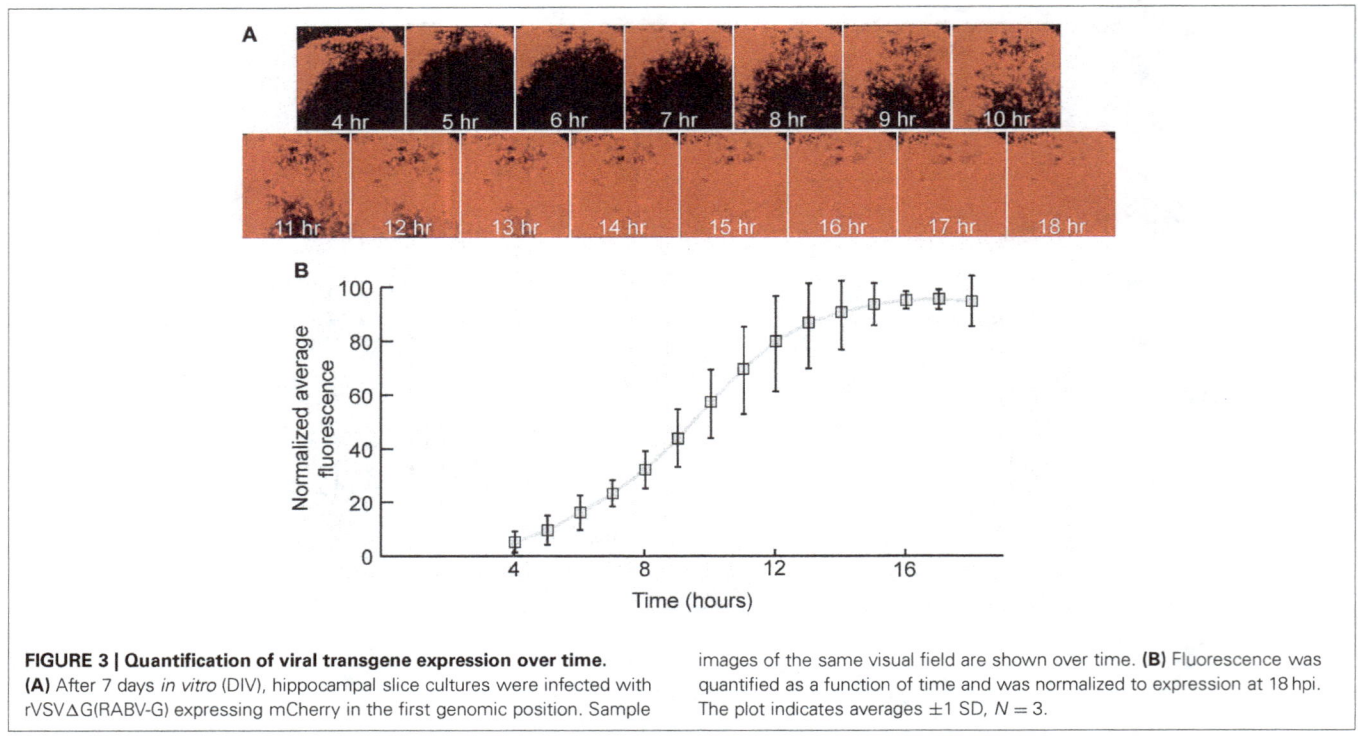

FIGURE 3 | Quantification of viral transgene expression over time.
(A) After 7 days *in vitro* (DIV), hippocampal slice cultures were infected with rVSVΔG(RABV-G) expressing mCherry in the first genomic position. Sample images of the same visual field are shown over time. **(B)** Fluorescence was quantified as a function of time and was normalized to expression at 18 hpi. The plot indicates averages ±1 SD, N = 3.

layers 3 and 5 of the cortex, consistent with infection at the axon terminal and retrograde labeling of cell bodies of neurons known to project directly to the CP (**Figure 5C**) (Albin et al., 1995). Areas labeled by CP injection are indicated in **Figure 5B**.

The patterns of spread for the replication-competent rVSV(RABV-G) were characterized over the course of 1–5 dpi (**Figures 5D–H**). During this interval, progressively more cells in infected regions were labeled by rVSV(RABV-G), including within the CP, nucleus basalis, cortex, and GP (listed in **Figure 5B**). In addition, more cortical cells were labeled in clusters near cortical pyramidal neurons, both ipsilateral and contralateral to the injected side, including neurogliaform cells (data not shown). These data are in contrast to those observed following infection with an anterograde transsynaptic tracing virus, such as rVSV with its own G gene, rVSV(VSV-G) (**Figure 5B**). At 3 dpi following rVSV(VSV-G) injection into the CP, the cerebral cortex was not labeled, but regions receiving projections from the CP, such as the STn, GP, and SN, were labeled (Beier et al., 2011).

In order to investigate other areas for evidence of cell-to-cell retrograde transsynaptic spread, the nucleus basalis was examined following infection of the CP with replication-competent rVSV(RABV-G). The nucleus basalis was labeled by 2 dpi (**Figures 5E–H**), consistent with at least a single transsynaptic jump, as this area does not directly project to the CP. The virus appeared to travel transsynaptically at the rate of roughly 1 synapse per day, as evidenced by the lack of labeled neurogliaform cells in the cortex, and lack of neurons in the nucleus basalis at 1 dpi, and label appearing in these cell types/areas at 2 dpi, as previously observed (Beier et al., 2011). Labeling remained well-restricted to the expected corticostriatal circuits at 5 dpi,

suggesting that viral spread becomes less efficient after crossing one or two connections, consistent with injections into V1 (**Figure 4**). While glial cells can be infected and were observed near the injection site (van den Pol et al., 2002; Chauhan et al., 2010), infected glial cells away from the injection site generally were not observed.

POLYSYNAPTIC TRACERS CAN BE COMBINED *in vivo*

One advantage of having both anterograde and retrograde forms of the same virus is that they can be used in parallel, or in tandem, to trace circuitry to and from a single or multiple sites of injection, with each virus having similar kinetics of spread and gene expression. In fact, if different fluorophores are used in different viruses, e.g., rVSV(VSV-G) and rVSV(RABV-G), then the viruses can be co-injected into the same site and their transmission can be traced independently (**Figure 6A**). This is most straightforward if there are no cells at the injection site that are initially infected by both viruses. Co-infected cells can be easily detected, as they would express both fluorescent proteins shortly after injection.

In order to determine whether two viruses would allow simultaneous anterograde and retrograde transsynaptic tracing from a single injection site, a rVSV(VSV-G) expressing Venus and a rVSV(RABV-G) expressing mCherry were injected individually (**Figures 6B–D**) or co-injected (**Figures 6E–G**) into the motor cortex, and brains were examined 3 dpi. The pattern of labeling from the co-injected brains was equivalent to the patterns observed when each virus was injected individually: rVSV(VSV-G) was observed to infect neurons in the cortex, CP, and downstream nuclei, whereas the rVSV(RABV-G) was not observed to infect neurons in the CP, but rather in the thalamus and nucleus basalis (N = 4). The initial co-infection rate is dependent upon

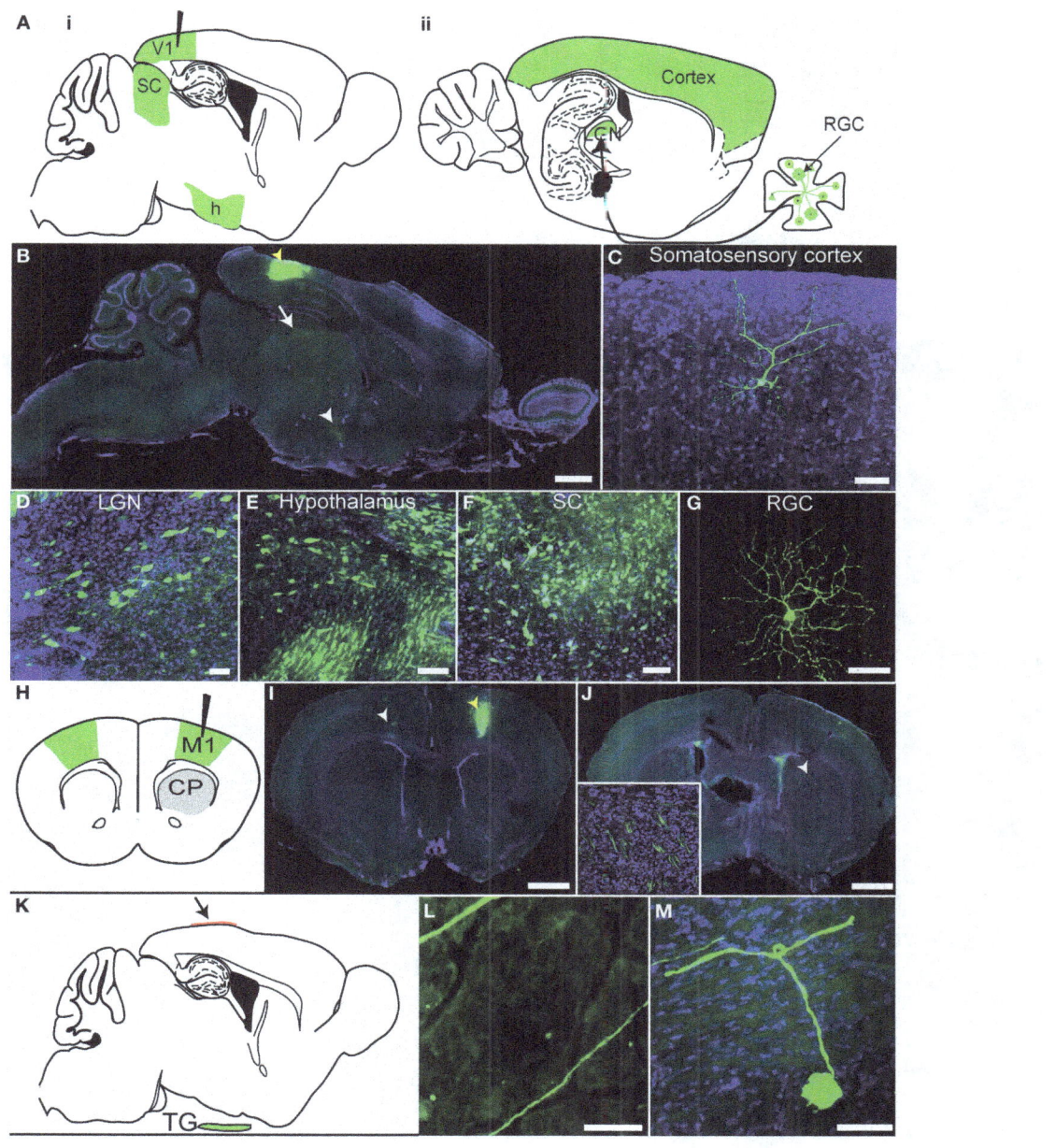

**FIGURE 4 | rVSV(RABV-G) exhibits polysynaptic retrograde spread
in vivo. (A)** Schematics of two parasaggital sections separated by 1.3 mm
are shown. rVSV(RABV-G) injected into V1 (black needle) should yield
infected cells in the labeled areas shown in green, including RGCs in the
retina (panel **ii**). Areas projecting directly to V1, such as the hypothalamus
(h), LGN, as well as other cortical areas, can be labeled by direct
retrograde uptake of injected virions, whereas RGCs, which project to the
LGN, can only be labeled by secondary viral spread. **(B)** rVSV(RABV-G) was
injected into V1 (yellow arrowhead), and both the brain and retina
examined 7 dpi. Infection in the brain appeared to be primarily in directly
projecting areas, including the surrounding cortices, the LGN (white arrow),
and hypothalamus (white arrowhead). Higher magnifications of labeled
cells from a V1 injection are shown in panels **(C–G)**. **(C)** somatosensory
cortex, 7 dpi; **(D)** LGN, 3 dpi; **(E)** hypothalamus, 3 dpi; **(F)** SC, 3 dpi; **(G)**
RGC, 3 dpi. **(H)** Schematic of a coronal section showing rVSV(RABV-G)
injected into M1 (black needle). The contralateral cortex (green) should be
labeled by this virus, while at early time points such as 2 dpi, the CP,
which receives projections from the cortex but does not itself send
projections to the cortex, should not (gray). **(I)** Coronal section showing
GFP-labeled neurons in M1, imaged 4 dpi. The injection site was in M1,
indicated by a yellow arrowhead, with neurons projecting to the injection
site indicated by the white arrowhead. **(J)** CP neuronal cell bodies were
not labeled, but labeled cortical axon bundles running through the CP were
observed (inset shows axon bundles in the area demarcated by the white
arrowhead). **(K–M)** rVSV(RABV-G) can trace circuits into the CNS from a
peripheral site. **(K)** Parasaggital schematic showing a predicted area of
infection following infection of the dura with a retrogradely transported
virus. rVSV(RABV-G) was applied to the intact dura (arrow) and if
retrograde uptake and transport can occur, trigeminal ganglion neurons that
project to the dura (green) should become labeled. **(L)** Examples of axons
located on the dura, 3 dpi. Infected neuronal cell bodies were not located
on the dura, **(M)** but instead were observed in the trigeminal ganglion. No
infection of the brain was observed in these animals. Scale bars: **(B,I,J)** =
1 mm, **(L)** = 100 μm, **(C–G,M)** = 50 μm.

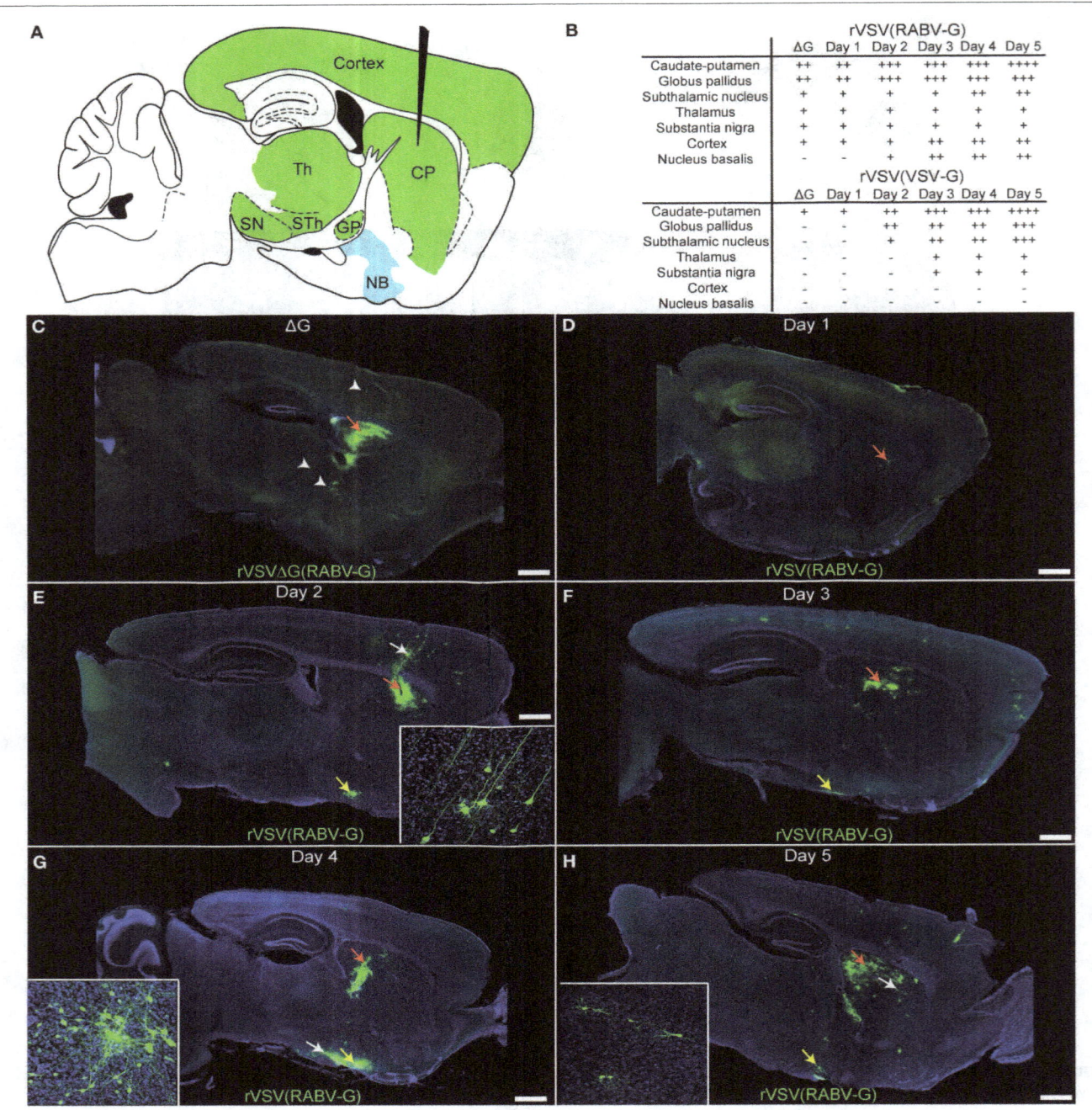

FIGURE 5 | Time course of rVSV(RABV-G) spread from the CP recapitulates the connectivity of known basal ganglia-thalamo-cortical circuits. (A) A parasaggital schematic showing the relevant projections into and from the injection site in the CP. Black needle points to injection site, green = primary projecting regions, blue = secondary projecting region. CP, caudate-putamen; GP, globus pallidus; SN, substantia nigra; STh, subthalamic nucleus; Th, thalamus; NB, nucleus basalis. **(B)** Assessment of viral spread from rVSV(RABV-G) and rVSV(VSV-G) injections into the CP. The presence or absence of labeling is indicated by (+) and (−), respectively. The extent of labeling is indicated by the number of (+). Some animals were infected with ΔG viruses to determine which areas were labeled by direct uptake of the virions, rather than by replication and transmission. These were sacrificed at

3 dpi. **(C)** Parasaggital section of a brain infected with VSV[greek delta]G(RABV-G). The injection site is marked by a red arrow. Several areas that project directly to the CP were labeled due to direct uptake of the virions, including the cortex, thalamus, and GP (arrowheads), 3 dpi. **(D–H)** Replication-competent rVSV(RABV-G) was injected into the CP (red arrows), and the time course of labeling was monitored for 5 days [**(D)** 1 day, **(E)** 2, **(F)** 3, **(G)** 4, and **(H)** 5 days]. Insets show high magnifications of areas indicated by white arrows. Sections from animals at 1 dpi show labeling consistent with the initial infection [compare to rVSVΔG(RABV-G), panel **C**], while spread to secondarily connected areas, such as the nucleus basalis, was observed at 2 dpi (yellow arrows). Viral spread was relatively restricted to the basal ganglia circuit, even out to 5 dpi. Scale bars = 1 mm.

Vesicular stomatitis virus with the rabies virus glycoprotein directs retrograde transsynaptic transport...

93

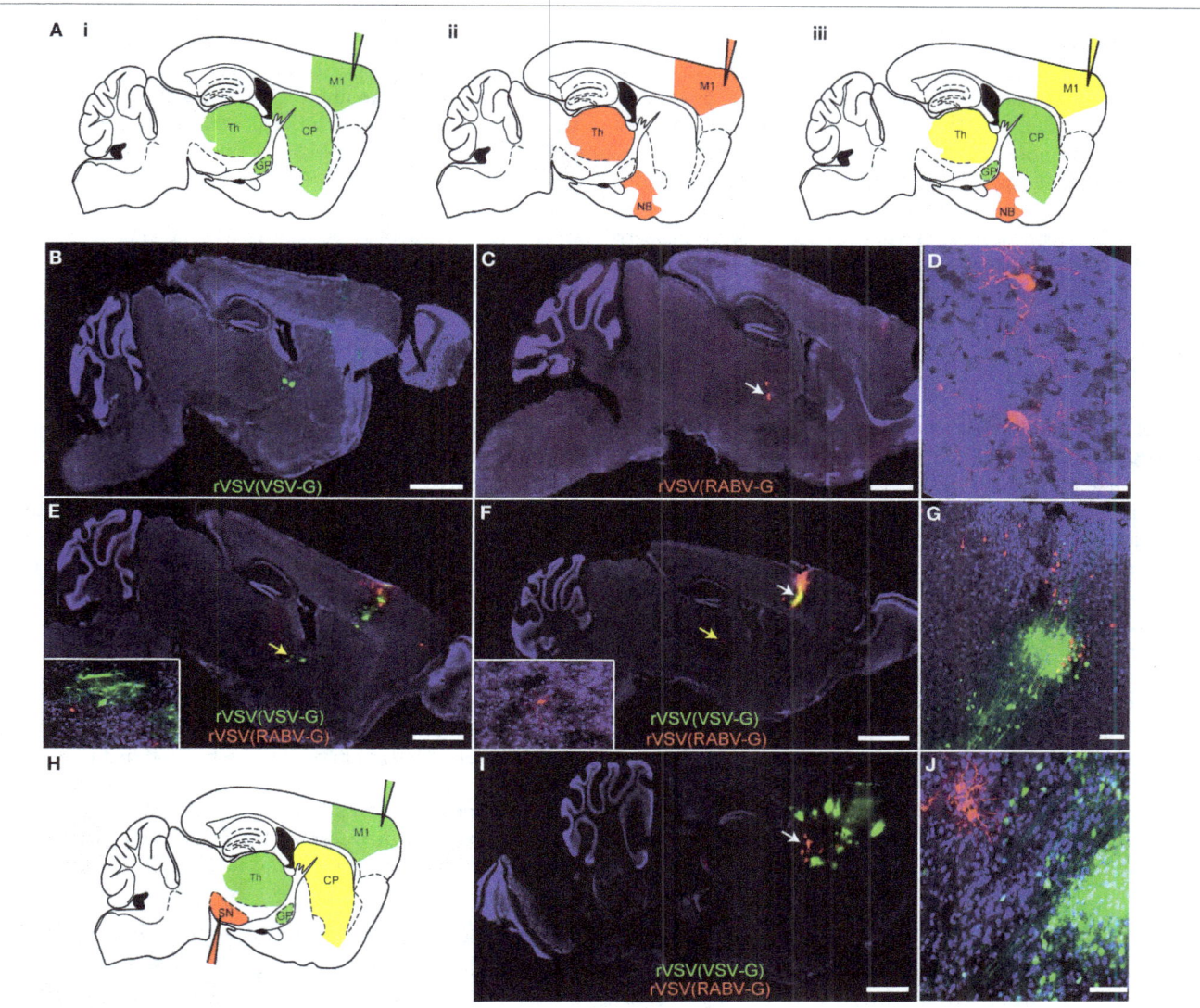

FIGURE 6 | Simultaneous anterograde and retrograde transsynaptic circuit tracing using rVSV. (A) Connectivity schematics of parasaggital sections indicating patterns of spread from injection of M1 (injection needles) with a polysynaptic virus transmitting across synapses in the **(i)** anterograde or **(ii)** retrograde directions. Panel **(iii)** shows the pattern from co-injection of two polysynaptic viruses, one anterograde and one retrograde. Green represents the anterograde virus, red the retrograde virus, and yellow, both. Note that yellow indicates that the area is predicted to host infection by both viruses, with potentially some individual cells showing infection with both viruses. **(B)** The anterograde transsynaptic virus rVSV(VSV-G), when injected alone, labeled M1 as well as anterograde projection areas, such as the CP, GP, and thalamus, whereas **(C)** the retrograde virus rVSV(RABV-G) labeled M1 as well as areas projecting to the cortex, including the thalamus. **(D)** High magnification of thalamic cells shown in **(C)** (white arrow). **(E,F)** Examples taken from a series of parasaggital sections from the same brain of an animal injected with both viruses simultaneously into M1. Co-infection of cells in M1 was not observed, **(G)**, and no spurious labeling of anterograde or retrograde projection regions was observed—i.e., the combination of viruses was equal to the sum of each virus injected individually. Insets show high magnifications of thalamic neurons in **(E)** and **(F)** labeled by the two viruses (indicated by the yellow arrows) demonstrating no co-labeling. **(G)** A high magnification view of the injection site in the cortex shown in panel **(F)** (white arrow), showing independent labeling of neurons by each virus. **(H)** A schematic of a parasaggital section depicting the pattern of transmission of an anterograde (green) and retrograde (red) virus injected into two different areas of the basal ganglia circuit. This strategy can be used to connect multiple elements in a circuit. The rVSV(VSV-G) that expressed Venus (labeled cells depicted in green) was injected into M1, while the rVSV(RABV-G) that expressed mCherry was injected into the SN, where it labeled direct pathway MSNs in the CP (yellow). **(I)** Using these coordinates, largely non-overlapping regions of the CP were labeled by these viruses, as shown in **(J)**. Scale bars: **(B,C,E,F,I)** = 1 mm; **(D,G,J)** = 50 μm.

the dose of the initial inocula. When injecting 3×10^3 focus forming units (ffu) rVSV(VSV-G) and 3×10^4 ffu rVSV(RABV-G), no co-infection was observed at the injection site. Thus, co-infection of the same brain region, without co-infection of the same cells, does not alter the spreading behavior of either rVSV(VSV-G) or rVSV(RABV-G).

One example of how this dual retrograde and anterograde transsynaptic tracing system can be used is to determine if three distinct regions are connected and the directionality of any connections. For example, the anterograde transsynaptic virus can be injected into one region, the retrograde into another, and a third region can then be examined for evidence of labeling by either or both viruses (e.g., **Figure 6H**). To test this possibility, rVSV(VSV-G) was injected into the motor cortex, rVSV(RABV-G) was injected into the substantia nigra pars reticulara (SNr), and animals were sacrificed at 3 dpi. We observed that cells were singly labeled, either with Venus [rVSV(VSV-G)] or with mCherry [rVSV(RABV-G)], and were located largely in different regions of the CP (**Figures 6I,J**) ($N = 3$). These results suggest that the anterograde connections from the cells infected with rVSV(VSV-G) in the M1 were with CP MSNs that did not project to the region of the SNr injected with rVSV(RABV-G) ($N = 3$ animals).

VSV CAN TRACE MONOSYNAPTICALLY CONNECTED CIRCUITS IN THE RETROGRADE DIRECTION

In addition to polysynaptic tracing, VSV can be modified to trace circuits monosynaptically (Beier et al., 2011). With RABV, this was achieved *in vivo* by first infecting with an adeno-associated virus (AAV) expressing TVA, a receptor for an avian retrovirus, and RABV-G (Wall et al., 2010). This was followed 3 weeks later by infection with a ΔG RABV with an EnvA/RABV-G chimeric glycoprotein on the virion surface (Wickersham et al., 2007b), which allowed infection specifically of the cells expressing TVA. A similar strategy was used to test rVSV's ability to monosynaptically trace retrogradely connected neurons *in vivo*. Inputs to choline acetyltransferase (ChAT)-expressing neurons in the striatum were used for this test. These neurons primarily receive input from the cortex and the thalamus (Thomas et al., 2000; Bloomfield et al., 2007) (**Figure 7A**). In order to mark this population, we crossed ChAT-Cre mice to Ai9 mice, which express tdTomato in cells

with a Cre expression history (Madisen et al., 2010). Six-week-old mice from this cross were injected in the CP with two AAV vectors: one expressing a Cre-conditional ("floxed") TVA-mCherry fusion protein, and another expressing a floxed RABV-G. Two weeks later, the mice were injected in the same coordinates with rVSVΔG with the EnvA/RABV-G chimeric glycoprotein on the virion surface [rVSVΔG(A/RG)] (Beier et al., 2011). Cells successfully infected with these two AAV vectors could host infection by a rVSV and should be able to produce rVSV virions with RABV-G on the surface. Such starter cells should also express tdTomato and GFP. If rVSV were to be produced, and if it were to transmit across the synapse retrogradely, cortical and thalamic neurons should be labeled by GFP.

Mice injected with these AAV and rVSV viruses were sacrificed 5 days after rVSV infection, and brains analyzed for fluorescence. As expected for starter cells, some neurons in the CP expressed both tdTomato and GFP (**Figure 7B**). Outside of the CP, small numbers of GFP+ neurons that were not mCherry+ were observed in the cortex (**Figures 7C,D**) and thalamus (**Figure 7E**), consistent with retrograde spread. Control animals not expressing Cre, or not injected with AAV encoding RABV-G, did not label cells in the cortex or thalamus ($N = 3$ for both controls and experimental condition).

DISCUSSION

rVSV(RABV-G) IS A RETROGRADE TRACER IN THE CNS

Here, we report on the use of rVSV as a retrograde transsynaptic tracer for CNS circuitry. VSV can be modified to encode the RABV-G protein in the viral genome, allowing the virus to replicate and transmit across multiple synaptically connected cells, i.e., as a polysynaptic tracer. Alternatively, if the virus has the G gene deleted from its genome and RABV-G is provided *in trans*,

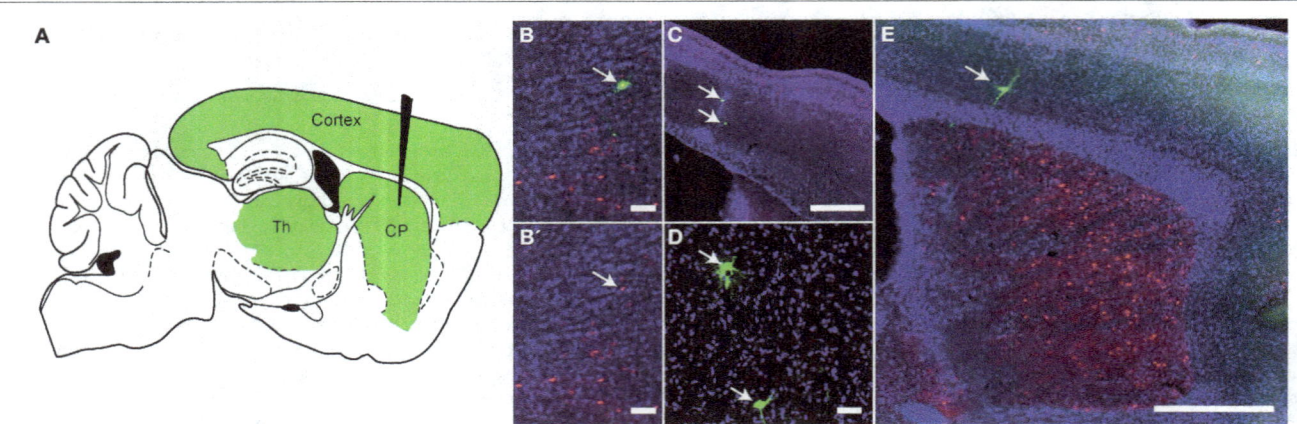

FIGURE 7 | Monosynaptic retrograde tracing using rVSV *in vivo*.
(A) A schematic of a parasaggital section showing the predicted pattern of monosynaptic retrograde spread from Choline Acetyltransferase (ChAT)-expressing neurons in the CP to directly connected cells. A combination of two Cre-dependent adeno-associated viruses (AAVs), one expressing a TVA-mCherry fusion protein and the other RABV-G, were injected into the CP of ChAT-Cre/Ai9 animals. This permits expression of the transgenes encoded in the AAVs in cells with a ChAT expression history. Two weeks later, rVSVΔG(A/RG), a G-deleted virus that only infects TVA-expressing neurons, was injected into the same region, and the brain

was observed 5 days later. The injection of rVSV into the CP (black needle) should result in infection of TVA-expressing neurons in the CP. From these starter cells, monosynaptic spread could occur only to directly connected inputs such as those in the cortex and thalamus (green). **(B,B')** Initially infected cells in the CP were both red (TVA-expressing) and green (rVSV infected) (arrow). **B'** shows the red and blue channels only, blue = DAPI. **(C–E)** Examples of rVSV-infected cells in the cortex **(C,E)** and thalamus **(D)** that were infected by monosynaptic transmission from the starter cells, (arrows indicate cells infected by transmission), $N = 3$. Scale bars: **(B,D)** = 50 μm, **(C,E)** = 500 μm.

it behaves as a monosynaptic tracer (Beier et al., 2011). Although it has been known for many years that RABV travels retrogradely among neurons (Astic et al., 1993; Ugolini, 1995; Kelly and Strick, 2003), and pseudotyping lentiviruses with RABV-G is sufficient for axonal transport (Mazarakis et al., 2001), the retrograde transmission specificity among neurons had not been clearly shown to be a property of the G protein itself, as it might have been due to other viral proteins in addition to, or instead of, the viral G protein. Since native VSV does not have these retrograde transsynaptic properties (van den Pol et al., 2002; Beier et al., 2011), and the only alteration to the VSV genome was the substitution of the VSV G gene with the G gene of RABV, it is clear that the RABV glycoprotein is responsible for retrograde direction of viral transmission across synapses, at least in the case of rVSV.

VSV AS A VIRAL VECTOR FOR THE CNS: RAPID GENE EXPRESSION AND GENOME CAPACITY

The early onset of gene expression from VSV relative to RABV (one hour vs. multiple hours) makes it beneficial in experimental paradigms in which the experiment needs to be done within a narrow window of time, such as tissue slices and explants. In addition, more than one transgene can be encoded in the viral genome without the need of a 2A or IRES element. The use of the first position of the genome enhances the expression level of the transgene inserted at that location, since VSV (and RABV) express genes in a transcriptional gradient; therefore, the first gene is the most highly transcribed (Knipe, 2007). This leads to rational predictions of expression levels so that one can choose the position of insertion of a transgene, or transgenes, according to this gradient and the desired level of expression. The size of the viral capsid is apparently not rigid, allowing for the inclusion of genomes that are substantially larger than the native genome, unlike the rigid capacity for some other viral vectors, such as AAV (Duan et al., 2000; Yan et al., 2000).

SUFFICIENCY OF GLYCOPROTEINS TO CONFER DIRECTIONALITY OF rVSV SPREAD ENABLES NOVEL APPLICATIONS

The fact that VSV can be made to spread anterogradely (Beier et al., 2011) or retrogradely across synapses with the change of a single gene affords several advantages over viral tracers that heretofore have not shown such flexibility in the directionality of tracing. In addition to the obvious application of tracing anterograde connections, combinations can be made to exploit the different forms of the virus. One example that employs the simultaneous infection with an anterograde and retrograde form of VSV is demonstrated in **Figure 6**. This experiment was designed to address whether the anterograde projections from the cortex to the CP would label the same brain regions as were labeled by a retrograde virus injected into the SN. Although a block of super-infection by the virus may preclude infection of the same cell with multiple rVSVs, adjacent cells could still become labeled by different viruses (Whitaker-Dowling et al., 1983). The observed results could be due to a preferential labeling by the anterograde transsynaptic virus of indirect pathway MSNs in this experiment, which then synapse onto the GP, thereby reflecting a viral bias. Alternatively, it could indicate that the cortical neurons in the injected region largely do not label the MSNs that project to the

area of the SN injected with the retrograde virus. One further possibility is that too little virus was used to observe co-labeling of a given region. However, given the density of infection (i.e., **Figures 6I,J**), the latter possibility seems unlikely. Additionally, the spread of the polysynaptic rVSV(RABV-G) appears to attenuate with increasing numbers of synapses crossed, permitting an analysis of more restricted viral spread. This is quite fortuitous, as if spread were to continue, it would lead to widespread infection and lethality. In addition, reconstruction of connectivity would be more difficult. This reduced efficiency appears to also hold for the monosynaptic form of VSV complemented with RABV-G, as the efficiency of transmission appeared lower than the comparable experiment with RABV (Watabe-Uchida et al., 2012). This is likely due to viral attenuation when VSV-G is replaced with RABV-G.

ADVANTAGES OF VSV OVER OTHER VIRAL TRACERS: SAFETY

We were attracted to the use of VSV as a viral tracer due to its long track record as a safe, replication-competent laboratory agent. Laboratory workers using VSV have not contracted any diseases, and natural VSV infections among human populations in Central America and the southwestern United States (Rodríguez, 2002) occur without evident pathology (Johnson et al., 1966; Brody et al., 1967). VSV was thus an attractive candidate for its use as a polysynaptic tracer for CNS studies, which requires an ability to replicate through multiple transmission cycles. Both replication-competent and incompetent forms of VSV are in use under Biosafety Level 2 containment. Replication-competent RABV is Biosafety Level 3, due to the fact that infection with replication-competent RABV is almost always fatal to humans and in mice when infected intracerebrally (Smith, 1981; Knipe, 2007).

Differences in pathogenicity between VSV and RABV are likely due to the ability of RABV to evade the innate immune system, particularly interferon (Hangartner et al., 2006; Junt et al., 2007; Lyles and Rupprecht, 2007; Rieder and Conzelmann, 2009; Iannacone et al., 2010). VSV infection efficiently triggers an interferon response, and it has not evolved a method of escape from this response, unlike RABV (Brzózka et al., 2006). In fact, VSV is being pursued as a vaccine for other viruses, including RABV (Lichty et al., 2004; Publicover et al., 2004; Kapadia et al., 2005; Schwartz et al., 2007; Iyer et al., 2009; Geisbert and Feldmann, 2011). VSV does not typically spread beyond the initially infected site in the periphery (Kramer et al., 1983; Vogel and Fertsch, 1987). This likely is the cause of the minor or absent symptoms in humans and animals infected in nature. Polysynaptic VSV vectors are thus predicted to be much safer than polysynaptic RABV vectors. We have tested this prediction by injecting a series of mice in the footpads and hind leg muscles with rVSV(RABV-G), with the result that no injected animals showed any evidence of morbidity or mortality (Beier, Goz et al., in preparation).

While safer for laboratory workers than RABV, the main drawback to using VSV is its rapid cellular toxicity (van den Pol et al., 2009; Beier et al., 2011). Toxicity is due to suppression of cellular transcription and a block in the export of cellular RNAs from the nucleus to the cytoplasm (Black and Lyles, 1992; Her et al., 1997; Ahmed and Lyles, 1998; Petersen et al., 2000; von Kobbe et al., 2000), as well as inhibition of the translation of cellular mRNAs (Francoeur et al., 1987; Jayakar et al., 2000; Kopecky et al.,

2001). VSV is much quicker to enact its gene expression program than is RABV, such that cells suffer the toxic effects more quickly than after RABV infection. One aspect of VSV that can be exploited in the future to ameliorate the speed of toxicity is the use of VSV mutants and variants. One such mutant is the M51R, which permitted us to conduct physiological analyses of pre-and post-synaptic cells (Beier et al., 2011). We are in the process of examining the transmission properties of this mutant *in vivo*, as well as the effects of other mutations or viral variants on prolonging the health of neurons after infection.

SUMMARY

rVSV vectors can be used to study the connectivity of neuronal circuitry. In addition to combinations of replication-competent forms of VSV, the replication-incompetent, monosynaptic forms of the virus can be easily combined, without the need to change viruses (Beier et al., 2011). This allows a straightforward way to study both the projections into, and out from, a genetically defined cell population. This can be done with the same viral genome, with the only change needed being the glycoprotein, for the selection of the direction of transmission. This flexibility of VSV makes it a powerful, multi-application vector for studying connectivity in the CNS.

MATERIALS AND METHODS
VIRUS CONSTRUCTION AND PRODUCTION

All rVSV clones were cloned from the rVSVΔG backbone (Chandran et al., 2005). mCherry, Kusabira orange, Venus, and CFP were cloned into the first (GFP) position using XhoI and MscI sites, and VSV-G (a gift from Richard Mulligan, Harvard Medical School, Boston, MA) and RABV-G (a gift from Ed Callaway, Salk Institute, San Diego, CA) were cloned into the fifth (G) position using the MluI and NotI restriction sites. Genes for fluorescent proteins were obtained from Clontech.

Viruses were rescued as previously described (Whelan et al., 1995). At 95% confluency, eight 10 cm plates of BSR cells were infected at an MOI of 0.01. Viral supernatants were collected at 24-h time intervals and ultracentrifuged at 21,000 RPM using a SW28 rotor and resuspended in 0.2% of the original volume. For titering, concentrated viral stocks were applied in a dilution series to 100% confluent BSR cells and plates were examined at 12 hpi. Viral stocks were stored at −80°C.

For ΔG viruses, 293T cells were transfected with PEI (Ehrhardt et al., 2006) at 70% confluency on 10 cm dishes with 5 µg of pCAG-RABV-G. Twenty-four hours post-infection, the cells were infected at an MOI of 0.01 with rVSVΔG expressing either GFP or mCherry. Viral supernatants were collected for the subsequent 4 days at 24 h intervals.

Virus preparations are now available from the Salk GT3 viral core (http://vectorcore.salk.edu/). All plasmids are available from Addgene (http://www.addgene.org/).

AAV VECTORS

AAV-FLEx-RABV-G and AAV-FLEx-TVA-mCherry plasmids originated from the Lab of Naoshige Uchida (Watabe-Uchida et al., 2012), and virus stocks were generous gifts from Brad Lowell, Harvard Medical School.

INJECTIONS OF MICE

ChAT-Cre (B6;129S6-Chat$^{tm1(cre)Lowl}$/J) and Ai9 (B6.Cg-Gt(ROSA)26Sor<tm9(CAG-tdTomato)Hze>/J) mice were obtained from the Jackson Laboratory (Madisen et al., 2010).

Eight-week-old CD-1 mice were injected using pulled capillary microdispensers (Drummond Scientific, Cat. No: 5-000-2005), using coordinates from The Mouse Brain in Stereotaxic Coordinates (Franklin and Paxinos, 1997). Injection coordinates (in mm) used were:

Primary Motor Cortex: A/P +1.34 from bregma, L/M 1.7, D/V −1 from pial surface
LGN: A/P −2.46 from bregma, L/M 2, D/V −2.75
Superior Colliculus: A/P −3.88 from bregma, L/M 0.5, D/V −1
CP: A/P +1 from bregma, L/M 1.8, D/V −2.5
Primary Visual Cortex (V1): A/P −3.4 from bregma, L/M 2.5, D/V −0.8.
SNr: A/P −3.28 from bregma, L/M 1.5, D/V −4.25

For multi-color analysis (**Figures 1C,D**), 3×10^9 ffu/mL rVSV was injected into various regions. For CP injections, 100 nL of rVSV(RABV-G) or rVSV(VSV-G) at 3×10^7 ffu/mL was injected at a rate of 100 nL/min. For the replication-incompetent viruses, 100 nL of 1×10^7 ffu/mL rVSVΔG(RABV-G) or rVSVΔG (VSV-G) was injected. In the motor cortex, 100 nL of 1×10^7 ffu/mL rVSV(RABV-G) was injected, and mice harvested 2 dpi. For V1 injections, 100 nL of 3×10^{10} ffu/mL rVSV(RABV-G) was injected, and mice were examined 3 or 7 dpi.

For infections of the dura mater, 1 µL of 3×10^{10} ffu/mL rVSV(RABV-G) was applied to the surface of the dura. The virus was allowed to absorb, and the surface was subsequently covered in bone wax, and the wound sutured.

For co-injections of virus into the same animal, 100 nL of a combination of 3×10^7 ffu/mL rVSV(VSV-G) and 3×10^8 ffu/mL rVSV(RABV-G) were co-injected into the motor cortex, and brains examined 3 dpi. For injections of the viruses into different regions, 100 nL of 3×10^7 ffu/mL rVSV(VSV-G) was injected into M1, and 100 nL of 3×10^8 ffu/mL rVSV(RABV-G) into the SNr, and brains examined 3 dpi. A lower titer of rVSV(VSV-G) was used, as rVSV(RABV-G) is attenuated.

All mouse work was conducted in biosafety containment level 2 conditions and was approved by the Longwood Medical Area Institutional Animal Care and Use Committee.

SLICE PREPARATION AND PHARMACOLOGY

Recordings were made from cortical pyramidal neurons in slices taken from postnatal day 12–18 mice, inoculated in the CP 12–18 h prior with rVSV(RABV-G). Coronal slices (300 µm thick) were cut in ice-cold external solution containing (in mM): 110 choline, 25 NaHCO$_3$, 1.25 NaH$_2$PO$_4$, 2.5 KCl, 7 MgCl$_2$, 0.5 CaCl$_2$, 25 glucose, 11.6 Na-ascorbate, and 3.1 Na-pyruvate, bubbled with 95% O$_2$ and 5% CO$_2$. Slices were then transferred to artificial cerebrospinal fluid (ACSF) containing (in mM): 127 NaCl, 25 NaHCO$_3$, 1.25 NaH$_2$PO$_4$, 2.5 KCl, 1 MgCl$_2$, 2 CaCl$_2$, and 25 glucose, bubbled with 95% O$_2$ and 5% CO$_2$. After an incubation period of 30–40 min at 34°C, slices were stored at room temperature. All experiments were conducted at room temperature (25°C). In all experiments, 50 µM picrotoxin, 10 µM 2,3-Dioxo-6-nitro-1,2,3,4-tetrahydrobenzo [f] quinoxaline-7-sulfonamide (NBQX), and 10 µM 3-((R)-2-Carboxypiperazin-4-yl)-propyl-1-phosphonic acid (CPP) were present in the ACSF to block GABAA/C, AMPA, and NMDA receptor-mediated transmission, respectively. All chemicals were from Sigma or Tocris.

ELECTROPHYSIOLOGY AND IMAGING

Whole-cell recordings were obtained from infected and uninfected deep layer cortical pyramidal neurons identified with video-IR/DIC and GFP fluorescence was detected using epifluorescence illumination. With the deep layers of the cortex, 2-photon laser scanning microscopy (2PLSM) was used to confirm the cell types based on morphology. Deep layer pyramidal neurons had large cell bodies, classic pyramidal shape and dendritic spines. Glass electrodes (2–4 MΩ) were filled with internal solution containing (in mM): 135 KMeSO$_4$, 5 KCl, 5 HEPES, 4 MgATP, 0.3 NaGTP, 10 Na$_2$HPO$_4$, 1 EGTA, and 0.01 Alexa Fluor-594 (to image neuronal morphology) adjusted to pH 7.4 with KOH. Current and voltage recordings were made at room temperature using a AxoPatch 200B or a Multiclamp 700B amplifier. Data was filtered at 5 kHz and digitized at 10 kHz.

DATA ACQUISITION AND ANALYSIS

Imaging and physiology data were acquired and analyzed as described previously (Carter and Sabatini, 2004). Resting membrane potential was determined by the average of three 5-s sweeps with no injected current. Passive properties of the cell, membrane (Rm) and series resistance (Rs) and capacitance (Cm), were measured while clamping cells at −65 mV and applying voltage steps from −55 to −75 mV. The current—firing relationship was determined in current clamp with 1-s periods of injected current from 100 to 500 pA.

HIPPOCAMPAL SLICE CULTURES

The time course of viral gene expression experiments were carried out in organotypic hippocampal slice cultures prepared from postnatal day 5–7 Sprague-Dawley rats as described previously (Stoppini et al., 1991). Slices were infected after 7 days *in vitro*, and images were acquired on a two-photon microscope.

ACKNOWLEDGMENTS

We are grateful for technical assistance from Vanessa Kainz in the laboratory of Rami Burstein at the Beth Israel Deaconess Medical Center. This work was supported by HHMI (Constance L. Cepko and Bernardo L. Sabatini), and #NS068012-01 (Kevin T. Beier).

REFERENCES

Ahmed, M., and Lyles, D. S. (1998). Effect of vesicular stomatitis virus matrix protein on transcription directed by host RNA polymerases, I, II, and III. *J. Virol.* 72, 8413–8419.

Albin, R. L., Young, A. B., and Penney, J. B. (1995). The functional anatomy of disorders of the basal ganglia. *Trends Neurosci.* 18, 63–64.

Astic, L., Saucier, D., Coulon, P., Lafay, F., and Flamand, A. (1993). The CVS strain of rabies virus as transneuronal tracer in the olfactory system of mice. *Brain Res.* 619, 146–156.

Balachandran, S., and Barber, G. N. (2000). Vesicular stomatitis virus (VSV) therapy of tumors. *IUBMB Life* 50, 135–138.

Beier, K. T., Saunders, A., Oldenburg, I. A., Miyamichi, K., Akhtar, N., Luo, L., et al. (2011). Anterograde or retrograde transsynaptic labeling of CNS neurons with vesicular stomatitis virus vectors. *Proc. Natl. Acad. Sci. U.S.A.* 108, 15414–15419.

Black, B. L., and Lyles, D. S. (1992). Vesicular stomatitis virus matrix protein inhibits host cell-directed transcription of target genes *in vivo*. *J. Virol.* 66, 4058–4064.

Bloomfield, C., O'Donnell, P., French, S. J, and Totterdell, S. (2007). Cholinergic neurons of the adult rat striatum are immunoreactive for glutamatergic N-methyl-d-aspartate 2D but not

N-methyl-d-aspartate 2C receptor subunits. *Neuroscience* 150, 639–646.

Bock, D., Lee, W. C., Kerlin, A., Andermann, M., Hood, G., Wetzel, A., et al. (2011). Network anatomy and *in vivo* physiology of visual cortical neurons. *Nature* 471, 177–182.

Brandly, C. A., and Hanson, R. P. (1957). Epizootiology of vesicular stomatitis. *Am. J. Public Health Nations Health* 47, 205–209.

Briggman, K. L., Helmstaedter, M., and Denk, W. (2011). Wiring specificity in the direction-selectivity circuit of the retina. *Nature* 471, 183–188.

Brody, J. A., Fischer, G. F., and Peralta, P. H. (1967). Vesicular stomatitis virus in Panama. Human serologic patterns in a cattle raising area. *Am. J. Epidemiol.* 86, 158–161.

Brzózka, K., Finke, S., and Conzelmann, K.-K. (2006). Inhibition of interferon signaling by rabies virus phosphoprotein P: activation-dependent binding of STAT1 and STAT2. *J. Virol.* 80, 2675–2683.

Carter, A. G., and Sabatini, B. L. (2004). State-dependent calcium signaling in dendritic spines of striatal medium spiny neurons. *Neuron* 44, 483–493.

Chandran, K., Sullivan, N. J., Felbor, U., Whelan, S. P., and Cunningham, J. M. (2005). Endosomal proteolysis of the Ebola virus glycoprotein is

necessary for infection. *Science* 308, 1643–1645.

Chauhan, V. S., Furr, S. R., Sterka, D. G., Nelson, D. A., Moerdyk-Schauwecker, M., Marriott, I., et al. (2010). Vesicular stomatitis virus infects resident cells of the central nervous system and induces replication-dependent inflammatory responses. *Virology* 400, 187–196.

Coulon, P., Rollin, P., Aubert, M., and Flamand, A. (1982). Molecular basis of rabies virus virulence. I. Selection of avirulent mutants of the CVS strain with anti-G monoclonal antibodies. *J. Gen. Virol.* 61(Pt 1), 97–100.

Duan, D., Yue, Y., Yan, Z., and Engelhardt, J. F. (2000). A new dual-vector approach to enhance recombinant adeno-associated virus-mediated gene expression through intermolecular cis activation. *Nat. Med.* 6, 595–598.

Ehrhardt, C., Schmolke, M., Matzke, A., Knoblauch, A., Will, C., Wixler, V., et al. (2006). Polyethylenimine, a cost-effective transfection reagent. *Sig. Transduct.* 6, 179–184.

Francoeur, A. M., Poliquin, L., and Stanners, C. P. (1987). The isolation of interferon-inducing mutants of vesicular stomatitis virus with altered viral P function for the inhibition of total protein synthesis. *Virology* 160, 236–245.

Franklin, K., and Paxinos, G. (1997). *The Mouse Brain in Stereotaxic Coordinates*. San Diego, CA: Academic Press.

Geisbert, T. W., and Feldmann, H. (2011). Recombinant vesicular stomatitis virus-based vaccines against Ebola and Marburg virus infections. *J. Infect. Dis.* 204(Suppl. 3), S1075–S1081.

Hangartner, L., Zinkernagel, R. M., and Hengartner, H. (2006). Antiviral antibody responses: the two extremes of a wide spectrum. *Nat. Rev. Immunol.* 6, 231.

Her, L.-S., Lund, E., and Dahlberg, J. E. (1997). Inhibition of Ran guanosine triphosphatase-dependent nuclear transport by the matrix protein of vesicular stomatitis virus. *Science* 276, 1845–1848.

Iannacone, M., Moseman, E. A., Tonti, E., Bosurgi, L., Junt, T., Henrickson, S. E., et al. (2010). Subcapsular sinus macrophages prevent CNS invasion on peripheral infection with a neurotropic virus. *Nature* 465, 1079–1083.

Iyer, A. V., Pahar, B., Boudreaux, M. J., Wakamatsu, N., Roy, A. F., Chouljenko, V. N., et al. (2009). Recombinant vesicular stomatitis virus-based west Nile vaccine elicits strong humoral and cellular immune responses and protects mice against lethal challenge with the virulent west Nile virus strain LSU-AR01. *Vaccine* 27, 893–903.

Jayakar, H. R., Murti, K. G., and Whitt, M. A. (2000). Mutations in the PPPY motif of vesicular stomatitis virus matrix protein reduce virus budding by inhibiting a late step in virion release. *J. Virol.* 74, 9818–9827.

Johnson, K. M., Vogel, J. E., and Peralta, P. H. (1966). Clinical and serological response to laboratory-acquired human infection by Indiana type vesicular stomatitis virus (VSV). *Am. J. Trop. Med. Hyg.* 15, 244–246.

Junt, T., Moseman, E. A., Iannacone, M., Massberg, S., Lang, P. A., Boes, M., et al. (2007). Subcapsular sinus macrophages in lymph nodes clear lymph-borne viruses and present them to antiviral B cells. *Nature* 450, 110.

Kandel, E. J. (2000). *Principles of Neural Science.* New York, NY: McGraw Hill Professional.

Kapadia, S. U., Rose, J. K., Lamirande, E., Vogel, L., Subbarao, K., and Roberts, A. (2005). Long-term protection from SARS coronavirus infection conferred by a single immunization with an attenuated VSV-based vaccine. *Virology* 340, 174–182.

Kelly, R. M., and Strick, P. L. (2000). Rabies as a transneuronal tracer of circuits in the central nervous system. *J. Neurosci. Methods* 103, 63–71.

Kelly, R. M., and Strick, P. L. (2003). Cerebellar loops with motor cortex and prefrontal cortex of a non-human primate. *J. Neurosci.* 23, 8432–8444.

Knipe, D. M. (2007) *Fields Virology.* Philadelphia, PA: Lippincott Williams and Wilkins.

Kopecky, S. A., Willingham, M. C., and Lyles, D. S. (2001). Matrix protein and another viral component contribute to induction of apoptosis in cells infected with vesicular stomatitis virus. *J. Virol.* 75, 12169–12181.

Kramer, M. J., Dennin, R., Kramer, C., Jones, G., Connell, E., Rolon, N., et al. (1983). Cell and virus sensitivity studies with recombinant human alpha interferons. *J. Interferon Res.* 3, 425–435.

Lichty, B. D., Power, A. T., Stojdl, D. F., and Bell, J. C. (2004). Vesicular stomatitis virus: re-inventing the bullet. *Trends Mol. Med.* 10, 210–216.

Lyles, D. S., and Rupprecht, C. E. (2007). Rhabdoviridae. *Virology* 1, 1363–1408.

Madisen, L., Zwingman, T., Sunkin, S., Oh, S., Zariwala, H., Gu, H., et al. (2010). A robust and high-throughput Cre reporting and characterization system for the whole mouse brain. *Nat. Neurosci.* 13, 133–140.

Mayberg, M. R., Zervas, N. T., and Moskowitz, M. A. (1984). Trigeminal projections to supratentorial pial and dural blood vessels in cats demonstrated by horseradish peroxidase histochemistry. *J. Comp. Neurol.* 223, 46–56.

Mazarakis, N. D., Azzouz, M., Rohll, J. B., Ellard, F. M., Wilkes, F. J., Olsen, A. L., et al. (2001). Rabies virus glycoprotein pseudotyping of lentiviral vectors enables retrograde axonal transport and access to the nervous system after peripheral delivery. *Hum. Mol. Genet.* 10, 2109–2121.

Penfield, W., and McNaughton, F. (1940). Dural headache and innervation of the dura mater. *Arch. Neurol. Psychiatry* 44, 43–75.

Petersen, J. M., Her, L. S., Varvel, V., Lund, E., and Dahlberg, J. E. (2000). The matrix protein of vesicular stomatitis virus inhibits nucleocytoplasmic transport when it is in the nucleus and associated with nuclear pore complexes. *Mol. Cell. Biol.* 20, 8590–8601.

Publicover, J., Ramsburg, E., and Rose, J. K. (2004). Characterization of nonpathogenic, live, viral vaccine vectors inducing potent cellular immune responses. *J. Virol.* 78, 9317–9324.

Rieder, M., and Conzelmann, K.-K. (2009). Rhabdovirus evasion of the interferon system. *J. Interferon Cytokine Res.* 29, 499–510.

Rodríguez, L. L. (2002). Emergence and re-emergence of vesicular stomatitis in the United States. *Virus Res.* 85, 211–219.

Schwartz, J. A., Buonocore, L., Roberts, A., Suguitan, A., Kobasa, D., Kobinger, G., et al. (2007). Vesicular stomatitis virus vectors expressing avian influenza H5 HA induce cross-neutralizing antibodies and long-term protection. *Virology* 366, 166–173.

Smith, J. S. (1981). Mouse model for abortive rabies infection of the central nervous system. *Infect. Immun.* 31, 297–308.

Standish, A., Enquist, L. W., and Schwaber, J. S. (1994). Innervation of the heart and its central medullary origin defined by viral tracing. *Science* 263, 232–234.

Stojdl, D., Lichty, B., Knowles, S., Marius, R., Atkins, H., Sonenberg, N., et al. (2000). Exploiting tumor-specific defects in the interferon pathway with a previously unknown oncolytic virus. *Nat. Med.* 6, 821–825.

Stojdl, D., Lichty, B., tenOever, B., Paterson, J., Power, A., Knowles, S., et al. (2003). VSV strains with defects in their ability to shutdown innate immunity are potent systemic anti-cancer agents. *Cancer Cell* 4, 263–275.

Stoppini, L., Buchs, P. A., and Muller, D. (1991). A simple method for organotypic cultures of nervous tissue. *J. Neurosci. Methods* 37, 173–182.

Thomas, T. M., Smith, Y., Levey, A. I., and Hersch, S. M. (2000). Cortical inputs to m2-immunoreactive striatal interneurons in rat and monkey. *Synapse* 37, 252–261.

Ugolini, G. (1995). Specificity of rabies virus as a transneuronal tracer of motor networks: transfer from hypoglossal motoneurons to connected second-order and higher order central nervous system cell groups. *J. Comp. Neurol.* 356, 457–480.

Ugolini, G., Kuypers, H. G., and Strick, P. L. (1989). Transneuronal transfer of herpes virus from peripheral nerves to cortex and brainstem. *Science* 243, 89–91.

van den Pol, A. N., Dalton, K. P., and Rose, J. K. (2002). Relative neurotropism of a recombinant rhabdovirus expressing a green fluorescent envelope glycoprotein. *J. Virol.* 76, 1309–1327.

van den Pol, A. N., Ozduman, K., Wollmann, G., Ho, W. S. C., Simon, I., Yao, Y., et al. (2009). Viral strategies for studying the brain, including a replication-restricted self-amplifying delta-G vesicular stomatis virus that rapidly expresses transgenes in brain and can generate a multicolor golgi-like expression. *J. Comp. Neurol.* 516, 456–481.

Vogel, S. N., and Fertsch, D. (1987). Macrophages from endotoxin-hyporesponsive (Lpsd) C3H/HeJ mice are permissive for vesicular stomatitis virus because of reduced levels of endogenous interferon: possible mechanism for natural resistance to virus infection. *J. Virol.* 61, 812–818.

von Kobbe, C., van Deursen, J. M., Rodrigues, J. P., Sitterlin, D., Bachi, A., Wu, X., et al. (2000). Vesicular stomatitis virus matrix protein inhibits host cell gene expression by targeting the nucleoporin Nup98. *Mol. Cell* 6, 1243–1252.

Wall, N. R., Wickersham, I. R., Cetin, A., De La Parra, M., and Callaway, E. M. (2010). Monosynaptic circuit tracing in vivo through Cre-dependent targeting and complementation of modified rabies virus. *Proc. Natl. Acad. Sci. U.S.A.* 107, 21848–21853.

Watabe-Uchida, M., Zhu, L., Ogawa, S. K., Vamanrao, A., and Uchida, N. (2012). Whole-brain mapping of direct inputs to midbrain dopamine neurons. *Neuron* 74, 858–873.

Whelan, S. P., Ball, L. A., Barr, J. N., and Wertz, G. T. (1995). Efficient recovery of infectious vesicular stomatitis virus entirely from cDNA clones. *Proc. Natl. Acad. Sci. U.S.A.* 92, 8388–8392.

Whitaker-Dowling, P., Youngner, J. S., Widnell, C. C., and Wilcox, D. K. (1983). Superinfection exclusion by vesicular stomatitis virus. *Virology* 131, 137–143.

Wickersham, I. R., Finke, S., Conzelmann, K.-K., and Callaway, E. M. (2007a). Retrograde neuronal tracing with a deletion-mutant rabies virus. *Nat. Methods* 4, 47–49.

Wickersham, I. R., Lyon, D. C., Barnard, R. J. O., Mori, T., Finke, S., Conzelmann, K. K., et al. (2007b). Monosynaptic restriction of transsynaptic tracing from single, genetically targeted neurons. *Neuron* 53, 639–647.

Yan, Z., Zhang, Y., Duan, D., and Engelhardt, J. F. (2000). Trans-splicing vectors expand the utility of adeno-associated virus for gene therapy. *Proc. Natl. Acad. Sci. U.S.A.* 97, 6716–6721.

7

Sub-millisecond closed-loop feedback stimulation between arbitrary sets of individual neurons

Jan Müller*, Douglas J. Bakkum and Andreas Hierlemann

Bio Engineering Laboratory, ETH Zürich, Basel, Switzerland

Edited by:
Steve M. Potter, Georgia Institute of Technology, USA

Reviewed by:
Antonio Novellino, ETT s.r.l., Italy
Jürg Streit, University of Bern, Switzerland

*Correspondence:
Jan Müller, Bio Engineering Laboratory, ETH Zürich, Basel, Switzerland.
e-mail: 217534@gmail.com

We present a system to artificially correlate the spike timing between sets of arbitrary neurons that were interfaced to a complementary metal–oxide–semiconductor (CMOS) high-density microelectrode array (MEA). The system features a novel reprogrammable and flexible event engine unit to detect arbitrary spatio-temporal patterns of recorded action potentials and is capable of delivering sub-millisecond closed-loop feedback of electrical stimulation upon trigger events in real-time. The relative timing between action potentials of individual neurons as well as the temporal pattern among multiple neurons, or neuronal assemblies, is considered an important factor governing memory and learning in the brain. Artificially changing timings between arbitrary sets of spiking neurons with our system could provide a "knob" to tune information processing in the network.

Keywords: closed-loop, high-density microelectrode array, STDP, acausal stimulation, LTD, sub-millisecond

INTRODUCTION

Different theories describing learning and memory in the brain have been developed, and converging evidence shows that the precise activity timing of individual or groups of neurons may play a paramount role in plasticity of neuronal circuits. The well-known spike timing dependent plasticity (STDP) rule states that if two synaptically connected neurons fire within tens of milliseconds of each other, the connectivity strength of the involved synapses gets potentiated or depressed depending on the firing order. In pioneering studies, STDP rules were discovered (Markram et al., 1997) and further characterized (Bi and Poo, 1998; Song et al., 2000) by observing the effect of correlated firing of two neurons either artificially induced by stimulating a pre-and a post-synaptic neuron with two patch-clamps or by applying trains of paired-pulse stimuli to one neuron in the network (Bi and Poo, 1999). Furthermore, computation in a network is likely due not only to the relative timing of two individual neurons but also to the correlated activity of different neurons forming an associated group, i.e., assembly (Chang et al., 2000; Izhikevich, 2006). In this vein, different studies reported the existence of precise time-locked activity patterns of multiple neurons, both *in vivo* and *in vitro* (Abeles and Gerstein, 1988; Bienenstock, 1995; Ikegaya et al., 2004; Rolston et al., 2007). Having a system to generate feedback stimulation quickly and accurately to interact with such activity patterns would expand such studies beyond finding rules governing the plasticity between two cells toward finding rules governing the spatio-temporal dynamics of whole networks or assemblies (Froemke and Dan, 2002; Izhikevich et al., 2004).

In recent years, different systems to artificially control such feedback stimulation in a closed-loop manner, and thus study neuronal plasticity, have been developed for both *in vivo* (Jackson et al., 2006b; Bontorin et al., 2007; Venkatraman et al., 2009) and *in vitro* applications (Bontorin et al., 2007; Hafizovic et al., 2007; Novellino et al., 2007; Rolston et al., 2010; Zrenner et al., 2010; Wallach et al., 2011). In turn, activity-dependent feedback

stimulation was shown to modify the functional connectivity of neuronal networks, both *in vivo* and *in vitro*, as done by reprogramming the motor output of freely behaving primates (Jackson et al., 2006a), changing the functional connectivity in rat forelimb sensorimotor cortex (Rebesco et al., 2010), or shaping *in vitro* neocortical networks into predefined activity states (Bakkum et al., 2008b). *In vivo* systems usually record from needles inserted into a certain location of the brain and subsequently stimulate the same or another site upon the detection of activity. These systems usually comprise the implanted needles, a head stage to amplify the signals, and some means to transmit the acquired signals to a PC. In the case of closed-loop feedback stimulation, these systems usually feature a dedicated very-large-scale-integrated application-specific circuit (VLSI ASIC) (Chen et al., 2009; Rizk et al., 2009; Lee et al., 2010; Azin et al., 2011), or use a general-purpose microcontroller to achieve the respective goals (Mavoori et al., 2005; Zanos et al., 2011). Most *in vitro* systems, on the other hand, use a data acquisition card (DAQ) to sample data for analysis on a PC; feedback stimulation is typically returned through a DAQ card as well.

In order to accurately control the timing of feedback stimulation loops within the timescales relevant for STDP to occur, the delays introduced by a system must be understood. A generic description is given in **Figure 1**. Different system implementations will have different sources for and values of delays. Signal-processing algorithms introduce an inherent delay in the processing itself. Systems, which rely on general-purpose computers, might introduce latencies and jitter through the presence of data buffers, interrupts, shared resources, or user interactions, etc. In **Figure 1**, the time points t_{0-3} and t_S specify the occurrence of important events. At $t_0 = 0$, the trigger neuron emits an action potential, which is recorded by the acquisition system. After entering the signal-processing stages, it is ready to be detected as a spike event at time t_1. From there, the system emits a stimulation pulse hitting the electrode at time t_2. Conventionally,

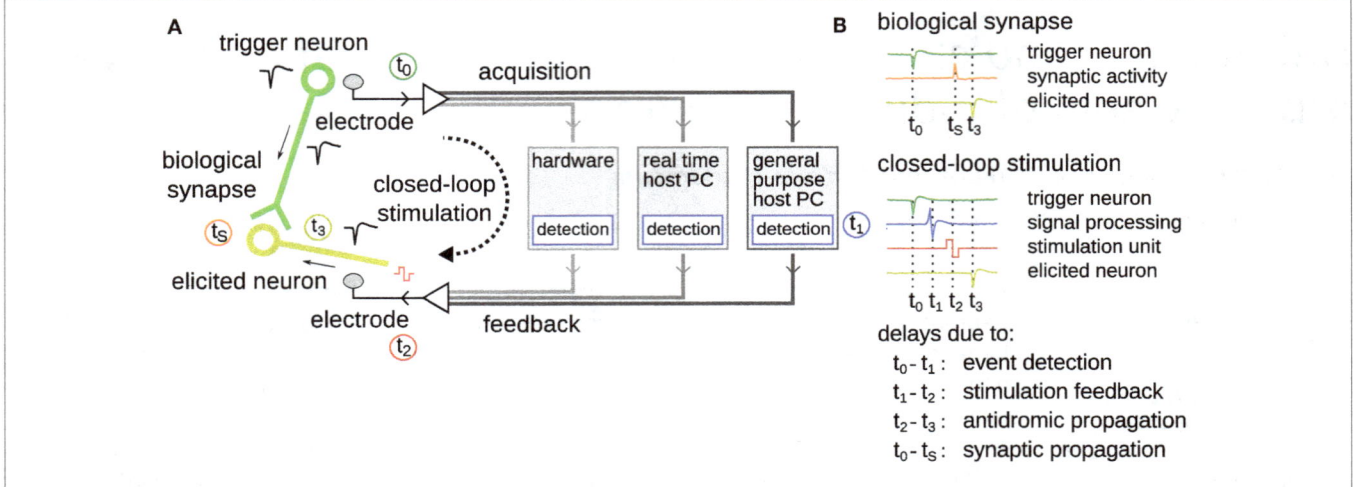

FIGURE 1 | Schematic overview of latencies in feedback stimulation systems. (A) The different components making up a closed-loop feedback stimulation system are shown. The green circle represents the "trigger neuron" whose action potential initiates the start of the loop. The green line represents an axon connecting to synapses of the elicited neuron drawn in yellow. The black dashed arrow shows the closed-loop feedback stimulation path. Between data acquisition and stimulation feedback, different components, over which the feedback-loop can be closed, are possible,

including digital signal-processing hardware, a real-time host PC, or a general purpose host PC. The time points t_{0-3} and t_S correspond to different events as listed in **(B)**, such as the occurrence of the spike; its detection after signal-processing; the stimulation feedback; and the antidromic propagation of an action potential back into the soma of the elicited neuron. At time t_S, the synapse activates due to pre-synaptic activity of the trigger neuron. The color of the traces corresponds to the color of the timings of $t_{0-3, S}$ and schematically shows the timeline of the respective signals.

the loop is considered "closed" at this point. The stimulation pulse evokes neuronal activity, frequently activating nearby axons (Bakkum et al., 2008a) whose signals propagate antidromically toward the soma until eliciting an action potential at time t_3. In the case depicted in **Figure 1**, where the trigger neuron is synaptically connected to the elicited neuron, an additional biological time, t_S, denotes the duration of an action potential propagation through the axon of the trigger neuron until synaptic activation of the elicited neuron. In case where $t_0 - t_1 - t_2$ is faster than $t_0 - t_S$, that is when the signal propagates faster through the artificial feedback-loop than down the axon toward the biological synapse, acausal stimulation, and thus the introduction of long-term depression (LTD) according to the STDP rule, is possible.

In order to apply closed-loop stimulation feedback precise and fast enough to study plasticity at the timescales of STDP or acausal stimulation, and flexible enough to interact with cell assemblies, we developed a field-programmable gate array (FPGA)-based system, interfaced with a complementary metal–oxide–semiconductor high-density microelectrode array (CMOS-MEA). The CMOS-MEA features a total of 126 readout and 42 stimulation channels, which can be connected to an almost arbitrary subset of 11,011 $5 \times 7 \, \mu m^2$ electrodes, arranged in a $2 \times 1.75 \, mm^2$ array. The feedback stimulation loop is closed around the CMOS-MEA using an FPGA that performs signal-processing, such as spike-detection and feedback generation. The system functionality was verified using cultured networks of cortical neurons and glia. The minimum programmable latency of the closed-loop stimulation feedback ($t_0 - t_1 - t_2$) was $400 \, \mu s$ with jitter below $50 \, \mu s$, suitable to induce STDP. This is faster than many axonal propagation delays ($t_0 - t_S$), rendering it possible to

conduct acausal stimulation experiments. An "event engine" was designed and implemented to trigger feedback stimulation at the occurrence of activity patterns, such as those described in Ikegaya et al. (2004) and Rolston et al. (2007). Patterns could be of almost arbitrary length and could consist of up to 1000's of individual elements, only limited by the available resources of the FPGA. Configurations for the event engine could be (re)loaded within milliseconds. Unique to this system is the possibility to enable low-latency, high-throughput, STDP-like experiments as well as acausal stimulations across many individual neurons, or neuronal assemblies in parallel through the simultaneous application of many feedback stimulation loops. To infer changes in synaptic strengths, correlations between putative mono-synaptically connected neurons (Fujisawa et al., 2008) can be monitored using extracellular spikes. In the future, high-throughput STDP experiments will be possible by adding a patch electrode to the system in order to monitor changes in intracellular post-synaptic currents.

METHODS
SYSTEM ARCHITECTURE
The main design goals were to implement (1) multiple feedback stimulation loops (2) to match arbitrary spike patterns with (3) short latencies (<1 ms) and (4) high accuracy (<50 μs) (5) while still recording from all available 126 channels. A main component of the presented system is an FPGA, used to hijack signals traveling between the analog-to-digital converter on the CMOS device and the host PC. Due to the inherent parallel nature of FPGAs, signal-processing and feedback generation using data from additional recording channels can be done without introducing additional delays or jitter.

The system consists of three main parts as shown in **Figure 2**. The first is a high-density CMOS-MEA device featuring on chip signal-conditioning, stimulation, and analog-to-digital conversion (ADC) units (Frey et al., 2010), described in more detail in the next section. It is plugged into a custom printed circuit board (PCB) that provides reference voltages and clock signals. The digital data as provided by the CMOS-MEA are transmitted through a low-voltage differential link to reduce sensitivity to electromagnetic interferences as caused, for example, by a nearby incubator. The second part is an FPGA, which reads in the differential signals and subsequently performs signal-processing, spike-detection, and feedback stimulation, as well as compression and framing of the data to be sent via TCP/IP over Ethernet to a host PC, the third main part. On the host PC, further data analysis can be performed online or offline. It is also used to program and control the CMOS-MEA device during experimentation with different settings, like amplifier gain or electrode-to-amplifier routing, in order to be adopted for use in different experimental sessions.

CMOS DEVICE

The CMOS-MEA includes 126 readout channels with programmable amplification (0 dB to 80 dB), on chip ADCs sampling at 20 kHz, and stimulation capabilities (see below). It features a sensor area of $2 \times 1.75\,\text{mm}^2$ with a total of 11,011 electrodes, each with a size of $5 \times 7\,\mu\text{m}^2$ and a pitch of $18\,\mu\text{m}$. Beneath the electrodes resides a sophisticated analog-switching matrix to connect an almost arbitrary subset of the 11,011 electrodes to the 126 readout channels. The readout electronics were placed

outside of the sensor array, instead of directly below the electrodes as done in active-pixel sensor devices (APS) (Berdondini et al., 2009), to provide space for larger circuitry elements that produce less noise. This scheme also allows for reducing the pitch of the electrodes below the spatial requirements of the readout electronics. See Frey et al. (2010) for more details.

FPGA

A reprogrammable Virtex II pro FPGA (Xilinx Inc., San Jose, USA) was used as an intermediate signal-processing device between the CMOS-MEA and the host PC to perform real-time signal-processing, decision-making and feedback generation. The FPGA acquires digital data coming from the differential link and forwards it to a PC over Ethernet. The Virtex II pro features an embedded PowerPC microprocessor running at 300 MHz that operates a Linux kernel with a Busybox operating system. The TCP/IP stack of the Linux kernel handles the network communication and data transfer. As the embedded PowerPC microprocessor is relatively slow, compared to modern CPUs, this provides a bottleneck for fast data transmission. We measured the latency between the TCP/IP stack of the FPGA and the host PC to be $83 \pm 21\,\text{ms}$ (mean $\pm$ SD, $N = 308$) at full-frame data transmission, which is larger than the STDP window of up to tens of milliseconds. One solution to this problem might be to stop streaming of the full data readout, while performing a closed-loop experiment and to only route out the data channels strictly needed for the closed-loop feedback stimulation. This would free some of the bandwidth of the Ethernet link and make it available for faster feedback stimulation. Crucially, however,

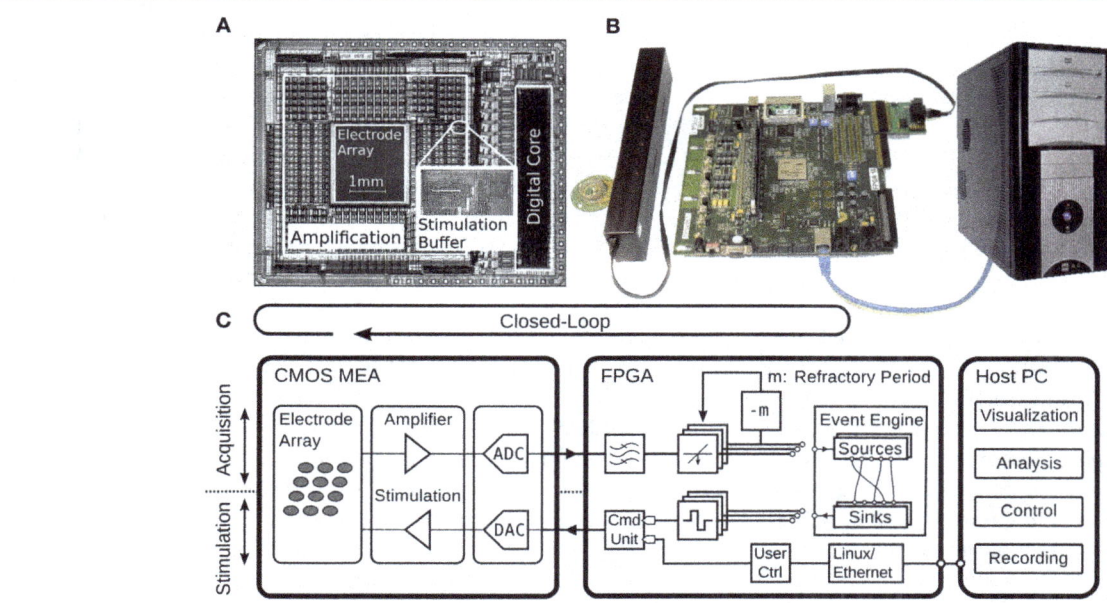

FIGURE 2 | Overview of the presented closed-loop system, implemented with a CMOS-MEA, an FPGA, and a host PC. (A) Micrograph of the CMOS-MEA highlighting the electrode array, amplification and stimulation units, and the digital core with an inset showing a close-up of the stimulation buffer. **(B)** Photograph of the CMOS-MEA plugged into the custom printed-circuit board, which is connected through an LVDS link to the Xilinx

Virtex II pro FPGA board from Digilent Inc., Pullman, USA. The host PC running data acquisition and visualization software is connected to the FPGA through Ethernet. **(C)** Schematic diagram of the setup. The diagram shows the acquisition (upper part) and stimulation path (lower part). The feedback stimulation loop is closed around the CMOS-MEA and the FPGA. The components are described in detail in the text.

we would lose the possibility to simultaneously monitor neural activity elsewhere in the cultured network by applying such a paradigm. Another option might be to bypass the Ethernet link by streaming the data directly to a DAQ card, attached to the host PC, and to send stimulation information back through a second link to the FPGA. All these methods are less practical than using the universal TCP/IP connection, which plugs into almost every kind of host PC and does not require additional hardware. An attractive alternative for achieving low latencies was to implement all needed signal-processing and feedback generation directly on the FPGA. The next paragraphs highlight the different building blocks needed to implement such a scheme. Although the FPGA can be reprogrammed at will, this is time-consuming and error prone and, therefore, not suitable during an experimental session. To accommodate reprogramming, a more flexible, module-based design was developed in VHDL and programmed into the FPGA logic together with a software interface to quickly reconfigure the connectivity of the individual modules (see "Event Engine").

SPIKE-DETECTION

One such signal-processing building block is spike-detection, which extracts spiking events from the raw voltage traces, recorded at the electrodes. Spike-detection is implemented as a threshold crossing. The signals are first digitally band-pass filtered with a two-tab Butterworth filter (500 Hz–3 kHz) to suppress DC offset components and higher frequency noise; this will emphasize the action potential frequency components. The detection threshold level is user-programmable and typically set around 4.5 times the noise standard deviation. During experimentation, this value can be determined by software running online on the host PC. After an identified spike event, we set a programmable refractory period to 3 ms. After stimulation, detection was disabled for 3 ms as well, to avoid oscillating loops due to feedback stimulation artifacts being falsely classified as spikes.

EVENT ENGINE

To avoid time-consuming reprogramming of the FPGA fabric, a more flexible and modular event-based scheme for feedback generation (Event Engine) was designed and implemented. The event engine consists of small building blocks, called modules, each of which implements a specific simple function. Each module has one or more event sinks as inputs and one event source as an output. By connecting the event sources to the appropriate event sinks, different, almost arbitrary pattern matching, and event handling algorithms can be achieved. **Table 1** summarizes the implemented modules. **Figure 3** shows different basic configurations to achieve defined pattern matching. In **Figure 3A**, the simplest closed-loop configuration is depicted, where the source of a spike-detection module gets connected to the sink of a delay unit and from there to a stimulation function generator. Whenever the source produces an event (i.e., in this case detects a spike), the sink triggers a stimulation pulse after a defined time delay. By means of software, the sources can be connected to sinks dynamically and rapidly within milliseconds while running an experiment such that pattern matching can adapt to ongoing activity in the living culture. One notable property is the lack of time binning. Each spike gets represented as a single pulse with a

temporal resolution set by the sampling frequency, i.e., 20 kHz. As a consequence, certain desired operations might not make sense, as the biological neurons have some inherent variability in when they spike. For example, the user might want to match a pattern, where two neurons spike together (see **Figure 3E**). To achieve this, a SPREADING module "spreads" the spike pulse in time in order to compensate for jitter. This way, the subsequent AND module can generate an output event whenever the two neurons fire together within a specified range of time. As discussed in Ikegaya et al. (2004) and Rolston et al. (2007), 2 ms is suitable for most recurring patterns. Another module can be used to convert the spread-out spike pulse back into a single one-shot event, which then can be used, for example, to trigger the stimulation unit only once per spread-out pulse. The particular selection of implemented modules (as listed in **Table 1**) represents a minimal set, which, if combined in the appropriate way, allows for matching different kinds of events, such as specific spatio-temporal activity patterns, time sequences, network bursts, local bursts, etc. In order to keep the event engine as flexible as possible and adaptable to different, possibly unforeseen pattern matching sequences, the implementation of a minimal set of small building blocks has been chosen over the approach, where each envisioned pattern would require a single, but more complex, and less flexible building block. Thus, available modules can be combined together in almost infinite different ways, limited only by the available FPGA memory that keeps track of all source-sink associations.

STIMULATION/FUNCTION GENERATOR

The CMOS-MEA has 42 on-chip integrated stimulation units, which are driven by two 10bit DACs. On the FPGA is a function generator implemented to achieve arbitrary stimulation waveforms. A defined waveform has to be programmed at the start of the experiment. We used biphasic, first positive then negative voltage pulses of 200 μs duration per phase and ±300 or 400 mV amplitude. The stimulation buffers can be chosen to operate in voltage- or current mode (Livi et al., 2010). Whenever the event engine outputs an event, the appropriate stimulation buffer, located on the CMOS-MEA, gets connected, and the function generator starts its operation. Stimulation artifacts on the readout channels could result in falsely detected spikes and cause a reverberation problem for low-latency feedback-loops. Therefore, spike-detection is blanked during a time period of a few milliseconds after stimulation onset.

CULTURES

The performance of the closed-loop system was tested with cortical neurons and glia grown over the CMOS-MEA. Animal handling protocols were approved by the Basel-Stadt Veterinary office according to Swiss federal laws on animal welfare. Briefly, a time-pregnant rat was anesthetized using isoflurane, then decapitated to gain E18 embryos. Cortices were extracted from the embryos and dissociated enzymatically in trypsin (Invitrogen) followed by mechanical trituration. A layer of laminin (Sigma) over a layer of poly(ethyleneimine) (Sigma) was used to adhere between 20 and 40 k cells. Plating media consisted of 850 μL of Neurobasal, supplemented with 10% horse serum (HyClone), 0.5 mM GlutaMAX (Invitrogen), and 2% B27 (Invitrogen). After

Table 1 | A minimal set of modules making up the event engine.

z^{-1}	DELAY(t, **A**)	Delays the event **A** by a defined amount of time t.
&	AND(**A**, **B**)	Emits an event, when both of the two input events, **A** and **B** occurred simultaneously.
≥1	OR(**A**, **B**)	Emits an event, when either of the two input events **A** or **B** occurred.
$\bar{\&}$	INH(t, **A**, **B**)	Emits an event, when an event on **A**, however, no event on **B** occurred in a defined time window, t, in order to create inhibitory feedback-loops.
❋	RAND(p, **A**)	Propagates the event **A** to the output or drops it after a Bernoulli-distributed pseudo-random variable with a definable probability, p.
±	ACCU(n, **A**, **B**)	Increments (event **A**) or decrements (event **B**) an internal accumulator and emits an event after a definable threshold, n, has been reached, after which it is reset to zero.
⊓	SPREAD(t, **A**)	Spreads the event **A** in time for a defined time, t.
⊔	SPREAD^{-1}(**A**)	Converts the onset of a spread-out event **A** back into a single event.
⊿	DETECTION(c)	Emits an event, when the specified channel, c, detected a spike.
⊓ᴸ	STIMULATION(c, **A**)	Generates a stimulation pulse on the specified channel, c, whenever input event **A** happened.
t_0	START	Single pulse after system start-up, which can be used to start repetitive stimulation protocols.

Configurable parameters are represented in italics (t, p, n, c), and input events are denoted in bold letters (A, B).

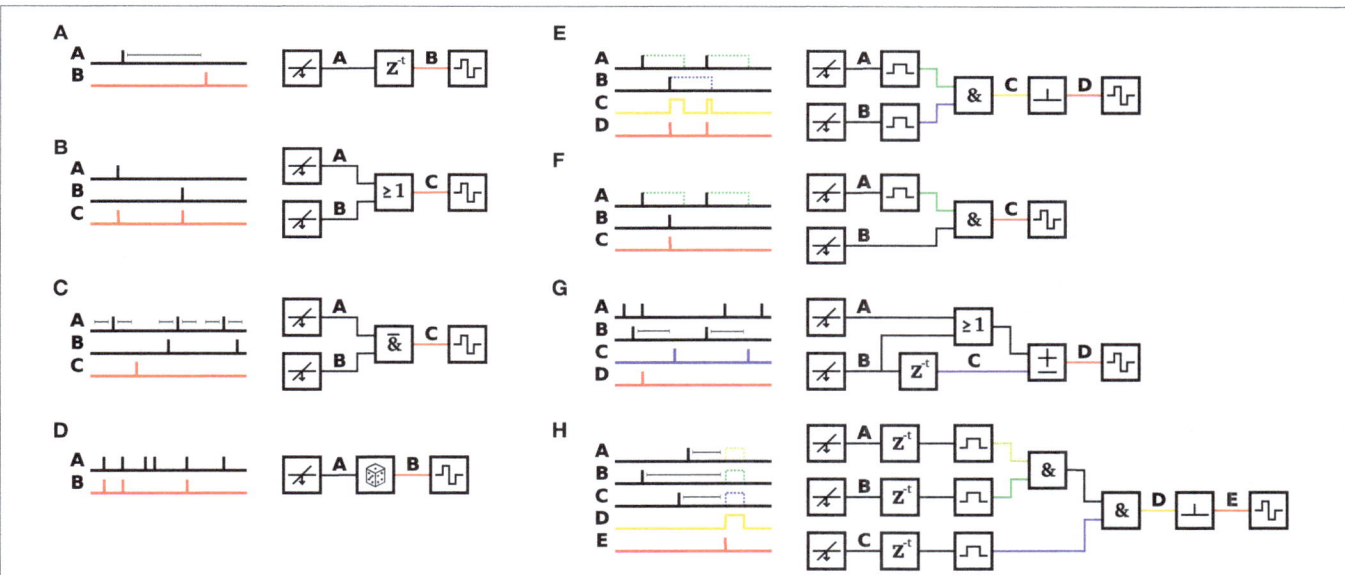

FIGURE 3 | Example configurations of the event engine. Stitching together the appropriate set of modules allows the event engine to be configured to match a variety of patterns in order to trigger feedback stimulation. Different minimal examples are shown. **(A)** A DELAY element is inserted after a DETECTION module to trigger STIMULATION after a programmable delay. This configuration, with the delay set to zero, was used for the experiments shown in **Figures 5**, **7**. **(B)** Either an event on channel **A** OR an event on channel **B** triggers stimulation. **(C)** In a programmable time window before and after an event on channel **A**, there may not be any event on channel **B** in order to trigger stimulation (trace **C**). **(D)** A RAND module propagates or discards the events, in this case with a probability of ½. **(E)** Events on channel **A** and channel **B** are fed through SPREAD modules into an AND module, which outputs events (on trace **C**), when both inputs are active. The intermediate trace **C** is fed into a SPREAD^{-1} module to trigger stimulation at the onset of the event. **(F)** When the event on channel **B** happens subsequently to an event on channel **A**, an event **C** is generated **(G)** An ACCU module is set to increment, when either an event on channel **A** OR channel **B** happened, and to decrement, when a delayed event from channel **B** (trace **C**) arrived. In this example, the ACCU threshold is set to three events. Once the threshold is reached, the internal counter gets reset to zero. When the three input events happen shortly after each other, a stimulation event gets emitted. As shown in the example, the delayed channel **B** (trace **C**) decrements the accumulator and thus delays or prohibits crossing of the threshold. **(H)** All modules can be combined together to achieve almost arbitrarily complex pattern matching. For example, this configuration was used to match the pattern of **Figure 6**. The formula describing this pattern is: STIMULATION(*1*, SPREAD^{-1}(AND(AND(SPREAD(*2 ms*, **A**), SPREAD(*2 ms*, **B**)), SPREAD(*2 ms*, **C**)))).

24 h, the plating media was changed to growth media: 850 μL of DMEM (Invitrogen), supplemented with 10% horse serum, 0.5 mM GlutaMAX, and 1 mM sodium pyruvate (Invitrogen). Cultures matured for 3–4 weeks prior to experimentation, and experiments were conducted inside an incubator to control environmental conditions (34.5°C and 5% CO_2). For further details see Hales et al. (2010).

EVALUATION AND RESULTS

This section begins with data characterizing the suitability of our setup to perform closed-loop feedback stimulation experiments, using cultures of cortical neurons and glia for validation. First, the process of identifying neurons to be used in closed-loop feedback stimulation will be described. Then the system's loop speed and jitter performance will be quantified. An example event engine was run to provide stimulation feedback, triggered by an activity pattern. Preliminary data and techniques to analyze the consequences of such stimulation on the functional connectivity between neurons will be presented and discussed. Finally, an experimental session to induce LTD through acausal stimulation will be sketched, and its implications discussed. Data in the figures demonstrate proof-of-principle experiments from individual cultures, the setup has, however, been successfully applied to many tens of cultures.

RECORDING/STIMULATION SELECTIVITY

High-density CMOS-MEAs can potentially sample from complete neuronal populations. Due to the high-density (18 μm pitch) of the CMOS electrode array, every neuron lying on the 2×1.75 mm^2 array can be bidirectionally addressed. On the other hand, when stimulating one electrode, a defined subset of neurons is often directly activated in response (Bakkum et al., 2008a). **Figure 4** shows such a scenario. In **Figure 4A**, one electrode, marked with a black cross, was stimulated multiple times, and the evoked activity was recorded during a window of 12 ms after stimulation onset. The median calculated over all voltage traces filters out noise and spontaneously spiking neurons/traces. Reliable activity (usually with a jitter on the order of 100 μs or below) is considered due to an antidromic action potential initiated at the neuron's axon (Lipski, 1981). Since only a subset of 126 out of the 11,011 electrodes can be readout simultaneously, the stimulation sequence was repeated multiple times, each time with a different subset of electrodes, until all electrodes were covered. After recording all sequences, the traces of the individual recordings were aligned in time. To highlight the electrodes that recorded elicited action potentials, the negative peak of the recorded voltage level during 12 ms after stimulation is color-coded and clipped at −100 μV. The red circles around the exemplified 11 spots highlight neurons that fired directly elicited action potentials. Their traces are individually shown in **Figure 4B**, demonstrating that the elicited action potentials were reliably and precisely fired after a given time, and only in a few cases (traces 2, 4, 6, 9), activity with different timing occurred. These could stem from a different neuron that happened to sit near the same electrode and/or from action potentials occurring within a coincident network burst.

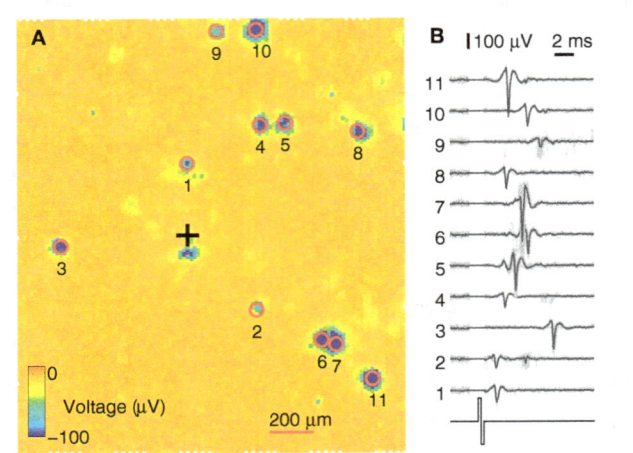

FIGURE 4 | Identification of directly evocable action potentials.
(A) Data recorded in response to repeated stimulation of one electrode (black cross) from the whole 2×1.75 mm^2 sensor area of the CMOS-MEA (each pixel is one electrode). Recording electrode configurations were scanned across the array in sets of 126 electrodes at a time. For every configuration, data were recorded for 12 ms after stimulation onset. The amplitude of the negative voltage peak within these 12 ms is color-coded and clipped at −100 μV. Blue indicates the detection of directly evoked somatic action potentials. **(B)** Example traces from 11 somas and the stimulation pulse are shown on the right. Traces from 30 stimulation trials are overlaid, with the median trace highlighted in black. The stimulation artifact was blanked prior to recording. Numbers are ordered by increasing distance from the stimulation site.

As shown, recording and stimulation with the CMOS-MEA feature high spatial resolution and, therefore, are locally very confined. However, the facts that one electrode can detect signals from more than one neuron, and that the stimulation through one electrode can directly evoke action potentials of more than one neuron have to be considered when planning closed-loop feedback stimulation experiments. In this case, the feedback-loop is not closed between two neurons, but includes two sets of neurons.

FEEDBACK LATENCIES

According to the rules of STDP, the timing window to induce long-term potentiation (LTP) at synapses is between less than a few milliseconds and up to tens of milliseconds post-synaptic activation before and after pre-synaptic activity. Thus, even though feedback cycles of 5–10 ms are fast enough to induce LTP, we aimed at reaching cycle-times below 1 ms to enable the system to perform acausal stimulations, as explained in the respective section below.

Figure 5 shows the overlay of 128 traces of the feedback-loop. Here, the event engine was configured to detect events on only one channel and stimulate immediately after detection, i.e., without any further delays in order to test the system performance (cf. **Figure 3A**). The traces are aligned at the onset-time of the stimulation pulse, and time zero is set to be at the negative peak of the spike of the trigger neuron. In red are the traces from the trigger neuron, and in black, the traces from the elicited neuron. The timing between a trigger neuron spike and the onset

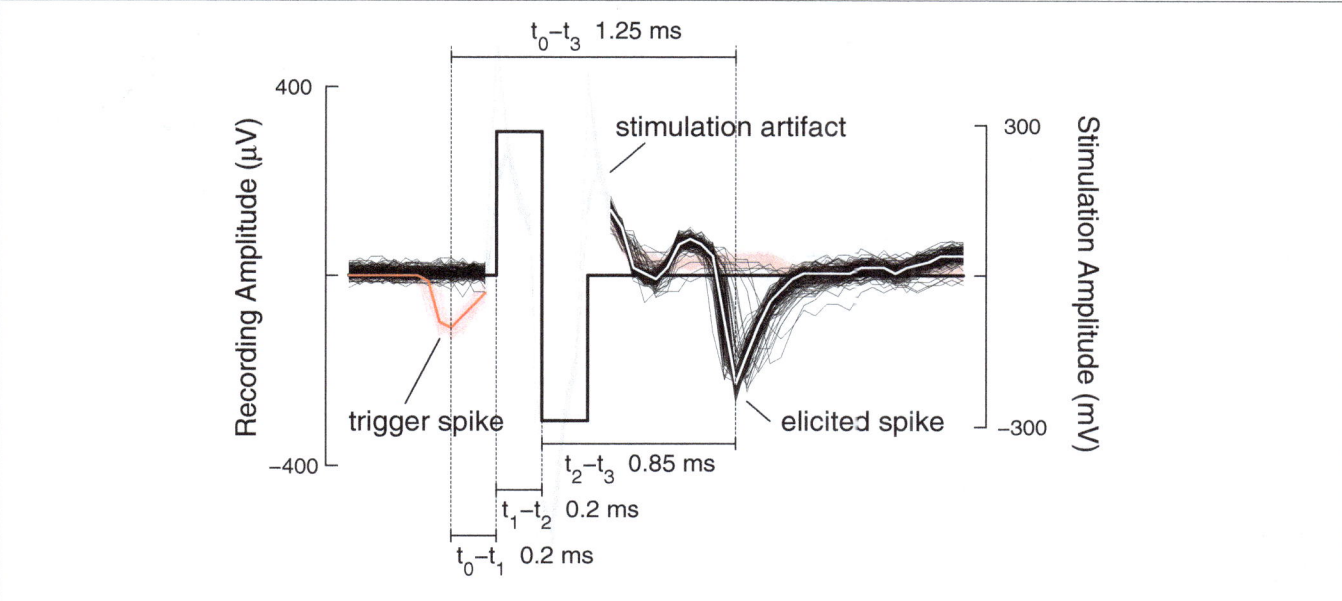

FIGURE 5 | Feedback stimulation performance. One hundred and twenty-eight traces from a closed-loop stimulation sequence are aligned at the stimulation onset-time and overlaid. Traces in red show the trigger spikes with the median over all trigger traces shown in bold red. The stimulation artifact is grayed-out for better visual clarity. The traces in black show spikes, elicited in all but four cases after stimulation. The median over all elicited traces is shown in bold white. The antidromic propagation delay for the elicited spikes was around 0.85 ms. The different timings, detection delay, stimulation delay, and antidromic propagation delay sum up to the full loop delay of 1.25 ms.

of the stimulation pulse was 200 µs, i.e., 4 sampling periods. This delay arises as follows: 50 µs (1 sampling period) was used to buffer the incoming data in the FPGA; 100 µs accounted for the delay of the two-tab Butterworth filter and the last 50 µs account for all other delays, such as synchronizing the stimulation pulse with the recording sampling time. Delays for sending digital data between the CMOS device and the FPGA were on the order of nanoseconds and thus are negligible. When stimulating with biphasic voltage pulses, the steep negative transition, which injects negative current ($I = C \times dV/dt$), is the time point, when a cell is activated (Wagenaar et al., 2004; Bakkum et al., 2008b). Thus, this time point was taken to measure the latency between stimulation and an elicited spike. In the case depicted in **Figure 5**, this timing is 0.85 ms, and the overall latency between trigger neuron activity and a spike on the elicited neuron was 1.25 ms.

As can be seen in **Figure 5**, besides achieving short feedback cycles, another advantage of using digital hardware (in this case FPGAs) for feedback generation is that no additional jitter is introduced, as such a system is fully deterministic. Sources of jitter in other systems (Hafizovic et al., 2007; Rolston et al., 2010) that close the feedback-loop around general-purpose or real-time personal computers are, for example, system interrupts that might disrupt the data processing, or buffer sizes of the USB, TCP/IP, or DAQ cards, which have to be set large enough in order to guarantee full data throughput. Usually these buffers have a size larger than one sample period. Depending on when an event happened inside this buffer, the latency could be larger or smaller and thus introduce jitter. This can be avoided by using digital hardware to hijack the data stream. In our case, the jitter was below

±50 µs and arose from the fact that neural activity is, of course, not aligned to the sampling period of the CMOS-MEA (50 µs). The exact time of the threshold crossing relative to the negative spike peak depends, among other things, on the slope of the spike waveform. Since the recorded signal was not interpolated between samples, this was an unavoidable source for jitter.

PATTERN MATCHING

To demonstrate the event engine in operation, feedback stimulation, triggered by an activity pattern, was performed. For the dataset presented in **Figure 6**, the event engine was programmed according to **Figure 3H** and classified spontaneous activity patterns as follows: A neuron recorded on electrode N2 fires an action potential; then an action potential is recorded from a neuron on electrode N3 after 3 ms; finally an action potential is recorded on electrode N1 after another 1.5 ms. Each individual event occurrence was allowed to have a jitter of ±1 ms. After successful identification of such a pattern, a stimulation pulse was emitted to elicit action potentials on a different neuron, NE. The cell cultures under investigations typically expressed bursting behavior, and this was when almost all of the patterns occurred. During bursts, the cells usually fired more than once at an elevated frequency, and this explains why the neurons on electrodes N1–N3 showed additional spikes "outside" of the detected pattern. Nevertheless, the pattern matching event engine identified 22 activity pattern occurrences during 12 min of recording.

CORRELATION ANALYSIS

To assess the connectivity between different neurons and the efficacy of change, induced by the closed-loop feedback

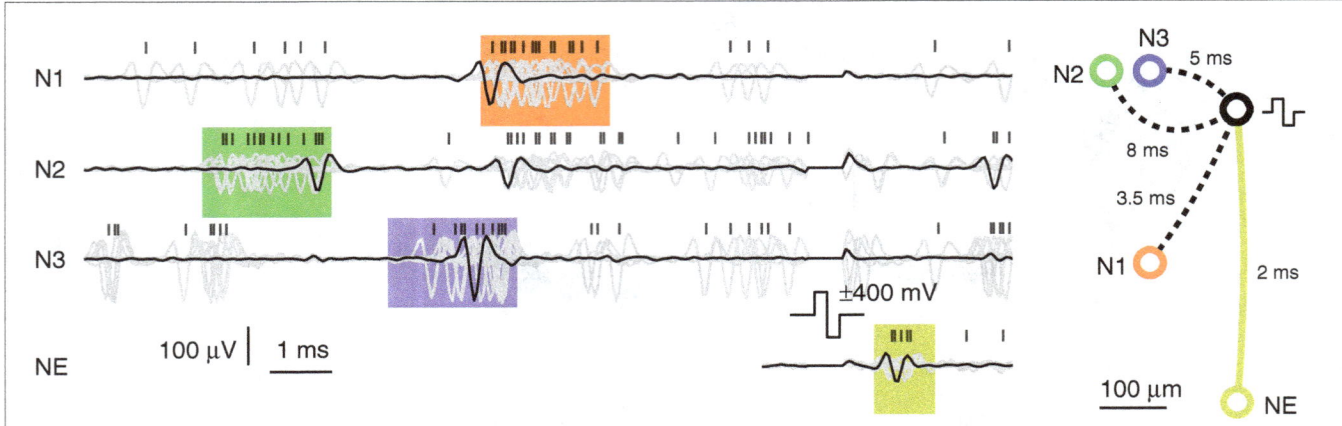

FIGURE 6 | Pattern-matching feedback stimulation. Electrode traces were recorded from neurons sitting on three different electrodes N1–N3 while performing pattern matching. The pattern was matched 22 times within 12 min, all overlaid and drawn in light-gray color. One arbitrary pattern is highlighted with black traces. The 12 ms before and 4 ms after stimulation pulse are shown. The orange, green, and blue colored boxes represent the spread-out-windows set in the event engine. A yellow box of arbitrary width is drawn around the elicited activity of neuron NE. Above the traces, negative peak times are marked with black vertical bars, showing spikes clustered within the colored boxes. The figure on the right shows electrode locations and the timings making up the pattern to match as well as the antidromic propagation delay of 2 ms to the elicited neuron.

stimulation, cross-correlation curves (Perkel et al., 1967) were computed between spike trains of the trigger neuron and the elicited neurons. When exceeding a 95% confidence interval (Brillinger, 1976), correlation is considered significant. **Figure 7** shows three descriptive cases, comparing the cross-correlation curves from 1 h of spontaneous activity before and after closed-loop feedback stimulation was applied for 1 h. To evaluate significance of the change, a similar procedure as in Fujisawa et al. (2008) was used. Briefly, the two times 1 h of spontaneous activity recordings were divided into smaller bins of 10 min duration and were randomly assigned to be before or after the closed-loop stimulation. Cross-correlation from this shuffled data was computed for both "before" and "after" and the difference was evaluated. This procedure was repeated 1000 times to generate a surrogate data set. Points on the x-axis, where the true difference is larger than 95% of the surrogate data, were assigned to be significant and are marked with an orange bar in **Figure 7**. Assessing the true connectivity of neuronal networks by means of extracellular measurements is difficult, and using the cross-correlation to that end is not ideal, as effects like common inputs or firing rate changes cannot be easily explained. However, in our context of evaluating the effect of feedback stimulation, we do not necessarily seek to precisely explain the changes in network connectivity, but to rather demonstrate that a change occurred at all and to what extent.

ACAUSAL STIMULATION

One motivation for very short feedback cycles is to open the possibility of acausal stimulation. If the closed-loop stimulation ($t_0 - t_2$) is faster than the time it takes the action potential to travel along the axon and hit the synapses ($t_0 - t_S$), acausal stimulation and, therefore, induction of LTD by means of closed-loop feedback stimulation is possible. The time that it takes for an action potential, initiated at the axonal hillock, to propagate

down the axonal arbor to the synapses depends on the propagation velocity of action potentials along axons and the length of the axons. Action potential conduction velocities in unmyelinated axons were reported around 0.2–0.4 ms^{-1} (Debanne et al., 2011). As demonstrated in **Figure 5**, the closed-loop stimulation ($t_0 - t_2$) can be as fast as 0.4 ms, meaning acausal stimulation is possible for trigger neurons (t_0) with unmyelinated axons that synapse to an elicited neuron ($t_{3/S}$) after a minimum axial length of 80–160 µm. **Figure 8** shows such an acausal stimulation procedure. First, before applying a closed-loop, the activity between different neurons was measured then evaluated by computing the cross-correlation. In the example in **Figure 8**, the firing activity of the second neuron B with respect to the first neuron A was elevated around a delay of 2.5 ms, implying neuron A has a functional connection with neuron B. Integrating the cross-correlation curve, where it exceeds the confidence intervals around 2–3 ms after the reference time zero, reveals an integral probability of around 40% chance for neuron B to spike 2–3 ms after neuron A had fired. Once two such neurons could be identified, closed-loop stimulation can be applied between them with a very short feedback cycle. In the presented example, the delay from the trigger neuron to the elicited spike was around 1 ms, smaller than the average delay between the occurrence of their spontaneous action potentials. The closed-loop feedback stimulation was applied for 20 min, and, afterwards, the correlation was measured again. Now, the correlation no longer exceeded the confidence intervals at around 2–3 ms after the trigger neuron. Note, however, that Bi and Poo (1998) have shown that LTD can only be induced, if the spontaneous synaptic efficiency is not strong enough to evoke a post-synaptic action potential. Otherwise, the post-synaptic Ca^{2+} influx dominates, and LTP will occur. For the experiment shown in **Figure 8**, the elicited neuron spiked only a fraction of the time, and provided an intermediary synapse; in all

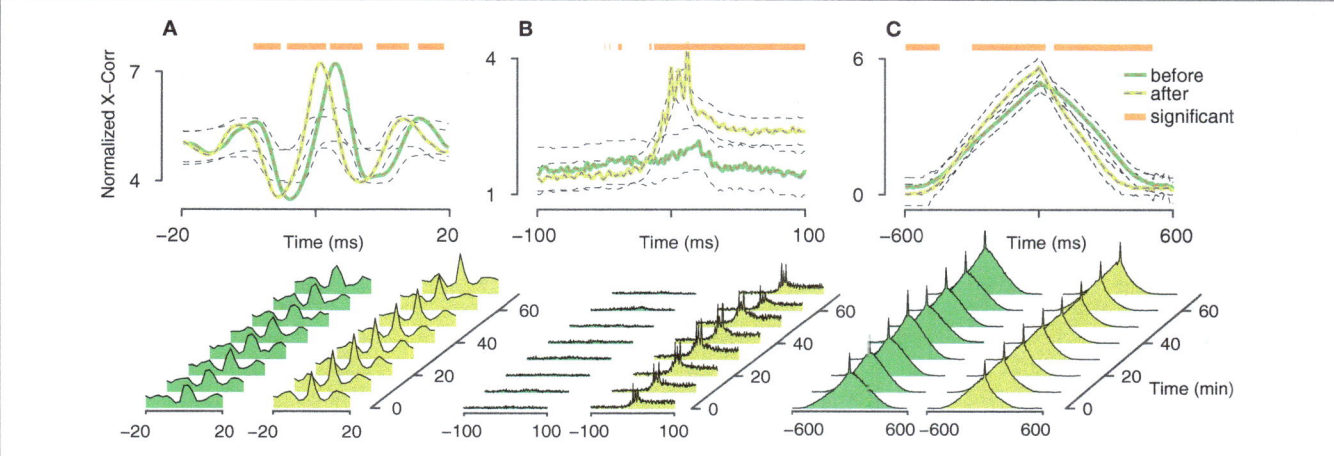

FIGURE 7 | Cross-correlation analysis. Three descriptive cases of changes in correlated firing between trigger neurons and elicited neurons. Spontaneous activity was recorded 1 h before and 1 h after the application of closed-loop feedback stimulation. Periods, where the difference exceeded a confidence bound (see text), were assigned to be significant and are indicated with an orange bar. The 95% confidence intervals are indicated with black dashed lines. Cross-correlation is computed based on trains with 9000–13000 spikes per neuron. **(A)** Relative probability remained constant, but the timing between trigger neuron and elicited neuron changed and became more synchronous. **(B)** The elicited neuron became more likely to fire in concert with the trigger neuron. **(C)** Relative timing within a network burst changed.

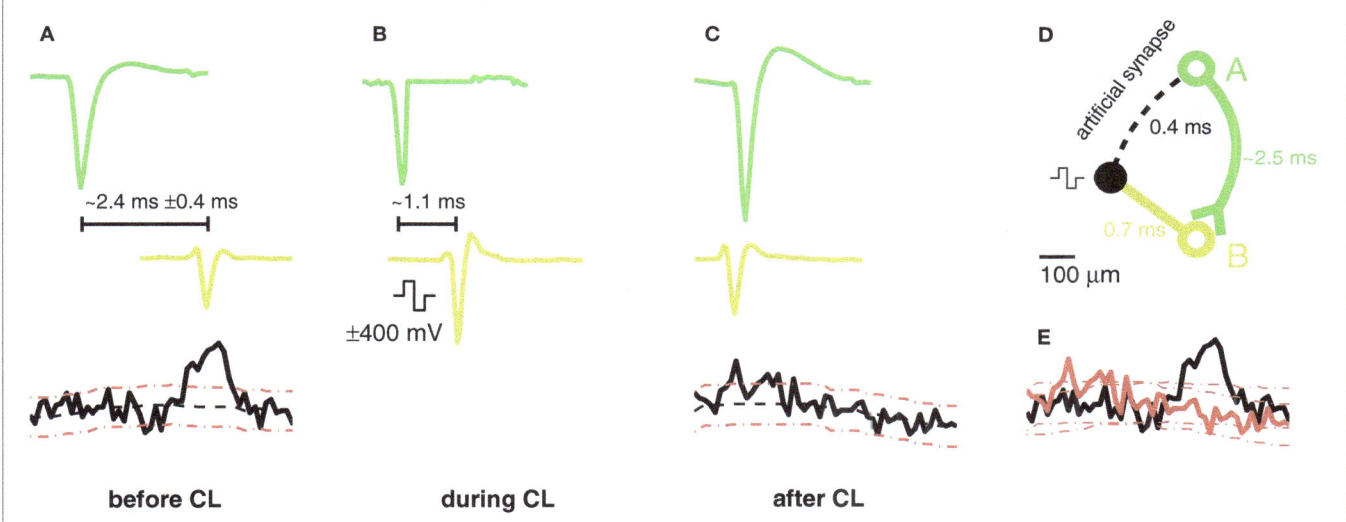

FIGURE 8 | Schematic of an acausal stimulation sequence.
(A) Spontaneous activity before application of the closed-loop. Shown spike traces are the median waveform of several spikes aligned at the negative peak. Top: Spike trace of the trigger neuron, A, in green. Middle: Example spike trace of a correlated neuron, B, drawn in yellow. The time delay between the plotted spikes of neuron A and neuron B was chosen to align with the maximum peak of the cross-correlation curve. Bottom: Cross-correlation curve of spike-times of neuron B with respect to neuron A. 95% confidence intervals are drawn with dotted red lines. Cross-correlations were computed with trains having 2000–3000 spikes. Significantly elevated correlated activity of neuron B can be detected around 2.4 ± 0.4 ms after neuron A fired an action potential. **(B)** Same situation as in **(A)** but with a closed-loop feedback stimulation applied. Due to the low-latency loop, the time delay of the yellow spikes with respect to the green ones was reduced by about 1.3 ms. For neuron A, the trace was zeroed at the start of the stimulation pulse. **(C)** Same as **(A)** but after the application of the closed-loop feedback stimulation. The cross-correlation no longer shows a significant peak for latencies larger than zero. The time delay between the plotted spikes of neuron A and neuron B was again chosen to align with the maximum peak of the cross-correlation. **(D)** Geometric sketch of the situation. The trigger neuron A and its axon are shown in green and the elicited neuron B in yellow. **(E)** Comparison of the two cross-correlation curves before (black) and after (red) the acausal stimulation with their 95% confidence intervals.

other cases, evoked excitatory post-synaptic currents (EPSCs) remained below the threshold. Further experiments are required before drawing conclusions. Additionally, to explore LTD and LTP in more depth, and advantageously, across many synapses simultaneously, extracellular recordings targeted to many trigger neurons, and an elicited neuron on the CMOS-MEA could be combined with an intracellular patch-clamp, attached to the elicited neuron and measuring the incoming EPSCs.

DISCUSSION

With the presented system, capable of applying multiple flexible feedback-loops simultaneously, many different experiments will be possible. The dynamic clamp technique proved to be a valuable tool for investigating the membrane dynamics involved in action potential generation (Destexhe and Bal, 2009; Economo et al., 2010). In such systems, intracellularly applied closed-loop-controlled voltage feedback enables the manipulation of cell membrane functions. Similarly, extracellularly applied closed-loop stimulation feedback, as presented in this work, might provide a useful tool for investigating cellular and network level plasticity and enable the manipulation of neuronal network functions. Potential questions include how information processing and the amount of memory that can be stored in a cultured network are influenced by adding one or more feedback-loops. Further experiments might involve more detailed studies of both LTP and LTD of individual sets of neurons by implementing causal and acausal feedback-loops between them. Using the pattern matching capabilities of the event engine will allow for extending plasticity studies to the network level. For example, investigations of the temporal order and history of spike trains, similar to those reported by Froemke and Dan (2002) and Ikegaya et al. (2004), could be performed, however, in parallel on multiple different neurons and pathways and, in addition, the respective pathways could be dynamically altered by targeted closed-loop feedback stimulations. Further rules governing plasticity beyond the classical STDP could be investigated.

An inherent limitation of extracellular recording systems is the inability to directly measure EPSCs. Conventional plasticity studies rely on patch-clamp to directly measure the EPSC to assess synaptic connectivity strength. Since these currents are not accessible with extracellular measurement techniques, indirect methods to assess synaptic connectivity have to be employed. Although cross-correlation seems attractive and is commonly used to assess connectivity, either between different brain regions or networks, or even between individual cells, it remains to be investigated to what extent correlation analysis unveils the direct synaptic strength between neurons. A combination of patch-clamp techniques and MEAs would provide a more direct way to measure the EPSC than through the computation of cross-correlation curves. By patching the post-synaptic neuron, EPSC strengths can be directly measured and related to extracellularly recorded pre-synaptic activity. Combining the advantages of both techniques, i.e., the precise EPSC measurements through patch-clamp, and the large-scale parallel, extracellular measurements and stimulations through CMOS-MEAs with flexible feedback-loops programmed by the event engine, would greatly expand experimental horizons. One could study the plasticity of hundreds of synapses in parallel. Furthermore, by hooking up the patch-clamp system to the event engine through dedicated spike-detection and stimulation modules, feedback-loops could be applied through the patch-clamp between extracellularly recorded and intracellularly stimulated (or vice versa) neurons.

Although, due to the high-density of electrodes, potentially all neurons can be read out individually, the recorded signals from two different neurons, located close to each other, are sometimes difficult to separate. A spike-sorting step, incorporated prior to event detection, can help to sort, and separate even neurons recorded from with the same electrodes. This holds in particular for using high-density electrode arrays (Franke et al., 2012). The spike-sorting might enable the identification of neurons with smaller spiking amplitudes, close to the noise level, and the identification of more neurons or cell assemblies. However, a drawback of more sophisticated spike-sorting algorithms is an additional time delay in the detection phase ($t_0 - t_1$). Spike-sorting, together with intracellular stimulation through patch-clamp as described above, could eliminate the aforementioned limitations in section "Recording/stimulation selectivity": Trigger spikes can be assigned to an individual neuron through spike-sorting, and stimulation pulses will only activate action potentials in the patched neuron.

CONCLUSION

By using an FPGA to perform signal-processing, as well as feedback generation, fast, and flexible loop cycles have been realized. Our approach using reconfigurable digital hardware to perform computationally intensive tasks, such as signal filtering, spike identification, decision-making, and feedback generation, is a compromise between traditionally employed methods either using a general-purpose (micro-) processor, which introduces additional latencies, and jitter, and the highly integrated application-specific circuits (VLSI ASICs), which are much less flexible in terms of adaptations to new experimental paradigms. Our achieved closed-loop feedback latencies are lower than many axonal propagation delays and thus enable acausal stimulation. Due to the flexible event engine, high-throughput experiments applying many feedback-loops in parallel are conceivable.

ACKNOWLEDGMENTS

We thank Milos Radivojevic and Marta Lewandowska for culturing assistance and Felix Franke, Michele Fiscella, Ian Jones, and David Jäckel for helpful discussions. This work was financially supported through the ERC Advanced Grant 267351 "NeuroCMOS" and the Swiss National Science Foundation Ambizione Grant PZ00P3_132245.

REFERENCES

Abeles, M., and Gerstein, G. L. (1988). Detecting spatiotemporal firing patterns among simultaneously recorded single neurons. *J. Neurophysiol.* 60, 909–924.

Azin, M., Guggenmos, D. J., Barbay, S., Nudo, R. J., and Mohseni, P. (2011). A battery-powered activity-dependent intracortical microstimulation ic for brain-machine-brain interface. *IEEE J. Solid-State Circ.* 46, 731–745.

Bakkum, D. J., Chao, Z. C., and Potter, S. M. (2008a). Long-term activity-dependent plasticity of action potential propagation delay and amplitude in cortical networks. *PLoS ONE* 3:e2088. doi: 10.1371/journal.pone.0002088

Bakkum, D. J., Chao, Z. C., and Potter, S. M. (2008b). Spatio-temporal electrical stimuli shape behavior of an embodied cortical network in a goal-directed learning task. *J. Neural Eng.* 5, 310–323.

Berdondini, L., Imfeld, K., Maccione, A., Tedesco, M., Neukom, S., Koudelka-Hep, M., et al. (2009). Active pixel sensor array for high spatio-temporal resolution electrophysiological recordings from single cell to large scale neuronal networks. *Lab Chip* 9, 2644–2651.

Bi, G., and Poo, M. (1999). Distributed synaptic modification in neural networks induced by patterned stimulation. *Nature* 401, 792–796.

Bi, G. Q., and Poo, M. M. (1998). Synaptic modifications in cultured hippocampal neurons: dependence on spike timing, synaptic strength, and postsynaptic cell type. *J. Neurosci.* 18, 10464–10472.

Bienenstock, E. (1995). A model of neocortex. *Netw. Comput. Neural Syst.* 6, 179–224.

Bontorin, G., Renaud, S., Garenne, A., Alvado, L., Le Masson, G., and Tomas, J. (2007). A real-time closed-loop setup for hybrid neural networks. *Conf. Proc. IEEE Eng. Med. Biol. Soc.* 2007, 3004–3007.

Brillinger, D. R. (1976). Measuring the association of point processes: a case history. *Am. Math. Mon.* 83, 16–22.

Chang, E. Y., Morris, K. F., Shannon, R., and Lindsey, B. G. (2000). Repeated sequences of interspike intervals in baroresponsive respiratory related neuronal assemblies of the cat brain stem. *J. Neurophysiol.* 84, 1136–1148.

Chen, T.-C., Chen, K., Yang, Z., Cockerham, K., and Liu, W. (2009). "A biomedical multiprocessor SoC for closed-loop neuroprosthetic applications," in *IEEE International Solid-State Circuits Conference Digest of Technical Papers.* (San Francisco, CA).

Debanne, D., Campanac, E., Bialowas, A., Carlier, E., and Alcaraz, G. (2011). Axon physiology. *Physiol. Rev.* 91, 555–602.

Destexhe, A., and Bal, T. (eds.). (2009). *Dynamic-Clamp: From Principles to Applications.* Springer Series in Computational Neuroscience. Vol. 1. XIV, 429, 60 illus. ISBN: 978-0-387-89278-8.

Economo, M. N., Fernandez, F. R., and White, J. A. (2010). Dynamic clamp: alteration of response properties and creation of virtual realities in neurophysiology. *J. Neurosci.* 30, 2407–2413.

Franke, F., Jäckel, D., Dragas, J., Müller, J., Radivojevic, M., Bakkum, D. J., et al. (2012). High density microelectrode array recordings and real-time spike sorting for closed-loop experiments: an emerging tool to study neural plasticity. *Front. Neural Circuits* 6:105. doi: 10.3389/fncir.2012.00105

Frey, U., Sedivy, J., Heer, F., Pedron, R., Ballini, M., Mueller, J., et al. (2010). Switch-matrix-based high-density microelectrode array in CMOS technology. *IEEE J. Solid-State Circ.* 45, 467–482.

Froemke, R. C., and Dan, Y. (2002). Spike-timing-dependent synaptic modification induced by natural spike trains. *Nature* 416, 433–438.

Fujisawa, S., Amarasingham, A., Harrison, M. T., and Buzsaki, G. (2008). Behavior-dependent short-term assembly dynamics in the medial prefrontal cortex. *Nat. Neurosci.* 11, 823–833.

Hafizovic, S., Heer, F., Ugniwenko, T., Frey, U., Blau, A., Ziegler, C., et al. (2007). A CMOS-based microelectrode array for interaction with neuronal cultures. *J. Neurosci. Methods* 164, 93–106.

Hales, C. M., Rolston, J. D., and Potter, S. M. (2010). How to culture, record and stimulate neuronal networks on micro-electrode arrays (MEAs). *J. Vis. Exp.* 39:e2056. doi:10.3791/2056

Ikegaya, Y., Aaron, G., Cossart, R., Aronov, D., Lampl, I., Ferster, D., et al. (2004). Synfire chains and cortical songs: temporal modules of cortical activity. *Science* 304, 559–564.

Izhikevich, E. M. (2006). Polychronization: computation with spikes. *Neural Comput.* 18, 245–282.

Izhikevich, E. M., Gally, J. A., and Edelman, G. M. (2004). Spike-timing dynamics of neuronal groups. *Cereb. Cortex* 14, 933–944.

Jackson, A., Mavoori, J., and Fetz, E. E. (2006a). Long-term motor cortex plasticity induced by an electronic neural implant. *Nature* 444, 56–60.

Jackson, A., Moritz, C. T., Mavoori, J., Lucas, T. H., and Fetz, E. E. (2006b). The Neurochip BCI: towards a neural prosthesis for upper limb function. *IEEE Trans. Neural Syst. Rehabil. Eng.* 14, 187–190.

Lee, J., Rhew, H.-G., Kipke, D. R., and Flynn, M. P. (2010). A 64 channel programmable closed-loop neurostimulator with 8 channel neural amplifier and logarithmic, ADC. *IEEE J. Solid-State Circ.* 45, 1935–1945.

Lipski, J. (1981). Antidromic activation of neurones as an analytic tool in the study of the central nervous system. *J. Neurosci. Methods* 4, 1–32.

Livi, P., Heer, F., Frey, U., Bakkum, D. J., and Hierlemann, A. (2010). Compact voltage and current stimulation buffer for high-density microelectrode arrays. *IEEE Trans. Biomed. Circuits Syst.* 4, 372–378.

Markram, H., Lubke, J., Frotscher, M., and Sakmann, B. (1997). Regulation of synaptic efficacy by coincidence of postsynaptic APs and EPSPs. *Science* 275, 213–215.

Mavoori, J., Jackson, A., Diorio, C., and Fetz, E. (2005). An autonomous implantable computer for neural recording and stimulation in unrestrained primates. *J. Neurosci. Methods* 148, 71–77.

Novellino, A., D'Angelo, P., Cozzi, L., Chiappalone, M., Sanguineti, V., and Martinoia, S. (2007). Connecting neurons to a mobile robot: an *in vitro* bidirectional neural interface. *Comput. Intell. Neurosci.* 2007, 13.

Perkel, D. H., Gerstein, G. L., and Moore, G. P. (1967). Neuronal spike trains and stochastic point processes. II. Simultaneous spike trains. *Biophys. J.* 7, 419–440.

Rebesco, J. M., Stevenson, I. H., Kording, K. P., Solla, S. A., and Miller, L. E. (2010). Rewiring neural interactions by micro-stimulation. *Front. Syst. Neurosci.* 4:39. doi: 10.3389/fnsys.2010.00039

Rizk, M., Bossetti, C. A., Jochum, T. A., Callender, S. H., Nicolelis, M. A., Turner, D. A., et al. (2009). A fully implantable 96-channel neural data acquisition system. *J. Neural Eng.* 6:026002. doi: 10.1088/1741-2560/6/2/026002

Rolston, J. D., Gross, R. E., and Potter, S. M. (2010). Closed-loop, open-source electrophysiology. *Front. Neurosci.* 4:31. doi: 10.3389/fnins.2010.00031

Rolston, J. D., Wagenaar, D. A., and Potter, S. M. (2007). Precisely timed spatiotemporal patterns of neural activity in dissociated cortical cultures. *Neuroscience* 148, 294–303.

Song, S., Miller, K. D., and Abbott, L. F. (2000). Competitive Hebbian learning through spike-timing-dependent synaptic plasticity. *Nat. Neurosci.* 3, 919–926.

Venkatraman, S., Elkabany, K., Long, J. D., Yao, Y., and Carmena, J. M. (2009). A system for neural recording and closed-loop intracortical microstimulation in awake rodents. *IEEE Trans. Biomed. Eng.* 56, 15–22.

Wagenaar, D. A., Pine, J., and Potter, S. M. (2004). Effective parameters for stimulation of dissociated cultures using multi-electrode arrays. *J. Neurosci. Methods* 138, 27–37.

Wallach, A., Eytan, D., Gal, A., Zrenner, C., and Marom, S. (2011). Neuronal response clamp. *Front. Neuroeng.* 4:3. doi: 10.3389/fneng.2011.00003

Zanos, S., Richardson, A. G., Shupe, L., Miles, F. P., and Fetz, E. E. (2011). The Neurochip-2: an autonomous head-fixed computer for recording and stimulating in freely behaving monkeys. *IEEE Trans. Neural Syst. Rehabil. Eng.* 19, 427–435.

Zrenner, C., Eytan, D., Wallach, A., Thier, P., and Marom, S. (2010). A generic framework for real-time multi-channel neuronal signal analysis, telemetry control, and sub-millisecond latency feedback generation. *Front. Neurosci.* 4:173. doi: 10.3389/fnins.2010.00173

8

The iso-response method: measuring neuronal stimulus integration with closed-loop experiments

Tim Gollisch[1]* and Andreas V. M. Herz[2]

[1] Department of Ophthalmology and Bernstein Center for Computational Neuroscience Göttingen, University Medical Center Göttingen, Göttingen, Germany
[2] Department Biology II and Bernstein Center for Computational Neuroscience Munich, Ludwig-Maximilians-Universität München, Munich, Germany

Edited by:
*Ahmed El Hady, Max Planck
Institute for Dynamics and Self
Organization, Germany*

Reviewed by:
*C. J. Heckman, Northwestern
University, USA
Ronen Segev, Ben-Gurion
University, Israel*

*Correspondence:
*Tim Gollisch, Department of
Ophthalmology and Bernstein
Center for Computational
Neuroscience Göttingen, University
Medical Center Göttingen,
Waldweg 33, 37073
Göttingen, Germany.
e-mail: tim.gollisch@
med.uni-goettingen.de*

Throughout the nervous system, neurons integrate high-dimensional input streams and transform them into an output of their own. This integration of incoming signals involves filtering processes and complex non-linear operations. The shapes of these filters and non-linearities determine the computational features of single neurons and their functional roles within larger networks. A detailed characterization of signal integration is thus a central ingredient to understanding information processing in neural circuits. Conventional methods for measuring single-neuron response properties, such as reverse correlation, however, are often limited by the implicit assumption that stimulus integration occurs in a linear fashion. Here, we review a conceptual and experimental alternative that is based on exploring the space of those sensory stimuli that result in the *same* neural output. As demonstrated by recent results in the auditory and visual system, such *iso-response stimuli* can be used to identify the non-linearities relevant for stimulus integration, disentangle consecutive neural processing steps, and determine their characteristics with unprecedented precision. Automated closed-loop experiments are crucial for this advance, allowing rapid search strategies for identifying iso-response stimuli during experiments. Prime targets for the method are feed-forward neural signaling chains in sensory systems, but the method has also been successfully applied to feedback systems. Depending on the specific question, "iso-response" may refer to a predefined firing rate, single-spike probability, first-spike latency, or other output measures. Examples from different studies show that substantial progress in understanding neural dynamics and coding can be achieved once rapid online data analysis and stimulus generation, adaptive sampling, and computational modeling are tightly integrated into experiments.

Keywords: neural computation, sensory systems, stimulus integration, closed-loop experiment, isoresponse, neuron models

INTRODUCTION

Mapping high-dimensional input streams into low-dimensional output spike trains is a core operation of almost every neuron in the brain. No auditory neuron is sensitive to only one frequency of a time-varying sound signal, no visual neuron responds to only one wavelength in a light stimulus. Both types of neurons rather integrate inputs over a range of frequencies. Similarly, strong dimensional reduction also occurs when retinal ganglion cells integrate signals over space via tens to hundreds of bipolar cells with smaller receptive fields, when pyramidal cells combine input from 10,000 other cortical neurons, or when cerebellar Purkinje cells are innervated by 200,000 parallel fibers to cause well-orchestrated movement patterns. In all these cases, huge amounts of information are lost—and need to be lost, or rather discarded, so that those particular stimulus combinations can be distilled that are indeed important for behavior.

Extracting the specific rule of how a given neuron combines its inputs is a prerequisite for understanding its computational function. Consider, for example, the responses of auditory neurons to a sound pressure wave $s(t)$ with several frequency components, $s(t) = \Sigma_i\, s_i \cos(2\pi\nu_i t)$. A neuron whose firing rate r is

some function f of the summed amplitudes, $r = f(\Sigma_i s_i)$, encodes the maximal sound amplitude whereas another neuron whose activity depends on the summed squares of these components, $r = g(\Sigma_i s_i^2)$, encodes sound energy. In both cases, it is a particular scalar quantity, $\Sigma_i s_i$ or $\Sigma_i s_i^2$, respectively, that matters for the neuron's firing rate, whereas the detailed composition of the vector $(s_1, s_2, s_3, \ldots)$ is irrelevant. Similarly, the shapes of the output non-linearities f and g are of no importance for the fact that the two neurons encode sound amplitude and energy, respectively, as long as the cells' firing thresholds, saturation levels, and input sensitivities are such that behaviorally important signal ranges can be encoded. Moreover, this simple example demonstrates that measuring a cell's input-output relation by changing the total input strength—as often done in electrophysiological experiments—will provide information about the output non-linearity, but will typically *not* reveal which computation is represented by the cell's activity.

This observation calls for alternative methods to investigate the principles and mechanisms of stimulus integration and to reveal the potential non-linearities involved in this process. Here, we review recent advances to this end, based on closed-loop measurements of iso-response stimuli. Iso-response stimuli are defined as those combinations of the individual stimulus components that yield the same predefined neuronal response. To efficiently search for sets of such stimulus combinations in neurophysiological experiments, closed-loop experiments with automated data analysis and appropriate feedback to the applied stimulation provide an essential ingredient. As discussed and exemplified below, this iso-response approach has already led to new fundamental insights into the function of neurons and neural circuits in different sensory modalities and provides a large potential for future developments and advances in a wide range of systems.

MODEL FRAMEWORK FOR INVESTIGATING STIMULUS INTEGRATION

A common methodology for analyzing a neuron's stimulus-response relation is based on system identification theory and applies the framework of cascade models (see e.g., Marmarelis and Marmarelis, 1978; Korenberg and Hunter, 1986). These models aim at describing input-output systems in a phenomenological way by a sequence of mathematical primitives, such as linear filters and non-linear transformations. The most prominent member of the cascade model family is arguably the LN model (Hunter and Korenberg, 1986; Sakai, 1992; Meister and Berry, 1999; Chichilnisky, 2001; Paninski, 2003; Schwartz et al., 2006), which comprises a stage of linear filtering of the stimulus, followed by a non-linear transformation of the filter output.

The appeal of this model stems from its simple interpretation; the linear filter describes how different stimulus components are integrated and thus represents the neuron's receptive field structure, whereas the non-linearity captures the output transformation induced by spike generation. In addition, the model elements can be derived in physiological experiments with relative ease. The linear filter, for example, can readily be found through calculating the spike-triggered average (STA) in response to broad-band stimulation, such as white-noise input (de Boer and Kuyper, 1968; Bryant and Segundo, 1976; Eggermont et al., 1983; Chichilnisky, 2001; Paninski, 2003). In using a single linear filter for the stimulus integration stage, however, the LN model implicitly assumes that the entire stimulus integration occurs in a linear fashion. All non-linear effects are relegated to the output non-linearity. The LN model is thus of limited use as soon as the true processing chain contains non-linear operations before stimulus integration is complete. A prominent example are complex cells in visual cortex, whose input stage corresponds to the sum of two squared Gabor filter signals—resulting in the well-known energy model (Adelson and Bergen, 1985)—so that the cells' input-output function corresponds to an LNLN instead of an LN cascade.

A step forward is made by analyzing the spike-triggered covariance (STC) matrix (Bryant and Segundo, 1976; de Ruyter van Steveninck and Bialek, 1988; Brenner et al., 2000; Schwartz et al., 2006; Samengo and Gollisch, 2012), an extension of the STA. STC analysis allows one to extract multiple linear filters whose contributions are non-linearly combined. This works well for assessing whether a neuron can be described as a linear integrator (STC then yields just one filter) or is better described by non-linear stimulus integration (STC yields multiple filters).

Furthermore, this analysis can thereby identify those stimulus components (i.e., filters) whose non-linear integration underlies a neuron's response characteristics. Yet, STC analysis by itself is typically not sufficient for quantitatively assessing the functional form of non-linear stimulus integration, in particular because several parallel filters have to be considered and non-linear effects of stimulus integration and of the output stage need to be separated. We will return to this aspect later and discuss the complementary nature of STC and iso-response analysis.

Given the above considerations, let us thus consider a model that goes beyond the LN model by incorporating an explicit separation between non-linear operations before and after stimulus integration has taken place (**Figure 1A**). The input to this model is provided by two or more stimulus components $s_1, \ldots, s_n$ that separately undergo some non-linear transformation $N_1(\cdot)$. The linear sum of these terms then serves as input to a second non-linearity $N_2(\cdot)$. This results in a sequence of non-linear, linear, and again non-linear operations and is thus correspondingly called an NLN cascade (Marmarelis and Marmarelis, 1978; Korenberg and Hunter, 1986). In what follows, the NLN cascade model serves as a canonical framework for studying stimulus integration and helps us formalize the relevant challenges and strategies. More complex cascades can be obtained by extending the linear sum to a linear filter operation or by combining more elementary building blocks. For example, auditory signal transduction has been described by an LNLN cascade (**Figure 1D**; Gollisch and Herz, 2005).

The important feature of the canonical model of **Figure 1A** is that it separates non-linear transformations occurring after stimulus integration has taken place (function N_2) from non-linear transformations occurring just before or in the course of stimulus integration (function N_1). Thus, it is the function N_1 that determines the nature of stimulus integration and dictates which scalar measure is distilled out of the combination of stimulus components s_i. N_2, on the other hand, provides a transformation that determines how this scalar measure is represented, but does not affect what is represented in the neuron's output. Hence, the benefit of the canonical model of **Figure 1A** is to provide a framework for separating non-linearities that are relevant for stimulus integration from those that are irrelevant for this purpose, even if they strongly influence the neural output, for example in the form of an all-or-none spike generation threshold or pronounced response saturation.

THE ISO-RESPONSE METHOD

As seen in the discussion above, a fundamental challenge to studying neuronal information processing is that non-linearities relevant for stimulus integration need to be separated from subsequent non-linearities, in particular those at the output stage. To approach this challenge, an experimental design is needed that directly reflects these different non-linear processing stages. Crucial insight is provided by a strategy known from measuring threshold curves in neurobiology (Evans, 1975) or using equivalence criteria in psychophysics (Jameson and Hurvich, 1972): instead of estimating the full input-output relation, stimulus parameters are varied such that the neuron's response stays at a *constant level* (Gollisch et al., 2002; Gollisch and Herz, 2003).

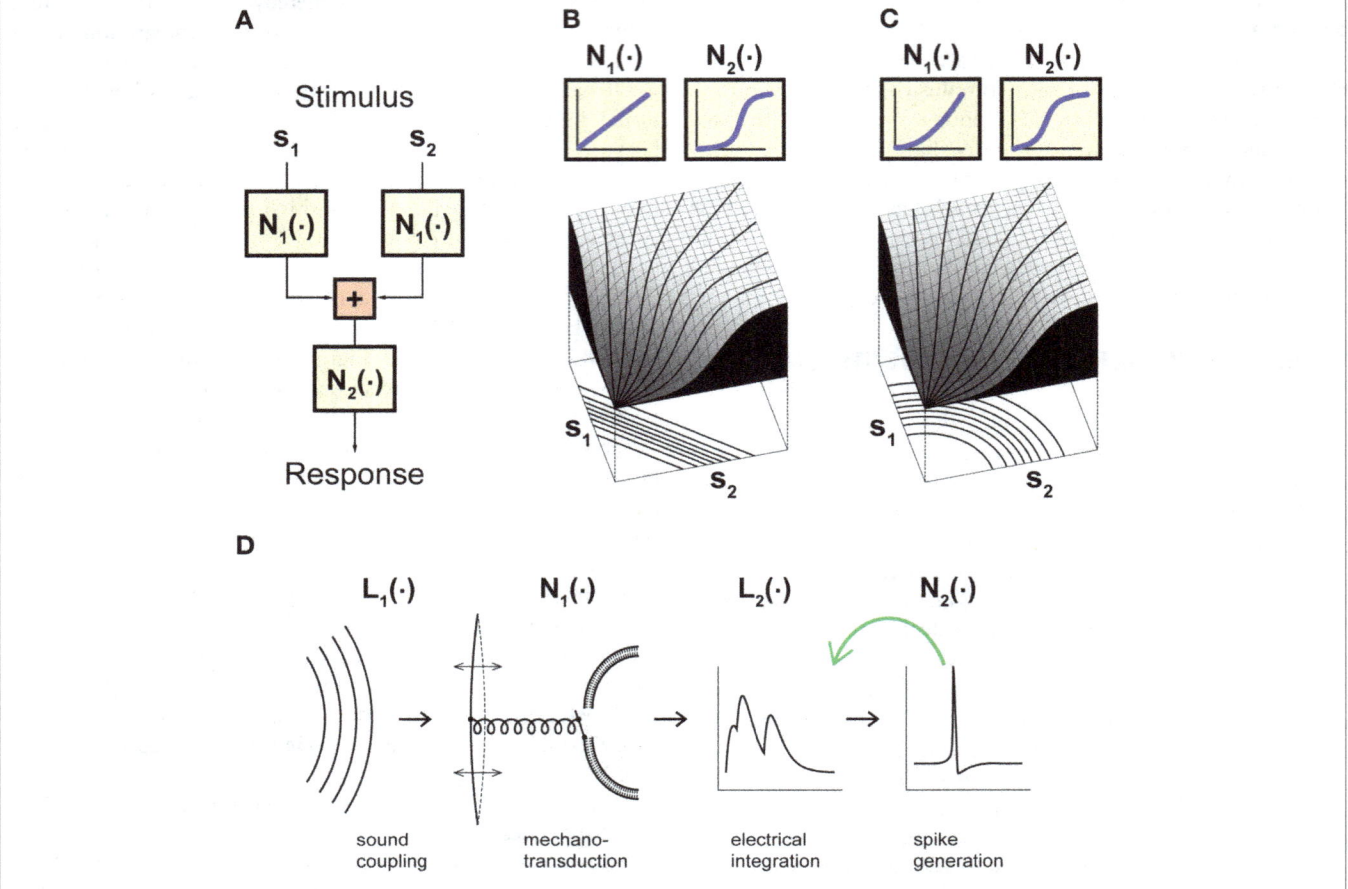

FIGURE 1 | Model framework for analyzing neuronal stimulus integration with iso-response measurements. (A) A canonical model for separating non-linear effects before and after stimulus integration. The model considers two (or more) separate inputs $s_1 \ldots s_n$, which each undergo a non-linearity N_1 before summation, and a final output non-linearity N_2. Stimulus integration is governed by the non-linearity N_1, whereas N_2 provides a transformation of the integrated signal. Assessing the nature of stimulus integration thus amounts to measuring N_1 independently of N_2. **(B)** Model responses obtained with linear stimulus integration and sigmoidal output transformation. The response surface is dominated by the sigmoidal shape of the output non-linearity, but the iso-response curves shown below the surface plot are straight lines and thus reveal the linear nature of stimulus integration in this model. **(C)** Same as **(B)**, but with a quadratic non-linearity N_1 and thus non-linear stimulus integration. While the response surface is still dominated by a sigmoidal shape, the iso-response curves are now circles and thus reveal the quadratic non-linearity relevant for stimulus integration. The non-linearities N_2 in **(B)** and **(C)** were adjusted such that if s_1 or s_2 are presented alone, the input-output relations are identical in the two models. **(D)** A cascade model for sound transduction, consisting of two linear filters L_1 and L_2 and two non-linear transformations N_1 and N_2. The green arrow indicates that the cascade may also include a feedback mechanism, corresponding to adaptation induced by the neuron's spiking activity. Panels **(B)** and **(C)** adapted from Gollisch and Herz (2003) with permission, Copyright (2003), Frankfurt Institute for Advanced Studies. Panel **(D)** adapted from Gollisch and Herz (2005) according to the Creative Commons Attribution License.

The key idea behind this concept is that staying at a constant response level removes the effect of the output non-linearity in the canonical model of stimulus integration (**Figure 1A**). How different stimulus components have to be combined to reach this response level thus serves as a direct signature of the nature of stimulus integration. This is most easily seen when considering a system with two independent input channels s_1 and s_2. In the two-dimensional stimulus space spanned by s_1 and s_2, iso-response stimuli are typically located on one-dimensional curves, which we call iso-response curves. Linear integration, for example, is characterized by iso-response curves that are straight lines, even if the overall response function of the neuron is strongly non-linear because of the output non-linearity (**Figure 1B**). Deviations from

linearity in the integration process, on the other hand, lead to differently shaped curves. As a simple example, integration in the form of a sum of squares yields circular iso-response curves, defined by the circle equation $s_1^2 + s_2^2 = \text{const}$ (**Figure 1C**).

In higher dimensional stimulus spaces, the iso-response curves become iso-response manifolds. Linear integration then corresponds to an iso-response manifold whose shape is a hyperplane. The iso-response manifolds represent the invariances of a neuron's input-output relation and therefore provide an important characterization of the neuron's computational role, even when considering only low-dimensional stimulus subspaces. These still supply a signature of the neuron's invariances; for example, if a neuron has ellipsoids as iso-response manifolds in a high-dimensional stimulus space, an investigation of a two-dimensional planar subspace will display elliptic iso-response curves. High-dimensional hyperplanes, on the other hand, always yield simple straight lines in a two-dimensional projection.

The prime advantage of the method lies in the fact that the iso-response manifolds are independent of the potentially highly non-linear operation occurring at the final output stage; the iso-response approach relies solely on comparisons of stimuli for which this output stage has identical effects. This focus on a particular response range also makes the approach experimentally efficient, which is of special importance when data acquisition time is limited. Furthermore, by their very definition, iso-response stimuli are "perceived" as identical by the neuron under investigation. The shape of an iso-response manifold thus has a direct functional interpretation, whereas it is often difficult to assign a particular meaning to the specific shape of a neuron's traditional stimulus-response curve. Finally, as the full stimulus-response curve need not be determined within the iso-response paradigm, strong stimulation can be obviated so that experimental artifacts caused by activity-dependent cellular fatigue are not an issue.

Depending on the investigated neuron or on the considered stimuli, different neuronal output characteristics may be relevant for information transmission. Accordingly, the iso-response concept is not limited to "iso-firing rate" but can also be implemented as "iso-first-spike latency" (Bölinger and Gollisch, 2012), "iso-firing phase," or other iso-response variants. In fact, *every* neural response feature that depends on input stimuli can serve as an iso-response dimension, including the value of the probability that a single spike occurred at all (Gollisch and Herz, 2005). Other useful target response measures could be the firing phase relative to some underlying large-scale rhythm or a specific temporal discharge pattern. This goes along with a freedom of choice regarding the dynamics of the chosen stimulus. Iso-response methods can be applied with extremely brief, highly non-stationary stimuli down to the sub-millisecond range (Gollisch and Herz, 2005) as well as with longer, stationary stimuli (Gollisch et al., 2002; Horwitz and Hass, 2012). The first paradigm provides a chance to disentangle rapid biophysical processes that subserve temporally precise stimulus integration, whereas the second setting allows one to focus on the system's spectral or spatial integration properties, independently of temporal dynamics. Furthermore, a given neuron may use different coding schemes for different stimulus attributes. To cover such multiplexing of information (or rule it out for the neuron under study), one can apply different iso-response measures within one experiment (Bölinger and Gollisch, 2012).

HISTORICAL BACKGROUND OF ISO-RESPONSE MEASUREMENTS

The concept of measuring different stimuli that yield the same response also underlies the measurements of threshold tuning curves, which are widely used, for example, to characterize auditory neurons (Tasaki, 1954; Holton and Weiss, 1983; Harris and Dallos, 1984; Geisler et al., 1990). Here, the predefined response is typically set to be the minimal notable difference from baseline activity, and these thresholds are obtained along the axis of varying sound frequency. The measurements of threshold—as compared to measuring the response strengths for a given stimulus amplitude at different sound frequencies—has the advantage that it avoids overly strong stimulation, which would trigger non-linear suppression mechanisms, blurring the tuning characteristics (Eustaquio-Martín and Lopez-Poveda, 2011).

Other early applications of iso-response measurements have been carried out in the visual system. In the frog retina, threshold intensities of spots in the receptive field center of a recorded ganglion cell were obtained for different light intensity in the surround (Barlow, 1953). This was used to study whether signals in the center and surround of the receptive field were combined in a linear or non-linear fashion. For neurons in primary visual cortex, the combined direction and spatial frequency selectivity was characterized by measuring responses to different combinations of motion direction and spatial frequency and then extracting iso-response curves in the 2D direction–frequency space (Jones et al., 1987). The purpose of these iso-response curves was to provide an easy visualization of the data, which were then analyzed to determine whether motion direction and frequency affected the response independently of each other or whether an interaction between these stimulus dimensions became apparent.

These early applications of the iso-response paradigm, however, did not aim at detailed characterizations of the non-linearities involved in stimulus integration. This requires high-precision measurements of iso-response stimuli, despite the limited recording time in physiological experiments. A key development for providing the required efficiency in the assessment of iso-response stimuli has been the possibility to use closed-loop experiments, benefiting from the recent colossal advancements in computer hardware and software.

MEASURING ISO-RESPONSE STIMULI WITH CLOSED-LOOP EXPERIMENTS

From an experimental viewpoint, the iso-response methodology suggests a conceptual change in the design of a neurophysiological experiment—instead of measuring how responses vary for different predefined stimuli, the goal is to manipulate stimuli such that the recorded cell's output stays at the same level, or at least remains within a small predefined range. This challenging task can only be accomplished efficiently within a closed-loop setting (Benda et al., 2007) so that information about changes in the neural output can immediately be fed back to the stimulus generator (**Figure 2A**).

In a first, exploratory phase of an iso-response experiment, the closed-loop setting is highly useful to determine which stimulus dimensions should be explored at all (e.g., which spatial locations or spectral components). In the second phase, the actual iso-response stimuli are determined. To do so, the closed-loop setup is used to implement a search algorithm. The search for a particular stimulus that provides a predefined response can, for example, proceed radially outwards from stimulus origin in different directions (**Figure 2B**). Alternatively, the search can move along an iso-response curve (**Figure 2C**) by starting at some stimulus and then searching in its vicinity for stimuli leading to the same response. The search for a stimulus that yields a predefined response is essentially a root-finding problem, for which many

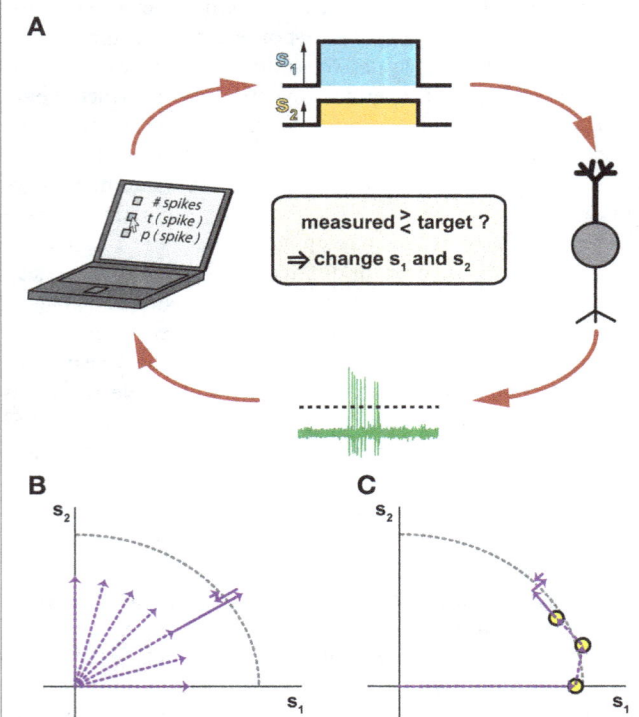

FIGURE 2 | Closed-loop methods for measuring iso-response stimuli.
(A) Closing the loop by tuning stimulus parameters according to measured responses. In response to a stimulus with two components s_1 and s_2 (top), a recorded neuron (right) responds with spikes that are automatically detected, for example by a threshold criterion (bottom). The spike response is then compared to a chosen target criterion (left), which may be the number of spikes, the timing of the first spike, the probability of spiking, or any other accessible response feature. According to this comparison, the values of s_1 and s_2 are adjusted for the next stimulus presentation in order to approach the target response. **(B)** Potential search strategy in radial directions of the stimulus space. This combines several linear searches, which can be performed sequentially or interleaved, typically starting near the origin so that overly strong stimulation is avoided. **(C)** Potential search strategy by tracking iso-response curves. Here, previously measured iso-response stimuli are used as starting conditions for searching nearby stimuli that yield the same response. This can be done, for example, by changing the ratio of s_1 and s_2 while keeping the same radial distance as for a previously measured iso-response stimulus and then tuning this radial distance until the desired response is obtained. As compared to the strategy of pure radial searches in **(B)**, this sequential search can provide higher recording efficiency, but does not allow interleaving multiple searches.

algorithms of varying efficiency and complexity exist (Press et al., 1992). Essentially, however, the search amounts to comparing the measured response to a target and deciding whether increasing or decreasing the strength of the stimulus components reduces the deviation. As it is not always possible to exactly reach the desired response value, the parameter values for these stimuli are often determined through interpolation from stimuli that led to responses within a small region around the set response. To save precious experimental time, this can also be done offline.

In either phase of the iso-response experiments, precise, flexible, and fast stimulus control is needed, as well as good control over the data acquisition, in particular regarding spike detection and spike sorting (Lewicki, 1998; Quiroga et al., 2004; Santhanam et al., 2004; Wood et al., 2004; Rutishauser et al., 2006). The rapid detection of iso-response stimuli through efficient closed-loop approaches can then not only be used to obtain high-accuracy measurements, but also allows one to measure and compare different variations of iso-response curves from the same cells. For example, it may help elucidate the mechanisms underlying the non-linearities of stimulus integration to repeat iso-response measurements in the presence of pharmacological blockers, for different response measures, or using different stimulus components as the inputs s_1 and s_2. To illustrate the power and potential of closed-loop methods for iso-response measurements, we will, in the following, summarize some key ideas and results of recent applications of this method in different sensory systems.

EXAMPLE I: THE AUDITORY PERIPHERY OF LOCUSTS

We begin with the integration of acoustic stimuli in locust auditory receptor cells. In this model system, three different types of iso-response experiments have been performed to address several distinct questions. In a first study, iso-firing rate stimuli were used to discriminate between rival hypotheses for spectral integration of sound signals (Gollisch et al., 2002). In a second study, iso-spike probability experiments revealed temporal integration mechanisms on a sub-millisecond scale (Gollisch and Herz, 2005). In a third study, iso-firing rate stimuli were used once more, but they were now designed such that different adaptation mechanisms could be discerned (Gollisch and Herz, 2004). Together, the three iso-response studies led to new insights and quantitative results far beyond the scope of traditional experiments.

Locust auditory receptor neurons are directly attached to the animal's eardrum via short dendrites. When the eardrum vibrates in response to incident sound, mechanosensory ion channels in the neurons open (Gillespie and Walker, 2001). The transduction currents cause depolarizations of the neuronal membrane and thereby trigger spikes, which can be recorded from the receptors' axons in the auditory nerve (Hill, 1983a). Individual receptor cells are broadly tuned to sound frequencies above a few kilohertz and do not phase-lock to the sound's carrier frequency (Hill, 1983b).

Returning to the example from the introduction, let us consider sound pressure waves s(t) that consist of superimposed pure tones, $s(t) = \Sigma_i s_i \cos(2\pi\nu_i t)$. How the cells' average firing rate r depends on sound intensity is subject to three rival hypotheses, in which r is considered to be a non-linear function $r = f(J)$ of the "effective stimulus intensity" J, which in turn represents a different fundamental measure of sound intensity according to each hypothesis (Garner, 1947; Tougaard, 1996; Heil and Neubauer, 2001): *Amplitude Hypothesis*: J is proportional to a weighted sum of the tone amplitudes, $J_{AH} = \Sigma_i \lambda_i s_i$, where the factors λ_i represent the relative sensitivities of the eardrum to different sound frequencies. Thus, J reflects the maximum amplitude of the eardrum vibration. *Energy Hypothesis*: J corresponds to the energy of the eardrum oscillations, $J_{EH} = \Sigma_i \lambda_i^2 s_i^2$. *Pressure Hypothesis*: J corresponds to the temporal mean of the absolute value of the oscillation, $J_{PH} = <|\hat{s}(t)|>$, where $\hat{s}(t)$ describes the sound pressure wave after taking the sensitivities λ_i into account.

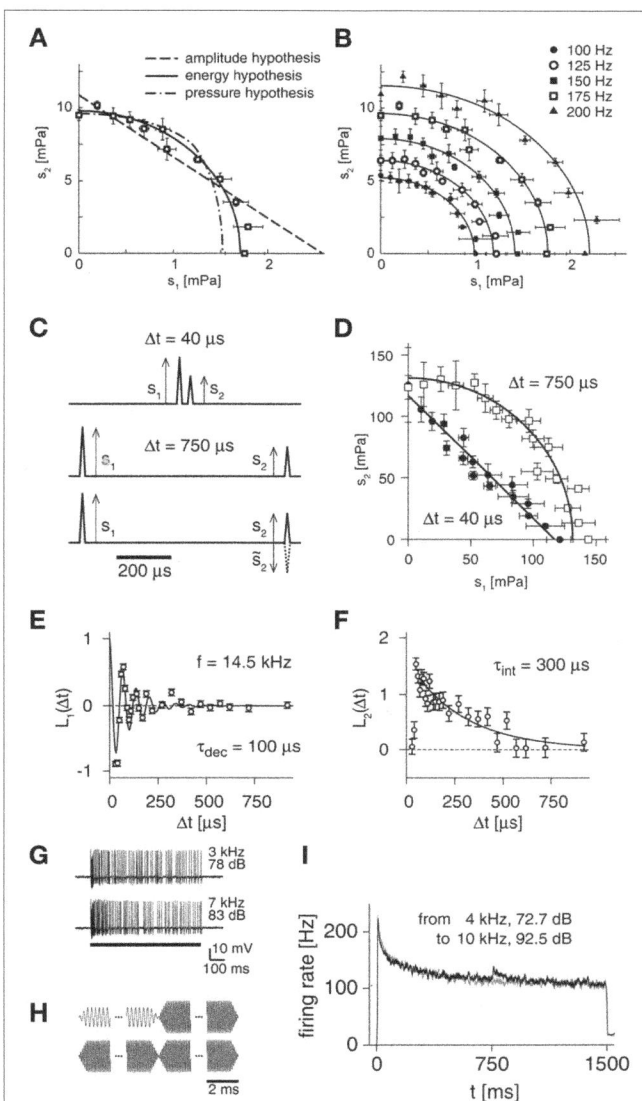

FIGURE 3 | Iso-response measurements for locust auditory receptors. (A) Iso-response curve of spectral integration to distinguish between three rival hypotheses of sound transduction. Stimuli consisted of superpositions of two pure tones with amplitudes s_1 and s_2, respectively. The data points show such combinations that yielded a firing rate of 175 Hz. These are well fitted by an ellipse, corresponding to the energy hypothesis, but not by iso-response curves of the other two model hypotheses. **(B)** Comparison of iso-response curves from the same cell as in **(A)** for different target response levels. The iso-response curves are ellipses that are scaled versions of each other, confirming the energy hypothesis. **(C)** Click stimuli used to probe temporal integration. The clicks can be presented with short (top) or long (middle) inter-click intervals, and the second click can have the same or opposite sign as compared to the first (bottom). **(D)** Iso-response curves for pairs of clicks at different inter-click intervals, corresponding to a spike probability of 70%. Short inter-click intervals yield straight lines, longer inter-click intervals result in circles, corresponding to linear and quadratic temporal integration, respectively. **(E)** Linear filter L_1 for a sample receptor cell obtained from iso-response measurements with different signs of the second click. The filter corresponds to the first stage of the LNLN model of sound transduction (**Figure 1D**). The filter shape can be fitted by an impulse response function of a damped oscillator (black line) with oscillation frequency f and (mechanical) decay time constant τ_{dec} as indicated in the plot. **(F)** Linear filter L_2 for the same receptor cell as in **(E)**. The filter shape can be fitted by an exponential function (black line) with (electrical) integration time constant τ_{int} as indicated in the plot. **(G)** Sample spike trains recorded from a locust auditory receptor neuron for presentations of pure tones, showing the adaptation of the firing rate during the course of stimulation. **(H)** Acoustic stimuli used to test for input-driven adaptation. Amplitudes of a high-frequency tone and a low-frequency tone were tuned with closed-loop experiments so that they evoked the same steady state firing rates. Stimuli then consisted of switches between the tones (top) as well as of repetitions of the same tone as control condition (bottom). **(I)** Firing-rate profile for a sample receptor neuron. For the switch from one tone to another, the firing rate displays a transient increase (black line), which is absent in the control condition (gray line). This indicates that besides the strong feedback adaptation driven by the neuron's spikes, an additional adaptation component exists before signals are integrated over sound frequencies. Panels **(A)** and **(B)** reprinted from Gollisch et al. (2002) with permission, Copyright (2002), *Journal of Neuroscience*, Society for Neuroscience. Panels **(C–F)** adapted from Gollisch and Herz (2005) according to the Creative Commons Attribution License. Panels **(G–I)** reprinted from Gollisch and Herz (2004) with permission, Copyright (2004), *Journal of Neuroscience*, Society for Neuroscience.

Which of these three hypotheses applies to locust auditory receptors? Answering this question about the true physical cause of output activity is complicated by the strongly non-linear dependence of r on J through the output non-linearity f and because J cannot be determined directly since the locust auditory system is very delicate so that one cannot reliably measure sound transduction prior to the receptor cells' spike generation. Thus, to investigate stimulus integration independently of f, the iso-response paradigm was implemented, using superpositions of two sine-wave stimuli in order to identify those amplitude combinations that led to the same firing rate. Note that for each of the three hypotheses, the stimulus-response relation takes on the form of the canonical model of **Figure 1A**: the output non-linearity N_2 is always given by the function f, whereas N_1 is either just a linear function (amplitude hypothesis), a squaring relation (energy hypothesis), or a more complicated non-linearity that has to be determined numerically (pressure hypothesis). The iso-response curves can thus distinguish

between the three hypotheses independently of the non-linear relation between the effective stimulus strength and the firing rate.

As indicated in **Figure 3A** for an exemplary receptor neuron, the amplitude and pressure hypotheses were rejected by the measured shapes of iso-response curves, whereas the energy hypothesis provided a good fit to the data (Gollisch et al., 2002). To test the generality of this conclusion, a useful extension is to investigate how iso-response curves for different response levels are related to one another (**Figure 3B**). For locust auditory receptor neurons, iso-firing rate curves obtained for the same neuron at different firing rates turned out to lie on ellipses that are scaled versions of one another. Again, this finding is in accordance with the energy hypothesis, which predicts that the ratio of the ellipses' half-axes should always equal the ratio of the constants λ_1 and λ_2. In addition, the energy model also holds for the initial transient response at stimulus onset as well as for superpositions of multiple pure tones and even accurately predicts receptor responses to broad-band noise stimulation (Gollisch et al., 2002).

These observations led to the conclusion that sound-intensity coding in this insect model system is well captured by a cascade model (**Figure 1D**), in which the sound wave is first mechanically filtered by the eardrum and the transduction stage then provides a squaring non-linearity prior to temporal integration of the electrical signals in the receptor neuron. A non-linear output stage finally describes the firing-rate encoding of the effective sound intensity J_{EH}, resulting in an LNLN-cascade. The temporal dynamics of this cascade, in particular of the different filtering stages, however, were beyond the reach of this first set of experiments with stationary stimuli.

Instead, disentangling the characteristics of temporal integration in sound encoding requires the application of highly dynamic stimuli. Accordingly, the iso-response paradigm was extended to a response measure appropriate for such a dynamic scenario, namely the probability of occurrence of a single spike following a brief stimulus (Gollisch and Herz, 2005). Thus, iso-response curves were measured for double-click stimuli with inter-click intervals of less than one millisecond. The two click amplitudes s_1 and s_2 were again adjusted via a closed-loop search algorithm during an experiment such that a recorded cell responded to repeated stimulation with a fixed spike probability.

When the inter-click intervals were sufficiently large (**Figure 3C**, middle panel), the iso-response curves were approximately circular (**Figure 3D**, open squares). This finding further corroborates the energy hypothesis, as the circular iso-response curve shows that equal spike probability was obtained for equal sound energy, $s_1^2 + s_2^2$. When very short inter-click intervals were chosen (**Figure 3C**, top panel), however, the iso-response curves were nearly straight lines (**Figure 3D**, filled circles). Thus, on short times scales, the sum of the two click amplitudes, $s_1 + s_2$, determines the spike probability. This is readily explained if one assumes that the two stimulus components are already mechanically integrated by the oscillation of the eardrum, which is expected to act as a linear filter for the sound-pressure wave (Schiolten et al., 1981).

The different shapes of the iso-response curves on different time scales imply that different integrative steps are relevant during the mechanosensory transduction process. This is expected, as the sound pressure wave is first mechanically filtered by the eardrum. After conversion into electrical signals, these are integrated by the capacitive properties of the neuron's cell membrane. In the LNLN cascade of sound transduction (**Figure 1D**), the two temporal integration steps are captured by the linear filters L_1 and L_2, respectively. How can the temporal structure of these two filters, separated by the squaring non-linearity of mechanosensory transduction, be disentangled? The solution again lies in properly designed iso-response measurements, here by comparing the click amplitudes necessary to evoke the same spike probability when the pressure deflection of the second click either has the same or the opposite sign of the pressure deflection of the first click (**Figure 3C**, bottom panel). The rationale behind this approach is that the linear integration before the squaring non-linearity is sensitive to a change in sign, whereas the integration following the squaring transformation is not.

Using the mathematical description of the LNLN cascade, this reasoning can be cast into formulas for extracting filter shapes of L_1 and L_2 at different time points, which correspond to the applied inter-click intervals (Gollisch and Herz, 2005).

This approach showed that L_1 resembles the filter of a damped oscillator (**Figure 3E**). In fact, the measured resonance frequencies of these oscillators corresponded to the receptor cells' maximal spectral sensitivity, which typically lies in the range of several kilohertz (Gollisch and Herz, 2005). In addition, these measurements revealed damping time constants of typically few hundred microseconds, thus providing insight into the mechanical eardrum properties at the different sites where the receptor cells are attached. By contrast, the second filter L_2 rather had the shape of a leaky integrator with exponential decay characteristics, thus showing the time scales of electrical integration at the cell membrane (**Figure 3F**). Typically, the decay of L_2 was slower than that of L_1. Thus, long inter-click intervals surpass the mechanical integration and rather reveal the quadratic integration characteristics of electrical signals as evident in the approximately circular iso-response curves for sufficiently long inter-click intervals (**Figure 3D**).

Note that the assessment of the integration dynamics on time scales as short as few tens of microseconds could be achieved by measuring the spike probability with comparatively large temporal windows of several milliseconds. This makes the approach insensitive to variability in spike timing, which mars the temporal resolution of traditional correlations techniques (Aldworth et al., 2005; Dimitrov and Gedeon, 2006; Gollisch, 2006). By contrast, the temporal resolution in these iso-response measurements is limited only by the accuracy of stimulus delivery, which may easily reach the microsecond range with appropriate hardware and software.

On much longer time scales, many neurons exhibit spike-frequency adaptation (**Figure 3G**). An initially high firing rate slowly decreases over time, even though the stimulus stays constant. There is a wide range of different biophysical mechanisms known to be involved in spike-frequency adaptation. In many neurons, a major contribution stems from output-driven components that are triggered by the spiking activity of the neuron. Adaptation may, however, also contain components that are driven by the sensory or synaptic input in a feed-forward way. The different dependences of adaptation on the sensory input and neural output will have distinct effects on the coding properties of a sensory neuron. For a functional characterization of adaptation, we therefore have to identify the causal relationships between sensory input, neural activity, and the level of adaptation.

To tackle this problem, one needs to measure input-driven adaptation, which is triggered by the strength of a stimulus component s_i, independently of output-driven adaptation, which follows the total response level of the neuron. Applying again the iso-response approach to auditory receptor neurons, this can be done by tuning the intensities for different sound frequencies in such a way that the steady-state firing rate is the same (Gollisch and Herz, 2004). Consequently, the level of output-driven adaptation must be equal. Switching between these sounds (**Figure 3H**) can then reveal input-driven components, because these need to approach a new equilibrium value after such a switch. This process results in transient deflections of the firing rate, which can be observed in electrophysiological recordings of the spiking activity (**Figure 3I**). The careful tuning of the sounds leads to a high sensitivity of the method that allows one to detect input-driven adaptation components even when they are far smaller in effect than simultaneously present output-driven components.

EXAMPLE II: RETINA

The vertebrate retina is a neural network at the back of the eyeball that constitutes the first stage of visual processing. The processed visual signals are encoded by retinal ganglion cells into patterns of spikes for transmission along the optic nerve to various brain regions. As in many other sensory systems, the network of the retina features a great deal of convergence; a single ganglion cell can collect signals from tens to hundreds of excitatory bipolar cells (Freed and Sterling, 1988), which in turn each collect signals from many photoreceptors. Inhibitory interactions mediated by horizontal cells and amacrine cells influence which signals are transmitted in this processing chain and how they are modified.

The spikes from an individual retinal ganglion cell thus reflect the processing of this complex upstream circuit. What the circuit computes follows to a large degree from the nature of the non-linearities associated with the ganglion cell's integration over its collection of inputs (Gollisch and Meister, 2010). That this integration can occur in a non-linear fashion has been known for more than fifty years, since ganglion cells were first categorized as linear X cells and non-linear Y cells (Enroth-Cugell and Robson, 1966). Yet, the classical experiments for identifying non-linear stimulus integration with reversing spatial gratings only indicate whether or not a non-linearity is present and do not directly reveal its functional form. Moreover, it is likely that the class of non-linearly integrating cells is composed of various types of ganglion cells, which may express different types of non-linear characteristics, serving different visual functions.

Based on the iso-response paradigm, the nature of stimulus integration in the receptive field can be analyzed by subdividing the receptive field into two halves (**Figure 4A**) and using the values of the visual contrast in each half as inputs, analogous to the canonical model of **Figure 1A**. This approach

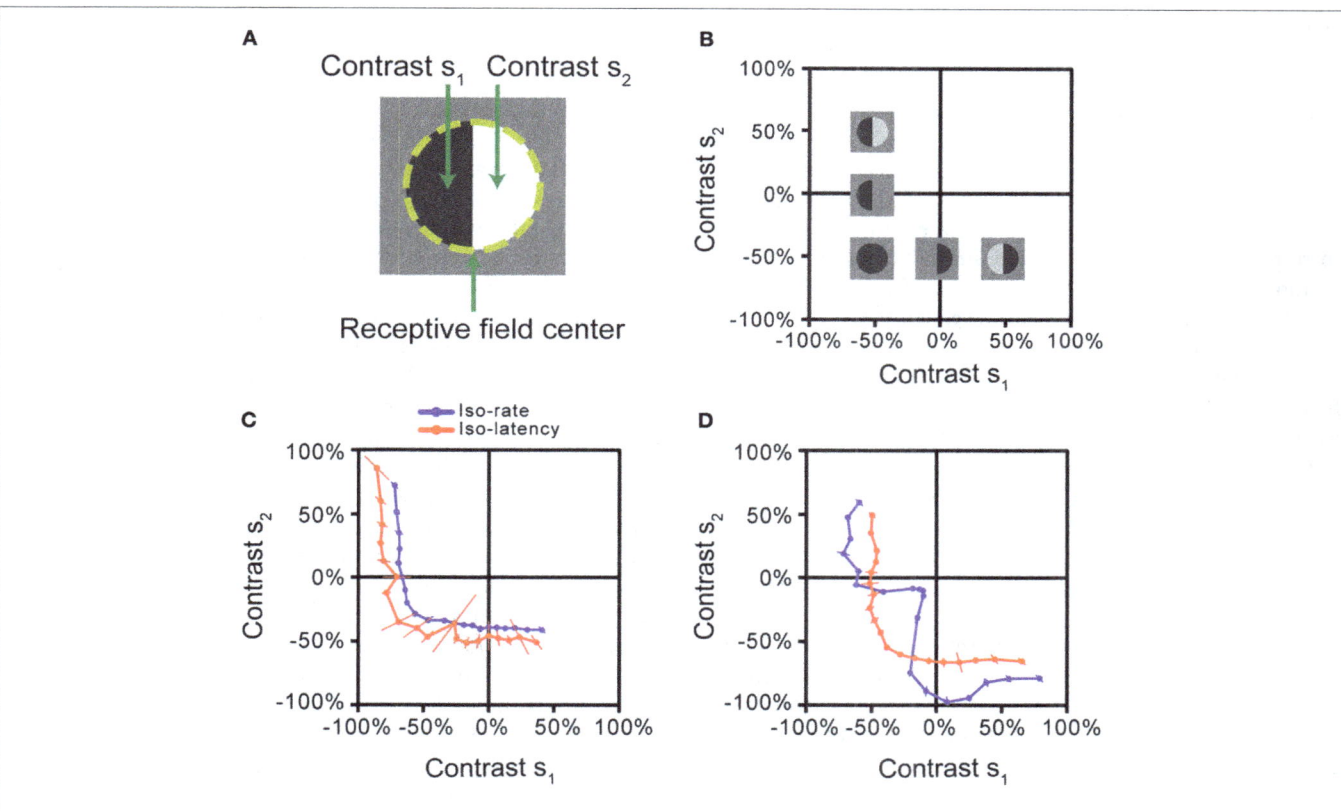

FIGURE 4 | Iso-response measurements of spatial stimulus integration by retinal ganglion cells. (A) Stimulus pattern used in the measurements. After determining the receptive field center of a retinal ganglion cell (dashed line), different contrast levels s_1 and s_2 were simultaneously displayed for 500 ms, each in one half of the receptive field. **(B)** Stimulus space. Iso-response stimuli were measured in the space spanned by s_1 and s_2. Experiments were performed on Off-type ganglion cells, which best respond to negative contrast. Several sample stimulus patterns are shown at their respective locations in stimulus space. The origin corresponds to the gray level of background illumination. **(C)** Iso-rate and iso-latency curves for a sample ganglion cell, corresponding to the majority of recorded cells in the salamander retina. Both iso-response curves have similar shapes that indicate a threshold-quadratic non-linearity of stimulus integration. **(D)** Iso-rate and iso-latency curves for a different ganglion cell from a subpopulation in the salamander retina. While the iso-latency curve has a similar shape as the curves in **(C)**, the iso-rate curve shows a notch along the lower-left diagonal, corresponding to particular sensitivity to homogeneous stimulation of the receptive field. This follows from a dynamic local gain control mechanism, mediated by inhibitory interactions. All panels reprinted from Bölinger and Gollisch (2012), Copyright (2012), with permission from Elsevier.

has recently been applied to measuring stimulus integration by Off-type ganglion cells in the salamander retina (Bölinger and Gollisch, 2012). The contrast combinations (s_1, s_2) were flashed briefly onto the receptive field of a ganglion cell, whose spikes were recorded extracellularly. Closed-loop experiments were then used to find such combinations that either gave the same spike count (iso-rate curves) or the same first-spike latency (iso-latency curves). As the stimulus started from an intermediate gray illumination, both positive contrast (brightening) as well as negative contrast (dimming) could be applied, and iso-response stimuli were therefore measured beyond just one quadrant of stimulus space (**Figure 4B**).

The iso-response curves revealed that all measured ganglion cells in the salamander retina featured non-linear stimulus integration. For the majority of cells, iso-rate curves and iso-latency curves had the same general shape, as shown by an example in **Figure 4C**. The curves were approximately circular in the region where both contrast values were negative (corresponding to the preferred contrast for these Off-type cells). In this region, the curves thus resembled the circular iso-response curves seen in a simple model (**Figure 1C**) and in the previous example (**Figure 3A**), suggesting that a sum of squares determines the response of these ganglion cells. Combinations of negative contrast in one half of the receptive field and positive contrast in the other, however, yielded sections of the iso-response curves that were nearly parallel to the axes of the plot. This suggests that the amount of positive contrast had little or no effect on the response strength, corresponding to a thresholding mechanism that implements a half-wave rectification. Together, the shape of these iso-response curves indicates that a threshold-quadratic transformation is the fundamental non-linearity of stimulus integration over the receptive field center of these ganglion cells.

Other recorded ganglion cells, however, showed a fundamentally different shape of the iso-rate curves (**Figure 4D**). Instead of the circular shape in the region where both contrast values are negative, the curves show a pronounced notch, indicating that particularly small contrast levels were required to reach the target spike count when both receptive field halves were stimulated with the same negative contrast. Accordingly, the cells were named "homogeneity detectors," as they appear particularly suited to detect large, homogeneous objects, even at low contrast (Bölinger and Gollisch, 2012).

Both types of ganglion cells, those with threshold-quadratic non-linearities as well as homogeneity detectors, are strongly non-linear in their integration characteristics. They would thus both be classified as Y-type cells according to a conventional investigation of linear vs. non-linear stimulus integration with reversing grating stimuli (Enroth-Cugell and Robson, 1966; Bölinger and Gollisch, 2012). The assessment of integration characteristics with iso-response curves, on the other hand, allowed an analysis of the particular type of non-linearity in a quantitative and detailed fashion and thus provided a distinction between different types of non-linear stimulus integration that had not been apparent before.

Interestingly, the iso-latency curves of homogeneity detectors did not display the characteristic notch, but rather showed the circular region, similar to the majority of measured iso-rate curves.

The comparison between iso-rate and iso-latency curves thus already provides insights regarding the mechanism responsible for the characteristics of homogeneity detectors; it suggests that sensitivity to homogeneous stimuli is obtained through a process that acts only after the first spike is initiated and thus has a dynamic nature. Further investigations showed that this phenomenon is brought about by local inhibitory circuitry, acting as a local gain control and coming into effect with a slight delay because of the additional synaptic stage involved in the inhibitory pathway (Bölinger and Gollisch, 2012).

EXAMPLE III: VISUAL CORTEX

A further recent application of iso-response measurements has shed light onto the integration of color information by neurons in primate visual cortex (Horwitz and Hass, 2012). This study was motivated by the puzzle that neuronal responses in visual cortex to color stimuli often appeared incongruent with representing linear sums and differences of cone signals, an expectation that had been developed on the basis of psychophysical color perception experiments (Hering, 1920; Hurvich and Jameson, 1957). To resolve this issue and test whether non-linear integration of cone signals had been a missing ingredient in the models with which the data had been analyzed, Horwitz and Hass (2012) measured iso-response surfaces of macaque V1 neurons in a three-dimensional color stimulus space, defined by the activation of the three types of cones in the retina (**Figure 5**). Using drifting chromatic gratings as stimuli, the iso-response stimuli were defined as those combinations of cone activation that elicited the same firing rate over the stimulus duration.

The iso-response stimuli define two-dimensional surfaces in this three-dimensional stimulus space. For some cells, the iso-response surfaces were simple planes (**Figure 5A**), indicating that these cells represent indeed a linear combination of cone activation strengths. Other cells, however, showed strong deviations from linear integration; for those cells, the iso-response data points were much better fitted by quadratic models, either corresponding to a hyperboloid (**Figure 5B**) or to an ellipsoid (**Figure 5C**). Taken together, the data show that iso-response surfaces of individual cells are generally well described by either a linear or a quadratic integration model. This finding demonstrates that the previous lack of a coherent description of cortical responses to color stimuli in terms of cone activations resulted from not taking non-linear integration into account.

Interestingly, the hyperboloid iso-response surface of **Figure 5B** is similarly non-convex as the iso-response curve of homogeneity detectors measured in the retina (**Figure 4D**). This shape suggests that the cells are especially sensitive to one particular stimulus dimension—homogeneous stimulation of the receptive field in the case of the retinal neuron; a particular cone activation pattern in the case of the cortical neuron—whereas responses in other directions appear suppressed; in the case of the cortical neuron, this means that for certain combinations of cone activation, the desired response is never reached. One may thus hypothesize that the hyperboloid shape of the iso-response surface in cortical neurons is brought about by a similar active suppression mechanism as mediated by local inhibition in the case of the retinal homogeneity detectors.

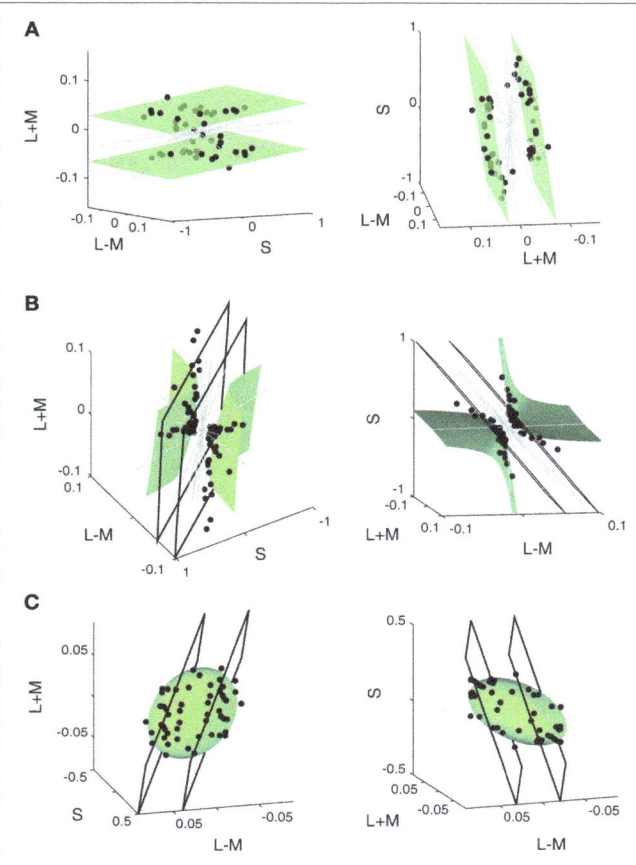

FIGURE 5 | Iso-response measurements of integration of cone signals by neurons in macaque primary visual cortex. The panels show iso-response stimuli (black circles) obtained with drifting chromatic gratings for three representative sample cells in **(A)**, **(B)**, and **(C)**, respectively. Stimuli that yielded the same firing rate are plotted in the space spanned by S-cone activation (S) and by the sum and difference of L-cone and M-cone activation (L + M and L − M, respectively). For each cell, the data are shown in the 3D plots for two different viewpoints (left and right column, respectively). Gray lines indicate directions in stimulus space along which the predefined response criterion could not be reached. As shown by the green surface plots, iso-response stimuli are well fitted by a linear plane for the cell in **(A)**, by a hyperboloid for the cell in **(B)**, and by an ellipsoid for the cell in **(C)**. Panels **(B)** and **(C)** also show best fits of linear planes (black quadrangles), which do not provide good descriptions of the iso-response stimuli. Reprinted by permission from Macmillan Publishers Ltd: Nature Neuroscience (Horwitz and Hass, 2012), copyright (2012).

The iso-response surface in the shape of an ellipsoid (**Figure 5C**), on the other hand, indicates that the cell represents a sum of squares, similar to findings in both the locust auditory system (**Figure 3A**) and the salamander retina (**Figure 4C**) as well as in the energy model for complex cells in visual cortex (Adelson and Bergen, 1985). The ubiquity of this type of non-linear stimulus integration may indicate a general-purpose representation, providing invariance under rotations in stimulus space.

MULTIPLE STAGES OF STIMULUS INTEGRATION

The canonical model of **Figure 1A** suggests that the iso-response method is most easily applied to systems with two non-linear

stages, one before stimulus integration has taken place and one afterwards. Yet, valuable insight can also be obtained for systems with more successive non-linearities. First, from a functional point of view it may not be necessary to disentangle all non-linear stages; rather, it may be of interest to determine the total, combined non-linear transformation before stimulus integration takes place and separate it from the total non-linearity afterwards. This procedure aims at casting the investigated system again into the form of the canonical NLN cascade of **Figure 1A**, but will fail for systems that deviate strongly from this simplified structure.

Second, one may profit from the fact that many neural systems, in particular sensory systems, are organized in a hierarchical fashion so that the relevant temporal, spatial, and spectral scales increase from processing layer to processing layer. This allows one to choose the stimulus layout—by appropriately defining what is represented by the two components s_1 and s_2—in such a way that the relevant stimulus integration occurs at a certain stage along the processing chain, dividing the chain into the total non-linear transformation before and after this stage. By varying the stimulus scale used in the analysis, one can thus distinguish between successive non-linear stages.

To illustrate this strategy, let us consider a model with three non-linear stages N_1, N_2, and N_3, separated by successive stages of stimulus integration, which first only pool over sets of neighboring inputs and subsequently integrate over these sets (**Figure 6A**). To separate these integration stages, we now first choose a "coarse" stimulus layout, in which the four input channels are combined into pairs so that "nearby" channels, which are pooled together already in the first integration stage, receive the same stimulus intensity s_1 or s_2, respectively (stimulus pattern inside the blue box in **Figure 6A**). For this stimulus layout, s_1 and s_2 remain separate through both N_1 and N_2 and are combined only prior to the output non-linearity N_3. This means that the iso-response curve of s_1 and s_2 will reflect the concatenation of N_1 and N_2, but is not influenced by N_3. Now, let us consider a "finer" stimulus layout, in which "nearby" input channels already receive different stimulus components s_1 and s_2 (stimulus pattern inside the green box in **Figure 6A**). For this layout, s_1 and s_2 are combined directly after N_1 and before N_2, which means that the iso-response curve of s_1 and s_2 will now only reflect the non-linearity N_1 and be insensitive to both N_2 and N_3. Investigating and comparing the shapes of iso-response curves on a fine and coarse scale thus can be used to derive both non-linearities N_1 and N_2. Finally, for completeness, N_3 could simply be obtained by homogeneously stimulating all four input channels with the same, varying stimulus intensity, thus measuring the combined effect of all three non-linear stages, and comparing this to the effect of N_1 and N_2 alone.

The strategy of comparing iso-response curves measured with coarse and fine stimulus layouts has been used to track the origin of the non-linearities in the receptive fields of retinal ganglion cells that were described in **Figure 4** (Bölinger and Gollisch, 2012). Spatial stimulus integration in the retina occurs successively from photoreceptor cells via biopolar cells to ganglion cells. These integration stages cover different spatial scales; photoreceptor cells integrate light over a distance of about 10 μm (Mariani, 1986; Sherry et al., 1998), whereas bipolar cells have receptive

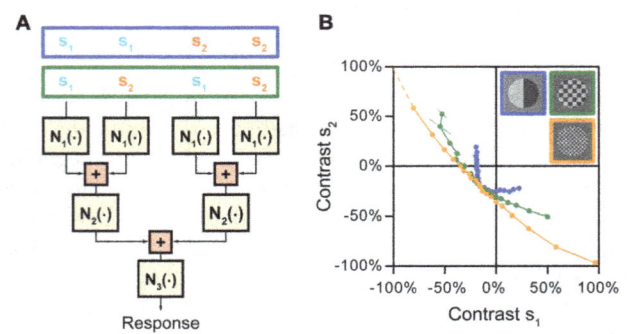

FIGURE 6 | Approach for disentangling non-linearities at multiple stages of stimulus integration in hierarchical models. (A) Cascade model with three consecutive non-linear stages, N_1, N_2, and N_3, separated by two integration stages. The model assumes that first nearby stimulus components are integrated, whose results are then combined in a subsequent stage. Different stimulation schemes that can be used to separate the effects of the non-linearities are shown on top. When nearby input channels are stimulated with the same stimulus component s_1 or s_2, respectively (stimulus pattern in blue box), the iso-response curve is affected by the combination of N_1 and N_2. When the two stimulus components s_1 and s_2 are placed so that they are combined already by the first integration stage (stimulus pattern in green box), only non-linearity N_1 is relevant for the shape of the iso-response curve. **(B)** Application of the strategy to separate different integration stages of spatial integration by retinal ganglion cells. When nearby spatial locations receive the same contrast (blue data points), the iso-rate curve shows the standard threshold-quadratic non-linearity as in **Figure 4C**. When the two contrast components s_1 and s_2 are interleaved so that presynaptic bipolar cells typically already start integrating the two components, but individual photoreceptors only receive either one of the components (green and orange data points, corresponding to squares in the stimulus layout with 150 and 60 μm side length, respectively), the iso-rate curves approach straight lines, showing that the integration stage from photoreceptors to bipolar cells can be approximated as linear integration. Panel **(B)** reprinted from Bölinger and Gollisch (2012), Copyright (2012), with permission from Elsevier.

fields of roughly 50–100 μm diameter (Wu et al., 2000; Baccus et al., 2008) and ganglion cells in the range of 200–600 μm. Thus, analyzing whether the non-linear structures of iso-response curves persist or change on spatial scales below several tens of micrometers allows one to test whether the site of the non-linearity is before or after stimulus integration by bipolar cells. This concept has been applied by arranging the stimulus components in a checkerboard-like fashion with different sizes of the individual checkerboard fields. Measurements of iso-response stimuli then showed that, as the scale of the fields fell roughly below 100 μm, the shapes of iso-response curves approached straight lines (**Figure 6B**). This meant that no relevant non-linearity occurred between photoreceptor cells and bipolar cells; to good approximation, stimuli were integrated linearly by bipolar cells.

Essentially the same principle was also behind the separation of different integration stages in locust auditory receptor neurons, as discussed above, by probing the system with pairs of acoustic clicks at different inter-click intervals (**Figure 3C**; Gollisch and Herz, 2005). For very short inter-click intervals, iso-response curves showed linear integration of the two clicks, corresponding

to the linear mechanical integration at the eardrum; for longer inter-click intervals that surpassed the mechanical integration time, the quadratic non-linearity of transduction became apparent (**Figure 3D**).

COMPARISON WITH SPIKE-TRIGGERED COVARIANCE ANALYSIS

The iso-response method aims at identifying non-linear interactions in consecutive stages of neuronal processing. This relates the method conceptually to cascade models and reverse-correlation techniques, such as STA and STC analysis. As already discussed above, STA analysis fails to capture non-linear integration, because all stimulus integration is assumed to occur linearly in the single-filter LN model. STC analysis and related information-theoretic techniques (Paninski, 2003; Sharpee et al., 2004; Pillow and Simoncelli, 2006), on the other hand, provide multiple filters and a corresponding multi-dimensional non-linearity. While the popularity of STC analysis primarily rests on its ability to determine the number and shapes of relevant filters, it also, in principle, allows studying non-linear stimulus integration by analyzing the features of the multi-dimensional non-linearity. A primary challenge for this is again the need to separate non-linearities of stimulus integration from the non-linearity at the output stage. If no explicit models of the output non-linearity are available, calculating iso-response curves within the multi-dimensional stimulus subspace that is spanned by the identified filters (Rust et al., 2005) appears to be the method of choice for identifying non-linearities of stimulus integration, even if these iso-response curves must be computed in an offline fashion.

Note, however, that there are important practical differences between analyzing non-linear stimulus integration with STC analysis or with closed-loop iso-response measurements. STC analysis is based on continuous, stationary stimulation, typically with white-noise statistics. The closed-loop iso-response method, on the other hand, can also be applied under non-stationary presentation of individually analyzed stimulus segments and can thus be used also for fairly brief stimuli, such as flashed visual images or short sound bursts. This difference in stimulus statistics can have interesting consequences for the processing features of the investigated system. For example, high-threshold inhibition from amacrine cells in the retina (Bölinger and Gollisch, 2012) may be effectively absent in white-noise experiments, but contribute to ganglion cell processing for flashed or saccade-like image presentations.

Second, STC analysis can yield a fairly large number of filters, and the high dimensionality of the associated stimulus subspace may impede a detailed analysis of the non-linear stage (Rust et al., 2005). Unless spiking is well described by a Poisson process, the temporal dynamics of spike generation alone can lead to a collection of several relevant filters (Agüera y Arcas and Fairhall, 2003; Agüera y Arcas et al., 2003). Along the same line, STC analysis of retinal ganglion cells with purely temporal stimuli has been shown to yield multiple temporal filter components (Fairhall et al., 2006). When on top of temporal variations, stimuli have further structure, such as spatial dimensions, one obtains additional filters, including filter combinations that mix temporal effects with other stimulus dimensions. A detailed analysis of the full non-linear stage then easily becomes impractical, in particular for more than two or three dimensions, both for reasons of graphical display and required amounts of data. As a feasible alternative, one may aim at analyzing non-linearities in low-dimensional subspaces, for example, spanned by just two selected filters (Rust et al., 2005). However, all other relevant filters then effectively act as noise sources, reducing the efficiency of this analysis. The closed-loop iso-response approach circumvents this problem by focusing on a chosen, small-dimensional set of stimulus components, such as two spectral or spatial stimulus components. This becomes particularly useful when combined with prior closed-loop identification of appropriate stimulus components, for example, by matching the components to the location and size of a receptive field. The possibility to focus on few purposefully selected stimulus components as well as on a narrow response regime is the benefit of the technically more demanding closed-loop approach. Yet, the selected components remain a choice of the experimenter under the assumption that these correspond to meaningful, separate input channels for the neuron under study.

In this view, STC analysis and iso-response measurements are complementary. While the strength of the STC analysis lies mostly in determining—with relatively few prior assumptions—the number and nature of stimulus features that are non-linearly integrated, the iso-response method assumes certain stimulus components to be relevant features and aims at determining their non-linear integration in detail. For systems with little prior expectation about the relevant input channels, it may well make sense to base a closed-loop measurement of iso-response stimuli on the results of a prior STC analysis for guiding the choice of the applied stimulus components.

NEXT STEPS AND FUTURE CHALLENGES

As shown by the above examples, the iso-response method provides a powerful concept for studying how neurons integrate sensory inputs. Using different types of stimuli allows one to focus on spectral, spatial, temporal, or spatio-temporal integration. Exploring and comparing different output measures, such as firing-rate or first-spike latency, provides valuable insight into potential coding schemes. Furthermore, unlike correlation-based approaches, the temporal resolution of the iso-response method is *not* limited by the precision with which the output signal can be measured. This is best illustrated by the experiments where click-stimuli were presented to auditory receptor neurons whose output was measured in terms of the probability that a single, isolated spike is generated within a window stretching several milliseconds (Gollisch and Herz, 2005). The temporal filters L_1 and L_2 of the corresponding LNLN cascade were determined at a temporal resolution below 20 microseconds, restricted only by the precision of the acoustic stimulus generator. The stochastic nature of neural responses did not cause any limitations—in fact, the iso-spike-probability paradigm is only feasible because of a nonzero intrinsic noise level so that a single spike is generated in some, but not all trials. The critical, beneficial role of a neural characteristic that is usually considered an experimental nuisance was an interesting observation in these studies. In addition, one may think that the iso-response paradigm applies to conventional feedforward chains only; but as demonstrated by the study on input-

vs. output-driven adaptation, certain feedback loops can also be studied with iso-response methods (Gollisch and Herz, 2004). We are thus confident that the iso-response paradigm will see further conceptual and methodological extensions in the future.

On the practical side, ongoing advances in soft- and hardware technology will increase the closed-loop interaction speed and also make it possible to include second-level analyses into the very design of iso-response experiments. This concern, for example, automated stopping rules in the search algorithms and automated selection of search directions, two developments of key importance for extending the iso-response approach to higher-dimensional search spaces. Closed-loop experiments have already been used to determine stimulus *ensembles* that are optimal from an information theoretical point of view (Machens et al., 2005). This is a computationally highly demanding task. With ever-rising computer power, however, it might be interesting to extend this concept and search for iso-information stimulus ensembles.

A prominent research area that could also benefit strongly from the iso-response methodology concerns the computations carried out by dendrites and dendritic trees. Synaptic integration along dendrites is often assumed to be linear, although it has been known for a long time that non-linearities exist and that they can have substantial consequences for neuronal computation (Koch et al., 1983; Mel, 1994; Poirazi et al., 2003; Katz et al., 2009; Abrahamsson et al., 2012). Based on traditional measurement paradigms, however, electrophysiological as well as imaging experiments can only address the question whether synaptic integration is linear, sublinear, or perhaps superlinear. Characterizing these non-linearities using the iso-response method would be an important step toward understanding dendritic computation. To investigate the scope and limits of such an approach, one could first focus on single-cell models of increasing complexity (Herz et al., 2006) with which one can test the method under well-defined and easily modifiable control conditions.

As demonstrated by the examples presented in this review, the iso-response method opens a new vista on neural dynamics and information processing. By focusing on one key question—"Which input combinations generate the *same* neural output?"—the method automatically reveals the invariance classes of the neuron (or neural substructure) under study. This feature should prove particularly helpful for studying sensory systems with complex and poorly understood stimulus spaces, such as olfaction, as well as for understanding multi-sensory integration and higher cortical processing. Note in this context that neural responses in the cortical area MST have been explained using a LNLN cascade model (Mineault et al., 2012). As shown in this review, the iso-response method is ideally suited to explore such models and determine their parameters with high precision. This suggests that even neural processing levels far from the sensory periphery can be studied quantitatively using the iso-response method.

At least conceptually, one could also extend this method beyond the single-neuron level and study multi-neuronal activity patterns. As a simple example, one may explore iso-synchrony stimuli that keep the level of synchronous activity between two or more neurons constant. Searching for multi-neuronal response patterns will require some conceptual developments regarding the applied search algorithm, that is, how to systematically tune stimuli toward eliciting a given multi-neuronal spike pattern. On the technological side, the necessary methods for fast and reliable online spike detection and sorting of multiple spike trains have already begun to become available (Quiroga et al., 2004; Santhanam et al., 2004; Wood et al., 2004; Rutishauser et al., 2006), but still need to be further explored for practical applications of closed-loop experiments.

At a larger scale, network activity could be characterized by identifying iso-population-response stimuli, using local-field-potential, MEG, or even fMRI signals. As for single neurons, one may learn far more by carefully analyzing those stimulus combinations that cause the same large-scale response than by observing that certain stimuli lead to more activation than others—without really knowing how to interpret differences in the activation levels. Within the iso-response framework, the tricky task of construing activity changes can be circumvented, and one can directly focus on one of the most important functional characteristics of a specific neuron or neural population: How are sensory or synaptic inputs integrated over space, frequencies, and time?

ACKNOWLEDGMENTS

This work was supported by the German Initiative of Excellence, the International Human Frontier Science Program Organization, and the Deutsche Forschungsgemeinschaft (DFG) through the Collaborative Research Center 889 (Tim Gollisch) as well as by the German Ministry for Science and Education (BMBF) through the Bernstein Center for Computational Neuroscience Munich (FKZ 01GQ1004A) (Andreas V. M. Herz).

REFERENCES

Abrahamsson, T., Cathala, L., Matsui, K., Shigemoto, R., and Digregorio, D. A. (2012). Thin dendrites of cerebellar interneurons confer sublinear synaptic integration and a gradient of short-term plasticity. *Neuron* 73, 1159–1172.

Adelson, E. H., and Bergen, J. R. (1985). Spatiotemporal energy models for the perception of motion. *J. Opt. Soc. Am. A* 2, 284–299.

Agüera y Arcas, B., and Fairhall, A. L. (2003). What causes a neuron to spike? *Neural Comput.* 15, 1789–1807.

Agüera y Arcas, B., Fairhall, A. L., and Bialek, W. (2003). Computation in a single neuron: Hodgkin and Huxley revisited. *Neural Comput.* 15, 1715–1749.

Aldworth, Z. N., Miller, J. P., Gedeon, T., Cummins, G. I., and Dimitrov, A. G. (2005). Dejittered spike-conditioned stimulus waveforms yield improved estimates of neuronal feature selectivity and spike-timing precision of sensory interneurons. *J. Neurosci.* 25, 5323–5332.

Baccus, S. A., Ölveczky, B. P., Manu, M., and Meister, M. (2008). A retinal circuit that computes object motion. *J. Neurosci.* 28, 6807–6817.

Barlow, H. B. (1953). Summation and inhibition in the frog's retina. *J. Physiol.* 119, 69–88.

Benda, J., Gollisch, T., Machens, C. K., and Herz, A. V. M. (2007). From response to stimulus: adaptive sampling in sensory physiology. *Curr. Opin. Neurobiol.* 17, 430–436.

Bölinger, D., and Gollisch, T. (2012). Closed-loop measurements of iso-response stimuli reveal dynamic nonlinear stimulus integration in the retina. *Neuron* 73, 333–346.

Brenner, N., Bialek, W., and de Ruyter van Steveninck, R. (2000). Adaptive rescaling maximizes information transmission. *Neuron* 26, 695–702.

Bryant, H. L., and Segundo, J. P. (1976). Spike initiation by transmembrane current: a white-noise analysis. *J. Physiol.* 260, 279–314.

Chichilnisky, E. J. (2001). A simple white noise analysis of neuronal light responses. *Network* 12, 199–213.

de Boer, R., and Kuyper, P. (1968). Triggered correlation. *IEEE Trans. Biomed. Eng.* 15, 169–179.

de Ruyter van Steveninck, R., and Bialek, W. (1988). Realtime performance of a movement-sensitive neuron in the blowfly visual system: coding and information transmission in short spike sequences. *Proc. Soc. Lond. B Biol. Sci.* 234, 379–414.

Dimitrov, A. G., and Gedeon, T. (2006). Effects of stimulus transformations on estimates of sensory neuron selectivity. *J. Comput. Neurosci.* 20, 265–283.

Eggermont, J. J., Aertsen, A. M., and Johannesma, P. I. (1983). Quantitative characterisation procedure for auditory neurons based on the spectro-temporal receptive field. *Hear. Res.* 10, 167–190.

Enroth-Cugell, C., and Robson, J. G. (1966). The contrast sensitivity of retinal ganglion cells of the cat. *J. Physiol.* 187, 517–552.

Eustaquio-Martín, A., and Lopez-Poveda, E. A. (2011). Isoresponse versus isoinput estimates of cochlear filter tuning. *J. Assoc. Res. Otolaryngol.* 12, 281–299.

Evans, E. F. (1975). "Cochlear nerve and cochlear nucleus," in *Handbook of Sensory Physiology, Auditory Systems, Vol. 5.2*, eds W. D. Keidel and W. D. Neff (Berlin: Springer), 1–108.

Fairhall, A. L., Burlingame, C. A., Narasimhan, R., Harris, R. A., Puchalla, J. L., and Berry, M. J. 2nd. (2006). Selectivity for multiple stimulus features in retinal ganglion cells. *J. Neurophysiol.* 96, 2724–2738.

Freed, M. A., and Sterling, P. (1988). The ON-alpha ganglion cell of the cat retina and its presynaptic cell types. *J. Neurosci.* 8, 2303–2320.

Garner, W. R. (1947). The effect of frequency spectrum on temporal integration of energy in the ear. *J. Acoust. Soc. Am.* 19, 808–814.

Geisler, C. D., Yates, G. K., Patuzzi, R. B., and Johnstone, B. M. (1990). Saturation of outer hair cell receptor currents causes two-tone suppression. *Hear. Res.* 44, 241–256.

Gillespie, P. G., and Walker, R. G. (2001). Molecular basis of mechanosensory transduction. *Nature* 413, 194–202.

Gollisch, T. (2006). Estimating receptive fields in the presence of spike-time jitter. *Network* 17, 103–129.

Gollisch, T., and Herz, A. V. M. (2003). "Uncovering the functional dynamics of biological signal-transduction modules," in *Idea-Finding Symposium for the Frankfurt Institute for Advanced Studies*, eds G. Greiner and J. Reinhardt (Debrecen: EP Systema Bt.), 75–84.

Gollisch, T., and Herz, A. V. M. (2004). Input-driven components of spike-frequency adaptation can be unmasked *in vivo*. *J. Neurosci.* 24, 7435–7444.

Gollisch, T., and Herz, A. V. M. (2005). Disentangling sub-millisecond processes within an auditory transduction chain. *PLoS Biol.* 3:e8. doi: 10.1371/journal.pbio.0030008

Gollisch, T., and Meister, M. (2010). Eye smarter than scientists believed: neural computations in circuits of the retina. *Neuron* 65, 150–164.

Gollisch, T., Schütze, H., Benda, J., and Herz, A. V. M. (2002). Energy integration describes sound-intensity coding in an insect auditory system. *J. Neurosci.* 22, 10434–10448.

Harris, D. M., and Dallos, P. (1984). Ontogenetic changes in frequency mapping of a mammalian ear. *Science* 225, 741–743.

Heil, P., and Neubauer, H. (2001). Temporal integration of sound pressure determines thresholds of auditory-nerve fibers. *J. Neurosci.* 21, 7404–7415.

Hering, E. (1920). *Grundzüge der Lehre vom Lichtsinn*. Berlin: Springer.

Herz, A. V. M., Gollisch, T., Machens, C. K., and Jaeger, D. (2006). Modeling single-neuron dynamics and computations: a balance of detail and abstraction. *Science* 314, 80–85.

Hill, K. G. (1983a). The physiology of locust auditory receptors. I. Discrete depolarizations of receptor cells. *J. Comp. Physiol. A* 152, 475–482.

Hill, K. G. (1983b). The physiology of locust auditory receptors. II. Membrane potentials associated with the response of the receptor cell. *J. Comp. Physiol. A* 152, 483–493.

Holton, T., and Weiss, T. F. (1983). Frequency selectivity of hair cells and nerve fibres in the alligator lizard cochlea. *J. Physiol.* 345, 241–260.

Horwitz, G. D., and Hass, C. A. (2012). Nonlinear analysis of macaque V1 color tuning reveals cardinal directions for cortical color processing. *Nat. Neurosci.* 15, 913–919.

Hunter, I. W., and Korenberg, M. J. (1986). The identification of nonlinear biological systems: Wiener and Hammerstein cascade models. *Biol. Cybern.* 55, 135–144.

Hurvich, L. M., and Jameson, D. (1957). An opponent-process theory of color vision. *Psychol. Rev.* 64, 384–404.

Jameson, D., and Hurvich, L. M. (1972). *Handbook of Sensory Physiology, Visual Psychophysics, Vol. 7.4*. Berlin: Springer.

Jones, J. P., Stepnoski, A., and Palmer, L. A. (1987). The two-dimensional spectral structure of simple receptive fields in cat striate cortex. *J. Neurophysiol.* 58, 1212–1232.

Katz, Y., Menon, V., Nicholson, D. A., Geinisman, Y., Kath, W. L., and Spruston, N. (2009). Synapse distribution suggests a two-stage model of dendritic integration in CA1 pyramidal neurons. *Neuron 63,* 171–177.

Koch, C., Poggio, T., and Torre, V. (1983). Nonlinear interactions in a dendritic tree: localization, timing, and role in information processing. *Proc. Natl. Acad. Sci. U.S.A.* 80, 2799–2802.

Korenberg, M. J., and Hunter, I. W. (1986). The identification of nonlinear biological systems: LNL cascade models. *Biol. Cybern.* 55, 125–134.

Lewicki, M. S. (1998). A review of methods for spike sorting: the detection and classification of neural action potentials. *Network 9,* R53–R78.

Machens, C. K., Gollisch, T., Kolesnikova, O., and Herz, A. V. M. (2005). Testing the efficiency of sensory coding with optimal stimulus ensembles. *Neuron 47,* 447–456.

Mariani, A. P. (1986). Photoreceptors of the larval tiger salamander retina. *Proc. R. Soc. Lond. B Biol. Sci.* 227, 483–492.

Marmarelis, P. N., and Marmarelis, V. Z. (1978). *Analysis of Physiological Systems: the White-Noise Approach*. New York, NY: Plenum Press.

Meister, M., and Berry, M. J. 2nd. (1999). The neural code of the retina. *Neuron 22,* 435–450.

Mel, B. W. (1994). Information processing in dendritic trees. *Neural Comput.* 6, 1031–1085.

Mineault, P. J., Khawaja, F. A., Butts, D. A., and Pack, C. C. (2012). Hierarchical processing of complex motion along the primate dorsal visual pathway. *Proc. Natl. Acad. Sci. U.S.A.* 109, E972–E980.

Paninski, L. (2003). Convergence properties of three spike-triggered analysis techniques. *Network 14,* 437–464.

Pillow, J. W., and Simoncelli, E. P. (2006). Dimensionality reduction in neural models: an information-theoretic generalization of spike-triggered average and covariance analysis. *J. Vis.* 6, 414–428.

Poirazi, P., Brannon, T., and Mel, B. W. (2003). Arithmetic of subthreshold synaptic summation in a model CA1 pyramidal cell. *Neuron 37,* 977–987.

Press, W. H., Teukolsky, S. A., Vetterling, W. T., and Flannery, B. P. (1992). *Numerical Recipes*. Cambridge, UK: Cambridge University Press.

Quiroga, R. Q., Nadasdy, Z., and Ben-Shaul, Y. (2004). Unsupervised spike detection and sorting with wavelets and superparamagnetic clustering. *Neural Comput.* 16, 1661–1687.

Rust, N. C., Schwartz, O., Movshon, J. A., and Simoncelli, E. P. (2005). Spatiotemporal elements of macaque V1 receptive fields. *Neuron 46,* 945–956.

Rutishauser, U., Schuman, E. M., and Mamelak, A. N. (2006). Online detection and sorting of extracellularly recorded action potentials in human medial temporal lobe recordings, *in vivo. J. Neurosci. Methods 154,* 204–224.

Sakai, H. M. (1992). White-noise analysis in neurophysiology. *Physiol. Rev.* 72, 491–505.

Samengo, I., and Gollisch, T. (2012). Spike-triggered covariance: geometric proof, symmetry properties, and extension beyond Gaussian stimuli. *J. Comput. Neurosci.* doi: 10.1007/s10827-012-0411-y. [Epub ahead of print].

Santhanam, G., Sahani, M., Ryu, S., and Shenoy, K. (2004). An extensible infrastructure for fully automated spike sorting during online experiments. *Conf. Proc. IEEE Eng. Med. Biol. Soc.* 6, 4380–4384.

Schiolten, P., Larsen, O. N., and Michelsen, A. (1981). Mechanical time resolution in some insect ears. I. Impulse responses and time constants. *J. Comp. Physiol.* 143, 289–295.

Schwartz, O., Pillow, J. W., Rust, N. C., and Simoncelli, E. P. (2006). Spike-triggered neural characterization. *J. Vis.* 6, 484–507.

Sharpee, T., Rust, N. C., and Bialek, W. (2004). Analyzing neural responses to natural signals: maximally informative dimensions. *Neural Comput.* 16, 223–250.

Sherry, D. M., Bui, D. D., and Degrip, W. J. (1998). Identification and distribution of photoreceptor subtypes in the neotenic tiger salamander retina. *Vis. Neurosci.* 15, 1175–1187.

Tasaki, I. (1954). Nerve impulses in individual auditory nerve fibers of guinea pig. *J. Neurophysiol.* 17, 97–122.

Tougaard, J. (1996). Energy detection and temporal integration in the noctuid A1 auditory receptor. *J. Comp. Physiol. A 178,* 669–677.

Wood, F., Fellows, M., Donoghue, J. P., and Black, M. J. (2004). Automatic spike sorting for neural decoding. *Conf. Proc. IEEE Eng. Med. Biol. Soc.* 6, 4009–4012.

Wu, S. M., Gao, F., and Maple, B. R. (2000). Functional architecture of synapses in the inner retina: segregation of visual signals by stratification of bipolar cell axon terminals. *J. Neurosci.* 20, 4462–4470.

9

Dynamic control of modeled tonic-clonic seizure states with closed-loop stimulation

Bryce Beverlin II[1] and Theoden I. Netoff[2]*

[1] *Department of Physics, University of Minnesota, Minneapolis, MN, USA*
[2] *Department of Biomedical Engineering, University of Minnesota, Minneapolis, MN, USA*

Edited by:
Steve M. Potter, Georgia Institute of Technology, USA

Reviewed by:
John M. Beggs, Indiana University, USA
John D. Rolston, Emory University, USA
Robert E. Gross, Emory University School of Medicine, USA

*Correspondence:
Theoden I. Netoff, Department of Biomedical Engineering, University of Minnesota, 7-105 Nis Hasselmo Hall, 312 Church St SE, Minneapolis, MN 55455, USA.
e-mail: tnetoff@umn.edu

Seizure control using deep brain stimulation (DBS) provides an alternative therapy to patients with intractable and drug resistant epilepsy. This paper presents novel DBS stimulus protocols to disrupt seizures. Two protocols are presented: open-loop stimulation and a closed-loop feedback system utilizing measured firing rates to adjust stimulus frequency. Stimulation suppression is demonstrated in a computational model using 3000 excitatory Morris–Lecar (M–L) model neurons connected with depressing synapses. Cells are connected using second order network topology (SONET) to simulate network topologies measured in cortical networks. The network spontaneously switches from tonic to clonic as synaptic strengths and tonic input to the neurons decreases. To this model we add periodic stimulation pulses to simulate DBS. Periodic forcing can synchronize or desynchronize an oscillating population of neurons, depending on the stimulus frequency and amplitude. Therefore, it is possible to either extend or truncate the tonic or clonic phases of the seizure. Stimuli applied at the firing rate of the neuron generally synchronize the population while stimuli slightly slower than the firing rate prevent synchronization. We present an adaptive stimulation algorithm that measures the firing rate of a neuron and adjusts the stimulus to maintain a relative stimulus frequency to firing frequency and demonstrate it in a computational model of a tonic-clonic seizure. This adaptive algorithm can affect the duration of the tonic phase using much smaller stimulus amplitudes than the open-loop control.

Keywords: seizure model, deep brain stimulation, tonic-clonic, synchrony

INTRODUCTION

Approximately one third of patients with epilepsy do not have sufficient control of their seizures even with the use of antiepileptic drugs. The use of deep brain stimulation (DBS) to suppress or truncate seizures is an alternative approach for controlling seizures in drug refractory patients. However, DBS for seizure suppression has had mixed clinical success (Loddenkemper et al., 2001). The SANTE trial, a multi-center clinical trial, used open-loop DBS, and demonstrated a 35% reduction in seizures (significantly more than in the control group), but with very few seizure free patients (Fisher et al., 2010). Neuropace has developed a closed-loop stimulator that has been tested in multi-center clinical trials, resulting in a 37.9% decrease in seizures, which is also significant compared to a control group. Although some patients are reluctant to have a device implanted in their brain (Arthurs et al., 2010), there exists a population of patients who have exhausted other medical options and are willing to take surgical risks for any reduction in seizures. There is therefore a need to improve the efficacy of DBS.

We presume that DBS may be more effective if the stimulation parameters could be optimally tuned for each patient. However, improving the efficacy of DBS by tuning the stimulus parameters is difficult, particularly as the mechanism by which DBS suppresses seizures is poorly understood (Vonck et al., 2003). With a better understanding of the mechanisms by which DBS functions, we may be able to design and optimize stimulus parameters and develop a closed-loop stimulator that tunes the stimulus parameters. This paper illustrates how DBS stimulus parameters can be selected based on the dynamics of neurons within the targeted brain area in order to affect synchrony in different stages of a seizure.

There are several different working hypotheses about the underlying mechanism by which DBS is able to suppress seizures. In animal models indirect evidence suggests that stimulation in the anterior thalamic nuclear complex can induce a release of the inhibitory neurotransmitter GABA, which presumably depresses the activity of neurons and results in the observed increase of seizure threshold (Mirski et al., 1997). In brain slice experiments it is possible to directly measure the effect of DBS stimuli in neurons. It has been shown that high frequency stimulation can cause neurons to go into a depolarization blockade, where cells are unable to fire, that will truncate the seizure (Bikson et al., 2001). DC electric fields can be used to hyperpolarize neurons, in order to change the neuron's excitability and suppress seizures (Gluckman et al., 1996). It has also been suggested that the stimulation may prevent neuronal synchronization; under this hypothesis DBS stimuli with a Poisson train of pulses at the same frequency as the high frequency stimulation has been shown to suppress seizures (Wyckhuys et al., 2010).

TONIC-CLONIC SEIZURES

Grand-mal epileptic seizures consist of two major stages: the tonic and clonic phases. In the tonic phase patients lose consciousness and their muscles tense up, while in the clonic phase the patients begin to jerk (Fisch and Olejniczak, 2006; Bragin et al., 2010). High frequency oscillations (HFOs) (oscillations above 150 Hz) in the intracranial electroencephalogram (EEG) recordings are observed during these seizures (Schindler et al., 2007b) as well as using magnetoencephalogram (MEG) (Garcia Dominguez et al., 2005; Perez Velazquez et al., 2007). In human studies, it has been shown that firing rates at the onset of the seizure are very high and decrease over the course of the tonic-clonic seizure (Ward, 1961). EEG measurements suggest that population amplitude and coherence is greater in the clonic phase than the tonic phase (Quian Quiroga et al., 1997). Frequency sweeps observed in EEG during seizures are a biomarker that can be used to detect seizures (Schiff et al., 2000).

We have recently proposed a model explaining (1) a mechanism for the transition from tonic to clonic phases by slowing of firing of neurons over the seizure and (2) the differing ability of neurons to synchronize at high firing rates and low firing rates (Beverlin et al., 2011). The change in the firing rate in the model is due to due to synaptic depression of the neurons and spike rate adaptation of the neurons, both of which occur at high firing rates (Abbott et al., 1997; Manor and Nadim, 2001). When analyzing EEG, determining the transition between tonic to clonic is somewhat subjective to the epileptologist. In this paper we will simply define the tonic phase of the seizure as network activity with high firing rate and low synchrony, while the clonic phase is high firing rate with high synchrony.

FIRING RATE AND NETWORK SYNCHRONY

In previous brain slice experiments, it was found that while the firing rates of neurons were high during the tonic phase of the seizure, neurons exhibited a low degree of correlation. During the clonic phase the firing rate decreased and the population became highly synchronous (Netoff and Schiff, 2002). This transition from the tonic to clonic phases may be integral to the evolution of the seizure and its eventual termination. Based on this hypothesis, it has been shown that synchronizing populations with DBS pulses may promote seizure termination and truncate the seizure (Schindler et al., 2007a). We have recently developed a computational model that illustrates a mechanism by which synchrony changes during a seizure (Beverlin et al., 2011).

In our model, seizures start by the failure of inhibition. Without inhibition, the excitatory neurons increase their firing rate and excitatory drive within the network increases in a positive feedback loop resulting in very high firing rates. Over time, the firing rate slows down, and the network transitions to a synchronous high amplitude clonic phase of seizure. In the model the transition from tonic to clonic phases is caused by a change in the sensitivity of neurons to synaptic inputs as their firing rate slows; this leads to a shift in synchrony. We demonstrate how the transition occurs in a network of model neurons and explain the mechanisms using pulse-coupled oscillator theory. There are several ways in which network synchrony may change *in vivo*, including the reintroduction of activity from the inhibitory population

(provided they have entered depolarization block at the seizure onset) (Ziburkus et al., 2006), synaptic depression, and vesicle depletion. In our model, the change in firing rate is produced by including synaptic depression and a gradually decreasing input current to the model neurons, to simulate spike rate adaptation of the neurons.

PERIODIC STIMULATION IN EPILEPSY

DBS has been tested in models of epilepsy in order to disrupt seizures (Good et al., 2009; Fisher et al., 2010; Nelson et al., 2011; Rajdev et al., 2011). Stimuli designed to increase synchrony has been shown to effectively truncate seizures (Schindler et al., 2007a) and DBS has been employed in clinical trials with reasonable success (Morrell, 2006; Fisher et al., 2010; Morrell and On behalf of the RNS System in Epilepsy Study Group, 2011).

During a seizure the firing rate of neurons changes as the phases of the seizure progress. Therefore, we hypothesize that the influence of DBS on population synchrony will change if the stimulus does not adapt to the firing rate of the neuron. In this paper we first estimate the effects of periodic DBS on neuronal populations that are firing at high rates during the tonic phase, and then on the low firing rates during the clonic phase. To study the effects at each phase of the seizure, we fix the synaptic strengths and apply constant current and vary the DBS frequency and amplitude measuring the resulting increase or decrease in synchrony. We find that independent of firing rate, there are ratios of stimulus frequency to neuronal frequency that can either synchronize or desynchronize. Then, in the full model with changing firing rates, we demonstrate an adaptive algorithm that measures the firing rate of a neuron to adjust the stimulus frequency to maintain stimulation in the regime that promotes or decreases synchrony over the entire duration of the seizure. This exemplifies how an adaptive stimulus algorithm may be designed to disrupt synchrony in a population where the population oscillation is changing.

METHODS

We investigate the effectiveness of DBS within an epileptic model using computational simulations of excitatory neuronal networks. The neuron model captures the dynamics of a real neuron's sensitivity to synaptic inputs, current inputs, and periodic forcing from applied stimuli. Synaptic depression variables change the recurrent excitatory drive amongst the population, which changes the firing rates of the neurons. As the neuron's firing rate changes, the sensitivity to synaptic inputs also changes, allowing them to synchronize at slow firing rates, but not at high firing rates. Networks of neurons are connected using a second order network (SONET) that keeps the neurons at the edge of synchrony at the high firing rate.

MORRIS–LECAR MODEL NEURON

We use a modified version of the Morris–Lecar (M–L) model neuron (Morris and Lecar, 1981; Izhikevich, 2007), a 2-D reduction of the Hodgkin–Huxley model (Rinzel, 1985). DBS stimulation is simulated by applying periodic pulses of current input of varying strength and frequency, depending on the stimulation protocol. The conductance based M–L model calculates the change in voltage as a function of the membrane's ionic currents as described by the following equations:

$$C\dot{V} = I_{\text{input}} + I_{\text{DBS}} + I_{\text{noise}} - g_L(V - E_L)$$
$$- g_{Na}m^{\infty}(V)(V - E_{Na}) - g_K n(V - E_K)$$
$$- D(S - F)(V - E_{\text{syn}}),$$

$$\dot{n} = \frac{n_{\infty}(V) - n}{\tau(V)}$$

$$m_{\infty}(V) = \frac{1}{1 + e^{\frac{V_{1/2} - V}{k}}}$$

$$\tau(V) = C\, e^{\frac{-(V_{\max} - V)^2}{\sigma^2}}$$

$$\dot{S} = -\frac{S}{\tau_s} \sum_{j=1}^{M} \delta\left(t - t_{\text{syn}}^j\right)$$

$$\dot{F} = -\frac{F}{\tau_f} \sum_{j=1}^{M} \delta\left(t - t_{\text{syn}}^j\right)$$

where C is the membrane capacitance, V is the membrane voltage, I_{input} is an input current common to all neurons, I_{noise} is a white noise input proportional to the square root of the time step independent to each neuron, g are the maximal conductances of each current source, E are the reversal potentials for each ion, m and n are the ionic gating variables, where m_{∞} and n_{∞} are the steady-state activation for a given voltage, $V_{1/2}\,\text{m}$ satisfies $m_{\infty}(V_{1/2}) = 0.5$, $V_{\max}$ is the value of V at the maximum value of m, k is the degree of slope at $V_{1/2}$, τ is the voltage dependent time constant of the inactivation variable, σ determines the sensitivity of the time constant of V, S represents the slow variable of the synaptic input shape, with a time constant τ_s and F is the fast synaptic time constant. At times of synaptic input, 1 is added to both the S and F state variables for each presynaptic event at time t_{syn} for all M events. Synaptic depression, D, is defined as $D_{i+1,j} = D_{i,j}d$, updated for cell j after a synaptic input i as described in Varela et al. (1997) where the strength of depression is controlled by d.

The model is explained in more detail in our recent seizure model paper (Beverlin et al., 2011). The parameters of the M–L model were chosen so that the phase response curve (PRC) is similar to PRCs we have measured in hippocampal pyramidal neurons (Netoff et al., 2005); they are as follows: $C = 1.0\,\mu\text{F}$, $g_L = 8\,\text{nS}$, $E_L = -53.24\,\text{mV}$, $g_{Na} = 18.22\,\text{nS}$, $E_{Na} = 60\,\text{mV}$, $g_K = 4\,\text{nS}$, $E_K = -95.52\,\text{mV}$, $V_{1/2\,\text{m}} = -7.37\,\text{mV}$, $k_m = 11.97\,\text{mV}$, $V_{1/2\,n} = -16.35\,\text{mV}$, $k_n = 4.21\,\text{mV}$, $\tau = 1\,\text{ms}$, spikeWidth $= 0.03$, $E_{\text{syn}} = 0$, $\tau_f = 0.25\,\text{ms}$, $\tau_s = 0.5\,\text{ms}$. Matlab code for this model is available at http://neuralnetoff.umn.edu/public/TonicClonicControl and from Model DB website (http://senselab.med.yale.edu/modeldb).

NETWORK STRUCTURE

Directional networks of 3000 cells were generated with an average of 30 out-going excitatory synaptic connections using a second order network topology (SONET), which places additional correlated structure to random networks (Zhao et al., 2011). The specific network structure is determined by specifying the average connectivity (first order statistic) as well as the additional prevalence of two edge motifs, thus referred to as second order motifs. These second order structures are reciprocal, convergent, divergent, and chain connections, as illustrated in **Figure 1**. We generate large networks by specifying the first and second order statistics. It has been found that the prevalence of chains and convergent connections have a strong effect on the synchronizability of the network. Here we choose the network statistics which allow a network to both synchronize and desynchronize, depending on input current and firing rate. The network we use has statistics similar to that measured in rat visual cortex (Song et al., 2005). The specific SONET was chosen out of 186 candidates discussed in recently published results (Zhao et al., 2011). This network, which had 4 times the prevalence of reciprocal connections, 1.4 times the convergent connections, 1.3 times the divergent connections, and 1.2 times the chain connections compared to a random graph, was the closest to measured cortical networks in a rat model.

NETWORK SYNCHRONY MEASURE

Network synchrony is quantified using the Kuramoto order parameter (r) which ranges from 0 (neurons evenly distributed in phase) to 1 (neurons in coherent phase) and calculated as follows:

$$re^{i\phi} = \frac{1}{N} \sum_{j=1}^{N} e^{i\theta_j}$$

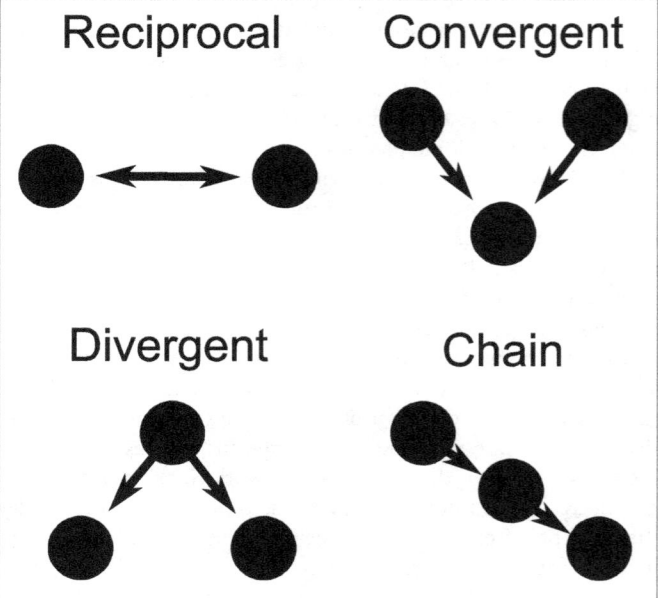

FIGURE 1 | Second order motifs. Connection motifs of two and three-cell combinations with two directional connections. The motifs are reciprocal, convergent, divergent, and chain motifs. The prevalence of these motifs within a larger network can be specified when generating the network.

where the phases of neurons (θ_j) are summed to create a population vector with magnitude (r) (Kuramoto, 1984; Strogatz, 2000).

RESULTS

The influence of DBS was tested in a network model that reproduces a tonic to clonic shift in network synchrony as a function of the firing rate of the neurons (Beverlin et al., 2011). In the simulations, at the seizure onset the firing rate of the neurons are very high, as might be expected with runaway excitation, and then over the duration of the seizure, the firing rate of the neurons slowly decreases, eventually bringing about a transition to the clonic phase of the seizure, seen in **Figure 2**. The tonic-clonic transition model reproduces the shift in synchrony observed in EEG. In this model, the firing rate was modulated by a combination of changes in tonic drive to all the neurons, representing drive of exogenous sources, and synaptic depression from neurons within the network. Simulations included 3000 M–L neurons connected using a second order network designed to be at the edge of synchrony when neurons were in the tonic phase of the seizure. Over the duration of the seizure we decreased the tonic drive to represent depression from the exogenous inputs, and the synapses within the network depress during the seizure due to the modeled synaptic depression. Decreased input from both the exogenous and endogenous sources results in a decrease in firing rate over the duration of the seizure.

In this paper we apply periodic stimulation to the seizure model. All cells receive the same stimulus input for a given set of stimulus parameters, assuming that the population is uniformly distributed from the electrode. To analyze the effects of the stimulation in each phase, we hold the applied current in the neurons constant and freeze the synaptic plasticity to study the effects of stimulation at each phase of the seizure separately. We analyze and model the effects at a high firing rate during the tonic phase and then again at a low firing rate during the clonic phase. Then, we restore the changing exogenous current and plasticity back into the model to measure the effects of periodic stimulation to the duration of the tonic and clonic phases.

OPEN-LOOP PERIODIC STIMULATION WITH FIXED DRIVE TO NEURONS

First, periodic stimulation was applied to a network simulation driven with high current input (6 nA), to model the tonic phase of the seizure. At this high firing rate the unstimulated network does not synchronize. Results of stimulation applied to all cells of the network at 5.5 ms intervals are shown in **Figure 3**. Stimulus at this interval during the tonic phase increases synchrony in the tonic phase.

Simulations were repeated while varying the stimulation frequency and amplitude. Synchrony was measured using the

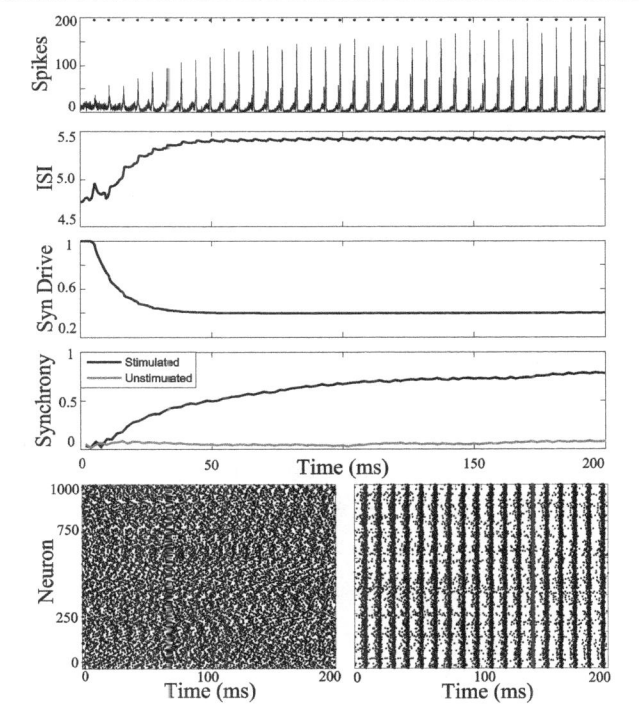

FIGURE 3 | Synchronizing a tonic phase model using periodic drive. Computational simulation of network activity with current set to 6 nA to simulate tonic phase of seizure. **Top**, population is entrained to periodic stimuli (points of stimulation as dots along top axis). ISI increases from 4.8 to 5.5 ms. Synaptic drive decreases from depression due to strong input from DBS. Synchrony of unstimulated network is low (gray) and stimulating with 5.5 ms pulses increases synchrony. **Below**, rasterplots of neuronal network spike times during unstimulated tonic activity and with network stimulation to synchronize. Spike times of 1000 model neurons from the 3000 cell network simulator. **Left**, unstimulated cells have low synchrony. **Right**, network stimulated with 5.5 ms pulses becomes coherent.

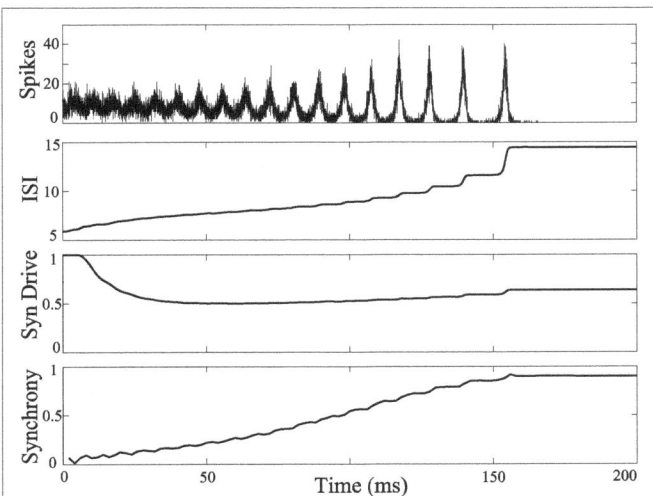

FIGURE 2 | Tonic-clonic transition in model network. Synchrony emerges in large scale networks with synaptic depression and ramped current from $I = 0$ nA to $I = -5$ nA and inclusion of synaptic depression. Average synaptic strength across the population is plotted against time in the 3rd panel labeled as "Syn Drive." Synchrony as a function of time is plotted at the bottom, measured using the Kuramoto order parameter. Synchrony emerges as interspike intervals of the neurons exceed about 7 ms. Synchrony will not occur if tonic current is held at 5 nA keeping interspike intervals shorter than about 7 ms.

Kuramoto order parameter, averaged over the last one quarter of the simulation to estimate the steady-state synchrony in the network. These simulations were repeated over a range of stimulus amplitudes and frequencies, results are shown in **Figure 4**. Darker areas indicate stimulus parameters that entrain the neurons, resulting in a synchronized population. These entrained regions are known as *Arnold Tongues* (Milton and Jung, 2003). These "tongues" of entrainment occur at integer ratios of stimulus period to the natural period of oscillation. The points on the map that are lightly shaded indicate those parameters where the network remains desynchronized.

The simulations were then repeated while applying a −2 nA current, in order to simulate a network during the clonic seizure phase, shown in **Figure 5**, where the unstimulated network would spontaneously synchronize. The network is then periodically stimulated with a 2 ms period, shown as dots along the top curve in **Figure 5**. This stimulation reduces the synchrony compared to the unstimulated simulation.

Simulations were run for a range of stimulus amplitudes and frequencies, while driving the network at −2 nA. A synchrony map for these results is shown in **Figure 6**. One notable difference is that the region of entrainment has shifted from 5.5 ms around the natural period when the system is driven with 6 nA, to a region of entrainment of 8.5 ms around the natural period when driven at −2 nA. Because the low current network synchronizes spontaneously, a wider range of stimulus parameters synchronize the network. There are several windows which desynchronize the population. In the example shown in **Figure 5**, we use 2 ms period for stimulation, but 4 ms or about 12.5 ms for example could be used as indicated by light bands in **Figure 6**.

CONTINUOUS CONTROL OF SEIZURES WITH VARIABLE STIMULUS FREQUENCY

Ultimately, control of seizure states may be most effectively achieved by implementing a closed-loop feedback system, in order to select the stimulus frequency from the measured neuronal frequency (Nelson et al., 2011). We have noticed that

the stimulus frequency that entrains the neurons occurs at frequencies just slightly faster than the firing rate of the neurons. Stimulus regimes that desynchronize the population are found to be slightly slower than the firing rate of the neurons. Based on this observation, we developed a simple feedback system

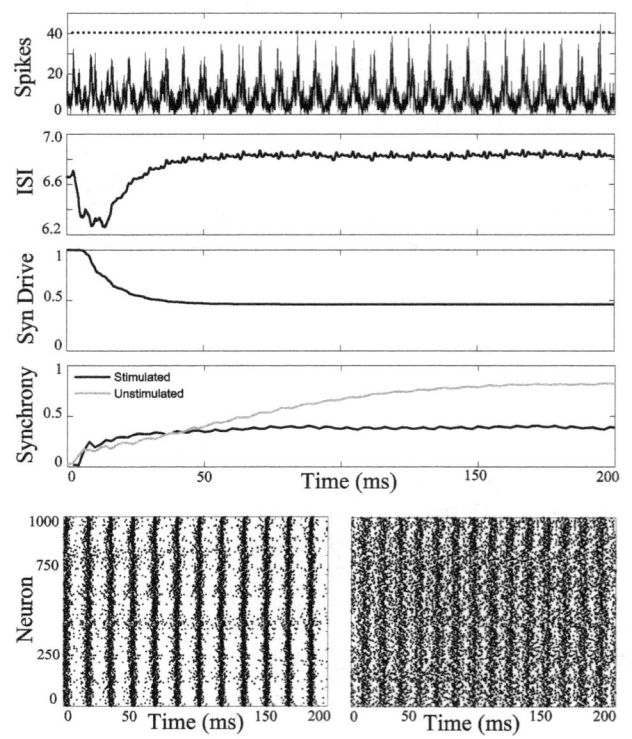

FIGURE 5 | Desynchronizing the clonic phase. Computational simulation of network activity with current set to −2 nA to simulate clonic phase of seizure. See **Figure 3** for general figure description. Synchrony of the unstimulated clonic network increases to a strong value near 0.8 (gray). When applying the 2 ms periodic DBS pulse, the network activity is desynchronized. Bottom Left, unstimulated cells have high synchrony. Bottom Right, network stimulated with 2 ms pulses. Less synchronous activity is observed in the stimulated network.

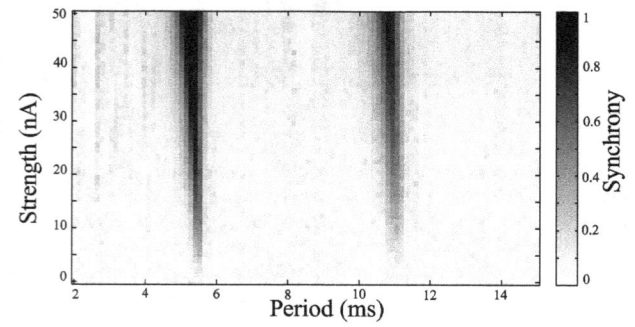

FIGURE 4 | Synchrony map of stimulated tonic networks. Current input of 6 nA applied to all cells. Grayscale indicates calculated synchrony as the Kuramoto order parameter averaged over the last 200 ms of individual simulation for a range of stimulus amplitudes and periods.

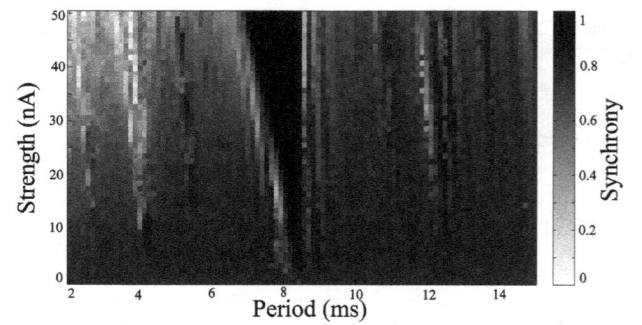

FIGURE 6 | Synchrony map of stimulated clonic networks. Current input of −2 nA applied to all cells. Grayscale indicates calculated synchrony as Kuramoto order parameter averaged over the last 200 ms of each simulation for a range of stimulus amplitudes and periods.

that modulates the stimulus period depending on the firing rate of one cell within the network. All other parameters are the same as previously used in the unstimulated tonic-clonic model, including the current ramp and network topology. Here, the feedback system selects the stimulus frequency based on a user chosen ratio of stimulus to measured frequencies. This ratio can be selected from the entrainment maps. A choice of 1:1, for example, would entrain a population, while a choice of 1:1.14 (stimulated to measured frequency ratio) may desynchronize a population.

Figure 7 shows the response of the network while stimulating at intervals 1.14 times the interspike intervals of neurons in the population. Synchrony emerges later in this stimulated case than the unstimulated network, prolonging the tonic phase. Eventually, the network slows sufficiently such that synchrony takes over, despite the dispersive effects of the stimulus. Conversely, by applying the stimulus at the same frequency as the firing rate of the neurons (1:1 ratio) we were able to bring about synchrony in much less time than in the unstimulated case, truncating the tonic phase, as shown in **Figure 8**. In both the synchronizing and desynchronizing closed-loop feedback experiments we used stimulus amplitude of 10 nA, one quarter the amplitude used in the open-loop conditions to achieve a similar effect.

DISCUSSION

Tonic-clonic seizures can be devastating to a patient with epilepsy. While there is evidence that DBS can reduce seizures, no clinical application has been found to be fully effective in truncating seizures. It is well known in oscillatory models that periodic forcing of a network of oscillators can synchronize or phase disperse the oscillators (Glass and Mackey, 1988; Elbert et al., 1994; Kaplan et al., 1996). It has previously been proposed

that this may be used to control seizures (Milton and Jung, 2003). In a recent paper, we proposed that this may be involved in treating Parkinsonian symptoms (Wilson et al., 2011). In this paper we use similar periodic stimulation theory to affect the tonic and clonic phases of a seizure in a computational model we have recently developed (Beverlin et al., 2011). Recently we proposed that the shift from the desynchronized tonic phase to the synchronous clonic phase occurs as the neuronal firing rate adapts over the duration of the seizure. At the high firing rates, the model neurons do not synchronize, but as the firing rates slow down, the cells become more sensitive to synaptic inputs and the network synchronizes. The change in spike rate is modeled by gradually decreasing the current drive to the neurons along with depressing synapses.

In this paper, we have added periodic stimulation to the tonic-clonic model to determine if periodic stimulation could be used to affect the duration of the seizure phases. We analyzed the effects of stimulus frequency and amplitude on the population synchrony at the tonic phase and again at the clonic phase. Depending on the stimulus frequency we were able to synchronize neurons during the asynchronous tonic phase, or desynchronize neurons in the synchronous clonic phase. Periodic stimulation at integer ratios of the stimulus frequency to the natural frequency was found to entrain and thereby synchronize the population. Conversely, periodic stimulation just slightly slower than the firing rates (and at some frequencies, faster than the firing rates of the neurons) could desynchronize the population. Our findings can be explained with PRC theory, which we previously used to explain the effects of the stimulus at different frequency amplitudes and its effect on population synchrony (Beverlin et al., 2011). The effect of firing rate shifting the peak of the PRC to the left in response to excitatory inputs is generally true and should therefore not be heavily

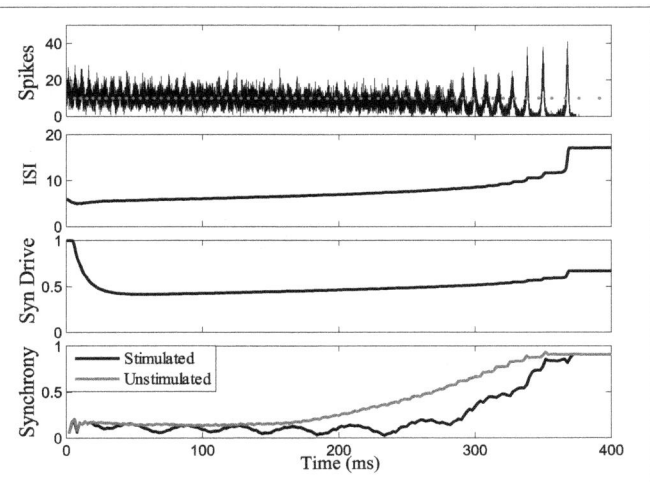

FIGURE 7 | Tonic phase prolonged. Stimulating at a desynchronizing frequency ratio of 1:1.14 where the stimulus is firing slightly slower than the measured frequency of one chosen cell. The tonic phase of low synchrony is prolonged when stimulating compared to the unstimulated model. Graphs labeled the same as **Figure 3**.

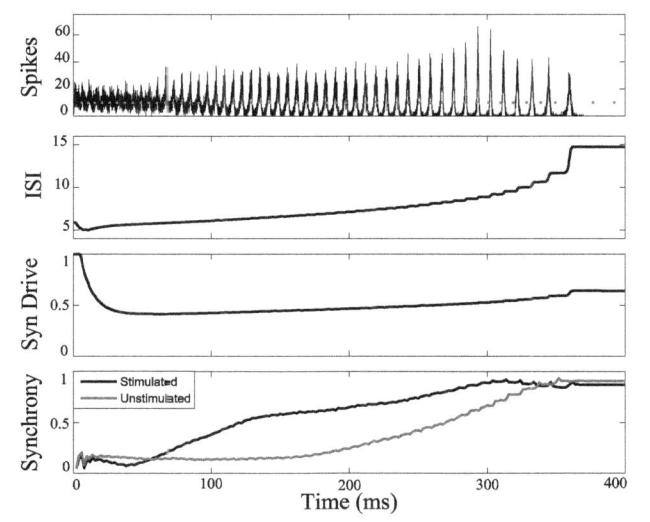

FIGURE 8 | Tonic phase truncation. Network of cells stimulated at 1:1 frequency ratio compared to one measured cell in the network. Bottom: Transition to synchronous clonic phase is earlier (black line) than the unstimulated model (gray line). Here the clonic phase is extended. Graphs labeled the same as **Figure 3**.

model dependent (Gutkin et al., 2005; Fink et al., 2011). We chose the M–L model because it is one of the simplest conductances based neuronal models that can demonstrate this effect.

Periodic stimulation of a network during a seizure with a fixed period would have a mixed effect; synchronizing at some phases of the seizure and desynchronizing at others, as the neurons are constantly changing their firing rate. However, the ratio of stimulus frequency to neuronal firing rate that entrains or desynchronizes the population is relatively consistent. Therefore, we created a closed-loop control system that adjusts the stimulus frequency to desynchronize or synchronize the population, holding the stimulus at a fixed rate relative to the neuronal firing rate. In this case the tonic phase of the seizure could effectively be shortened by applying a stimulus at the same frequency of the neurons, while the tonic phase could be prolonged by applying a stimulus frequency that is slightly slower than the firing rate of the neurons, effectively preventing the synchronization of the population.

This model illustrates the principle that periodic stimulation at certain ratios to the measured firing rate of neurons can be used to promote or decrease synchrony and this principle may be used in a closed-loop feedback system for seizure suppression. We are not suggesting that this model is an accurate model of the actual physiology in the brain. Instead, if PRCs can be measured during seizures, our theory may be tested experimentally. We plan to test these hypotheses in brain slice experiments in the near future.

In addition, the complicated structure and function of real neurons in real tissue are beyond the scope of this paper. Here we have investigated the applicability of DBS in a model network; naturally, there may be real world complications when implementing these protocols depending on the location of the electrode(s) and stimulus parameters. In addition, clinical applications of DBS thus far are typically less than 200 Hz. For example the SANTE trials studying the treatment of refractory epilepsy used a stimulation of 145 Hz (Fisher et al., 2010). Some of the frequencies in our model presented here exceed these typical frequencies, but the relative frequency between the stimulus and the neuronal firing rate is what we consider important. Our model is not designed to produce realistic firing rates, so we do not suggest based on this model that these are realistic stimulation frequencies for all brain regions that should be used clinically.

There are many aspects of this simulation which are not physiologically realistic which could be improved in future studies. First, the neurons are modeled as oscillators. Generally, neurons do not fire periodically. However, at the onset of a seizure with high rate of synaptic asynchronous synaptic inputs, neurons may fire close to periodically. All the neurons are also modeled as oscillators with the same parameters and the same firing rate, while it would be more realistic to model the neurons with a distribution of parameters and firing rates. Furthermore, in this model the stimulus was applied uniformly to all the neurons. In a real neuronal network there is geometry to the position of the neurons and a stimulus electrode will not uniformly stimulate all the neurons. All of these aspects of the model could be improved to make it more realistic, and will be the focus of further investigation, but we do not feel will change the fundamental approach we present here to desynchronizing populations.

How might this algorithm be implemented in practice, such as in a brain slice model of seizures and eventually in humans? First, a stimulation electrode and a recording electrode are needed. Then, it is necessary to determine the optimal stimulus frequency ratio with respect to the neuronal frequency. This can be determined from the neuron's PRC to the stimulus. The PRC is measured by open-loop stimulation at random intervals that are on average much longer than the period of the neuron on average. The phase of the oscillation is measured before and after the stimulation to estimate the phase advance of each stimulus. Generally, some model representing the phase advance as a function of the stimulus phase is fit to the resulting data. PRCs would need to be measured at different firing rates or phases of the seizure. From the measured PRCs the Lyapunov Exponents (LEs) of the population response at is estimated different stimulus amplitudes and frequencies (Wilson et al., 2011). Stimulus parameters are selected that maximize the LE to desynchronize the population, or minimize the LE to synchronize. To implement the algorithm, the recording electrode would be used to measure the firing rate of neurons in the population; the measured firing rate would then be used to modulate the frequency of the stimulating electrode.

An interesting finding is that the closed-loop controller could affect the duration of the tonic phase with equal efficacy at one quarter the stimulus amplitude than the open-loop control. This indicates that a simple measure of the neuronal firing rate may significantly improve the efficacy of DBS.

It is important to note that we do not propose that it is best to synchronize and shorten the duration of the tonic phase of the seizure, or to prolong it. We consider that the restructuring of the neuronal network by induction of synaptic plasticity by high firing rates of neurons during seizures may ultimately be the long term deleterious effect if seizures. The goal of the therapy may be to minimize the plasticity changes during a seizure. If neurons fire synchronously, plasticity may be greater than when neurons fire asynchronously. In this case, maximizing the tonic phase of the seizure and minimizing the clonic phase may result in less plasticity changes. However, if the synchronization of the population is integral to the termination of the seizure promoting synchrony may terminate the seizure earlier (Schindler et al., 2007a). For example, if seizures are sustained by recurrent excitation, increasing synchrony may decrease the excitable pool of neurons, thereby decreasing the likelihood of re-entry and terminating seizures earlier. Using a stimulus that can modulate the duration of the tonic phase may help us determine whether synchrony is just a network behavior that occurs at the termination of the seizure or whether it is integral to the termination.

HFOs are population oscillations that are seen between seizures. Suppressing these oscillations may be considered a target for DBS stimulation. The hope would be that disrupting these pathological oscillations may suppress epileptogenesis. The same approach used in this paper might be used to design a stimulus to suppress HFOs. HFOs might be a good target because they are observed to increase prior to a seizure in human and animal models (Worrell et al., 2004), and are thought to arise from synchronous bursts of neurons that occur in an epileptic focus (Bragin et al., 1999, 2010; Ibarz et al., 2010). There is also strong experimental evidence that synchrony amongst cortical regions is increased in epileptic patients (Bullock et al., 1995; Towle et al., 1999; Ben-Jacob et al., 2007; Schevon et al., 2007; Prusseit and Lehnertz, 2008; Zaveri et al., 2009) and that this synchrony changes in the lead up to a seizure (Lehnertz and Elger, 1995; Chavez et al., 2003; Le Van Quyen et al., 2005). In contrast, other evidence suggests that synchrony may decrease prior to a seizure (Mormann et al., 2003). We hypothesize that tuning DBS stimulators to desynchronize prominent pathological oscillations relevant to the generation of seizures interictally suppress seizures. However, we are not aware of any direct evidence that DBS affects these oscillations.

CONCLUSION

This work proposes a novel method to alter seizures using DBS. In a computational model we have demonstrated that the duration of the tonic-phase of a seizure may be extended or shortened by promoting synchrony using periodic stimulation. Promoting or decreasing synchrony depends on the relative frequency of the stimulation to the firing rate of the neurons. By using a closed-loop feedback to adjust the stimulation frequency dependent on the firing rate of the neurons, we are able to extend or decrease the duration of the tonic phase with much weaker stimulus pulses than was necessary in open-loop stimulation.

REFERENCES

Abbott, L. F., Varela, J. A., Sen, K., and Nelson, S. B. (1997). Synaptic depression and cortical gain control [see comments]. *Science* 275, 220–224.

Arthurs, S., Zaveri, H. P., Frei, M. G., and Osorio, I. (2010). Patient and caregiver perspectives on seizure prediction. *Epilepsy Behav.* 19, 474–477.

Ben-Jacob, E., Boccaletti, S., Pomyalov, A., Procaccia, I., and Towle, V. L. (2007). Detecting and localizing the foci in human epileptic seizures. *Chaos* 17:043113. doi: 10.1063/1.2805658

Beverlin, B. 2nd., Kakalios, J., Nykamp, D., and Netoff, T. I. (2011). Dynamical changes in neurons during seizures determine tonic to clonic shift. *J. Comput. Neurosci.* 33, 41.

Bikson, M., Lian, J., Hahn, P. J., Stacey, W. C., Sciortino, C., and Durand, D. M. (2001). Suppression of epileptiform activity by high frequency sinusoidal fields in rat hippocampal slices. *J. Physiol.* 531, 181–191.

Bragin, A., Engel, J. Jr., and Staba, R. J. (2010). High-frequency oscillations in epileptic brain. *Curr. Opin. Neurol.* 23, 151–156.

Bragin, A., Engel, J. Jr., Wilson, C. L., Fried, I., and Mathern, G. W. (1999). Hippocampal and entorhinal cortex high-frequency oscillations (100–500 Hz) in human epileptic brain and in kainic acid–treated rats with chronic seizures. *Epilepsia* 40, 127–137.

Bullock, T. H., McClune, M. C., Achimowicz, J. Z., Iragui-Madoz, V. J., Duckrow, R. B., and Spencer, S. S. (1995). EEG coherence has structure in the millimeter domain: subdural and hippocampal recordings from epileptic patients. *Electroencephalogr. Clin. Neurophysiol.* 95, 161–177.

Chavez, M., Le Van Quyen, M., Navarro, V., Baulac, M., and Martinerie, J. (2003). Spatiotemporal dynamics prior to neocortical seizures: amplitude versus phase couplings. *IEEE Trans. Biomed. Eng.* 50, 571–583.

Elbert, T., Ray, W. J., Kowalik, Z. J., Skinner, J. E., Graf, K. E., and Birbaumer, N. (1994). Chaos and physiology: deterministic chaos in excitable cell assemblies. *Physiol. Rev.* 74, 1–47.

Fink, C. G., Booth, V., and Zochowski, M. (2011). Cellularly-driven differences in network synchronization propensity are differentially modulated by firing frequency. *PLoS Comput. Biol.* 7:e1002062. doi: 10.1371/journal.pcbi.1002062

Fisch, J. F., and Olejniczak, P. W. (2006). "Generalized-tonic-clonic seizures," in *The treatment of Epilepsy: Principles and Practice*, eds E. Wyllie, A. Gupta, and D. K. Lachhwani (Philadelphia, PA: Lippincott Williams and Wilkins), 279.

Fisher, R., Salanova, V., Witt, T., Worth, R., Henry, T., Gross, R., et al. (2010). Electrical stimulation of the anterior nucleus of thalamus for treatment of refractory epilepsy. *Epilepsia* 51, 899–908.

Garcia Dominguez, L., Wennberg, R. A., Gaetz, W., Cheyne, D., Snead, O. C. 3rd., and Perez Velazquez, J. L. (2005). Enhanced synchrony in epileptiform activity? Local versus distant phase synchronization in generalized seizures. *J. Neurosci.* 25, 8077–8084.

Glass, L., and Mackey, M. C. (1988). *From Clocks to Chaos: the Rhythms of Life*. Princeton, NJ: Princeton University Press, 248.

Gluckman, B. J., Neel, E. J., Netoff, T. I., Ditto, W. L., Spano, M. L., and Schiff, S. J. (1996). Electric field suppression of epileptiform activity in hippocampal slices. *J. Neurophysiol.* 76, 4202–4205.

Good, L. B., Sabesan, S., Marsh, S. T., Tsakalis, K., Treiman, D., and Iasemidis, L. (2009). Control of synchronization of brain dynamics leads to control of epileptic seizures in rodents. *Int. J. Neural Syst.* 19, 173–196.

Gutkin, B. S., Ermentrout, G. B., and Reyes, A. D. (2005). Phase-response curves give the responses of neurons to transient inputs. *J. Neurophysiol.* 94, 1623–1635.

Ibarz, J. M., Foffani, G., Cid, E., Inostroza, M., and Menendez de la Prida, L. (2010). Emergent dynamics of fast ripples in the epileptic hippocampus. *J. Neurosci.* 30, 16249–16261.

Izhikevich, E. M. (2007). *Dynamical Systems in Neuroscience: the Geometry of Excitability and Bursting*. Cambridge, MA: MIT Press, 441.

Kaplan, D. T., Clay, J. R., Manning, T., Glass, L., Guevara, M. R., and Shrier, A. (1996). Subthreshold dynamics in periodically stimulated squid giant axons. *Phys. Rev. Lett.* 76, 4074–4077.

Kuramoto, Y. (1984). *Chemical Oscillations, Waves, and Turbulence*. Berlin; New York: Springer-Verlag, 156.

Lehnertz, K., and Elger, C. E. (1995). Spatio-temporal dynamics of the primary epileptogenic area in temporal lobe epilepsy characterized by neuronal complexity loss. *Electroencephalogr. Clin. Neurophysiol.* 95, 108–117.

Le Van Quyen, M., Soss, J., Navarro, V., Robertson, R., Chavez, M., Baulac, M., et al. (2005). Preictal state identification by synchronization changes in long-term intracranial EEG recordings. *Clin. Neurophysiol.* 116, 559–568.

Loddenkemper, T., Pan, A., Neme, S., Baker, K. B., Rezai, A. R., Dinner, D. S., et al. (2001). Deep brain stimulation in epilepsy. *J. Clin. Neurophysiol.* 18, 514–532.

Manor, Y., and Nadim, F. (2001). Synaptic depression mediates bistability in neuronal networks with recurrent inhibitory connectivity. *J. Neurosci.* 21, 9460–9470.

Milton, J., and Jung, P. (eds.). (2003). *Epilepsy as a Dynamic Disease*. New York, NY: Springer-Verlag, 417.

Mirski, M. A., Rossell, L. A., Terry, J. B., and Fisher, R. S. (1997). Anticonvulsant effect of anterior thalamic high frequency electrical stimulation in the rat. *Epilepsy Res.* 28, 89–100.

Mormann, F., Kreuz, T., Andrzejak, R. G., David, P., Lehnertz, K., and Elger, C. E. (2003). Epileptic seizures are preceded by a decrease in synchronization. *Epilepsy Res.* 53, 173–185.

Morrell, M. (2006). Brain stimulation for epilepsy: can scheduled or responsive neurostimulation stop seizures? *Curr. Opin. Neurol.* 19, 164–168.

Morrell, M. J., and On behalf of the RNS System in Epilepsy Study Group. (2011). Responsive cortical stimulation for the treatment of medically intractable partial epilepsy. *Neurology* 77, 1295–1304.

Morris, C., and Lecar, H. (1981). Voltage oscillations in the barnacle giant muscle fiber. *Biophys. J.* 35, 193–213.

Nelson, T. S., Suhr, C. L., Freestone, D. R., Lai, A., Halliday, A. J., McLean, K. J., et al. (2011). Closed-loop seizure control with very high frequency electrical stimulation at seizure onset in the GAERS model of absence epilepsy. *Int. J. Neural Syst.* 21, 163–173.

Netoff, T. I., Banks, M. I., Dorval, A. D., Acker, C. D., Haas, J. S., Kopell, N., et al. (2005). Synchronization in hybrid neuronal networks of the hippocampal formation. *J. Neurophysiol.* 93, 1197–1208.

Netoff, T. I., and Schiff, S. J. (2002). Decreased neuronal synchronization during experimental seizures. *J. Neurosci.* 22, 7297–7307.

Perez Velazquez, J. L., Garcia Dominguez, L., and Wennberg, R. (2007). Complex phase synchronization in epileptic seizures: evidence for a devil's staircase. *Phys. Rev. E Stat. Nonlin. Soft Matter Phys.* E75:011922. doi: 10.1103/PhysRevE.75.011922

Prusseit, J., and Lehnertz, K. (2008). Measuring interdependences in dissipative dynamical systems with estimated Fokker-Planck coefficients. *Phys. Rev.* E77, 041914-1–041914-10.

Quian Quiroga, R., Blanco, S., Rosso, O. A., Garcia, H., and Rabinowicz, A. (1997). Searching for hidden information with Gabor Transform in generalized tonic-clonic seizures. *Electroencephalogr. Clin. Neurophysiol.* 103, 434–439.

Rajdev, P., Ward, M., and Irazoqui, P. (2011). Effect of stimulus parameters in the treatment of seizures by electrical stimulation in the kainate animal model. *Int. J. Neural Syst.* 21, 151–162.

Rinzel, J. (1985). Excitation dynamics: insights from simplified membrane models. *Fed. Proc.* 44, 2944–2946.

Schevon, C. A., Cappell, J., Emerson, R., Isler, J., Grieve, P., Goodman, R., et al. (2007). Cortical abnormalities in epilepsy revealed by local EEG synchrony. *Neuroimage* 35, 140–148.

Schiff, S. J., Colella, D., Jacyna, G. M., Hughes, E., Creekmore, J. W., Marshall, A., et al. (2000). Brain chirps: spectrographic signatures of epileptic seizures. *Clin. Neurophysiol.* 111, 953–958.

Schindler, K., Elger, C. E., and Lehnertz, K. (2007a). Increasing synchronization may promote seizure termination: evidence from status epilepticus. *Clin. Neurophysiol.* 118, 1955–1968.

Schindler, K., Leung, H., Elger, C. E., and Lehnertz, K. (2007b). Assessing seizure dynamics by analysing the correlation structure of multichannel intracranial EEG. *Brain* 130, 65–77.

Song, S., Sjostrom, P. J., Reigl, M., Nelson, S., and Chklovskii, D. B. (2005). Highly nonrandom features of synaptic connectivity in local cortical circuits. *PLoS Biol.* 3:e68. doi: 10.1371/journal.pbio.0030068

Strogatz, S. H. (2000). From Kuramoto to Crawford: exploring the onset of synchronization in populations of coupled oscillators. *Phys. D* 143, 1.

Towle, V. L., Carder, R. K., Khorasani, L., and Lindberg, D. (1999). Electrocorticographic coherence patterns. *J. Clin. Neurophysiol.* 16, 528–547.

Varela, J. A., Sen, K., Gibson, J., Fost, J., Abbott, L. F., and Nelson, S. B. (1997). A quantitative description of short-term plasticity at excitatory synapses in layer 2/3 of rat primary visual cortex. *J. Neurosci.* 17, 7926–7940.

Vonck, K., Boon, P., Goossens, L., Dedeurwaerdere, S., Claeys, P., Gossiaux, F., et al. (2003). Neurostimulation for refractory epilepsy. *Acta Neurol. Belg.* 103, 213–217.

Ward, A. A. Jr. (1961). The epileptic neurone. *Epilepsia* 2, 70–80.

Wilson, C. J., Beverlin, B. 2nd., and Netoff, T. (2011). Chaotic desynchronization as the therapeutic mechanism of deep brain stimulation. *Front. Syst. Neurosci.* 5:50. doi: 10.3389/fnsys.2011.00050

Worrell, G. A., Parish, L., Cranstoun, S. D., Jonas, R., Baltuch, G., and Litt, B. (2004). High-frequency oscillations and seizure generation in neocortical epilepsy. *Brain* 127, 1496–1506.

Wyckhuys, T., Boon, P., Raedt, R., Van Nieuwenhuyse, B., Vonck, K., and Wadman, W. (2010). Suppression of hippocampal epileptic seizures in the kainate rat by Poisson distributed stimulation. *Epilepsia* 51, 2297–2304.

Zaveri, H. P., Pincus, S. M., Goncharova, I. I., Novotny, E. J., Duckrow, R. B., Spencer, D. D., et al. (2009). A decrease in EEG energy accompanies anti-epileptic drug taper during intracranial monitoring. *Epilepsy Res.* 86, 153–162.

Zhao, L., Beverlin, B., 2nd, Netoff, T., and Nykamp, D. Q. (2011). Synchronization from second order network connectivity statistics. *Front. Comput. Neurosci.* 5:28. doi: 10.3389/fncom.2011.00028

Ziburkus, J., Cressman, J. R., Barreto, E., and Schiff, S. J. (2006). Interneuron and pyramidal cell interplay during *in vitro* seizure-like events. *J. Neurophysiol.* 95, 3948–3954.

10

A translational platform for prototyping closed-loop neuromodulation systems

Pedram Afshar*, Ankit Khambhati, Scott Stanslaski, David Carlson, Randy Jensen, Dave Linde, Siddharth Dani, Maciej Lazarewicz, Peng Cong, Jon Giftakis, Paul Stypulkowski and Tim Denison*

Medtronic Neuromodulation, Minneapolis, MN, USA

Edited by:
Steve M. Potter, Georgia Institute of Technology, USA

Reviewed by:
Thomas DeMarse, University of Florida, USA
Douglas J. Bakkum, Georgia Institute of Technology, USA

*Correspondence:
Pedram Afshar and Tim Denison, Medtronic Neuromodulation, 7000 Central Avenue North, Minneapolis, MN 55432, USA.
e-mail: timothy.denison@ medtronic.com;
pedram.afshar@medtronic.com

While modulating neural activity through stimulation is an effective treatment for neurological diseases such as Parkinson's disease and essential tremor, an opportunity for improving neuromodulation therapy remains in automatically adjusting therapy to continuously optimize patient outcomes. Practical issues associated with achieving this include the paucity of human data related to disease states, poorly validated estimators of patient state, and unknown dynamic mappings of optimal stimulation parameters based on estimated states. To overcome these challenges, we present an investigational platform including: an implanted sensing and stimulation device to collect data and run automated closed-loop algorithms; an external tool to prototype classifier and control-policy algorithms; and real-time telemetry to update the implanted device firmware and monitor its state. The prototyping system was demonstrated in a chronic large animal model studying hippocampal dynamics. We used the platform to find biomarkers of the observed states and transfer functions of different stimulation amplitudes. Data showed that moderate levels of stimulation suppress hippocampal beta activity, while high levels of stimulation produce seizure-like after-discharge activity. The biomarker and transfer function observations were mapped into classifier and control-policy algorithms, which were downloaded to the implanted device to continuously titrate stimulation amplitude for the desired network effect. The platform is designed to be a flexible prototyping tool and could be used to develop improved mechanistic models and automated closed-loop systems for a variety of neurological disorders.

Keywords: **automation, closed-loop, neuromodulation, prototyping, hippocampus, seizure**

INTRODUCTION

Neuromodulation devices for deep brain stimulation (DBS) deliver targeted electrical stimulation to treat symptoms of diseases such as Parkinson's disease, essential tremor, and dystonia. To ensure benefit, these therapies require not only accurate placement of the stimulating electrode within neural tissue, but also proper selection of stimulation parameters (e.g., amplitude, pulse width, and frequency). These parameters can be used to mitigate side effects including hemiballism, gait and speech disturbances, and dyskinesias (Limousin et al., 1996, 1998; Hamani et al., 2005; Yu and Neimat, 2008; Bronstein et al., 2011). While many patients benefit from DBS, the parameter selection process is largely heuristic, and reprogramming sessions may be weeks or months apart.

Effort has been applied for more than a decade to build automated systems (**Figure 1**) that use patient state to adjust stimulation parameters, thereby reducing the delay between stimulation updates by many orders of magnitude compared to human intervention. Realizing these systems requires development of sensors to measure patient data and algorithms to translate the data to the appropriate stimulation parameters (Priori et al., 2012). Complexity in the nervous system motivates partitioning the algorithm into two components: one that translates sensor data into estimates of state (i.e., a classifier algorithm) and another that translates the state estimate into a stimulation parameter update (i.e., a control-policy algorithm). In this work, state is left intentionally ambiguous because its meaning depends on the application: examples include seizure versus non-seizure; Parkinson's ON versus OFF; asleep versus awake; or others. Regardless of the application, dividing the algorithm provides the following benefits:

- Matches clinical workflow: clinical practice often separates a patient assessment ("classification"), which translates clinical data into a diagnosis, and a treatment plan ("control policy"), which translates a diagnosis into a therapy. Designing the system to match this separation enables physicians to more easily validate and improve algorithms according to their existing workflow.
- Partitions complexity: algorithms can involve significant computational load, which is difficult for implantable systems due to power constraints (Lee Kyong et al., 2012). Partitioning the algorithm should enable more modular testing and prototyping; this is particularly useful when algorithm components can be externalized to allow greater computational freedom than the implanted device can provide. Once vetted, algorithms with

the desired trade-offs between performance, latency, and power consumption can be committed to embedded firmware for untethered operation.

The "agent-environment" model from artificial intelligence research is one model for describing the relationship between the physician and the automated neuromodulation system in learning and implementing algorithms (**Figure 2**). The goal of the agent is to develop a performance element (i.e., algorithm) to model the relationship between environmental percepts and actions taken by effectors. The informed critic (i.e., clinician-researcher) updates the performance element by learning from its input data (sensors) and intermediate processing (knowledge)

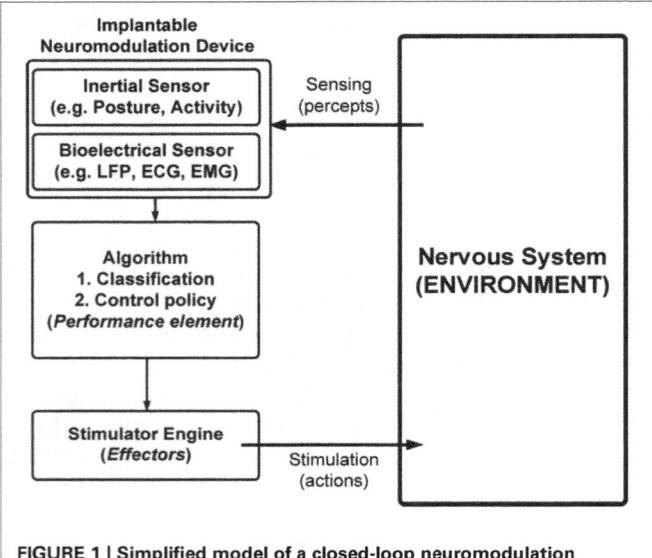

FIGURE 1 | Simplified model of a closed-loop neuromodulation system.

to develop new problems or hypotheses regarding the algorithm. Iterative testing allows the critic to simultaneously learn about the environment and develop the best performance element to modulate it.

The agent-environment model is suitable for the development of neuromodulation systems for several reasons. The model:

- Includes the physician-researcher's involvement to capture subject behavior to validate the algorithm.
- Describes the role of the performance element not only as a key element of the automated closed-loop.system, but also as the mechanism for the physician-researcher to learn about the nervous system.
- Captures the importance of developing better sensors and effectors to improve the ability to monitor and modulate the nervous system.
- Captures the iterative learning process needed to develop a first-principles understanding of the neurological diseases.
- Leaves the nature of the algorithm open, keeping free the choice of machine-learning techniques (e.g., support vector machine, Kalman filter) and data types (e.g., accelerometer, gyroscope, biopotential).

The translation of automated closed-loop systems has been helped by the development of more sophisticated neural sensors as well as improved understanding of the neural signals that underlie disease. Neurochip-2 (Zanos et al., 2011) and Hermes-D (Miranda et al., 2010) are two examples of technology to measure from the network. Neurochip-2 provides three channels of sensing and stimulation and allows for fast response loop closure to explore concepts like neural plasticity. The Hermes-D system allows for wireless, larger scale measurement (32 channels) of activity, but lacks stimulation capability. Both systems have the advantage of higher bandwidth, which allows for measurement of single unit activity, but draw greater than 1000× more

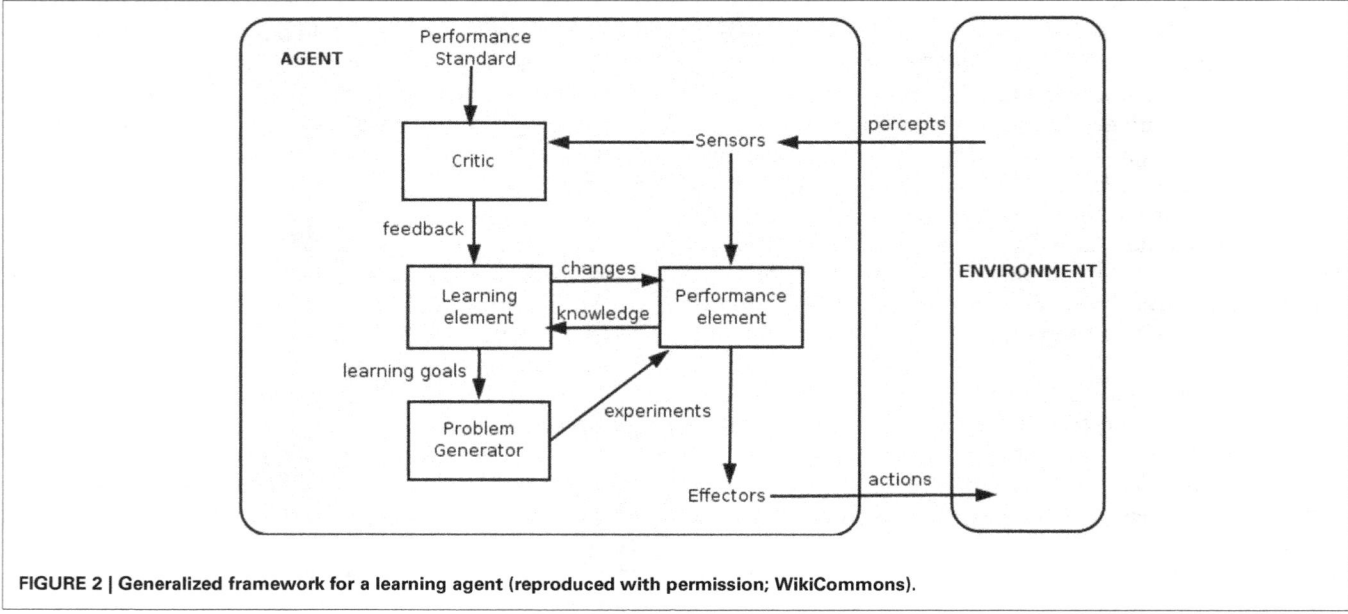

FIGURE 2 | Generalized framework for a learning agent (reproduced with permission; WikiCommons).

power for operation than a typical DBS implant, giving them longevity of at most a few days between recharges. Moreover, the limited biomarkers and control variables currently known for neurological diseases motivate the development of platform technologies to enable improved first-principles understanding, which may lead to more rapid clinical translation. A critical step in developing this understanding is the ability to provide simultaneous neural recording and therapeutic stimulation, which is lacking in many research tools today. This capability is needed to understand the system transfer function, which we define as the relationship between stimulation and network behavior.

The study of biopotential biomarkers has shown spectral power in local field potentials (LFP) to be a disease-relevant indicator in a variety of settings (Schnitzler and Gross, 2005; Uhlhaas and Singer, 2006). In particular, these signals are useful in studying networks of thalamo-cortical structures and their dynamic inter-relationships, where abnormal neural synchrony is believed to be a hallmark of disease states (Llinas and Ribary, 2001; Siegel et al., 2012). Furthermore, quantified differences in neural synchrony, which can be measured by calculating power $(uV/rtHz)^2$ in a particular frequency band (for example, "beta"), have been shown to correlate with symptom severity. For instance, power in the beta band (15–30 Hz) has been found to be related to cardinal Parkinson's symptoms such as bradykinesia and rigidity (Hammond et al., 2007; Eusebio and Brown, 2009; Kühn et al., 2009; Priori et al., 2012). Characteristic changes in power at the theta tremor frequency (Hellwig et al., 2001) and coherent activity in the 6–15 Hz frequency band (Raethjen et al.,

2002) have also been found in essential tremor. Synchronization in even lower frequencies (alpha and theta range) has been found in dystonia (Liu et al., 2002; Silberstein et al., 2003; Kühn et al., 2009; Sharott et al., 2008; Singh et al., 2011). Correlations between power in frequency bands as low as alpha (Zumsteg et al., 2006) and as high as 500 Hz (Blanco et al., 2011) have been reported in patients with epilepsy. Equally importantly, it has been shown that the effect of therapy can be correlated with LFP signals both in DBS (Eusebio et al., 2012; Priori et al., 2012) and levodopa therapy (Rossi et al., 2008). In aggregate, these studies suggest that LFP is a promising sensor input for automated systems treating a variety of neurological disorders.

In this work, we describe a platform for investigating these neural signals toward the development of an automated, closed-loop bioelectronic neuromodulation system. The platform comprises tools and a process flow to map the general learning agent to neuromodulation research and enables rapid prototyping of these tools in an implantable neuromodulation device. We use a preclinical, *in vivo* nervous system model to demonstrate the functional components of the system: collection of neural data, identification of relevant features (i.e., biomarkers), development of the algorithm, and consolidation of the algorithm into an implanted device.

SYSTEM STRATEGY AND INFRASTRUCTURE

To implement this system we mapped the general learning agent functional blocks into the neuromodulation domain (**Figure 3**). The interface is bi-directional, extracting measures of neural state

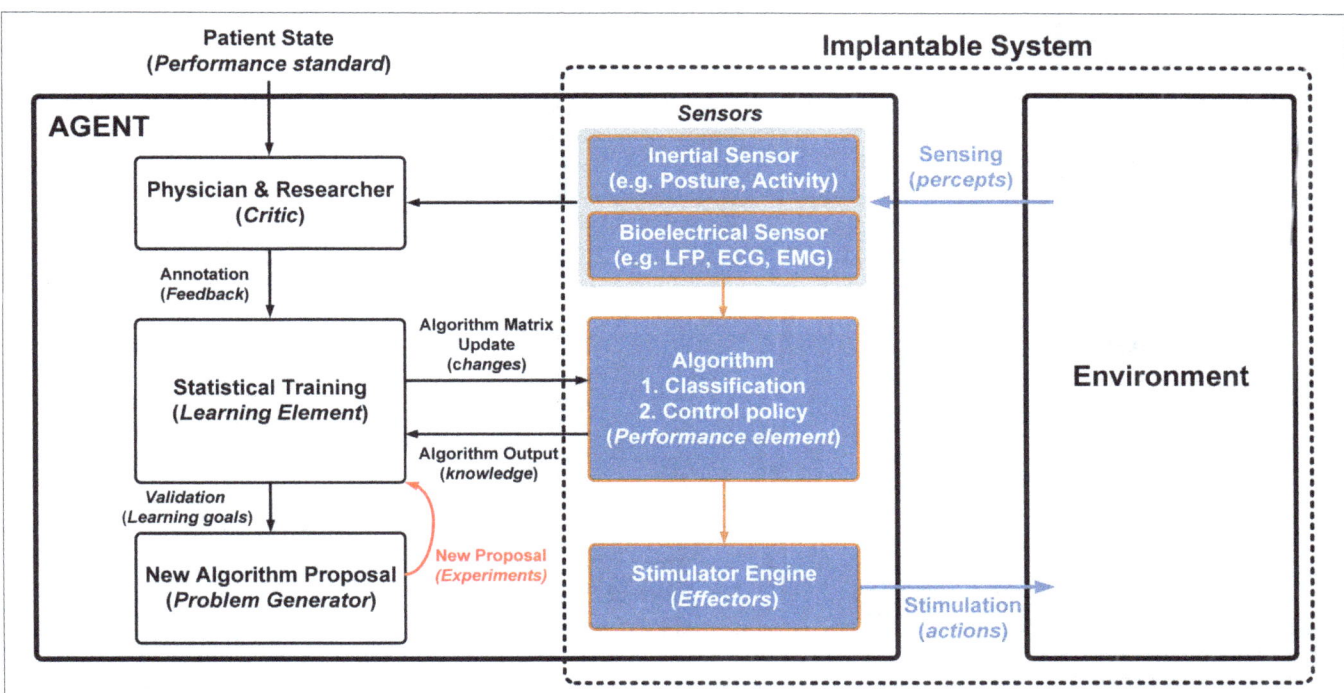

FIGURE 3 | Mapping a generalized learning model to the neuromodulation system; the components that are implanted are highlighted by the dashed box. The shaded boxes represent the implanted components that interface with the environment. Algorithm prototyping occurs in the agent where the physician and researcher can generate new algorithms based on historical data and algorithm performance.

through percepts and actuating states in the nervous system through effectors. Percepts are received through a combination of sensors that include bioelectrical sensing from electrodes (e.g., ECG, EMG, and LFP) and inertial sensing, (e.g., posture and activity). The effector pathway is defined by electrical stimulation pulse patterns, with parameters similar to approved therapy devices.

The challenge in designing the performance element is that characteristics of both percepts and effectors are still evolving. The algorithm addresses this ambiguity through use of classifier portion that maps sensed signals to estimates of state and a control-policy portion that maps state estimates into a desired stimulation.

We have implemented the learning system using an implantable research device and external application tool coupled with real-time telemetry; the system is illustrated in **Figure 4**. We call this partition of external learning elements that can be transferred to the implantable device performance element a "hybrid" design approach. The goal is to construct a complete platform (combining hardware, software, and firmware) for the learning procedure. The learning protocol includes four main steps from initial exploration to a chronic

prototype for validation: collection of sensed neural data; design of the performance element's classifiers based on biomarkers; development of the performance element control policy based on measured neural system identification; and embedding of the performance element into the device for chronic validation.

To do this, we designed a system with the following features:

o Implantable device for delivering stimulation including the following components:

- Bioelectric sensing with 4 bipolar sensing channels with 150 nV/rtHz noise floor without stimulation and 300 nV/rtHz noise floor with stimulation (nb: Stanslaski et al., 2012 describes constraints of sensing during stimulation).
- Inertial sensing with a custom three-axis accelerometer with a 10 mg-rms resolution floor drawing under 600 nW/axis (Denison et al., 2007).
- Stimulation using a commercially available neural simulator system with accepted therapy.
- Embedded algorithm with independently modifiable classifier and control-policy algorithms.

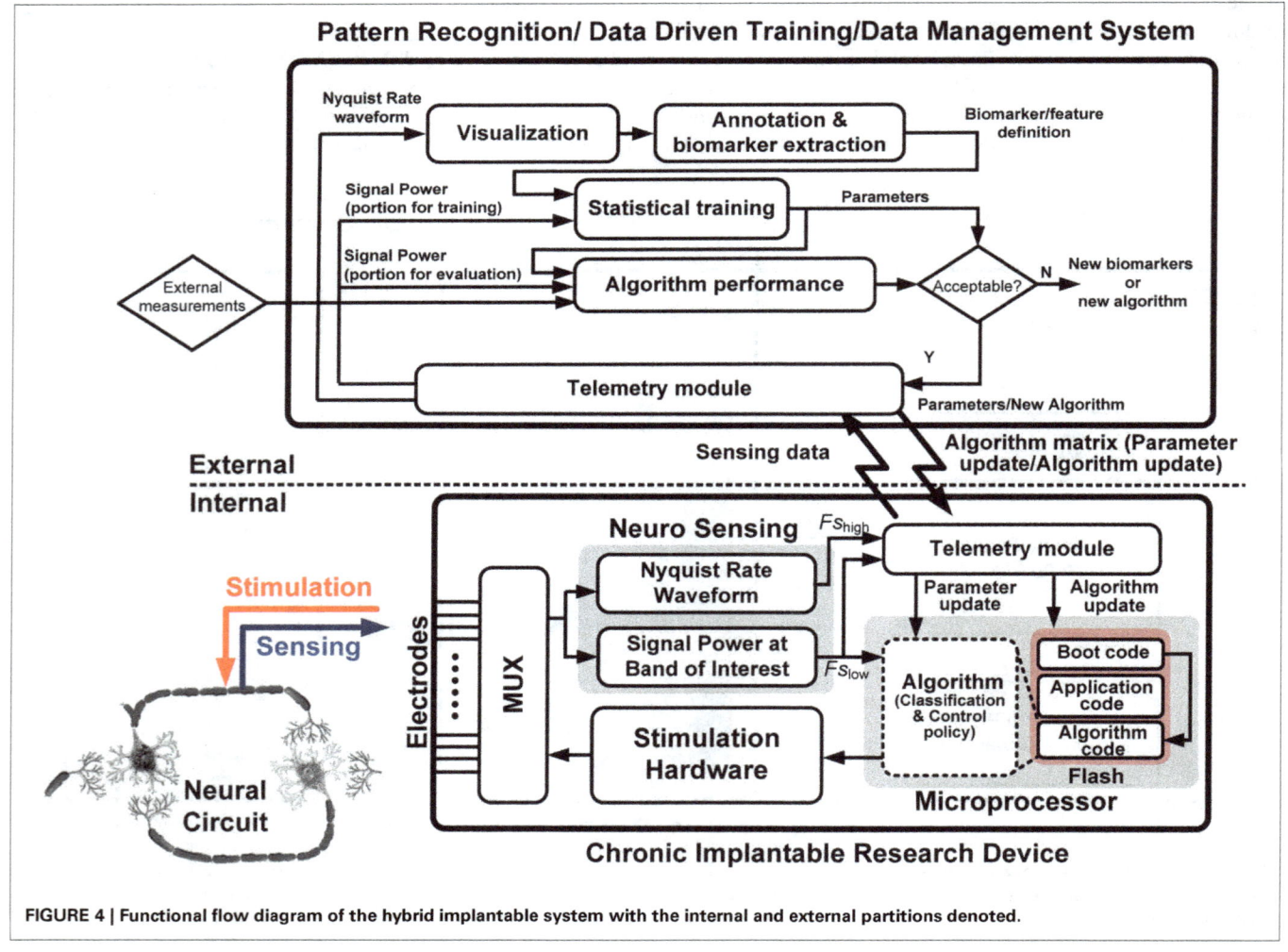

FIGURE 4 | Functional flow diagram of the hybrid implantable system with the internal and external partitions denoted.

○ External tool for learning and prototyping classifiers to translate sensor data to state estimates.

- Save, parse, and annotate data collected from implantable device.
- Implement, prototype, and compare machine learning algorithms.
- Develop and test classifiers for the implanted system.

○ External tool for learning and prototyping control policies to translate state to stimulation updates.

- Stream data directly from the implantable device to an external processor with latency less than 1 s (0.5 s typical).
- Send stimulation parameter updates to the implantable device with latency from command to stimulation at the electrode in less than 1 s (0.5 s typical).
- Monitor state transitions in classifier and control-policy algorithms.

○ Telemetry system for retrieving data, modifying classifiers, prototyping control policies, and rewriting device firmware.

The key for this system is to integrate all necessary elements to provide a complete platform for an accelerated learning procedure amenable to rapid-prototyping and clinical translation. The details of these steps follow below.

COLLECTION OF SENSED NEURAL DATA

The design of the performance element starts with data collection. While there are many methods to sense biopotential data, fully implanted devices offer the advantage of higher signal fidelity than fully external devices (e.g., EEG), reduced infection risk, and improved chronic, ambulatory data collection capability compared with implanted devices with external components (e.g., externalizing leads during DBS surgery or the Hermes-D system). We have previously described the design and implementation of our fully implanted, bi-directional neural interface (Rouse et al., 2011). In brief, the device contains both sensing and stimulation components. The stimulation feature embodies the capability of a commercial DBS system. Biopotential sensing is enabled with a custom-integrated interface chip that allows for measurements of LFP generated from EMG, ECoG, LFP, and ECG (Avestruz et al., 2008), with noise floor of 150 nV/rtHz without stimulation and 300 nV/rtHz with stimulation (nb: Stanslaski et al., 2012, gives details and constraints of sensing during stimulation). The custom integrated circuit (IC) provides data analysis for up to four bipolar channels, which are selectable between Nyquist-rate waveforms (i.e., time channels) and spectral power at specific frequency bands of interest (i.e., power channels). The time channels provide complete spectral information; however, they incur the penalty of much higher power consumption. Power channels, on the other hand, extract a power envelope that is down-sampled to 5 Hz prior to digital signal processing. The reduction of signal dynamic range prior to digitization is a common technique for saving energy in micropower systems. The design model is to use the time channels for neural system identification, including identifying biomarkers and to transfer to the power channels to optimize efficiency chronically. The inertial element uses a micromachined three-axis accelerometer that transduces capacitive fluctuations to a voltage output. The resolution floor of the inertial element is 10 mg rms, in a 20-Hz band of detection. The sensor draws a total of 2 uW during normal operation, which minimizes longevity impact in the device (Denison et al., 2007). The sensor inputs from bioelectric and inertial sensors can be fused together in the algorithm, if desired.

Data acquisition also provides an opportunity for optimizing efficiency. While the device supports streaming telemetry for time and power channels, it is limited to environments in which the subject is close to a telemetry system, and desired data sampling frequency is low. Event triggered recordings allow for timed segments of high sampling frequency data when the subject is ambulatory. Triggers include user programmable, timer-driven intervals; embedded classifiers; external subject button presses; or combinations thereof. For a typical event structure like motion or seizure onsets, an 8-s loop recording could be applied for two recording channels. With a typical data rate of 422 Hz, approximately 200 recordings can be stored by the embedded SRAM until it needs to be downloaded and cleared. To organize and manage the resulting number of files gathered over a longitudinal study, a file system was developed to provide data structure to researchers. Information such as event time stamps, parameter settings, and event type is embedded in the data during recording and automatically extracted as a companion file to the data. The combination of the custom integrated hardware, signal processing strategy, and data gathering infrastructure facilitates the design of the performance element.

LEARNING → PERFORMANCE ELEMENT I: CLASSIFICATION

The first subsystem of the performance element is a classifier to estimate the state of the nervous system from the sensed LFP biopotentials. Following the hybrid approach of our platform, we implement the classifier as both an internal function of the implantable device and as an external tool for learning and problem generation; the functional flow of the tool is illustrated in **Figure 5**. The external tool allows users to visualize time domain and spectral data, graphically annotate biomarkers of interest, and automatically generate classifiers using supervised machine-learning algorithms. In addition, classifier sensitivity and specificity can be adjusted manually to obtain the desired performance. The resulting classifiers can be stored and compared using automatically computed detection statistics. Beyond data manipulation, the key value of the tool is its relationship with the implanted device; the tool:

1. Serves as a data repository for grouping and sorting data files from different recording sessions.
2. Parses data collected from the implanted device, automatically accounting for differences in formatting and recording settings.
3. Creates algorithms that can be uploaded directly into the implantable device.

The default on-board classifier algorithm is a linear-discriminant using a modified Fischer-discriminant approach; it is a linear decision boundary in a user-selectable feature space that identifies

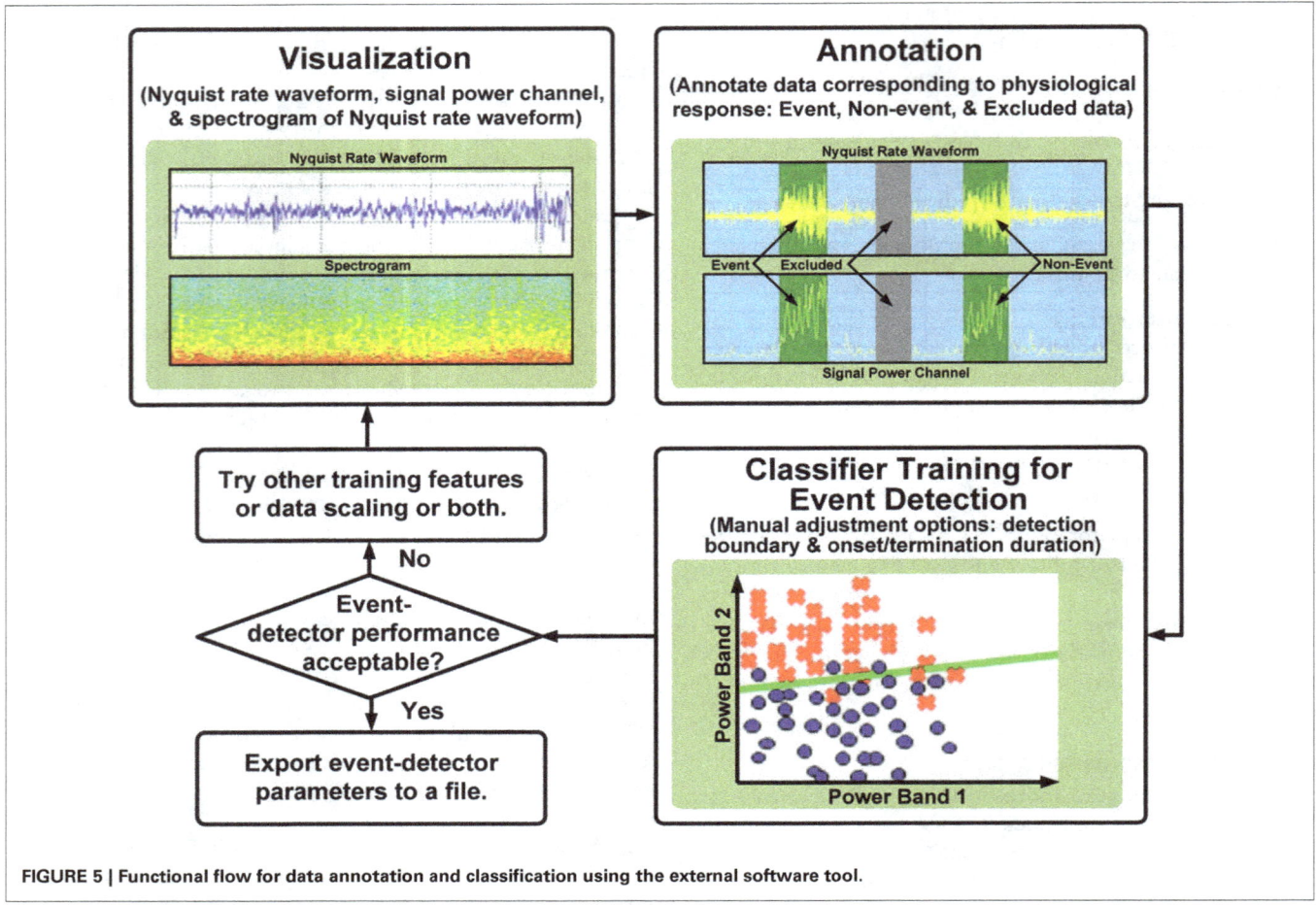

FIGURE 5 | Functional flow for data annotation and classification using the external software tool.

an event signal sample from other samples. The algorithm was designed using reduced set methods as described in (Shoeb et al., 2009). The use of the multi-dimensional linear boundary was found to optimize trade-offs in power consumption, latency, sensitivity, and specificity. Recent work by Lee describes a similar trade-off calculation and supports our design choices (Lee Kyong et al., 2012). The on-board algorithm can be used for detecting events, which are time-stamped and used to trigger recordings while the subject is ambulatory, thereby reducing current drain nearly 100-fold and reducing classification latency 5-fold, from ~1 s to ~200 ms. If the biomarker's characteristics warrant a more complex classifier or shorter latency, the algorithm can be updated, trading off power consumption.

LEARNING → PERFORMANCE ELEMENT II: CONTROL POLICY
The second algorithm subsystem is the control policy that maps the state estimate into an optimal stimulation sequence. Like the classifier algorithm, we implemented the control-policy algorithm both internal to the device and as an external system for learning and problem generation. Non-linearities in network dynamics heighten the need to sample many input–output pairs for system identification. This can be accomplished in two ways:

First, the external tool may be used to sweep any stimulation parameter (e.g., amplitude or frequency) while the implantable

device senses and saves biopotential data to the internal memory. Once retrieved from the device, system identification is performed by measuring the relationship between the stimulation parameters and biopotentials.

Second, the control policy may be adjusted in real-time on a researcher's device using an external device to wirelessly transfer data: sensed data is passed to the researcher's device and control-policy output is passed to the implantable device. This capability enables prototyping algorithms including the use of tapped-delay lines and time synchronizing with other sensors and hardware, and deriving a variety of signal features (e.g., phase amplitude coupling). The external device ensures data integrity in both directions through cyclic-redundancy checks and ensures patient safety by returning the device to safe, pre-programmed stimulation state should the researcher's control policy behave unexpectedly. Additional safety is ensured by allowing the control policy to select only among stimulation parameter boundaries that have been predetermined by the researcher.

For the platform design, particular attention was paid to the latency in the telemetry links, which is a key factor to effectively study the dynamics. In the first generation of development, we required that total latency through the channel be constrained to 1 s or less, and typically under 0.5 s. This degree of latency is suitable for many closed-loop algorithms that operate on timescales of seconds, hours, or days. The inherent latency of the links was dominated by two factors: the first is the data packet format and error correction handshakes using the 175 kHz ISM band, and the second is the internal packet transfer within the bioelectronic device, which, for safety reasons, are secondary interrupt priorities compared to the therapeutic stimulation. Although the latency can be much improved by running in the device, it limits flexibility during the initial learning phase. Therefore, for most cases, the new stimulation parameters are generated externally, where algorithms can be made arbitrarily complex and rapidly evaluated to see if they capture the desired behavior of the neural system. It is highly desirable to validate the behavior prior to committing to verification of embedded firmware due to regulatory constraints and requirements. For example, the platform can implement arbitrary control paradigms such as simple bang–bang controllers (modeled from early cardiac defibrillators) or more sophisticated proportional-integral-derivative and linear-quadratic-Gaussian controllers for achieving the optimal path to the desired state maintenance.

COMMITTING THE PERFORMANCE ELEMENT TO THE EMBEDDED DEVICE FOR VALIDATION

After learning and prototyping the classifier and control policy, the algorithm can be validated by embedding onto the implantable device firmware using telemetry. The firmware uses a dedicated boot loader that allows for a new series of code to be flashed to non-volatile memory inside the device in a few minutes. The firmware in the device is partitioned such that the classifier and control policy can be updated independently of the therapy code, thereby keeping the interaction to that necessary for real-time classification and closed-loop operation. To assist in validation, the firmware is capable of streaming out the classifier and control-policy states in addition to sensed signals in real-time, so that the user has visibility into the algorithm operation. For chronic operation, the state transition information is included in the data log for validation.

METHODS: DEMONSTRATION OF THE LEARNING AGENT ARCHITECTURE

As demonstration of the capabilities of our method and tools, we used the system to investigate, characterize and dynamically modulate the hippocampal dynamics within the circuit of Papez. The circuit of Papez is a thalamo-cortical circuit implicated in temporal lobe epilepsy and involves a reentrant loop involving the hippocampus (HC) and thalamus. The goal was to design from first principles a demonstrative "homeostatic" feedback loop, which would titrate stimulation dynamically to maintain network activity reflected in the field potentials; the intention was to show the capabilities of the technology, as opposed to demonstrate or claim a therapeutic algorithm *per se*. Design of the loop required that we address many issues of neuromodulation design: testing in an awake and freely moving subject, consideration for reliability and repeatability, and chronic implant stability and safety. Methods are detailed from the physiological preparation and technology points of view. The focus of this effort

was on exploring the bioelectrical properties of the network and building up a closed-loop system; the conceptual schema for developing inertial-based systems, classifiers and control policies was previously demonstrated with this architecture (Schultz et al., 2012).

PHYSIOLOGICAL METHODS

The *in vivo* device was chronically implanted in an ovine animal model conducted under an IACUC-approved protocol (Stypulkowski et al., 2011) and is summarized here. Following anesthesia, 1.5T MRIs were collected and transferred to a surgical planning station. Trajectories for a unilateral anterior nucleus (AN) DBS lead (Medtronic model 3389) and unilateral HC lead (Medtronic model 3387) were planned, and leads implanted using a frameless stereotactic system (NexFrame from Medtronic, Inc.). Once lead placement was confirmed based upon electrophysiological measures, Medtronic model 37083 extensions were connected to the DBS leads, tunneled to a post-scapular pocket, and connected to the prototype chronic implantable device. **Figure 6** illustrates the overall system placement and setup. Following closure of all incisions, anesthesia was discontinued, and the animal was transferred to surgical recovery.

All sensing and stimulation documented here were conducted in a single, awake sheep resting in a sling. In this particular work, all reported data were recorded from the HC with bipolar montage using contacts surrounding a monopolar stimulation contact (square, biphasic 300 μs pulse width on E1 with far-field return) to mitigate artifacts via common-mode rejection during stimulation (Stanslaski et al., 2012); functional network data from thalamic stimulation and sensing are not shown, but can be found in Stypulkowski et al. (2011). Neural data, stimulus trains and classifier detections were recorded and saved by PC software via wireless telemetry. Data were gathered over 15 months and represents over 18 months of operation with the device completely implanted.

As background to the analysis that follows, our physiological system relies on three qualitatively discernible states in the biological system:

1. *Resting*: defined as the state before any stimulation/neuromodulation has occurred.
2. *After-discharge (AD)*: defined as the state of high-energy LFP, similar to a seizure event, and by characteristic head movements of the subject. In our definition, the AD could occur at any time, independent of stimulation delivery.
3. *Suppression*: defined as the state with activity that is below the nominal resting state.

LEARNING FLOW METHODOLOGY

The system was deployed on the physiological preparation to develop an embedded closed-loop algorithm using our tools and processes. The technical methods applied the design flow outlined in the system architecture to the physiological preparation:

- **Collection of sensed neural data**
  Using the bi-directional telemetry link and embedded data gathering capabilities, we gathered baseline training data on

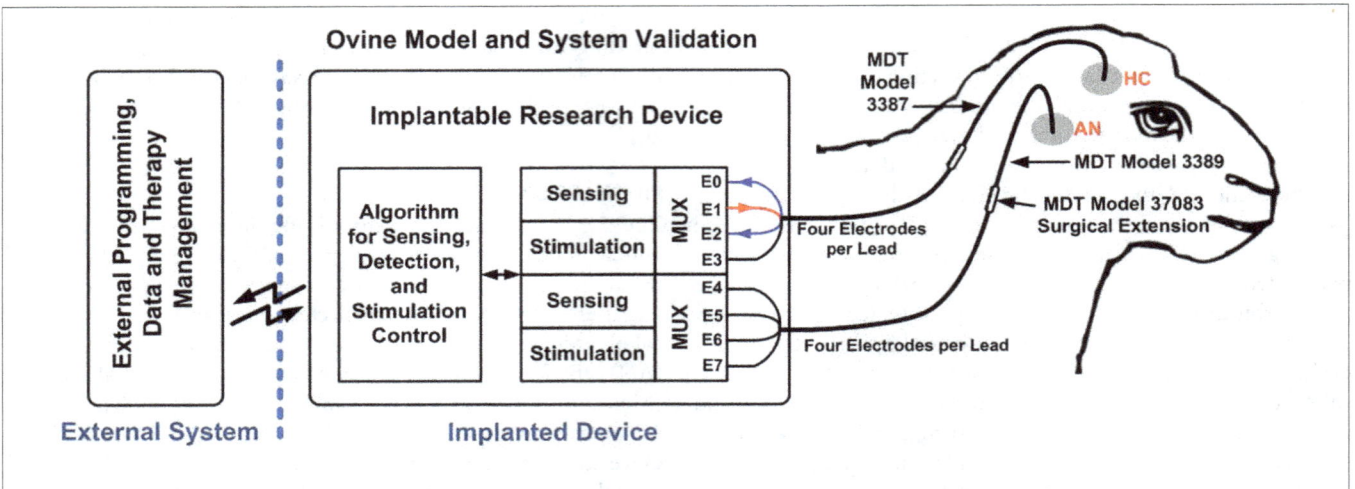

FIGURE 6 | Closed-loop neuromodulation system implanted in an ovine model. The figure is reproduced from Stanslaski et al. (2012) with permissions from the IEEE.

background network activity. We also used the stimulator and sensing functionality to identify useful biomarkers and understand system transfer functions required for closing the feedback loop.

- **Learning → Performance element I: design of classifier algorithm**

  The software algorithm tool was used to develop classifiers to support the after-discharge detection and verify suppression levels, which were validated using the real-time telemetry link.

- **Learning → Performance element II: development of the control policy**

  After development of the classifiers, the auto-detection of after-discharges and therapy titration was validated using off-line, real-time processing with the bi-directional telemetry link. Key parameters were verified to be acceptable for timing latency. An additional algorithm (data not shown) was tested to show the system could automatically search the parameter space to find acceptable suppression behavior.

- **Committing the performance element to the embedded device for validation**

  The final embedded algorithm implemented three sub-algorithms into a single-state machine: AD detection and mitigation; suppression detector; and parameter search. The code was then downloaded to the device through wireless telemetry, error checked for complete flash writes, and the implant was then activated with the closed-loop algorithm. All states were exercised in the algorithm routine to validate operation. State transitions were also recorded in the device data records for automated annotation of files, allowing for observational validation and algorithm refinement.

RESULTS

COLLECTION OF SENSED NEURAL DATA: IDENTIFICATION OF BIOMARKERS AND ALGORITHMS

We aimed to explore the states of the system to find relevant control-variable biomarkers *in vivo*. Analysis of the post-stimulation data showed decreasing mean beta band power

with increasing stimulation amplitude, suggesting suppression of activity, at least locally to the HC (**Figure 8**, right). To determine whether the network was truly suppressed, we performed a second series of transfer function experiments which measured the pre-stimulation baseline beta band power level followed with a high amplitude delivery (≥ 1.50 V) "probe pulse" capable of inducing AD. Because our experimental setup was not a seizure model, we used the post-stimulation AD duration as the desired output for assessment of network effect. Through spectral analysis of the data, we observed a potential control variable in the 20 ± 2.5 Hz band (approximately the beta band) that seemed correlated to the qualitatively observed states:

1. Resting state corresponded to relatively constant beta band power (approximately 2.7 uVrms).
2. AD state corresponded to increased beta band power (approximately 30 uVrms).
3. Suppression state corresponded to decreased beta band power (approximately 1.5 uVrms).

We characterized the biomarker over 15 months of data collection. For data shown, the units of spectral power in all data figures are (uV/rtHz)^2, with an arbitrary scale referred to as least significant bit (LSB). Results showed that AD generation was a probabilistic function of stimulation amplitude; stimulation below 1.5 V did not result in any AD, stimulation between 1.5 and 1.7 V resulted in occasional ADs, and stimulation above 1.7 V always resulted in ADs (data not shown). Furthermore, AD duration appeared to be a function of the beta band pre-stimulation state; the greater the pre-stimulation beta band power above the defined suppressed state, the greater the AD duration (**Figure 7**). Furthermore, these observations were robust: the suppressed state beta band power varied by less than 2LSB over the entire duration of the experiment. These results imply that spectral beta band power could be a control variable of interest when modulating network state.

To further understand the dynamic state of the system, we aimed to characterize the transfer function between our proposed biomarker—spectral beta band power—and stimulation patterns. To characterize the response of the biomarker to stimulation, we ran several titration sweeps. The recorded biomarker signals were captured at rest, during AD events, and during delivery of stimulation at several amplitudes (0.75–1.7 V) and frequencies (50, 120 Hz) in order to determine a reference value to discriminate both suppression and ADs. **Figure 8** shows the network response during stimulation (25 s, red) and between stimulation periods (25 s, blue). Importantly, the detection of AD induction required sensing neural activity in the presence of stimulation (Stanslaski et al., 2012) and would have been lost if channel blanking were employed.

The titration sweep for determining network-state response to stimulation is a critical step in designing the neural control algorithm. The data suggest that stimulation can have different effects on the network: while low and moderate stimulation amplitude appears to suppress the network excitability, high stimulation amplitude can induce an AD. Based on these results, we wanted to use our platform to implement a performance element to have two key features: (1) change stimulation amplitude to keep the network at the balance point of suppression and induction of AD and (2) due to the probabilistic nature of AD induction, allow for the detection of AD in real-time to abort stimulation and adjust the stimulation levels lower. To do this, we designed the performance element in two parts: states classification and control policy implementation.

LEARNING PERFORMANCE ELEMENT I: DESIGN OF CLASSIFIER ALGORITHMS

To automate a control loop, we used the observed qualitative correlations with a quantitative algorithm to detect the AD in real-time with a classifier constructed with the external classifier tool. To help mitigate stimulation artifact, we also used spectral band (approximately 70 Hz) to capture stimulation energy in the network without being confounded by observable changes in neural physiology. To achieve this, we applied a measure of stimulation artifact as a feature input within the algorithm to distinguish stimulation result and non-stimulation result as described in Stanslaski et al. (2012). We include the two power channel outputs in **Figure 9** for demonstration purposes, showing correlation between the amplitude of beta band power and AD in **Figures 9A,B**.

After annotation was supplied to the training data sets, we used the tool to develop a linear, binary classifier to detect AD with and without stimulation. The detection probability density plot, receiver operating characteristic (ROC) curves, and detection cross-validation result, which are directly generated

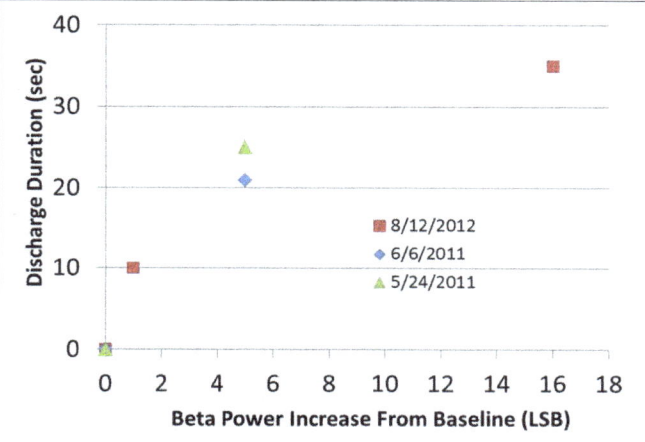

FIGURE 7 | After-discharge duration as a function of beta band power increase from suppressed baseline. High amplitude stimulation parameters were kept constant in a given session and were always determined to be sufficient to initiate an AD.

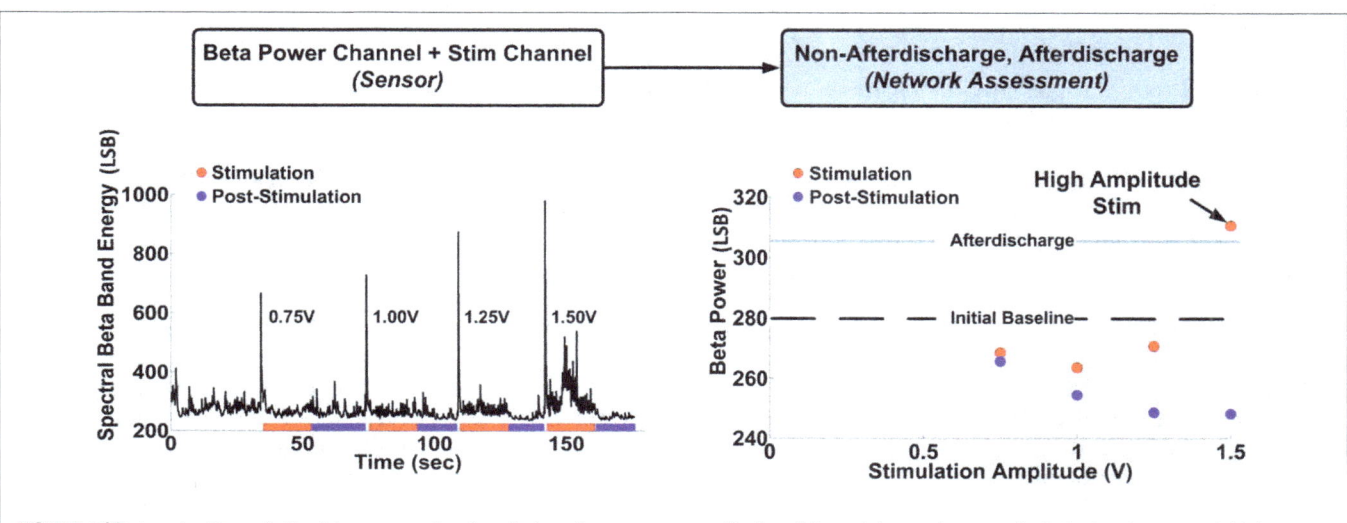

FIGURE 8 | Determination of the hippocampal network transfer function between stimulation and beta band spectral power. There is an initial reduction in beta band power at low stimulation

amplitudes, followed by an increase in beta band power at higher stimulation amplitudes, resulting in occasional AD during stimulation at 1.5 V.

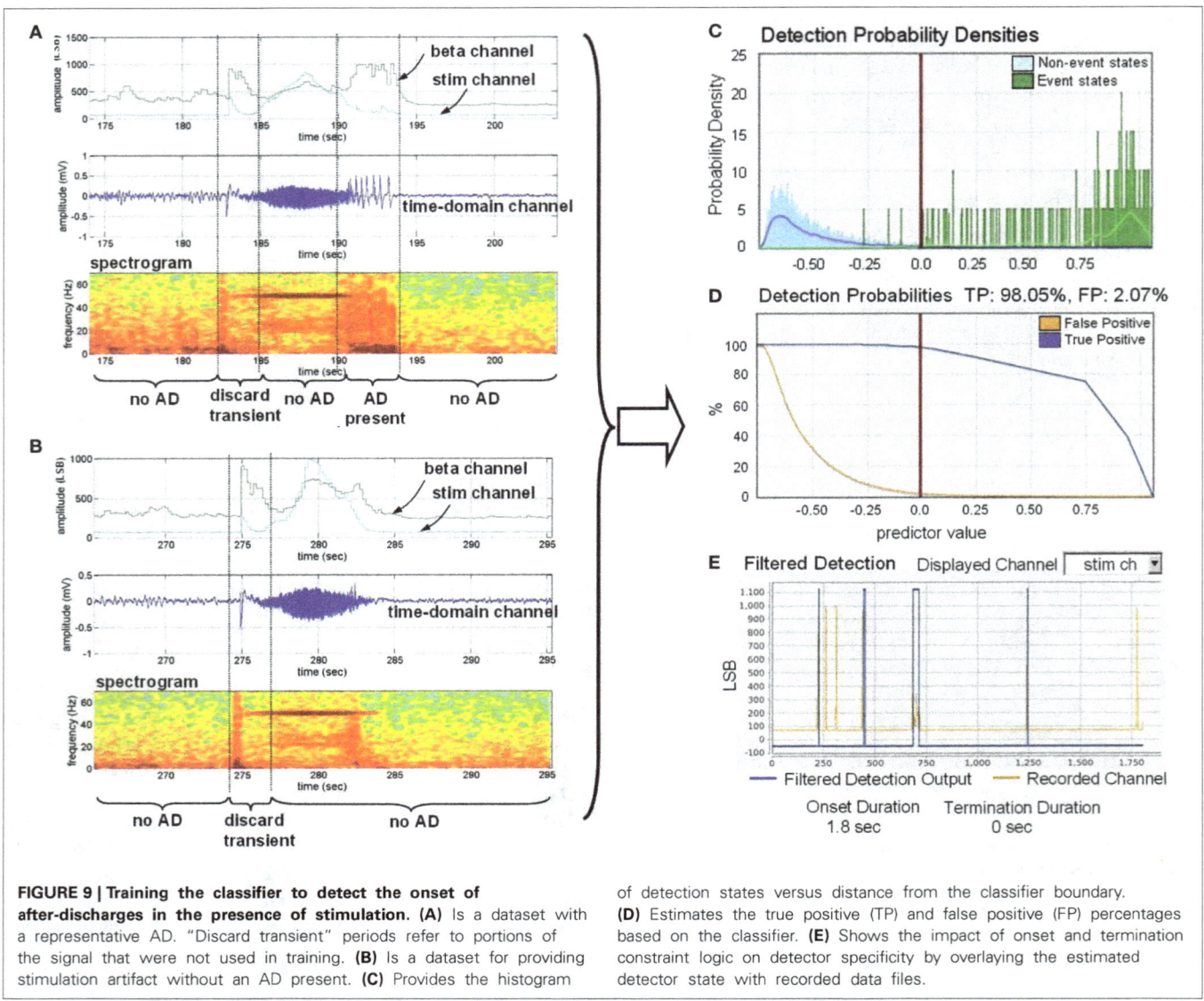

FIGURE 9 | Training the classifier to detect the onset of after-discharges in the presence of stimulation. (A) Is a dataset with a representative AD. "Discard transient" periods refer to portions of the signal that were not used in training. **(B)** Is a dataset for providing stimulation artifact without an AD present. **(C)** Provides the histogram of detection states versus distance from the classifier boundary. **(D)** Estimates the true positive (TP) and false positive (FP) percentages based on the classifier. **(E)** Shows the impact of onset and termination constraint logic on detector specificity by overlaying the estimated detector state with recorded data files.

by the software tool, are presented in **Figures 9C,D**, and **E**, respectively. The detection probability histogram (**C**) represents the magnitude of the state from the boundary, allowing for multiple dimensions of data to collapse to a single graph biomarker separation. The detection probabilities graph (**D**) provides an estimate of the true-positive and false-positive rates based on the derived classifier. The filtered detection summary graph (**E**) allows for the user to set onset and termination duration constraints (i.e., a minimum duration in a classified state before detection is determined) to help improve specificity at the expense of classifier latency. Graph (**E**) shows an overlay of the classification state over the data. We downloaded and embedded into the implanted device the classifier that optimized sensitivity, specificity, and latency trade-offs.

In addition, we used the tool to develop a separate classifier that could detect the presence of the suppression state based on the beta signal. This was also tested and similarly embedded in the implanted device. Thus, with these classifiers, the state of the neural system could be quantitatively classified on-line as suppression, AD, or resting.

LEARNING PERFORMANCE ELEMENT II: DEVELOPMENT OF THE CONTROL POLICY

With the classifier in place, we next determined the control policy. Given the unknown neural dynamic requirements and algorithm parameters, the control policy was first prototyped using the hybrid development partition to determine the stimulation amplitudes and changes that would be used for each state. **Figure 10** illustrates an example of this testing to show that stimulation can induce both the AD state and the suppression state. In this test, the controller logic uses two stimulation programs. In the cycle stim (CS) program, high amplitude stimulation (1.50 V) capable of inducing an AD is cycled on and off, while spectral power in critical bands and classifier state is continuously telemetered out of the device. If the classifier does not detect an AD, stimulation continues to cycle.

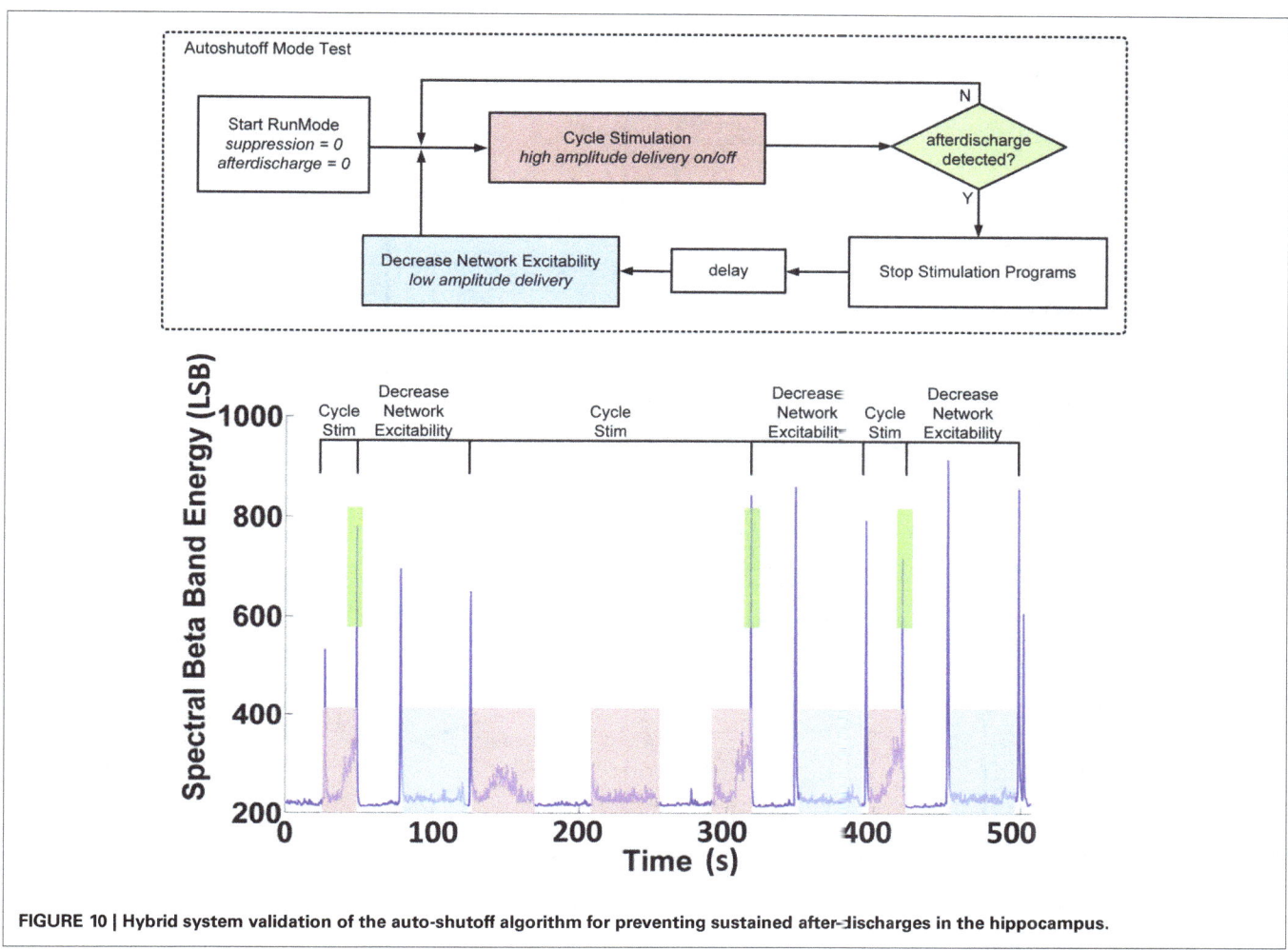

FIGURE 10 | Hybrid system validation of the auto-shutoff algorithm for preventing sustained after-discharges in the hippocampus.

When the AD state is detected, stimulation is stopped and an alternate setting is applied. The decreased network excitability (DNE) program delivers a lower stimulation level (1.25 V) after a programmed delay for one cycle, then returns to the CS program.

Figure 10 (bottom) shows typical results achieved with the hybrid algorithm. We ensured no false-positive detections occurred in both open-loop and closed-loop cases by examining the time-domain data. Our results demonstrate that open-loop stimulation leads to sustained ADs *post-stimulation* roughly 50% of the time when the cycle stimulation is applied without the algorithm enabled, whereas with the algorithm enabled, the sustained AD probability drops to 0% [$N = 12$, three monitor sessions, 15 months].

COMMITTING THE PERFORMANCE ELEMENT TO THE EMBEDDED DEVICE FOR VALIDATION

As a final prototyping phase, we desired a system capable of embedded operation to enable chronic, ambulatory data collection for long-term validation as well as improved response latency compared to subjects or other observers (e.g., researches, caregivers).

Based on findings with the hybrid system, the device was enabled to run a multi-branch algorithm for hippocampal network dynamics. The algorithms developed for the embedded detector were merged into a common state machine. As shown in **Figure 11**, this included the three critical loops for the algorithm corresponding to the states of the system, all of which share a common *stimulation sequence* forward loop. The beta band power threshold for determining the state classification was determined using the classifier. In addition, we prescribed an increment of 0.05 V and decrement of 0.1 V for stimulation controllers—i.e., slow attack, fast recovery for attempting to maximize safe searches of the parameter space.

- *Suppression loop*—detects suppression after stimulation and maintains defined suppression in the HC based on network activity within a broad beta band (10–30 Hz); the detector gates when stimulation pulses would occur based on measured spectral power.
- *After-discharge loop*—detects after-discharge and aborts stimulation, decrements stimulation amplitude, and sets a new "ceiling" on the stimulation level for future excitation patterns to avoid future AD events.

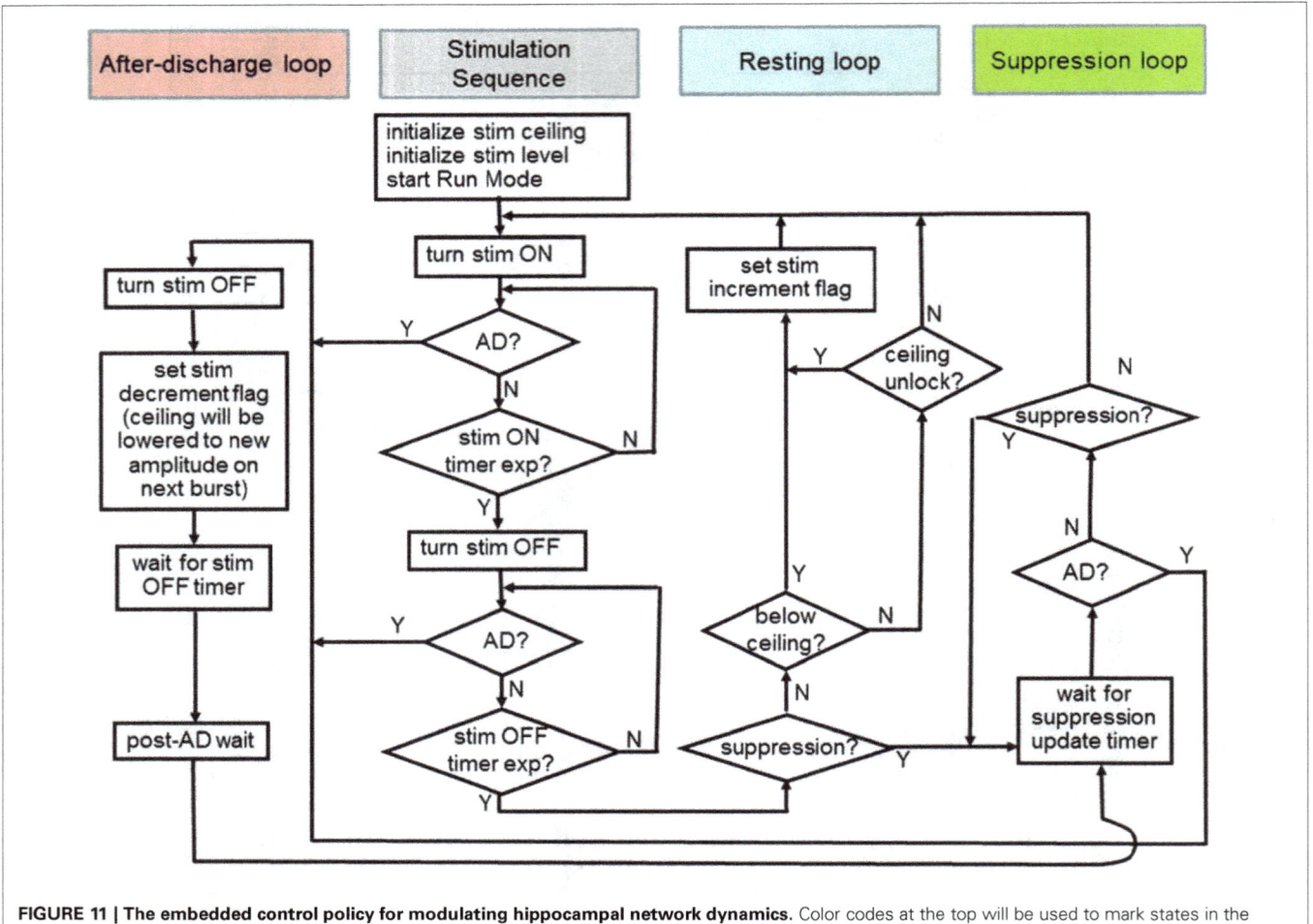

FIGURE 11 | The embedded control policy for modulating hippocampal network dynamics. Color codes at the top will be used to mark states in the resulting data summary.

- *Resting loop*—detects resting state and increments stimulation amplitude to verify the ceiling is still valid; this loop is activated when suppression is no longer being achieved with the suppression loop to counteract slowly changing behavior such as circadian patterns, medication dosing, etc.

Note: Additional parameters such as initialization variables and counters are also programmable through telemetry and could be refined as needed.

The algorithm firmware was downloaded into the device and validated with cyclic-redundancy checking.

The embedded algorithm was then evaluated with on-line processing in the ovine model. **Figure 12** presents a typical outcome of the standalone implantable device with the algorithm embedded; we demonstrate all possible states of the of the control policy in this data sample. We start by stimulating at an amplitude known to generate AD, resulting in appropriate stimulation shut-off. Then, stimulation is ON with reduced stimulation amplitude (from 1.7 to 1.6 V). Stimulation at this level produces suppression for one cycle, leading to maintenance of this stimulation level for 1 cycle. On the next cycle, however, suppression is not detected, resulting in stimulation increase to 1.65 V and then

again to 1.7 V. At 480 s, the 1.7 V stimulation again leads to an AD. The stimulation is again turned off due to the AD detection and the stimulation level is returned to 1.6 V. This testing showed that the learning procedure could result in a fully embedded solution, from initial identification of biomarkers and transfer functions to a fully-embedded control policy operating *in vivo*.

Several practical points are also worth noting. First, the algorithm is power efficient, because it runs reliably with total current drain less than $20\,\mu W$ with the addition of sensing and algorithm control. This represents roughly 10% of the nominal therapy power used in movement disorder neuromodulation system. Second, the algorithm shows robustness because signal power channel baseline is stable over 15 months with variation within 2 LSB, which is more than 20 times smaller than the AD detection threshold. Finally, the control policy is restricted to a bounded set of stimulation parameters with programmable inter-locks, thereby helping to ensure tolerability and safety.

DISCUSSION

Automated closed-loop control systems may potentially improve neuromodulation therapies by reducing latency for therapy adjustments and personalizing therapies to improve patient

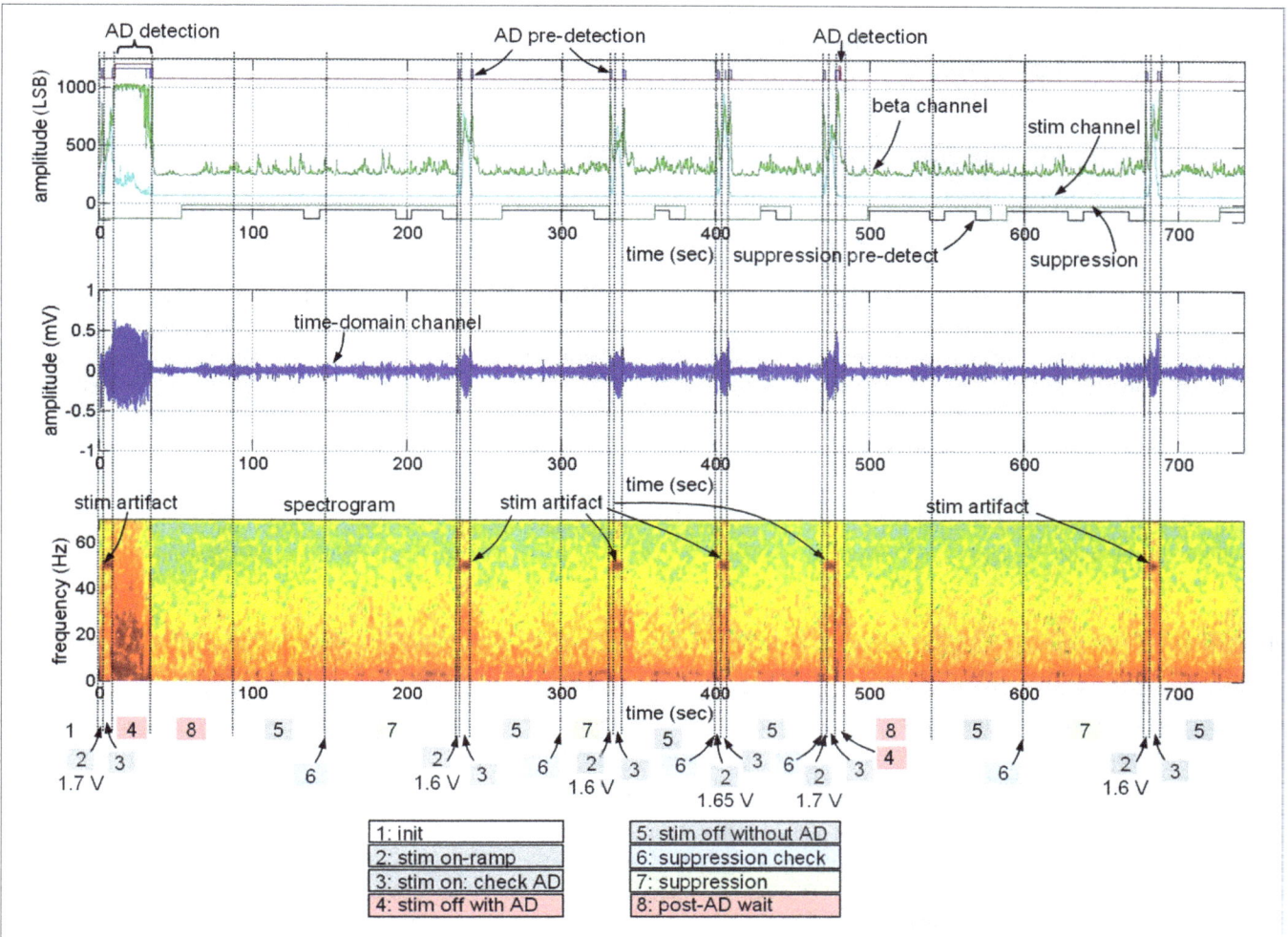

FIGURE 12 | Data sample from embedded algorithm (Figure 11). The sample demonstrates data associated with detection of seizure-like events in the presence and absence of stimulation and change stimulation parameters, resulting in no observed after-discharges. "Pre-detection" refers to the period of time when the onset or termination constraint has not yet been met.

health. These approaches rely on improved understanding of the nervous system dynamics and how they drive the mechanisms of action for neuromodulation. Mapping these concepts to a learning agent framework helps define key components that can lead to better characterization of the system: sensors for chronically collecting data; effectors for modulating the network; and algorithms for translating data into stimulation parameters. The investigational platform described here fills a gap in current technology by enabling a process methodology for designing and prototyping these algorithms and embedding them in an automated closed-loop neuromodulation device.

In this work, we demonstrated a platform consisting of an implantable device integrated with external tools for developing classifier and control-policy algorithms. We tested the platform in a system that exhibited contrasting behavior with respect to stimulation amplitude, motivating our algorithm design to find the fine balance point between over- and under stimulation. One of our significant findings was a potentially non-monotonic

relationship between stimulation amplitude and system response: beta band power was reduced from baseline at low stimulation amplitudes, while it was increased at higher stimulation amplitudes, resulting in occasional AD. These results imply that neural feedback may be an important consideration in determining the optimal stimulation amplitude.

While we performed our experiments in an *in vivo* ovine, our investigational approach could be applied to the study of other disease states, such as Parkinson's disease, essential tremor, epilepsy, or other neurological conditions. Preliminary exploration of the automated algorithm supports the design of other closed-loop systems using similar control policies to those described here (Eusebio and Brown, 2009; Priori et al., 2012). Furthermore, our system is not limited to neural biopotentials; we can theoretically record any biopotential of sufficient amplitude (e.g., EMG). These biopotentials, along with other sensor data, may be useful in prototyping and validating algorithms for future automated closed-loop systems (Yamamoto et al., 2012).

Our design involved several practical considerations. Perhaps most importantly, we designed the generalized learning system on a chassis that has received prior approval for select therapies. Building off an established foundation helps to lower the translational barriers to exploring advanced systems. An additional key design element is the ability to sense activity in the presence of stimulation (also described in Priori et al., 2012). Our results demonstrate the potential importance of network phenomena that occur while the network is being modulated—especially while characterizing transfer functions of the nervous system that might underlie mechanisms of action. In this work, this capability allowed us to monitor for evidence of AD during the stimulation as well as dynamically adjusting the stimulation ceiling as a function of suppression state. These phenomena may be missed by neural sensing architectures that blank out the signal chain during the stimulation (Sun et al., 2008).

Another practical consideration is that the learning pathway is amenable to chronic embedded algorithm operation, particularly in light of the trade-offs between complexity and performance versus simplicity and power consumption (Lee Kyong et al., 2012). The offline analysis and hybrid design approach allow for rapid prototyping of concepts before commitment to embedded firmware. Once embedded, the power draw with our system could be reduced to 20 uW, below 10% of existing nominal therapy power for Parkinson's disease, and latency can be reduced to approximately 200 ms. In the future, use of complementary sensors such as accelerometers and patient feedback may enable algorithms to maintain simplicity and efficiency without sacrificing performance. Ultimately, the ability to titrate stimulation to therapy using responsive algorithms (such as the suppression loop) could potentially yield a net energy savings of chronic responsive systems.

Finally, the experiments allowed us to observe overall reliability of the system. Observed signals of network states were stable over the course of the 15-month experiment, providing evidence of robustness in our detection algorithms (>20-fold margin) to detect state changes. This finding, combined with other results (Stypulkowski et al., 2011), provides initial confidence in the reliability of the system in an *in vivo* environment. In addition, our control-policy implementation used bounded stimulation parameters to ensure tolerability and safety. The chronic reliability and means of ensuring safety provide both a mechanism for longitudinal learning to occur within one subject and chronic validation of the methods, thereby greatly increasing the likelihood of clinical translation.

The study does suffer from limitations, mostly tied to the choice of animal model used for validation. First, the validation is tied to physiology measures and not a true disease model. The ultimate therapeutic utility of the algorithm will require additional testing in animal and clinical models which might drive refinement of the algorithm. In addition, the hybrid system is limited by telemetry latency. Future investigations characterizing the latency of the feedback loop may be needed to better understand this impact vis a vis neural dynamics. System latency may be particularly relevant when stimulating multiple neural regions, such as in stimulating pairs of neural targets or in functional electrical stimulation of muscle in response to sensed neural signals. Ultimately this latency is addressed when embedded in the system, but might limit the broader application of the hybrid design process.

In summary, we believe increased understanding of the nervous system with such platform systems may lead to improved technical capability to modulate the nervous system to address pathophysiology. As these systems mature, they can be embedded into devices to augment and potentially correct for a malfunctioning nervous system.

REFERENCES

Avestruz, A.-T., Santa, W., Carlson, D., Jensen, R., Stanslaski, S., Helfenstine, A., et al. (2008). A 5 μW/channel spectral analysis IC for chronic bidirectional brain machine interfaces. *IEEE J. Solid-State Circ.* 43, 3006–3024.

Blanco, J., Stead, M., Krieger, A., Stacey, W., Maus, D., Marsh, E., et al. (2011). Data mining neocortical high-frequency oscillations in epilepsy and controls. *Brain* 134, 2948–2959.

Bronstein, J. M., Tagliati, M., Alterman, R. L., Lozano, A. M., Volkmann, J., Stefani, A., et al. (2011). Deep brain stimulation for Parkinson disease: an expert consensus and review of key issues. *Arch. Neurol.* 68, 165.

Denison, T., Santa, W., Molnar, G., and Miesel, K. (2007). "Micropower sensors for neuroprosthetics," in *IEEE Sensors Conference* (Atlanta, GA).

Eusebio, A., and Brown, P. (2009). Synchronisation in the beta frequency-band: the bad boy of parkinsonism or an innocent bystander? *Exp. Neurol.* 217, 1–3.

Eusebio, A., Cagnan, H., and Brown, P. (2012). Does suppression of oscillatory synchronization mediate some of the therapeutic effects of DBS in patients with Parkinson's disease. *Front. Integr. Neurosci.* 6:47. doi: 10.3389/fnint.2012.00047

Hamani, C., Richter, E., Schwalb, J. M., and Lozano, A. M. (2005). Bilateral subthalamic nucleus stimulation for Parkinson's disease: a systematic review of the clinical literature. *Neurosurgery* 56, 1313–1321, discussion: 1314–1321.

Hammond, C., Bergman, H., and Brown, P. (2007). Pathological synchronization in Parkinson's disease: networks, models and treatments. *Trends Neurosci.* 30, 357–364.

Hellwig, B., Häussler, S., Schelter, B., Lauk, M., Guschlbauer, B., Timmer, J., et al. (2001). Tremor-correlated cortical activity in essential tremor. *Lancet* 357, 519–523.

Kühn, A., Tsui, A., Aziz, T., Ray, N., Brucke, C., Kupsch, A., et al. (2009). Pathological synchronisation in the subthalamic nucleus of patients with Parkinson's disease relates to both bradykinesia and rigidity. *Exp. Neurol.* 215, 380–387.

Lee Kyong, H., Kung, S.-Y., and Verma, N. (2012). Low-energy formulations of support vector machine kernel functions for biomedical sensor applications. *J. Signal Process. Syst.* 69, 339–349.

Limousin, P., Krack, P., Pollak, P., Benazzouz, A., Ardouin, C., Hoffmann, D., et al. (1998). Electrical stimulation of the subthalamic nucleus in advanced Parkinson's disease. *N. Engl. J. Med.* 339, 1105–1111.

Limousin, P., Pollack, P., Hoffmann, D., Benazzouz, A., Perret, J. E., and Benabid, A. L. (1996). Abnormal involuntary movements induced by subthalamic nucleus stimulation in parkinsonian patients. *Mov. Disord.* 11, 231–235.

Liu, X., Griffin, I., Parkin, S., Miall, C., Rowe, J. G., Gregory, R. P., et al. (2002). Involvement of the medial pallidum in focal myoclonic dystonia: a clinical and neurophysiological case study. *Mov. Disord.* 17, 346–353.

Llinas, R., and Ribary, U. (2001). Consciousness and the brain: the thalamocortical dialogue in health and disease. *Ann. N.Y. Acad. Sci.* 929, 166–175.

Miranda, H., Gilja, V., Chestek, C. A., Shenoy, K. V., and Meng, T. H. (2010). HermesD: a high-rate long-range wireless transmission system for simultaneous multichannel neural recording applications. *IEEE Trans. Biomed. Circuits Syst.* 4, 181–191.

Priori, A., Foffani, G., Rossi, L., and Marceglia, S. (2012). Adaptive deep brain stimulation (aDBS) controlled by local field potential oscillations. *Exp. Neurol.* pii: S0014–4886. doi: 10.1016/j.expneurol.2012.09.013. [Epub ahead of print].

Raethjen, J., Lindemann, M., Dümpelmann, M., Wenzelburger, R., Stolze, H., and Pfister, G. (2002). Corticomuscular coherence in the 6–15 Hz band: is the cortex involved in the generation of physiologic tremor? *Exp. Brain Res.* 142, 32–40.

Rossi, L., Marceglia, S., Foffani, G., Cogiamanian, F., Tamma, F., Rampini, P., et al. (2008). Subthalamic local field potential oscillations during on-going deep brain stimulation in Parkinson's disease. *Brain Res. Bull.* 76, 512–521.

Rouse, A. G., Stanslaski, S. R., Cong, P., Jensen, R. M., Afshar, P., Ullestad, D., et al. (2011). A chronic generalized bi-directional brain–machine interface. *J. Neural Eng.* 8, 036018.

Schnitzler, A., and Gross, J. (2005). Normal and pathological oscillatory communication in the brain. *Nat. Rev. Neurosci.* 6, 285–297.

Schultz, D. M., Webster, L., Kosek, P., Dar, U., Tan, Y., and Sun, M. (2012). Sensor-driven position-adaptive spinal cord stimulation for chronic pain. *Pain Physician* 15, 1–12.

Sharott, A., Grosse, P., Kühn, A. A., Salih, F., Engel, A. K., Kupsch, A., et al. (2008). Is the synchronization between pallidal and muscle activity in primary dystonia due to peripheral afferance or a motor drive? *Brain* 131, 473–484.

Shoeb, A., Carlson, D., Panken, E., and Denison, T. (2009). "A micropower support vector machine based seizure detection architecture for embedded medical devices," in *Annual International Conference of the IEEE Engineering in Medicine and Biology Society*.

Siegel, M., Donner, T., and Engel, A. (2012). Spectral fingerprints of large-scale neuronal interactions. *Nat. Rev. Neurosci.* 13, 121–134.

Silberstein, P., Kühn, A., Kupsch, A., Trottenberg, T., Krauss, J. K., Wohrle, J. C. et al. (2003). Patterning of globus pallidus local field potentials differs between Parkinson's disease and dystonia. *Brain* 126, 2597–2608.

Singh, A., Levin, J., Mehrkens, J., and Botzel, K. (2011). Alpha frequency modulation in the human basal ganglia is dependent on motor task. *Eur. J. Neurosci.* 33, 960–967.

Stanslaski, S., Afshar, P., Cong, P., Giftakis, J., Stypulkowski, P., Carlson, D., et al. (2012). Design and validation of a fully implantable, chronic, closed-loop neuromodulation device with concurrent sensing and stimulation. *IEEE Trans. Neural Syst. Rehabil. Eng.* 20, 410–421.

Stypulkowski, P. H., Giftakis, J. E., and Billstrom, T. M. (2011). Development of a large animal model for investigation of deep brain stimulation for epilepsy. *Strereotact. Funct. Neurosurg.* 89, 111–122.

Sun, F. T., Morrell, M. H., and Wharen, R. E. (2008). Responsive cortical stimulation for the treatment of epilepsy. *Neurotherapeutics* 5, 68–74.

Uhlhaas, P., and Singer, W. (2006). Neural synchrony in brain disorders: relevance for cognitive dysfunctions and pathophysiology. *Neuron* 52, 155–168.

Yamamoto, T., Katayama, Y., Ushiba, J., Yoshino, H., Obuchi, T., Koboyashi, K., et al. (2012). On-demand control system for deep-brain stimulation treatment of intention tremor. *Neuromodulation.* PMID: 23094990. doi: 10.1111/j.1525-1403.2012.00521.x. [Epub ahead of print].

Yu, H., and Neimat, J. S. (2008). The treatment of movement disorders by deep brain stimulation. *Neurotherapeutics* 5, 26–36.

Zanos, S., Richardson, A. G., Shupe, L., Miles, F. P., and Fetz, E. E. (2011). The Neurochip-2: an autonomous head-fixed computer for recording and stimulating in freely behaving monkeys. *IEEE Trans. Neural Syst. Rehabil. Eng.* 40, 427–435.

Zumsteg, D., Lozano, A., and Wennberg, R. (2006). Rhythmic cortical EEG synchronization with low frequency stimulation of the anterior and medial thalamus for epilepsy. *Clin. Neurophysiol.* 117, 2272–2278.

11

Creating new functional circuits for action via brain-machine interfaces

*Amy L. Orsborn[1] and Jose M. Carmena[1,2,3] ***

[1] UC Berkeley - UCSF Joint Graduate Program in Bioengineering, University of California Berkeley, Berkeley, CA, USA
[2] Department of Electrical Engineering and Computer Science, University of California Berkeley, Berkeley, CA, USA
[3] Helen Wills Neuroscience Institute, University of California Berkeley, Berkeley, CA, USA

Edited by:
John W. Krakauer, Johns Hopkins University, USA

Reviewed by:
Byron Yu, Carnegie Mellon University, USA
Lior Shmuelof, Ben Gurion University, Israel

***Correspondence:**
Jose M. Carmena, UC Berkeley - UCSF Joint Graduate Program in Bioengineering, University of California Berkeley, 644 Sutardja Dai Hall, Berkeley, CA, 94720-1764, USA
e-mail: carmena@eecs.berkeley.edu

Brain-machine interfaces (BMIs) are an emerging technology with great promise for developing restorative therapies for those with disabilities. BMIs also create novel, well-defined functional circuits for action that are distinct from the natural sensorimotor apparatus. Closed-loop control of BMI systems can also actively engage learning and adaptation. These properties make BMIs uniquely suited to study learning of motor and non-physical, abstract skills. Recent work used motor BMIs to shed light on the neural representations of skill formation and motor adaptation. Emerging work in sensory BMIs, and other novel interface systems, also highlight the promise of using BMI systems to study fundamental questions in learning and sensorimotor control. This paper outlines the interpretation of BMIs as novel closed-loop systems and the benefits of these systems for studying learning. We review BMI learning studies, their relation to motor control, and propose future directions for this nascent field. Understanding learning in BMIs may both elucidate mechanisms of natural motor and abstract skill learning, and aid in developing the next generation of neuroprostheses.

Keywords: brain-machine interfaces, motor learning, neural plasticity, volitional control, sensorimotor systems

Recent technological advances have made it possible to directly connect brains with machines. Recorded neural activity can be used to control external devices in real-time, and neural stimulation can be applied based on external events to convey information into the brain. These brain-machine interfaces (BMIs) have a wide range of potential applications, including rehabilitative and restorative therapies for patients with neurological deficits. Cochlear implants, for instance, are widely used to restore hearing to patients with severe hearing loss. Recently, there have been demonstrations of BMIs used to restore movement in paralyzed humans by using neural signals to control external devices (Hochberg et al., 2006, 2012; Collinger et al., 2012).

Much as there are many potential applications for BMI technology, there are a variety of possible implementations. BMIs can be used to replace motor or sensory systems, or both simultaneously. Motor (efferent) BMIs use recorded neural activity to control external devices, while sensory (afferent) BMIs use neural stimulation to transmit information to the brain. Many different types of neural signals can be used for efferent control including electroencephalography (EEG), electrocorticography (ECoG), local-field potentials (LFPs), or single- and multi-unit action potentials. Neural activity has been successfully used to control a variety of devices in real time, including virtual objects (Serruya et al., 2002; Taylor et al., 2002; Carmena et al., 2003; Leuthardt et al., 2004; Wolpaw and McFarland, 2004; Hochberg et al., 2006; Jarosiewicz et al., 2008; Kim et al., 2008; Schalk et al., 2008; Ganguly and Carmena, 2009; Suminski et al., 2010;

O'Doherty et al., 2011; Gilja et al., 2012; Engelhard et al., 2013; Rouse et al., 2013; Wander et al., 2013), robots (Carmena et al., 2003; Taylor et al., 2003; Millán et al., 2004; Velliste et al., 2008; Collinger et al., 2012; Hochberg et al., 2012), wheelchairs (Millán et al., 2009), or to drive movements of the user's body via muscle stimulation (Moritz et al., 2008; Ethier et al., 2012). Similarly, neural stimulation for sensory BMIs can be implemented using electrical approaches, such as intracortical microelectrode stimulation (ICMS), or via optogenetic methods. Stimulation at different levels of the central nervous system (CNS) has been used to convey auditory (Wilson et al., 1991), visual (Weiland and Humayun, 2008; Tehovnik et al., 2009), tactile (Romo et al., 2000; O'Doherty et al., 2011; Venkatraman and Carmena, 2011; Berg et al., 2013), and proprioceptive (London et al., 2008) feedback to users. Recent work also shows that sensory and motor BMIs can be combined (O'Doherty et al., 2011), which holds great promise for restoring function to paralyzed individuals lacking somatosensory feedback.

Decades of work in BMIs has produced impressive demonstrations, but also reveals that interfacing the brain with machinery is not a simple matter of restoring broken connections. Indeed, these interfaces create new systems that can engage learning and adaptation (Fetz, 2007). Interestingly, BMIs are distinct from the natural sensorimotor apparatus, yet still involve select components of the CNS. Understanding these unique systems may be particularly important for engineering development of successful neuroprosthetic systems (Ganguly and Carmena, 2009; Gilja et al.,

2012). They may also provide unique advantages for exploring fundamental questions in neuroscience. BMIs provide scientists a rare opportunity to create novel, well-defined functional circuits that are separate from, but parallel to, their natural counterparts.

BMIs may be particularly useful for studying questions of motor learning and skill formation. While studying the natural sensorimotor system has revealed significant insights, many questions about the neural mechanisms of skill learning remain (Wolpert et al., 2011). For instance, how are learned skills stored in the brain, and what brain areas facilitate their formation and recall? What are the neural underpinnings of performance optimization and refinement? BMIs create novel, functional circuits for action and/or sensation that can be used to study skill learning *de novo* and subsequent adaptation. Because these systems are defined by the experimenter, they may also reduce ambiguities inherent in neurophysiological motor learning studies caused by the complexities of the highly distributed natural motor control system. BMIs define a simpler, known mapping between neural activity and behavior, allowing for careful study of learning-related changes in neurons directly and in-directly contributing to behavior. BMI systems can be more readily interrogated and manipulated by the experimenter to provide new insights into the neurophysiological basis of learning.

Interestingly, BMIs can also be used to define systems that operate irrespective of the natural sensorimotor apparatus. Indeed, motor BMIs can be operated without movement (Taylor et al., 2002; Carmena et al., 2003; Ganguly and Carmena, 2009; Koralek et al., 2012). This property of BMIs might be useful for studying learning of more abstract, cognitive skills. Very little is known about how we acquire skills independent of movement, like solving puzzles. Closed-loop BMIs can be used to define new input-output relationships, or transforms, for the CNS to learn and solve irrespective of the natural sensorimotor system. Moreover, selection of different neural inputs for BMI could be used to study learning in a variety of brain areas and systems. We refer to skill learning in these novel systems controlled irrespective of movement as *neuroprosthetic skills*. Studying these neuroprosthetic skills may be particularly useful for understanding how abstract, non-physical skills are learned, and their neural representations.

Recent work in BMIs demonstrates the potential utility of this paradigm for studying learning, with a growing number of papers providing evidence about the neural mechanisms of adaptation and skill consolidation. Emerging work in sensory BMIs and other closed-loop interface systems also show great promise. Here, we discuss the interpretation of BMIs as novel closed-loop systems partially removed from the CNS. We review the key aspects of these systems that make them uniquely suited to motor learning studies, summarize work demonstrating their potential, and explore future avenues of research.

BMIs CREATE NOVEL CLOSED-LOOP CONTROL SYSTEMS

Despite variability in implementation, at their core, all sensorimotor neuroprostheses are simple closed-loop control systems (**Figure 1**). In motor BMIs, neural activity is recorded and an algorithm, "the decoder", is used to map the neural activity into a control signal to move the actuator. Feedback is provided to

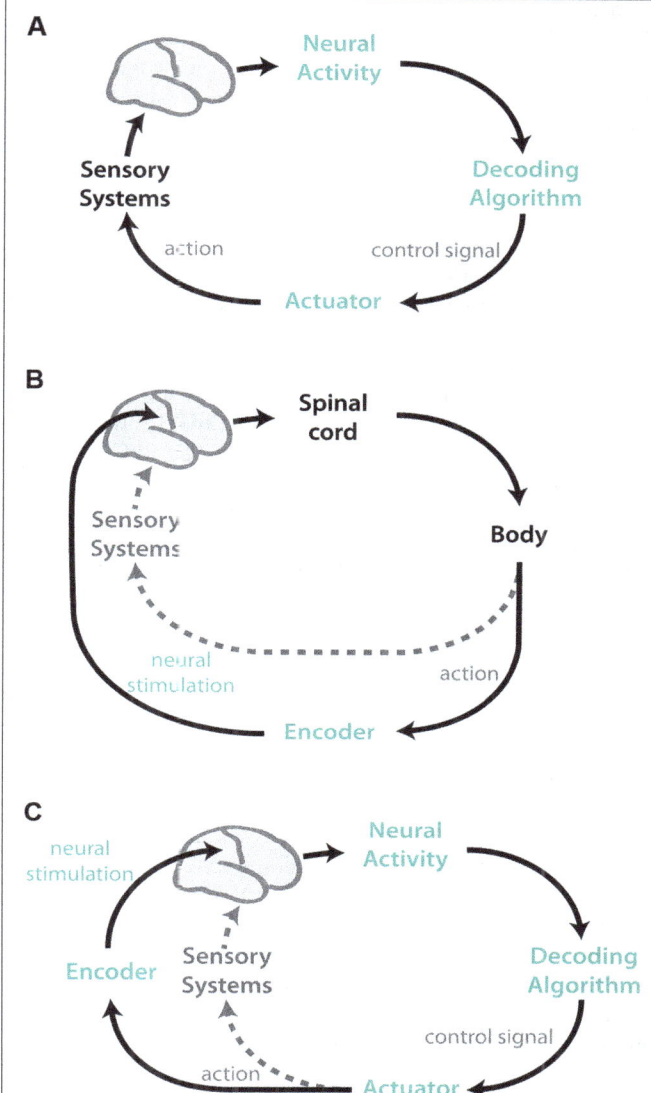

FIGURE 1 | Schematic representations of BMI systems. Components of the natural CNS are shown in black/grey; artificial, experimenter-controlled elements are colored. **(A)** Motor (efferent) BMIs map recorded neural activity into control signals for a device via a decoding algorithm. These systems typically use natural sensory systems, such as vision, to provide feedback to the user, creating a closed-loop system. **(B)** Sensory (afferent) BMIs use the natural motor apparatus to perform actions, but close the control loop using feedback conveyed via neural stimulation. Environmental variables are encoded into patterns of stimulation delivered to select brain regions. The artificial feedback can also be combined with natural sensory stimuli (grey dotted). **(C)** Afferent and efferent BMIs can be combined, where actions are decoded from neural activity and feedback is provided via encoded neural stimulation. Again, the artificial sensory feedback can be combined with natural sensory systems (grey dotted).

the user to create a closed-loop control system (**Figure 1A**). These systems typically use natural sensory systems, such as vision and/or audition, for feedback. Sensory BMI systems, in contrast, use algorithms to "encode" relevant information into neural stimulation patterns that are delivered to the brain (**Figure 1B**), and actions are implemented using the natural motor apparatus. This neural stimulation can also be combined with other native sensory feedback. These two approaches can be combined such that actions are implemented by a BMI controller, and feedback is provided using neural stimulation (**Figure 1C**).

The closed-loop nature of BMI systems is essential to their operation and makes them a particularly useful tool for studying learning. The feedback in BMI systems allow users to modify their behavior to achieve desired goals. Many studies show that rats, non-human primates and humans can learn to volitionally control neural activity using biofeedback at the level of single-unit action-potentials (Fetz, 1969, 2007; Fetz and Finocchio, 1971, 1975; Chapin et al., 1999; Gage et al., 2005; Cerf et al., 2010; Moritz and Fetz, 2011; Koralek et al., 2012), local field potentials (Engelhard et al., 2013; Flint et al., 2013), ECoG (Leuthardt et al., 2004; Schalk et al., 2008; Rouse et al., 2013), and EEG (reviewed in Wolpaw et al., 2002; McFarland and Wolpaw, 2011). Volitional control can also decouple single-unit activity from its typical functional roles (Fetz and Finocchio, 1971, 1975). Increasing research shows these volitional control plays a role in closed-loop BMI operation. For instance, subjects can learn to modulate neural activity in order to improve efferent BMI performance for a given decoder (Ganguly and Carmena, 2009).

It is also crucial to understand BMI systems' relation to the natural sensorimotor system. Consider motor BMIs for upper limb reaching. Natural arm movements are orchestrated by a host of brain areas, the spinal cord, and limb biomechanics; and somatosensory, proprioceptive and visual feedback play critical roles in the control. In BMI, subjects typically control an artificial device via visual observation alone, whose movements are governed by the activity of only a small subset of neurons in motor cortical areas (e.g., primary motor cortex). While BMIs can engage other cortical and subcortical areas (Ganguly et al., 2011; Koralek et al., 2012; Wander et al., 2013), the relationship between movement and neural activity imposed in BMI differs significantly from that of natural movements. These BMI systems may be able to replace motor function, but do so by creating a new control system that is distinct from natural arm movements. Yet, this novel system still incorporates elements of the natural system. For instance, motor BMIs (e.g., driven by activity from primary motor cortex) and arm movements both engage motor cortical areas. The control of BMI systems may, then, share key similarities to the control of natural movements. Research does suggest strong connections between natural motor learning and learning BMIs, as reviewed in Green and Kalaska (2011); Jackson and Fetz (2011) and the discussions below. BMI systems are separate from, but parallel to, the native functions they imitate.

Historically, work in BMIs have not fully appreciated the novel aspects of closed-loop BMI systems[1]. Many have focused on mimicking the natural system (reviewed in Jackson and Fetz, 2011), developing decoding algorithms to predict limb

movements or motor intentions from neural activity. However, increasing research shows that a decoder's prediction power does not necessarily translate to improved closed-loop performance (Koyama et al., 2009; Ganguly and Carmena, 2010; Cunningham et al., 2011). This has led some to re-examine BMI systems and the underlying assumptions of biomimetic approaches (Jackson and Fetz, 2011; Gilja et al., 2012). Recent work incorporating closed-loop perspectives shows great promise for improving BMI performance (Gilja et al., 2012). Understanding BMIs as closed-loop systems distinct from their natural counterparts may be essential for applications of BMI technology. Moreover, this insight opens up many possibilities for using it as a tool to study learning.

One of the most interesting and potentially valuable aspects of BMIs is that they allow experimenters to fully define functional circuits for action. The control system created by closed-loop BMIs are specified by the experimenter. Efferent BMIs define: (1) the neural activity used for control—i.e., the system input, (2) the mapping of how neural activity influences performance, manipulated via the decoder, (3) the variables controlled by the brain, and (4) the types of feedback provided to the user. Similarly precise control is available for afferent BMI systems, which stipulate what information is transmitted, how, and to what brain areas. This control also allows for more complete observation and analysis of the system during learning. For instance, neurophysiological studies during motor adaptation can feasibly monitor a small subset of the neurons within the highly distributed motor system (Wise et al., 1998; Gandolfo et al., 2000; Li et al., 2001; Paz et al., 2003; Padoa-Schioppa et al., 2004; Paz and Vaadia, 2004). Though informative, this captures only a portion of neural learning mechanisms. Moreover, the direct relationship between the activity of individual neurons in motor cortical areas and behavior is also still a topic of significant debate (e.g., reviewed in Shenoy et al., 2013), complicating mechanistic interpretations of neural activity changes with learning (Jarosiewicz et al., 2008). BMI systems artificially constrain the neural input and/or output, and in doing so provide full knowledge of the input-output mapping governing the system behavior. This may allow for more direct assessments of learning-related changes. The ability to create simplified control circuits could highlight principles and mechanisms that may be less clear in a more complex control system. However, leveraging the full potential of this aspect of BMIs also requires understanding how BMI relates to the natural motor system. We return to this critical question in the discussion below.

Finally, by creating new functional circuits, BMIs define novel tasks for the CNS to learn. Many classic sensorimotor learning paradigms apply perturbations to the natural motor system—for example, in the form of forces (e.g., Shadmehr and Mussa-Ivaldi, 1994) or visuomotor transformations (e.g., Krakauer et al., 2000)—and study how the nervous system learns these modifications (recently reviewed in Wolpert et al., 2011). How subjects learn these tasks may be shaped by prior experience, since these tasks modify the subjects' natural motor repertoire (Shadmehr et al., 2010; Wolpert et al., 2011). These paradigms have proven very useful for understanding how the motor system adapts, but may be less ideally suited to investigating how the CNS learns an entirely new skill, or how motor performance is refined in absence of perturbations (Shmuelof et al., 2012). For instance,

---

[1]There are, however, notable exceptions of researchers that recognized the importance of closed-loop BMI learning and adaptation early on (e.g. Taylor et al., 2002; Wolpaw et al., 2002; Carmena et al., 2003). The EEG community has also recognized and integrated these aspects more readily (Wolpaw et al., 2002; Millán and Mouriño, 2003).

how does the brain initially learn the dynamics of the motor system? How does the CNS learn to refine and optimize control? Because BMIs create a new control system distinct from the natural, well-learned sensorimotor apparatus, it is uniquely suited to studying these questions. The ability to define novel transforms removed from the natural sensorimotor apparatus also opens the possibility to study neuroprosthetic skills and learning beyond the sensorimotor system.

STUDYING LEARNING WITH BMI SYSTEMS

BMIs define novel functional circuits for action that actively engage subject learning and can be precisely manipulated in experiments. Recent studies in motor BMIs leveraged these unique properties to study skill learning and adaptation. Emerging work in afferent and efferent-afferent BMIs, as well as other interface systems also show the promise of BMI technology in learning studies.

Motor learning is thought to have distinct forms, including adaptation and skill formation, which may have different underlying neural mechanisms (Krakauer and Mazzoni, 2011). The same is likely true for BMI systems and abstract learning. While adaptation and skill can be separated in the natural motor system, these distinctions are currently less well-defined in BMI. Only a small number of studies have addressed learning in BMI, so information is limited, and few have attempted to model BMI learning processes. For the purposes of the proceeding discussion, we define "skill learning" as the process of learning to control a BMI system *de novo*, evidenced by the gradual formation of proficient performance. We use "adaptation" to refer to learning associated with compensating for perturbations to a previously-learned BMI system with proficient performance. Similarly, as noted above we use the term "neuroprosthetic skill" to refer to proficient BMI performance irrespective of physical movement. Such neuroprosthetic skills may be linked to more abstract forms of learning and skill. How our definitions of learning in BMI relate to adaptation and skill formation in the natural motor system, and the relationship of neuroprosthetic and abstract skills are fascinating and open questions we address in the discussion of future directions.

NEUROPROSTHETIC SKILL FORMATION

There are clear behavioral signatures of skill—robust, reliable performance that can be rapidly recalled. But the neural representations underlying skill formation remain uncertain. The motor cortices appears to be involved in the formation and retention of motor memories and skills (Krakauer and Shadmehr, 2006), but what is the substrate of that memory? How the brain forms and stores memories is a critical question in motor learning, and neuroscience at large.

Ganguly and Carmena investigated this question by examining how subjects learned skilled BMI control (Ganguly and Carmena, 2009). Non-human primate subjects operated a closed-loop cursor BMI using single-unit activity from the motor cortex without overt arm movements. Critically, the mapping between cursor movement and neural activity—the "neuroprosthetic circuit"—was held constant for many days. Subjects became proficient in BMI control over days. The behavior showed many similarities

to natural motor learning, with intra- and inter-session learning, and rapid recall of performance each day. Moreover, after achieving proficient control, a subject was able to learn a second decoder without disrupting the performance with the initial decoder. Together, these results suggest that BMI control was achieved via consolidation of a neuroprosthetic skill, identified by proficient, rapidly-recalled control of a disembodied actuator irrespective of natural movement.

The mapping between neural activity and output in BMI allows for thorough investigation of the neural underpinnings of neuroprosthetic skill. The direction tuning—relationship between firing rate and direction of target motion—of neurons contributing to the BMI decoder ("BMI neurons") shifted as subjects improved their BMI performance. Direction tuning changed significantly early during learning, but became more stable as performance reached a plateau. Skill consolidation resulted in the formation of a stable neural "map" of the decoder that could be rapidly recalled. Changing BMI decoders daily disrupted skill and neural map formation, suggesting they are specifically tied to learning the input-output transform defined by the neuroprosthetic circuit (Ganguly and Carmena, 2009).This map was significantly different from that of natural arm movements. Yet, subjects could readily switch between arm and neuroprosthetic control, and neural activity showed corresponding rapid shifts between two different maps (Ganguly et al., 2011).

BMI also allows observation of brain areas not directly contributing to the task. What occurs in other parts of the motor cortex as a subject learns a neuroprosthetic skill? Examining the activity of neurons in motor cortex but not contributing to the decoded output during transform learning revealed large-scale changes in their firing properties and relation to the task (Ganguly et al., 2011). Non-BMI neurons' preferred direction (cursor motion causing maximal firing) changed compared to arm movements, similar to BMI neurons. However, proficient neuroprosthetic control was associated with a reduction in non-BMI neurons' modulation depths compared to BMI-neurons. Interestingly, the reduction in modulation depth was dependent upon the non-BMI neurons' distance from BMI neurons. This effect was apparent in late, but not early, stages of learning, suggesting that it was linked to neuroprosthetic skill formation. Transform learning triggered a large-scale, reversible modification of the cortical network centered on the BMI neurons. Recent work in humans suggests that neuroprosthetic learning may also result in the formation of a more broadly distributed cortical network that extends well beyond the areas directly involved in control (Wander et al., 2013).

These results give tantalizing suggestions about the neural substrates of a skill. But where and how does this learning take place? Does neuroprosthetic learning involve similar brain structures as natural motor learning? To address these questions, Koralek et al. developed a BMI paradigm where rodents learned to control the pitch of an auditory cursor to reach one of two targets by modulating activity in primary motor cortex in the absence of physical movement (Koralek et al., 2012). They examined the activity of the dorsolateral striatum—a structure linked to motor skill learning—during learning of this abstract skill. Striatum neurons were modulated during neuroprosthetic control, and the activity in motor cortex—the output system—increased its coherence with the dorsolateral striatum as learning progressed. These coherence changes were also found to be specific to motor cortex neurons contributing to the decoder, consistent with the formation of a BMI-specific network (Koralek et al., 2013). Deletion of striatal N-methyl-aspartic acid (NMDA) receptors, which are necessary for corticostriatal long-term potentiation, severely impaired the development of this corticostriatal plasticity, and completely disrupted the subjects' ability to learn neuroprosthetic skills. These results suggest that corticostriatal circuits are involved in learning skills, even when they do not require physical movement. Moreover, these results show that the process of transform learning not only elicits changes in motor cortical networks, but also recruits elements of the natural motor system outside of the cortex, such as the basal ganglia. Neuroprosthetic skill learning, then, may utilize the built-in mechanisms for natural motor learning.

Together, these studies give preliminary evidence for cortical substrates of learning and the involvement of deep-brain structures in their formation. They also demonstrate that BMIs provide a platform to study the formation of skills. Many questions remain—for instance, the physiological mechanisms driving cortical network formation are uncertain. The relationship between this neuroprosthetic skill, natural motor learning and abstract skills also remains to be fully explored. Expansions of this long-term transform learning paradigm can be used to further probe how this learning occurs.

ADAPTATION IN BMI

BMIs can also be used to study adaptation to carefully controlled perturbations. A recent series of studies took advantage of the ability to manipulate the decoder to probe the behavioral and neural mechanisms of adaptation learning in BMI (Jarosiewicz et al., 2008; Chase et al., 2012; Golub et al., 2012). Non-human primates controlled a cursor-based BMI driven by single-unit activity. After subjects achieved proficient control, the researchers perturbed the decoder by rotating the resulting cursor velocity for a given neural input, and examined if and how neural activity changed. This is akin to visuomotor rotations commonly used in motor learning (Krakauer et al., 2000). What's more, they perturbed the input-output mapping of only a subset of units within the decoder to study if and how adaptation differed for perturbed and non-perturbed units. The behavioral responses to these decoder perturbations showed remarkable parallels to that of natural visuomotor rotations, with subjects initially producing curved trajectories that straighten over time. Removing the perturbation also revealed after-effects—curvature opposite that of the applied rotation—that quickly decayed.

The BMI paradigm allowed for careful examination of the adaptation strategies used by subjects and their neural correlates. While previous studies demonstrated shifts in motor cortex activity during natural motor adaptation, BMI provides knowledge of the precise mapping between neural activity and behavior, which can be used to more clearly interpret neural changes. There are several possible ways to solve a rotational perturbation task, including a global strategy of re-aiming to a new target, or local strategies to either reduce the contribution of perturbed units, or

selectively rotating the action-directions of the perturbed units. Analysis revealed evidence for both global and local adaptation. Interestingly, global re-aiming dominated and the degree to which the different strategies were employed showed some dependence on the number of units perturbed. This suggests that there may be limits to the degree of neural adaptation, at least in the short time-frame of these experiments (Chase et al., 2012).

Behavioral manipulations in BMI control and clever analyses also allowed for quantification of the subjects' control strategies and the time-scale of learning in this paradigm. Golub and colleagues removed visual feedback for the initial portion of reaches, and then used the timing of feedback corrections upon receiving visual feedback to quantify the control time-delay in BMI (Golub et al., 2012). This allowed the researchers to assess whether the subject based control operations on the perceived, delayed visual feedback or on estimates of the current cursor position, which would suggest the formation of an "internal model" of cursor movement. Their results suggest that subjects do indeed form internal predictions of cursor movement. Moreover, by analyzing the above-described decoder perturbation data, theses analyses also showed that learning may be accompanied by modification of this internal model and a method to quantify the time-scale of such adaptation.

By manipulating the decoding algorithm, these studies identified key neural components of learning and adaptation. However, additional work is needed to examine the underlying mechanisms. For instance, are changes in cortical firing driven by input to those areas or via synaptic plasticity? Are the different types of adaptation—global vs. local—achieved through the same or different means? What are the neural signatures of the "internal model" underlying BMI operation, and modified during adaptation? The ability to fully control the BMI system may prove extremely useful for answering these questions. Examination of non-BMI units in up-stream brain areas and within the same cortical area might shed light on the scale and specificity of adaptive mechanisms. Electrophysiology techniques could also be used to explore synaptic plasticity. The clear distinction between BMI and non-BMI units, and perturbed versus non-perturbed units will be essential for honing in on how physiological changes shape the circuit.

SENSORIMOTOR INTEGRATION AND SENSORY TRANSFORM LEARNING

The majority of learning-related BMI studies focus on efferent control. However, sensory BMIs can also be used to investigate key questions about sensorimotor learning and integration. Neural stimulation—via ICMS or optogenetic techniques—can be used to evoke percepts and influence cortical processing (Wilson et al., 1991; Romo et al., 2000; London et al., 2008; Weiland and Humayun, 2008; Tehovnik et al., 2009; Berg et al., 2013). Moreover, artificial neural stimulation can be integrated with natural sensory feedback to facilitate active-sensing tasks (O'Doherty et al., 2011; Venkatraman and Carmena, 2011). Emerging work also suggests that the integration of natural sensory information and artificial stimulation is modulated by the reliability of the sensory information (Dadarlat et al., 2012), in strong agreement with many observations of natural sensorimotor integration (Sabes,

2011). Together, these studies show that stimulation can convey useful information to subjects, making it possible to create closed-loop sensory BMI systems that operate parallel to the natural sensorimotor systems.

Interestingly, several studies suggest that the percepts evoked by artificial stimulation have only a slight similarity to their natural counterparts. For example, rats trained to respond to movement of the whiskers initially also responded to ICMS stimulation, but quickly learned to discern the two stimuli (Venkatraman and Carmena, 2011). Non-biomimetic approaches to neural stimulation have been shown to be effective (O'Doherty et al., 2011; Dadarlat et al., 2012). Thus, sensory BMIs also involve transform learning, where subjects learn a novel mapping between the artificially-evoked neural activity and environmental variables. However, studies of the underlying learning mechanisms involved in afferent BMIs are forthcoming. Closed-loop BMI studies have tremendous potential to illuminate the learning processes in sensory systems and the underlying neural mechanisms. Combining afferent and efferent BMIs (O'Doherty et al., 2011) is a similarly promising platform that may allow for careful study of how sensory inputs are transformed into actions.

BEYOND BRAIN-INTERFACING: TRANSFORM LEARNING TOOLS

The ability to create novel functional action circuits extends beyond BMI. Other signals from the CNS, such as muscle activity or limb kinematics, can be used to control artificially-defined systems. Myoelectric interfaces, for example, map electromyograms of select muscles to the motion of computer cursors via linear decoding algorithms (Radhakrishnan et al., 2008; Nazarpour et al., 2012). The joint angles of the human hand can also be artificially mapped to a cursor position (Mosier et al., 2005; Mussa-Ivaldi and Danziger, 2009; Liu et al., 2010). Much like BMI, these approaches create closed-loop control systems that are different from the natural sensorimotor system and can be used to investigate how the CNS learns to novel, abstract transforms. Subjects can readily learn to control these novel interfaces, even with arbitrary and non-intuitive mappings (Mosier et al., 2005; Radhakrishnan et al., 2008)

These two interface systems show tremendous potential for studying fundamental questions of motor learning and control. Myoelectric interfaces have been used to explore theories about muscle synergies and optimal control (Radhakrishnan et al., 2008; Nazarpour et al., 2012). Their work shows that subjects use coordinated patterns of muscle activity shaped to maximize task performance—hallmarks of optimal, synergy-based control—even in motor tasks disconnected from the natural sensorimotor apparatus. Kinematic interfaces have been used to explore how the motor systems deals with redundancy (Mosier et al., 2005; Mussa-Ivaldi and Danziger, 2009; Ranganathan et al., 2013). These mappings are highly redundant, and knowledge of the mapping's structure allowed researchers to separate subjects' movements into task-relevant and -irrelevant components. Transform learning was accompanied by significant reduction in task-irrelevant movements, suggesting that subjects learned to constrain their movements to those that contributed to cursor movements. Kinematic interfaces have also been used to study adaptation to perturbations, revealing previously unobserved distinctions

between adaptation to different types of manipulations (Liu et al., 2010). The authors suggest that the extensive experience with reaching may influence motor adaptation and learning studies. Novel interfaces may provide new and critical insights into motor learning that cannot be readily assessed by studying the natural motor system.

Subjects operating BMIs, myoelectric-, and kinematic-interfaces all show clear hallmarks of skill learning. However, several have noted differences in the learning rates and strategies of these systems (Green and Kalaska, 2011; Jackson and Fetz, 2011; Chase et al., 2012). The fundamental differences in the control inputs, and their relation to the natural motor system, may be a key factor in these learning differences (Jackson and Fetz, 2011). The mechanisms underlying learning may depend significantly upon the type of inputs the user controls. Moreover, learning and adaptation in the natural motor system may involve multiple learning mechanisms given its highly distributed and hierarchical nature. Exploring learning in these different types of interfaces may help elucidate plasticity, learning, and adaptation mechanisms at different levels of the CNS.

The differences in learning across interface types also highlights the importance of fully understanding subject-models and instructions used in BMIs and the systems they define. A variety of animal models have been used in motor BMI studies—some allow subjects to move unrestricted (Gilja et al., 2012), while others block movement either via restraints (Jarosiewicz et al., 2008; Velliste et al., 2008) or temporary paralysis (Moritz and Fetz, 2011; Ethier et al., 2012). This has caused debate in the community, primarily focused on identifying models that best inform translation to paralyzed individuals (Nuyujukian et al., 2011). However, these different models may also have an impact on BMI learning studies. Consider a motor BMI where the subject is allowed to move their body unrestricted during control. While the BMI system only uses neural activity to control the actuator, the subject can adopt a kinematic-level learning strategy. That is, they may learn the task as a transform mapping between their body's motion and the cursor, rather than learning the relationship between neural activity and cursor movement. Though both systems are interesting for studying learning, they may be solved in fundamentally different ways. Similarly, the context of BMI control, and its relationship to natural movement must also be considered. The presence of cognitive cues that distinguish BMI and natural movement contexts (e.g., movement restraints or removing the apparatus used for movement) could significantly shape learning strategies. Care must be taken to develop interface systems that are clearly defined.

FUTURE DIRECTIONS AND CONCLUSIONS

Use of BMI and other interface systems for studying learning is a nascent field. The latest developments clearly demonstrate their utility and potential. However, they only scratch the surface of many critical questions. There are many new avenues of exploration in BMI learning that have not yet been addressed.

RELATING BMI LEARNING TO MOTOR AND ABSTRACT LEARNING

One critical question is how the BMI learning observed in these early studies relates to well-documented types of motor learning, such as adaptation and skill-formation (Krakauer and Mazzoni, 2011). These types of learning are thought to have different underlying mechanisms and neural implementations. Connecting BMI learning to these well-documented and modeled forms of learning could both facilitate better understanding of the neural mechanisms driving different types of learning, as well as more formal study of BMI learning. Here, we have defined skill as learning proficient BMI control *de novo*, and adaptation as compensating for perturbations to a well-learned BMI system with proficient control. The underlying learning mechanisms in these systems, however, may not be directly associated with adaptation and skill as defined in the natural motor system. For instance, are tuning changes that accompanied neuroprosthetic skill acquisition in Ganguly and Carmena (2009) solely a reflection of the neural representations of skill? Or does learning neuroprosthetic skill involve multiple learning mechanisms? Early learning could be driven by adaptation, where subjects modify existing neural patterns from their natural motor repertoire, reflected by tuning changes. Later refinements of control, however, might be more similar to skill formation, with increased precision of recruited neural activity patterns, consistent with the highly stable tuning maps observed in late learning.

Addressing these questions will require better understanding of *how* subjects learn BMI transforms. A particularly important question is if and how BMI learning is linked to natural movement. While BMIs can be controlled without overt movements, their relationship to movement and the natural system is unclear. Are BMIs controlled by repurposing existing motor repertoires, or via direct operant conditioning of neural activity to create new neural networks—or some combination? Understanding BMI's relationship to the natural motor system will be critical for teasing apart the underlying mechanisms involved in BMI learning and relating them to those of natural motor learning. Better understanding this relationship is also crucial for relating neuroprosthetic skill (BMI learning irrespective of movement) to abstract skills.

Existing studies provide mixed evidence for how BMI control relates to the natural motor system. A recent study by Hwang et al. (2013) explored control strategies in a discrete-control BMI system driven by neural activity from the parietal reach region (PRR). The experimenters used the well-established visuomotor properties of PRR neurons to probe the strategy used to learn different decoders to select one of two possible actions. Their results suggested that subjects solved the task by aiming to alternate targets in order to select the desired target location. That is, BMI control relied explicitly on natural motor strategies. This strategy was further suggested by persistent activity of neurons not directly contributing to the target selection, which would not be expected by operant conditioning-based learning. Interestingly, these results differ substantially from studies with continuous-control BMIs, where long-term learning was accompanied by differential modulation of BMI units within motor cortex (Ganguly et al., 2011) and striatal interactions specific to BMI output neurons (Koralek et al., 2013). Similarly, decoder perturbation studies in motor cortices suggest that learning was not limited to global re-aiming strategies alone (Jarosiewicz et al., 2008; Chase et al., 2012). While these observations do not pre-clude the possibility that BMI learning is shaped by the natural motor repertoire, they strongly suggest that BMIs may create new neural networks rather than purely repurposing established ones. However, learning arbitrary decoders has been shown to require similar neural structures to that of natural motor learning, like the striatum (Koralek et al., 2012). BMI learning, then, may still leverage similar neural circuitry to that of the natural motor system.

Differences in learning across these studies highlights the need for careful consideration of the BMI system and task design, and how they may influence learning. These studies differed in both the brain areas used (PRR versus primary- and pre-motor cortex) and the types of feedback provided (discrete versus continuous), both of which may strongly influence learning. The type of feedback and subject instructions, in particular, can significantly influence learning in the natural motor system (Krakauer and Mazzoni, 2011; Taylor and Ivry, 2011). The type of feedback provided in BMI has also been shown to significantly impact learning, as rats were unable to learn a novel BMI task without continuous feedback (Koralek et al., 2012). If and how BMI learning is influenced by the brain area(s) used for control is also an open and interesting question—one that may be particularly important for understanding BMI learning's relationship to abstract skills. Much like natural motor tasks, BMI learning may be shaped by system properties such as the control signals, feedback, and subject instructions. Careful manipulations of these properties may be particularly important to fully elucidate the mechanisms of BMI learning.

FURTHER OPEN QUESTIONS IN BMI LEARNING

The brain can learn arbitrary transforms, as evidenced by many demonstrations of non-biomimetic interface learning (Fetz, 1969, 2007; Radhakrishnan et al., 2008; Ganguly and Carmena, 2009; O'Doherty et al., 2011). The limits of such transform learning, however, are unclear. The majority of neurons in motor cortices can be modulated via biofeedback (Moritz and Fetz, 2011), but it is unknown if there are constraints on coordinated network activity that might limit transform learning. Exploring the relationship between BMI decoders and neural changes during learning may shed light on these questions. Does neural activity reach an "optimal" solution to a decoder, or do network dynamics limit adaptation? Similarly, little is known about how the structure of a transform influences learning. Are some decoder or encoder structures more readily learned? Does the relationship to natural representations matter? Is learning dependent on the neural ensembles and brain areas used for control? Exploring the relationship between transform structure, neural inputs, and learning might further elucidate how the CNS learns such mappings. This may also be particularly important for relating BMI learning to that of the natural motor system and abstract learning as noted above.

Combining BMI transform learning with established motor learning paradigms and physiological techniques will also better elucidate the neural substrates of skills. Interference and disruption of partially-consolidated motor memories is a well-studied and fascinating phenomenon (Krakauer and Shadmehr, 2006). What are the physiological mechanisms of skill consolidation and disruption? Neuroprosthetic skill learning shows clear parallels to motor learning and consolidation (Ganguly and Carmena, 2009; Ganguly et al., 2011). Exploring the physiological differences— for instance, synaptic modifications—in networks between consolidated and non-consolidated BMI decoders may help identify the mechanisms of stable memory formation. Finding causal interventions that can perturb skill consolidation will also be essential. It may also be possible to use neural stimulation to modify and shape neural network structure (Jackson et al., 2006) and study the resulting effects on skill consolidation.

BMIs create novel functional circuits for action that can be carefully manipulated to study the mechanisms of skill learning. Exploring learning in BMIs can make great contributions to our understanding of motor and abstract skill learning. What's more, this knowledge may be particularly useful for developing rehabilitative and restorative therapies. For instance, understanding principles of transform learning and the underlying neural mechanisms may be particularly useful for developing rehabilitation strategies where subjects must relearn motor control (e.g., stroke). These insights will also help to design neuroprostheses that are easier to learn. Knowledge of the neural mechanisms of skill consolidation and disruption may also be essential for making BMIs that can be controlled in a variety of settings. The basic science and technological applications of BMI have a naturally symbiotic relationship.

REFERENCES

Berg, J. A., Dammann, J. F., Tenore, F. V., Tabot, G. A., Boback, J. L., Manfredi, L. R., et al. (2013). Behavioral demonstration of a somatosensory neuroprosthesis. *IEEE Trans. Neural Syst. Rehabil. Eng.* 21, 500–507. doi: 10.1109/tnsre.2013. 2244616

Carmena, J. M., Lebedev, M. A., Crist, R. E., O'Doherty, J. E., Santucci, D. M., Dimitrov, D. F., et al. (2003). Learning to control a brain-machine interface for reaching and grasping by primates. *PLoS Biol.* 1:e42. doi: 10.1371/journal. pbio. 0000042

Cerf, M., Thiruvengadam, N., Mormann, F., Kraskov, A., Quiroga, R. Q., Koch, C., et al. (2010). On-line, voluntary control of human temporal lobe neurons. *Nature* 467, 1104–1108. doi: 10.1038/nature09510

Chapin, J. K., Moxon, K. A., Markowitz, R. S., and Nicolelis, M. A. (1999). Real-time control of a robot arm using simultaneously recorded neurons in the motor cortex. *Nat. Neurosci.* 2, 664–670. doi: 10.1038/10223

Chase, S. M., Kass, R. E., and Schwartz, A. B. (2012). Behavioral and neural correlates of visuomotor adaptation observed through a brain-computer interface in primary motor cortex. *J. Neurophysiol.* 108, 624–644. doi: 10.1152/jn.00371. 2011

Collinger, J. L., Wodlinger, B., Downey, J. E., Wang, W., Tyler-Kabara, E. C., Weber, D. J., et al. (2012). High-performance neuroprosthetic control by an individual with tetraplegia. *Lancet* 381, 557–564. doi: 10.1016/s0140-6736(12)61816-9

Cunningham, J. P., Nuyujukian, P., Gilja, V., Chestek, C. A., Ryu, S. I., and Shenoy, K. V. (2011). A closed-loop human simulator for investigating the role of feedback control in brain-machine interfaces. *J. Neurophysiol.* 105, 1932–1949. doi: 10.1152/jn.00503.2010

Dadarlat, M., O'Doherty, J. E., and Sabes, P. N. (2012). Multisensory integration of vision and intracortical microstimulation for sensory substitution and augmentation. Presented at *Soc. Neurosci. Annual Meeting*, 2012, New Orleans, LA, Program No. 792.12/WW15.

Engelhard, B., Ozeri, N., Israel, Z., Bergman, H., and Vaadia, E. (2013). Inducing gamma oscillations and precise spike synchrony by operant conditioning via brain-machine interface. *Neuron* 77, 361–375. doi: 10.1016/j.neuron.2012.11. 015

Ethier, C., Oby, E. R., Bauman, M. J., and Miller, L. E. (2012). Restoration of grasp following paralysis through brain-controlled stimulation of muscles. *Nature* 485, 368–371. doi: 10.1038/nature10987

Fetz, E. E. (1969). Operant conditioning of cortical unit activity. *Science* 163, 955– 958. doi: 10.1126/science.163.3870.955

Fetz, E. E. (2007). Volitional control of neural activity: implications for braincomputer interfaces. *J. Physiol.* 579, 571–579. doi: 10.1113/jphysiol.2006. 127142

Fetz, E. E., and Finocchio, D. V. (1971). Operant conditioning of specific patterns of neural and muscular activity. *Science* 174, 431–435. doi: 10.1126/science.174. 4007.431

Fetz, E. E., and Finocchio, D. V. (1975). Correlations between activity of motor cortex cells and arm muscles during operantly conditioned response patterns. *Exp. Brain Res.* 23, 217–240. doi: 10.1007/bf00239736

Flint, R. D., Wright, Z. A., Scheid, M. R., and Slutzky, M. W. (2013). Long term, stable brain machine interface performance using local field potentials and multiunit spikes. *J. Neural Eng.* 10:056005. doi: 10.1088/1741-2560/10/5/ 056005

Gage, G. J., Ludwig, K. A., Otto, K. J., Ionides, E. L., and Kipke, D. R. (2005). Naive coadaptive cortical control. *J. Neural Eng.* 2, 52–63. doi: 10.1088/17412560/2/2/006

Gandolfo, F., Li, C., Benda, B. J., Schioppa, C. P., and Bizzi, E. (2000). Cortical correlates of learning in monkeys adapting to a new dynamical environment. *Proc. Natl. Acad. Sci. U S A* 97, 2259–2263. doi: 10.1073/ pnas.040567097

Ganguly, K., and Carmena, J. M. (2009). Emergence of a stable cortical map for neuroprosthetic control. *PLoS Biol.* 7:e1000153. doi: 10.1371/journal.pbio. 1000153

Ganguly, K., and Carmena, J. M. (2010). Neural correlates of skill acquisition with a cortical brain-machine interface. *J. Mot. Behav.* 42, 355–360. doi: 10. 1080/00222895.2010.526457

Ganguly, K., Dimitrov, D. F., Wallis, J. D., and Carmena, J. M. (2011). Reversible large-scale modification of cortical networks during neuroprosthetic control. *Nat. Neurosci.* 14 662–667. doi: 10.1038/nn.2797

Gilja, V., Nuyujukian, P., Chestek, C. A., Cunningham, J. P., Yu, B. M., Fan, J. M., et al. (2012). A high-performance neural prosthesis enabled by control algorithm design. *Nat. Neurosci.* 15, 1752–1757. doi: 10.1038/nn.3265

Golub, M. D., Yu, B. M., and Chase, S. M. (2012). Internal models engaged by braincomputer interface control. *Conf. Proc. IEEE Eng. Med. Biol. Soc.* 2012, 1327– 1330. doi: 10.1109/ EMBC.2012.6346132

Green, A. M., and Kalaska, J. F. (2011). Learning to move machines with the mind. *Trends Neurosci.* 34, 61–75. doi: 10.1016/j.tins.2010.11.003

Hochberg, L. R., Bacher, D., Jarosiewicz, B., Masse, N. Y., Simeral, J. D., Vogel, J., et al. (2012). Reach and grasp by people with tetraplegia using a neurally controlled robotic arm. *Nature* 485, 372–375. doi: 10.1038/ nature11076

Hochberg, L. R., Serruya, M. D., Friehs, G. M., Mukand, J. A., Saleh, M., Caplan, A. H., et al. (2006). Neuronal ensemble control of prosthetic devices by a human with tetraplegia. *Nature* 442, 164–171. doi: 10.1038/nature04970

Hwang, E. J., Bailey, P. M., and Andersen, R. A. (2013). Volitional control of neural activity relies on the natural motor repertoire. *Curr. Biol.* 23, 353–361. doi: 10. 1016/j.cub.2013.01.027

Jackson, A., and Fetz, E. E. (2011). Interfacing with the computational brain. *IEEE Trans. Neural Syst. Rehabil. Eng.* 19, 534–541. doi: 10.1109/TNSRE.2011. 2158586

Jackson, A., Mavoori, J., and Fetz, E. E. (2006). Long-term motor cortex plasticity induced by an electronic neural implant. *Nature* 444, 56–60. doi: 10. 1038/nature05226

Jarosiewicz, B., Chase, S. M., Fraser, G. W., Velliste, M., Kass, R. E., and Schwartz, A. B. (2008). Functional network reorganization during learning in a braincomputer interface paradigm. *Proc. Natl. Acad. Sci. U S A* 105, 19486–19491. doi: 10.1073/ pnas.0808113105

Kim, S.-P., Simeral, J. D., Hochberg, L. R., Donoghue, J. P., and Black, M. J. (2008). Neural control of computer cursor velocity by decoding motor cortical spiking activity in humans with tetraplegia. *J. Neural Eng.* 5, 455–476. doi: 10. 1088/1741-2560/5/4/010

Koralek, A. C., Costa, R. M., and Carmena, J. M. (2013). Temporally precise cell-specific coherence develops in corticostriatal networks during learning. *Neuron* 79, 865–872. doi: 10.1016/j. neuron.2013.06.047

Koralek, A. C., Jin, X., Long II, J.

D., Costa, R. M., and Carmena, J. M. (2012). Corticostriatal plasticity is necessary for learning intentional neuroprosthetic skills. *Nature* 483, 331–335. doi: 10.1038/nature10845

Koyama, S., Chase, S. M., Whitford, A. S., Velliste, M., Schwartz, A. B., and Kass, R. E. (2009). Comparison of brain–computer interface decoding algorithms in open-loop and closed-loop control. *J. Comput. Neurosci.* 29, 73–87. doi: 10. 1007/s10827-009-0196-9

Krakauer, J. W., and Mazzoni, P. (2011). Human sensorimotor learning: adaptation, skill, and beyond. *Curr. Opin. Neurobiol.* 21, 636–644. doi: 10.1016/j.conb.2011.06.012

Krakauer, J. W., Pine, Z. M., Ghilardi, M. F., and Ghez, C. (2000). Learning of visuomotor transformations for vectorial planning of reaching trajectories. *J. Neurosci.* 20, 8916–8924.

Krakauer, J. W., and Shadmehr, R. (2006). Consolidation of motor memory. *Trends Neurosci.* 29, 58–64. doi:10.1016/j.tins.2005.10.003

Leuthardt, E. C., Schalk, G., Wolpaw, J. R., Ojemann, J. G., and Moran, D. W. (2004). A brain-computer interface using electrocorticographic signals in humans. *J. Neural Eng.* 1, 63–71. doi:10.1088/1741-2560/1/2/001

Li, C. S., Padoa-Schioppa, C., and Bizzi, E. (2001). Neuronal correlates of motor performance and motor learning in the primary motor cortex of monkeys adapting to an external force field. *Neuron* 30, 593–607. doi:10.1016/s08966273(01)00301-4

Liu, X., Mosier, K. M., Mussa-Ivaldi, F. A., Casadio, M., and Scheidt, R. A. (2010). Reorganization of finger coordination patterns during adaptation to rotation and scaling of a newly learned sensorimotor transformation. *J. Neurophysiol.* 105, 454–473. doi: 10.1152/jn.00247.2010

London, B. M., Jordan, L. R., Jackson, C. R., and Miller, L. E. (2008). Electrical stimulation of the proprioceptive cortex (area 3a) used to instruct a behaving monkey. *IEEE Trans. Neural Syst. Rehabil. Eng.* 16, 32–36. doi: 10.1109/tnsre. 2007.907544

McFarland, D. J., and Wolpaw, J. R. (2011). Brain-computer interfaces for communication and control. *Commun. ACM* 54, 60–66. doi: 10.1145/1941487. 1941506

Millán, J. D. R., Galan, F., Vanhooydonck, D., Lew, E., Philips, J., and Nuttin, M. (2009). Asynchronous non-invasive brain-actuated control of an intelligent wheelchair. *Conf. Proc. IEEE Eng. Med. Biol. Soc.* 2009, 3361–3364. doi: 10. 1109/IEMBS.2009.5332828

Millán, J. del R., and Mouriño, J. (2003). Asynchronous BCI and local neural classifiers: an overview of the adaptive brain interface project. *IEEE Trans. Neural Syst. Rehabil. Eng.* 11, 159–161. doi: 10.1109/tnsre.2003.814435

Millán, J. D. R., Renkens, F., Mourino, J., and Gerstner, W. (2004). Noninvasive brain-actuated control of a mobile robot by human EEG. *IEEE Trans. Biomed. Eng.* 51, 1026–1033. doi: 10.1109/tbme.2004.827086

Moritz, C. T., and Fetz, E. E. (2011). Volitional control of single cortical neurons in a brain-machine interface. *J. Neural Eng.* 8:025017. doi: 10.1088/17412560/8/2/025017

Moritz, C. T., Perlmutter, S. I., and Fetz, E. E. (2008). Direct control of paralysed muscles by cortical neurons. *Nature* 456, 639–642. doi: 10.1038/nature07418 Mosier, K. M., Scheidt, R. A., Acosta, S., and Mussa-Ivaldi, F. A. (2005). Remapping hand movements in a novel geometrical environment. *J. Neurophysiol.* 94, 4362– 4372. doi: 10.1152/jn.00380.2005

Mussa-Ivaldi, F. A., and Danziger, Z. (2009). The remapping of space in motor learning and human-machine interfaces. *J. Physiol. Paris* 103, 263–275. doi: 10. 1016/j. jphysparis.2009.08.009

Nazarpour, K., Barnard, A., and Jackson, A. (2012). Flexible cortical control of taskspecific muscle synergies. *J. Neurosci.* 32, 12349–12360. doi: 10.1523/jneurosci.5481-11.2012

Nuyujukian, P., Fan, J. M., Gilja, V., Kalanithi, P. S., Chestek, C. A., and Shenoy, K. V. (2011). Monkey models for brain-machine interfaces: the need for maintaining diversity. *Conf. Proc. IEEE Eng. Med. Biol. Soc.* 2011, 1301–1305. doi: 10. 1109/IEMBS.2011.6090306

O'Doherty, J. E., Lebedev, M. A., Ifft, P. J., Zhuang, K. Z., Shokur, S., Bleuler, H., et al. (2011). Active tactile exploration using a brain-machine–brain interface. *Nature* 479, 228–231. doi: 10.1038/nature10489

Padoa-Schioppa, C., Li, C. R., and Bizzi, E. (2004). Neuronal activity in the supplementary motor area of monkeys adapting to a new dynamic environment. *J. Neurophysiol.* 91, 449–473. doi: 10.1152/jn.00876.2002

Paz, R., Boraud, T., Natan, C., Bergman, H., and Vaadia, E. (2003). Preparatory activity in motor cortex reflects learning of local visuomotor skills. *Nat. Neurosci.* 6, 882–890. doi: 10.1038/nn1097

Paz, R., and Vaadia, E. (2004). Learning-induced improvement in encoding and decoding of specific movement directions by neurons in the primary motor cortex. *PLoS Biol.* 2:E45. doi: 10.1371/journal.pbio.0020045

Radhakrishnan, S. M., Baker, S. N., and Jackson, A. (2008). Learning a novel myoelectric-controlled interface task. *J. Neurophysiol.* 100, 2397–2408. doi: 10. 1152/jn.90614.2008

Ranganathan, R., Adewuyi, A., and Mussa-Ivaldi, F. A. (2013). Learning to be lazy: exploiting redundancy in a novel task to minimize movementrelated effort. *J. Neurosci.* 33, 2754–2760. doi: 10.1523/jneurosci.1553-12. 2013

Romo, R., Hernández, A., Zainos, A., Brody, C. D., and Lemus, L. (2000). Sensing without touching: psychophysical performance based on cortical microstimulation. *Neuron* 26, 273–278. doi: 10.1016/s0896-6273(00)81156-3

Rouse, A. G., Williams, J. J., Wheeler, J. J., and Moran, D. W. (2013). Cortical adaptation to a chronic micro-electrocorticographic brain computer interface. *J. Neurosci.* 33, 1326–1330. doi: 10.1523/jneurosci.0271-12.2013

Sabes, P. N. (2011). Sensory integration for reaching: models of optimality in the context of behavior and the underlying neural circuits. *Prog. Brain Res.* 191, 195– 209. doi: 10.1016/B978-0-444-53752-2.00004-7

Schalk, G., Miller, K. J., Anderson, N. R., Wilson, J. A., Smyth, M. D., Ojemann, J. G., et al. (2008). Two-dimensional movement control using electrocorticographic signals in humans. *J. Neural Eng.* 5, 75–84. doi: 10.1088/17412560/5/1/008

Serruya, M. D., Hatsopoulos, N. G., Paninski, L., Fellows, M. R., and Donoghue, J. P. (2002). Instant neural control of a movement signal. *Nature* 416, 141–142. doi: 10.1038/416141a

Shadmehr, R., and Mussa-Ivaldi, F. A. (1994). Adaptive representation of dynamics during learning of a motor task. *J. Neurosci.* 14, 3208–3224.

Shadmehr, R., Smith, M. A., and Krakauer, J. W. (2010). Error correction, sensory prediction, and adaptation in motor control. *Annu. Rev. Neurosci.* 33, 89–108. doi: 10.1146/annurev-neuro-060909-153135

Shenoy, K. V., Sahani, M. A., and Churchland, M. M. (2013). Cortical control of arm movements: a dynamical systems perspective. *Annu. Rev. Neurosci.* 36, 337– 359. doi: 10.1146/annurev-neuro-062111-150509

Shmuelof, L., Krakauer, J. W., and Mazzoni, P. (2012). How is a motor skill learned? Change and invariance at the levels of task success and trajectory control. *J. Neurophysiol.* 108, 578–594. doi: 10.1152/jn.00856.2011

Suminski, A. J., Tkach, D. C., Fagg, A. H., and Hatsopoulos, N. G. (2010). Incorporating feedback from multiple sensory modalities enhances brain-machine interface control. *J. Neurosci.* 30, 16777–16787. doi: 10.1523/jneurosci.3967-10. 2010

Taylor, D. M., Helms-Tillery, S. I., and Schwartz, A. B. (2002). Direct cortical control of 3D neuroprosthetic devices. *Science* 296, 1829–1832. doi: 10.1126/science. 1070291

Taylor, J. A., and Ivry, R. B. (2011). Flexible cognitive strategies during motor learning. *PLoS Comp. Biol.* 7:e1001096. doi: 10.1371/journal.pcbi. 1001096

Taylor, D. M., Tillery, S. I. H., and Schwartz, A. B. (2003). Information conveyed through brain-control: cursor versus robot. *IEEE Trans. Neural Syst. Rehabil. Eng.* 11, 195–199. doi: 10.1109/tnsre.2003.814451

Tehovnik, E. J., Slocum, W. M., Smirnakis, S. M., and Tolias, A. S. (2009). Microstimulation of visual cortex to restore vision. *Prog. Brain Res.* 175, 347– 375. doi: 10.1016/s0079-6123(09)17524-6

Velliste, M., Perel, S., Spalding, M. C., Whitford, A. S., and Schwartz, A. B. (2008). Cortical control of a prosthetic arm for self-feeding. *Nature* 453, 1098–1101. doi: 10.1227/01. neu.0000335797.80384.06

Venkatraman, S., and Carmena, J. M. (2011). Active sensing of target location encoded by cortical microstimulation. *IEEE Trans. Neural Syst. Rehabil. Eng.* 19, 317–324. doi: 10.1109/tnsre.2011.2117441

Wander, J. D., Blakely, T., Miller, K. J., Weaver, K. E., Johnson, L. A., Olson, J. D., et al. (2013). Distributed cortical adaptation during learning of a brain-computer interface task. *Proc. Natl. Acad. Sci. U S A* 110, 10818–10823. doi: 10.1073/pnas. 1221127110

Weiland, J. D., and Humayun, M. S. (2008). Visual prosthesis. *Proc. IEEE* 96, 1076– 1084. doi: 10.1109/JPROC.2008.922589

Wilson, B. S., Finley, C. C., Lawson, D. T., Wolford, R. D., Eddington, D. K., and Rabinowitz, W. M. (1991). Better speech recognition with cochlear implants. *Nature* 352, 236–238. doi: 10.1016/0196-0709(91)90011-4

Wise, S. P., Moody, S. L., Blomstrom, K. J., and Mitz, A. R. (1998). Changes in motor cortical activity during visuomotor adaptation. *Exp. Brain Res.* 121, 285– 299. doi: 10.1007/s002210050462

Wolpaw, J. R., Birbaumer, N., McFarland, D. J., Pfurtscheller, G., and Vaughan, T. M. (2002). Brain-computer interfaces for communication and control. *Clin. Neurophysiol.* 113, 767–791. doi: 10.1016/S1388-2457(02)00057-3

Wolpaw, J. R., and McFarland, D. J. (2004). Control of a two-dimensional movement signal by a noninvasive brain-computer interface in humans. *Proc. Natl. Acad. Sci. U S A* 101, 17849–17854. doi: 10.1073/pnas.0403504101

Wolpert, D. M., Diedrichsen, J., and Flanagan, J. R. (2011). Principles of sensori-motor learning. *Nat. Rev. Neurosci.* 12, 739–751. doi: 10.1038/nrn3112

12

Control of breathing by interacting pontine and pulmonary feedback loops

Yaroslav I. Molkov[1,2], Bartholomew J. Bacak[1], Thomas E. Dick[3] and Ilya A. Rybak[1]*

[1] Department of Neurobiology and Anatomy, Drexel University College of Medicine, Philadelphia, PA, USA
[2] Department of Mathematical Sciences, Indiana University – Purdue University, Indianapolis, IN, USA
[3] Departments of Medicine and Neurosciences, Case Western Reserve University, Cleveland, OH, USA

Edited by:
Eberhard E. Fetz, University of Washington, USA

Reviewed by:
Ansgar Buschges, University of Cologne, Germany
Deborah Baro, Georgia State University, USA

*Correspondence:
Ilya A. Rybak, Department of Neurobiology and Anatomy, Drexel University College of Medicine, 2900 Queen Lane, Philadelphia, PA 19129, USA.
e-mail: ilya.rybak@drexelmed.edu

The medullary respiratory network generates respiratory rhythm via sequential phase switching, which in turn is controlled by multiple feedbacks including those from the pons and nucleus tractus solitarii; the latter mediates pulmonary afferent feedback to the medullary circuits. It is hypothesized that both pontine and pulmonary feedback pathways operate via activation of medullary respiratory neurons that are critically involved in phase switching. Moreover, the pontine and pulmonary control loops interact, so that pulmonary afferents control the gain of pontine influence of the respiratory pattern. We used an established computational model of the respiratory network (Smith et al., 2007) and extended it by incorporating pontine circuits and pulmonary feedback. In the extended model, the pontine neurons receive phasic excitatory activation from, and provide feedback to, medullary respiratory neurons responsible for the onset and termination of inspiration. The model was used to study the effects of: (1) "vagotomy" (removal of pulmonary feedback), (2) suppression of pontine activity attenuating pontine feedback, and (3) these perturbations applied together on the respiratory pattern and durations of inspiration (T_I) and expiration (T_E). In our model: (a) the simulated vagotomy resulted in increases of both T_I and T_E, (b) the suppression of pontine-medullary interactions led to the prolongation of T_I at relatively constant, but variable T_E, and (c) these perturbations applied together resulted in "apneusis," characterized by a significantly prolonged T_I. The results of modeling were compared with, and provided a reasonable explanation for, multiple experimental data. The characteristic changes in T_I and T_E demonstrated with the model may represent characteristic changes in the balance between the pontine and pulmonary feedback control mechanisms that may reflect specific cardio-respiratory disorders and diseases.

Keywords: **respiratory central pattern generator, brainstem, ventrolateral respiratory column, pre-Bötzinger complex, pontine-medullary interactions, pulmonary feedback, control of breathing, apneusis**

INTRODUCTION

The respiratory rhythm and motor pattern controlling breathing in mammals are generated by a respiratory central pattern generator (CPG) located in the lower brainstem (Cohen, 1979; Bianchi et al., 1995; Richter, 1996; Richter and Spyer, 2001). The pre-Bötzinger complex (pre-BötC), located within the ventrolateral respiratory column (VRC) in the medulla, contains mostly inspiratory neurons (Smith et al., 1991; Rekling and Feldman, 1998; Koshiya and Smith, 1999). The pre-BötC, interacting with the adjacent Bötzinger complex (BötC), containing mostly expiratory neurons (Cohen, 1979; Ezure, 1990; Jiang and Lipski, 1990; Bianchi et al., 1995; Tian et al., 1999; Ezure et al., 2003), represents a core of the respiratory CPG (Bianchi et al., 1995; Tian et al., 1999; Rybak et al., 2004, 2007, 2008, 2012; Smith et al., 2007, 2009; Rubin et al., 2009; Molkov et al., 2010, 2011). This core circuitry generates primary respiratory oscillations defined by the intrinsic biophysical properties of respiratory neurons, the architecture of network interactions within and between the pre-BötC and BötC, and the inputs and drives from

other brainstem compartments, including the pons, retrotrapezoid nucleus (RTN), raphé, and nucleus tractus solitarii (NTS). It has been suggested (Rybak et al., 2007, 2008; Smith et al., 2007) that these external inputs and drives may have a specific spatial mapping onto respiratory neural populations within the pre-BötC/BötC core network, so that changes in these inputs or drives can alter the balance in excitation between key populations within the core network, thereby affecting their interactions and producing specific changes in the respiratory motor patterns observed under different conditions.

Most CPGs controlling rhythmic motor behaviors in invertebrates and vertebrates operate under control of multiple afferent feedbacks and often provide feedback to the sources of their descending and afferent inputs hence allowing feedback regulation of the descending and afferent control signals (Dubuc and Grillner, 1989; Ezure and Tanaka, 1997; Blitz and Nusbaum, 2008; Buchanan and Einum, 2008), and this regulation often operates via presynaptic inhibition (Nushbaum et al., 1997; Ménard et al., 2002; Côté and Gossard, 2003; Blitz and Nusbaum, 2008).

As in other CPGs, afferent feedbacks are involved in the control of the mammalian respiratory CPG and the generation and shaping of the breathing pattern. Many peripheral mechano- and chemo-sensory afferents, including those from the lungs, tracheo-bronchial tree and carotid bifurcation, provide feedback signals involving in the homeodynamic control of breathing, cardiovascular function, and different types of motor behaviors coordinated with breathing, such as coughing (see Loewy and Spyer, 1990, for review). The NTS is the major integrative site of these afferent inputs. The present study focuses on the mechanoreceptor feedback mediated by pulmonary stretch receptors (PSRs). These mechanoreceptors respond to mechanical deformations of the lungs, trachea, and bronchi, and produce a burst of action potentials during each breath, thereby providing the central nervous system with feedback regarding rate and depth of breathing (see Kubin et al., 2006, for review). Activation of PSRs elicits reflex effects including inspiratory inhibition or expiratory facilitation (representing the so-called Hering-Breuer reflex), enhancement of early inspiratory effort, bronchodilatation, and tachycardia. PSR axons travel within the vagus nerve, and form excitatory synapses in NTS pump cells (Averill et al., 1984; Backman et al., 1984; Berger and Dick, 1987; Bajic et al., 1989; Anders et al., 1993; Kubin et al., 2006). Pharmacological microinjection and lesion studies (McCrimmon et al., 1987; Ezure et al., 1991, 1998; Ezure and Tanaka, 1996, 2004; Kubin et al., 2006) suggest that NTS pump cells mediate the Hering-Breuer reflex (lung-inflation induced termination of inspiration). Through pump cells, PSR-originating information alters the activity of CPG neurons in manners consistent with their proposed roles in rhythm generation.

The other feedback loop, important for the respiratory CPG operation, involves multiple pontine-medullary interactions. The pons (Kölliker-Fuse nucleus, parabrachial nucleus, A5 area, etc.) contains neurons expressing inspiratory (I)-, inspiratory-expiratory (IE)-, or expiratory (E)-modulated activity, especially in vagotomized animals (Bertrand and Hugelin, 1971; Feldman et al., 1976; Cohen, 1979; Bianchi and St. John, 1982; St. John, 1987, 1998; Shaw et al., 1989; Dick et al., 1994, 2008; Jodkowski et al., 1994; Song et al., 2006; Segers et al., 2008; Dutschmann and Dick, 2012). This modulation is probably based on reciprocal connections between medullary and pontine respiratory regions which were described in a series of morphological studies (Cohen, 1979; Bianchi and St. John, 1982; Nunez-Abades et al., 1993; Gaytan et al., 1997; Zheng et al., 1998; Ezure and Tanaka, 2006; Segers et al., 2008). The principal source of pontine influence on the medulla is thought to be the Kölliker-Fuse region in the dorsolateral pons, although other areas, including those from the ventrolateral pons, are also involved (Bianchi and St. John, 1982; Chamberlin and Saper, 1994, 1998; Dick et al., 1994; Fung and St. John, 1994a,b,c; Jodkowski et al., 1994, 1997; Morrison et al., 1994; St. John, 1998; Rybak et al., 2004; Dutschmann and Herbert, 2006; Mörschel and Dutschmann, 2009; Dutschmann and Dick, 2012). Pontine activity contributes to the regulation of phase duration as demonstrated by stimulation and lesion studies (Cohen et al., 1993; Jodkowski et al., 1994, 1997; Okazaki et al., 2002; Cohen and Shaw, 2004; Rybak et al., 2004; Dutschmann and Herbert, 2006; Mörschel and Dutschmann, 2009; Dutschmann

and Dick, 2012). Stimulation of the Kölliker-Fuse or medial parabrachial nuclei induced a premature termination of inspiration (I-E transition) and extended expiratory phase. These effects were similar to the effects of vagal stimulation (Cohen, 1979; Hayashi et al., 1996). Also, the effects of both vagal and pontine stimulation appear to be mediated by the same medullary circuits that control onset and termination of inspiration (Haji et al., 1999; Okazaki et al., 2002; Rybak et al., 2004; Mörschel and Dutschmann, 2009; Dutschmann and Dick, 2012). Finally, the respiratory pattern in vagotomized animals with an intact pons is similar to that in animals without the pons and vagi intact. The above observations support the idea that the pontine nuclei mediate a function similar to that of the Hering-Breuer reflex.

Bilateral injections of NMDA antagonists (MK-801 and AP-5) into the rostral pons reversibly increase the duration of inspiration in vagotomized rats, and this increase is dose-dependent (Fung et al., 1994). This suggests that the rostral pons contains neurons with NMDA-receptors participating in the inspiratory off-switch mechanism. Morrison et al. (1994) showed that lesions of the parabrachial nuclei in the decerebrate, vagotomized, unanesthetized rat produced a significant (4-fold) increase in the duration of inspiration and a doubling of the duration of expiration, supporting a role for this pontine area in the regulation of the timing of the phases of respiration. This abnormal breathing pattern is known as apneusis. Administration of MK-801 into the rostral dorsolateral pons was shown to induce apneusis in vagotomized ground squirrels (Harris and Milsom, 2003). Systemic injection of MK-801 increases the inspiratory duration or results in an apneustic-like breathing in vagotomized and artificially ventilated rats (Foutz et al., 1989; Monteau et al., 1990; Connelly et al., 1992; Pierrefiche et al., 1992, 1998; Fung et al., 1994; Ling et al., 1994; Borday et al., 1998). Similarly, Jodkowski et al. (1994) showed that electrical and chemical lesions in the ventrolateral pons produced apneustic breathing in vagotomized rats. At the same time, apneustic breathing is not usually developed if the vagi remained intact and can be reversed by vagal stimulation, suggesting that NMDA receptors are not involved in the pulmonary (vagal) feedback mechanism.

Feldman et al. (1976) recorded cells in the rostral pons that exhibited respiratory modulation only when lung inflation, via a cycle-triggered pump, was stopped. The emergence of this respiratory-modulated activity suggests that afferent vagal input may have an inhibitory effect on the respiratory modulated cells in the pons (see also Feldman and Gautier, 1976; Cohen and Feldman, 1977). In the same work, it was noticed that this activity had no apparent influence on the tonic discharge of pontine neurons, suggesting that this inhibition might be presynaptic. Dick et al. (2008) recorded several hundred cells in the dorsolateral pons of decerebrate cats, artificially ventilated by a cycle-triggered pump before and after vagotomy. In their experiments, vagotomy led to either an emergence or facilitation of respiratory modulation in the pons. Sustained electrical stimulation of the vagus nerve elicited the classic Hering-Breuer reflex. Systemic or local blockade of NMDA receptors can result in an apneustic breathing pattern (Foutz et al., 1989; Connelly et al., 1992; Pierrefiche et al.,

1992, 1998; Fung et al., 1994; Ling et al., 1994; Borday et al., 1998) similar to that demonstrated by pontine lesions or transections.

The specifics of feedback control in the brainstem respiratory CPG is that the latter operates under control of two control loops (pulmonary and pontine ones), which both regulate key neural interactions within the CPG, thereby affecting the respiratory rate, respiratory phase durations and breathing pattern, and, at the same time, interact with each other so that each of them may dominate in the control of breathing depending on the conditions and/or the state of the system. Such feedback interactions and a

state-dependent feedback control of the CPG may have broader implication in other CPGs in vertebrates and/or invertebrates.

Specifically, our study focuses on the following major feedback loops involved in the control of breathing (**Figure 1A**): (1) the peripheral, pulmonary (vagal) loop that controls the medullary rhythm-generating kernel via afferent inputs from PSRs mediated by the NTS circuits, and (2) the pontine control loop, that provides pontine control of the respiratory rhythm and pattern. Our central hypothesis is that both the peripheral afferent and pontine-medullary loops control the respiratory frequency and

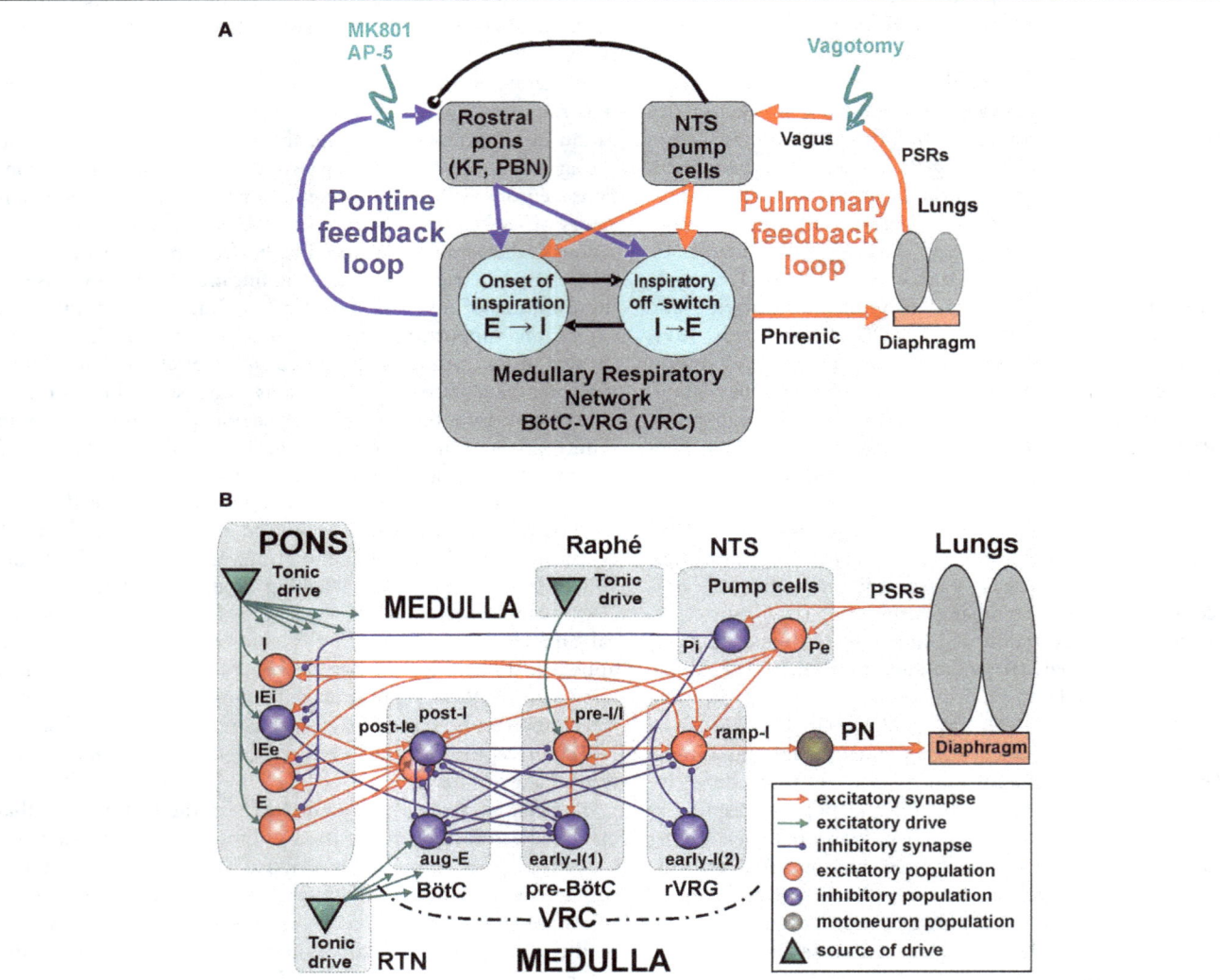

FIGURE 1 | The medullary respiratory network with pulmonary and pontine feedbacks. (A) A general schematic diagram representing the respiratory network with two interacting feedback. See text for details. **(B)** The detailing model schematic showing interactions between different populations of respiratory neurons within major brainstem compartments involved in the control of breathing (pons, BötC, pre-BötC, and rVRG) and the organization of pulmonary and pontine feedbacks. Each neural population (shown as a sphere) consists of 50 single-compartment neurons described in the Hodgkin-Huxley style. The model includes 3 sources of tonic excitatory drive located in the pons, RTN, and raphé—all shown as green triangles. These drives, project to multiple neural

populations in the model (green arrows; the particular connections to target populations are not shown for simplicity, but are specified in **Table A3** in the Appendix). See text for details. *Abbreviations:* AP-5, amino-5-phosphonovaleric acid, NMDA receptor antagonist; BötC, Bötzinger complex; e, excitatory; E, expiratory or expiration; i, inhibitory; I, inspiratory or inspiration; IE, inspiratory-expiratory; KF, Kölliker-Fuse nucleus; MK801, dizocilpine maleate, NMDA receptor antagonist; NTS, Nucleus Tractus Solitarii; P, pump cells; PBN, ParaBrachial Nucleus; PN, Phrenic Nerve; pre-BötC, pre-Bötzinger Complex; PSRs, pulmonary stretch receptors; RTN, retrotrapezoid nucleus; r, rostral; VRC, ventral respiratory column; VRG, ventral respiratory group.

phase durations via key medullary circuits responsible for the respiratory phase transitions (onset of inspiration, E-I, and inspiratory off-switch, I-E, see **Figure 1A**). In addition, these loops interact changing, balancing, and adjusting their control gain via interaction between NTS and VRC and pontine circuits. To investigate the involvement and potential roles of these feedback loops and their interactions with the medullary respiratory circuits we simulated the effects of suppression/elimination of each and both these feedbacks on the respiratory pattern and respiratory phase durations. The results of simulations were compared with the related experimental data and showed good qualitative correspondence hence providing important insights into feedback control of breathing.

METHODS
SIMULATION PACKAGE
All simulations in this study were performed using a neural simulation package NSM-3.0 developed at Drexel by Drs. Markin, Shevtsova, and Rybak and ported to the high-performance computer cluster systems running OpenMPI by Dr. Molkov. This simulation environment has been specifically developed and used for multiscale modeling and computational analysis of cross-level integration of: (a) the intrinsic biophysical properties of single respiratory neurons (at the level of ionic channel kinetics, dynamics of ion concentrations, synaptic processes, etc.); (b) population properties (synaptic interactions between neurons within and between populations with random distributions of neuronal parameters); (c) network properties (connectivity strength and type of synaptic interactions, with user-defined or random distribution of connections), (d) morpho-physiological structure (organization of interacting modules/compartments) (see Rybak et al., 2003, 2004, 2007, 2012; Smith et al., 2007; Baekey et al., 2010; Molkov et al., 2010, 2011). NSM-3.0 has special tools for simulation of various *in vivo* and *in vitro* experimental approaches, including suppression of specific ionic channels or synaptic transmission systems, various lesions/transections, application of various pharmacological, electrical and other stimuli to particular neurons or neural populations, etc.

MODELING BASIS: NEURONAL PARAMETERS AND IONIC CHANNEL KINETICS
The model presented in this paper continues a previously published series of models of neural control of respiration (Rybak et al., 2004, 2007; Smith et al., 2007; Baekey et al., 2010; Molkov et al., 2010, 2011) and, specifically, represents an extension of Smith et al. (2007) model. Following that model, each neuron type in the present model was represented by a population of 20–50 neurons. Each neuron was modeled as a single-compartment neuron described in the Hodgkin-Huxley (HH) style. These neuron models incorporated the currently available data on ionic channels in the medullary neurons and their characteristics. Specifically, the kinetic and voltage-gated and characteristics of fast (Na) and persistent (NaP) sodium channels in the respiratory brainstem were based on the studies of the isolated pre-BötC neurons in rats (Rybak et al., 2003). The kinetics and steady-state characteristics of activation and inactivation of high-voltage activated (CaL) calcium channels were based on the earlier

studies performed *in vitro* (Elsen and Ramirez, 1998) and *in vivo* (Pierrefiche et al., 1999). Temporal characteristics of intracellular calcium kinetics in respiratory neurons were drawn from studies of Frermann et al. (1999). Other descriptions of channel kinetics were derived from previous models (Rybak et al., 2007; Smith et al., 2007).

Heterogeneity of neurons within each population was set by a random distribution of some neuronal parameters and initial conditions to produce physiological variations of baseline membrane potential levels, calcium concentrations, and channel conductances. A full description of the model and its parameters can be found in the Appendix. All simulations were performed using the simulation package NSM 3.0 (see above). Differential equations were solved using the exponential Euler integration method with a step of 0.1 ms. We utilized the high-performance computational capabilities of the Biowulf Linux cluster at the National Institutes of Health, Bethesda, MD (http://biowulf.nih.gov).

MODEL ARCHITECTURE AND OPERATION IN NORMAL CONDITIONS
The main objective of this study was to investigate the mechanisms underlying control of the mammalian breathing pattern that is generated in the respiratory CPG circuits in the medulla and modulated by two major feedback loops, one involving interactions of medullary respiratory circuits with the lungs, and the other resulting from interactions of these circuits with the pontine circuits contributing to control of breathing (**Figure 1A**). We used an explicit computational modeling approach and focused on investigating the anticipated changes in the motor output (activity of the phrenic nerve, PN), specifically the changes in the duration of the inspiratory and expiratory phases under conditions of removal or suppression of the above feedback interactions (**Figure 1A**). The full schematic of our model is shown in **Figure 1B**. While developing this model, we used as a basis and extended the well-known large-scale computational model of the brainstem respiratory network developed by Smith et al. (2007). This basic model focused on the interactions among respiratory neuron populations within the medullary VRC. Similar to that model, the medullary respiratory populations in the present model (see **Figure 1B**) include (right-to-left): a ramp-inspiratory (ramp-I) population of pre-motor bulbospinal inspiratory neurons and an inhibitory early-inspiratory [early-I(2)] population—both in the rostral ventral respiratory group (rVRG); a pre-inspiratory/inspiratory (pre-I/I) and an inhibitory early-inspiratory [early-I(1)] populations of the pre-BötC; and an inhibitory augmenting-expiratory (aug-E) and inhibitory (post-I) and excitatory (post-Ie) post-inspiratory populations in the BötC. As suggested in the previous modeling studies (Rybak et al., 2004, 2007; Smith et al., 2007), these populations interact within and between the pre-BötC and BötC compartments and form a core circuitry of the respiratory CPG. In addition, multiple inputs and drives from other brainstem components, including the pons, RTN, NTS, and raphé affect interactions within this core circuitry and regulate its dynamic behavior and the motor output expressed in the activity of phrenic nerve (PN).

Respiratory oscillations in the basic and present models emerge within the BötC/pre-BötC core due to the dynamic interactions among: (1) the excitatory neural population, located in the pre-BötC and active during inspiration (pre-I/I); (2) the inhibitory population in the pre-BötC providing inspiratory inhibition within the network [early-I(1)]; and (3) the inhibitory populations in the BötC generating expiratory inhibition (post-I and aug-E). A full description of these interactions leading to the generation of the respiratory pattern can be found in previous publications (Rybak et al., 2004, 2007; Smith et al., 2007). Specifically, during expiration the activity of the inhibitory post-I neurons in BötC decreases because of their intrinsic adaptation properties (defined by the high-threshold calcium and calcium-dependent potassium currents) and augmenting inhibition from the aug-E neurons (**Figures 1B** and **2A,B**). At some moment, the pre-I/I neurons of pre-BötC release from the deceasing post-I inhibition and start firing (**Figure 2**) providing excitation to the inhibitory early-I(1) population of pre-BötC and the premotor excitatory ramp-I populations of rVRG (**Figure 1B**). The early-I(1) population inhibits all post-inspiratory and expiratory activity in the BötC leading to the

disinhibition of all inspiratory populations including the ramp-I hence completing the onset of inspiration (E-I transition). During inspiration early-I(1) inhibition of BötC expiratory neurons decreases due to intrinsic adaptation properties defined by the high-threshold calcium and calcium-dependent potassium currents (**Figure 2**). This decrease of inspiratory inhibition leads to the onset of expiration and termination of inspiration (inspiratory off-switch) (**Figure 2**). In the rVRG, the premotor ramp-I neurons receive excitation from the pre-I/I neurons and drive phrenic motoneurons and PN activity. The early-I(2) population shapes augmenting pattern of ramp-I neurons and PN. The PN projects to the diaphragm (**Figure 1B**) hence controlling changes in the lung volume (inflation/deflation) providing breathing.

The architecture of network interactions within the medullary VRC column (i.e., within and between the BötC, pre-BötC and rVRG compartments) in the present model is the same as in the preceding model of Smith et al. (2007). The extension of the basic model in the present study includes: (1) a more detailed simulation of the pontine compartment (in the Smith et al. model, the pontine compartment did not have neuron populations but

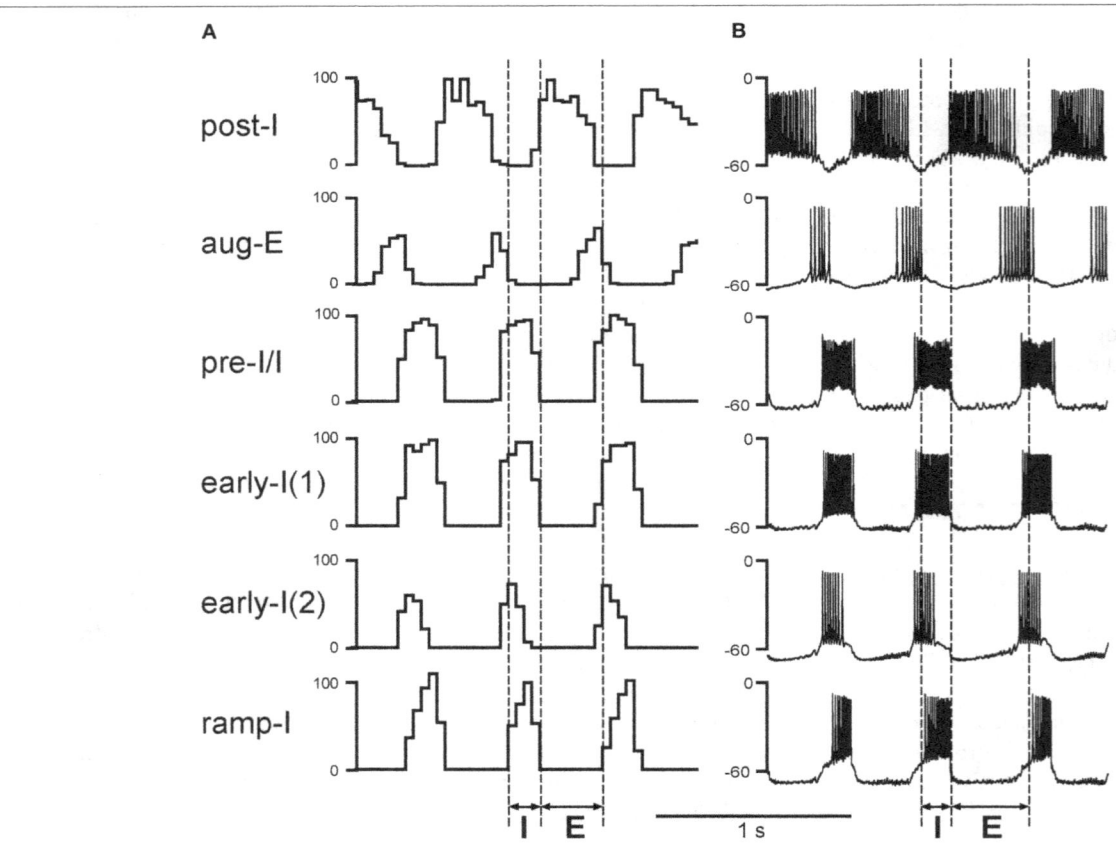

FIGURE 2 | Performance of the core medullary network under normal conditions (with both feedbacks intact). (A) The activity of main neural populations of the core respiratory network under normal conditions. The shown population activities include (top–down): post-inspiratory (post-I) and augmenting expiratory (aug-E) (both in BötC); pre-inspiratory/ inspiratory (pre-I/I) and early-inspiratory [early-I(1)] (both in pre-BötC);

early-inspiratory [early-I(2)] and ramp-inspiratory (ramp-I) (both in rVRG). The activity of each population is represented by the histogram of neuronal firing in the population (spikes/s; bin = 30 ms). **(B)** Traces of membrane potentials of the corresponding single neurons (randomly selected from each population). Vertical dashed line indicate the inspiratory (I) and expiratory (E) phases.

simply provided tonic drive to medullary respiratory populations), (2) incorporation of suggested interactions between the pontine and medullary populations that form the pontine control loop in the model (**Figures 1A,B**), and (3) incorporation of the pulmonary (vagal) control loop that included models of the lungs and pump cells in the NTS (**Figures 1A,B**).

PONTINE FEEDBACK LOOP

As shown in multiple studies in cats and rats, many pontine neurons (including those in the Kölliker-Fuse and parabrachial nuclei) exhibit respiratory modulated activity, specifically with I-, IE-, E-, or EI-related activity (Bertrand and Hugelin, 1971; Feldman et al., 1976; Cohen, 1979; Bianchi and St. John, 1982; St. John, 1987, 1998; Shaw et al., 1989; Dick et al., 1994, 2008; Jodkowski et al., 1994; Song et al., 2006; Segers et al., 2008; Dutschmann and Dick, 2012). These neurons may have respiratory modulated activity summarized with background tonic firing or may express a pure phasic respiratory activity (especially in rats, e.g., see Ezure and Tanaka, 2006; Song et al., 2006). These pontine respiratory-modulated activities are probably based on specific axonal projections and synaptic inputs from the corresponding medullary respiratory neurons (Cohen, 1979; Bianchi and St. John, 1982; Nunez-Abades et al., 1993; Gaytan et al., 1997; Zheng et al., 1998; Ezure and Tanaka, 2006; Segers et al., 2008). In turn, pontine neurons (including those in the Kölliker-Fuse and parabrachial nuclei) project back to the medullary respiratory neurons contributing to the control of the respiratory phase durations and phase switching (Okazaki et al., 2002; Cohen and Shaw, 2004; Rybak et al., 2004; Dutschmann and Herbert, 2006; Mörschel and Dutschmann, 2009; Dutschmann and Dick, 2012). These mutual interactions between pontine and medullary respiratory neurons form what we refer to as a pontine (or pontine-medullary) control loop.

To simulate the pontine feedback loop, we incorporated in the pontine compartment of the model the following populations (see **Figure 1B**): the excitatory populations of neurons with inspiratory-modulated (I), inspiratory-expiratory-modulated (IEe) and expiratory-modulated (E) activities, and the inhibitory population of neurons with an inspiratory-expiratory-modulated (IEi) activity. As described above, pontine neurons with such types of modulated activity were found in both rat and cat. However, the existing experimental data on intrapontine and pontine-medullary interactions are insufficient and do not provide exact information on the specific connections between these neuron types; they only suggest general ideas and principles for organization of these interactions, such as the possible reciprocal interconnections between the pontine and medullary neurons with similar respiratory-related patterns (see references in the previous paragraph) and the existence of pontine projections to key medullary neurons involved in the respiratory phase switching (such as post-I, see references above). Therefore in the model, respiratory modulation of neuronal activity in pontine populations was provided by excitatory inputs from the medullary respiratory neurons with the corresponding phases of activity within the respiratory cycle. Specifically, the inspiratory modulation activity in the pontine I population was provided by excitatory inputs from the medullary ramp-I population, the IE

modulation in the pontine IEe and IEi populations resulted from excitatory inputs from the medullary ramp-I and post-Ie populations, and the expiratory-modulation in the pontine E population was provided by inputs from the medullary post-Ie population. In addition, to simulate the presence of neurons with respiratory modulated phasic and tonic activities, each of the above four population was split into two equal subpopulations with neurons having the same properties and neuronal connections, but differed by tonic drive, which was received only by tonically active subpopulations (not shown in **Figure 1B**).

In turn, the pontine feedback in the model included (see **Figure 1B**): (1) excitatory inputs from the pontine I neurons (from both tonic and phasic subpopulations) to the medullary pre-I/I and ramp-I populations; (2) excitatory inputs from the pontine IEe neurons (both tonic and phasic subpopulations) to the medullary post-I population; (3) inhibitory inputs from the pontine IEi neurons (again both subpopulations) to the medullary early-I(1) population; and (4) excitatory inputs from the pontine E neurons (both subpopulations) to the medullary post-I, post-Ie, and aug-E populations. These neuronal connections from pons to medulla (especially pontine inputs to the medullary post-I and pre-I/I populations) allowed the pontine feedback to control operation of the respiratory network in the BötC/pre-BötC core and specifically to control the durations of the respiratory phases and phase switching. Specifically, the connection weights in the model were tuned so that (a) the durations of inspiration (T_I) and expiration (T_E) in the model without vagal feedback would be within the corresponding physiological ranges for the vagotomized rat *in vivo* ($T_I = 0.2$–0.55 s and $T_E = 0.8$–1.7 s, e.g., see Monteau et al., 1990; Connelly et al., 1992) and (b) after full suppression or removal of the pons, the value of T_I would dramatically increase (3–4 times or more) to be consistent with apneusis (Jodkowski et al., 1994; Morrison et al., 1994; Fung and St. John, 1995; St. John, 1998).

PULMONARY (VAGAL) FEEDBACK LOOP

The busting activity of phrenic motoneurons produces rhythmic inflation/deflation of the lungs, which in turn causes rhythmic activation of PSRs projecting back to the medullary respiratory network within the vagus nerve and hence providing pulmonary (vagal) feedback. The activity of pulmonary afferents in the medulla is relayed by the NTS pump (P) cells. To simulate pulmonary feedback loop, we incorporated simplified models of the lungs and PSRs, so that changes in the lung volume were driven by the activity of PN (see **Figures 1A,B**). The resultant lung inflation activates PSRs that projected back activating the excitatory (Pe) and inhibitory (Pi) pump cells populations in the NTS. The latter finally projected to the VRC and pons (**Figure 1B**). Hence in the model, both Pe and Pi populations were involved in the Hering-Breuer reflex preventing over-inflation of the lungs. Specifically (**Figure 1B**), the Pe population excited the post-I population, which was based on the previous experimental data that both lung inflation and electrical stimulation of the vagus nerve produced an additional activation of decrementing expiratory neurons (Hayashi et al., 1996). Following the previous model (Rybak et al., 2004) we suggested that vagal feedback inhibits the early-I(1) population (in this model, via the Pi population).

Both these interactions produced a premature termination of inspiration with switching to expiration and a prolongation of expiration.

INTERACTIONS BETWEEN THE LOOPS

As mentioned in the section "Introduction," the respiratory-modulated activity in the pons is usually much stronger in the absence of lung inflation and in vagotomized animals (e.g., see Feldman et al., 1976; Dick et al., 2008). One explanation for these effects is that the respiratory-modulated activity in the pons is suppressed by vagal afferents via NTS neurons projecting to the pons. There is indirect evidence that this suppression is based on presynaptic inhibition (Feldman and Gautier, 1976; Dick et al., 2008). Therefore in our model, this presynaptic inhibition is provided by the Pi population of NTS and affects all excitatory synaptic inputs from medullary to pontine neural populations (**Figure 1B**). Therefore, this presynaptic inhibition suppresses the respiratory modulation in the activities of pontine neurons and reduces the influence of pontine feedback on the medullary respiratory network operation and the respiratory pattern generated. Because of the lack of specific data, the synaptic weighs of connections from both pump cell populations (Pe and Pi) were set so that (a) significantly reduce the respiratory nodulation in all types of pontine neurons and (b) keep the durations of inspiration and expiration in simulations with vagal feedback intact within their physiological ranges for the rat *in vivo* ($T_I = 0.17$–0.3 s and $T_E = 0.3$–0.5 s, e.g., see Connelly et al., 1992).

SIMULATION OF VAGOTOMY (PULMONARY FEEDBACK REMOVAL)

Under normal conditions the "intact" model generated the respiratory pattern with the duration of inspiration $T_I = 0.189 \pm 0.046$ s and the duration of expiration $T_E = 0.388 \pm 0.064$ s (**Figures 2, 3A, 4A,** and **5A**). "Vagotomy" was simulated by breaking the pulmonary feedback, specifically by a removal of afferent inputs from PSRs to the pump cells in the NTS (**Figure 1A**). The resultant changes in the activity of different neural populations and in the output respiratory pattern in the model after simulated vagotomy are shown in **Figures 3B** and **4B**. As a result of vagotomy the pump cells (Pi and Pe populations) become silent (only the activity of Pi is shown in **Figures 3B** and **4B**; the activity of Pe population is similar, i.e., it also becomes silent). This eliminates the excitatory effect of lung inflation (PSR) on the post-I population (and post-Ie, pre-I/I, and ramp-I), mediated by Pe, and its inhibitory effect on the aug-E population, provided by Pi (**Figure 1B**). This also eliminates the pulmonary (vagal) control of respiratory phase switching and phase durations. However, this breaking of the pulmonary feedback also removes the presynaptic inhibition of all medullary inputs to pontine neural populations (provided in the intact case by the NTS's Pi population) hence increasing respiratory-modulated activities in the pontine neurons involved in the feedback control of the respiratory network operation (**Figures 1A,B**). This therefore increases the gain of pontine feedback and its role in the control of respiratory phase switching and phase durations. **Figure 3** shows that the vagotomy resulted in increases in the respiratory-modulated activity of pontine populations, a prolongation of inspiration ($T_I = 0.277 \pm 0.108$ s), and a dramatic increase in

the expiratory phase duration ($T_E = 0.938 \pm 0.065$ s). **Figure 4** shows that the applied vagotomy produced a significant increase of inspiratory (I), inspiratory-expiratory (IE), and expiratory (E) modulation in the activity of the corresponding pontine neurons with tonic activity and releases the corresponding firing in pontine neurons with phasic I, IE, and E activities not active in the intact case.

SIMULATION OF PONTINE FEEDBACK SUPPRESSION WITH AND WITHOUT PULMONARY FEEDBACK

A complete removal of the pons (i.e., a removal of pontine feedback) in the model with an intact pulmonary feedback produced a prolongation of inspiration ($T_I = 0.337 \pm 0.052$ s) and a slightly reduced in average (in comparison to the intact model) but highly variable expiratory duration ($T_E = 0.353 \pm 0.159$ s) characterized by occasional deletions of aug-E bursts (see **Figures 5B** and **6A**). To compare our simulations with the existing experimental data on the effects of pontine suppression by local injections of MK801, a blocker of NMDA receptors, that might not completely suppress the excitatory synaptic transmission in the pontine neurons and their activity, we also simulated a partial suppression of excitatory synaptic weights in the pontine compartment (e.g., by 25% see **Figure 6A**). Such partial suppression produced a visible prolongation of inspiration ($T_I = 0.262 \pm 0.028$ s with $T_E = 0.297 \pm 0.028$ s at 25% suppression, **Figure 6A**).

In contrast to pontine suppression with the intact pulmonary feedback, the same procedures after vagotomy led to a dramatic increase in the average duration of inspiration (making the inspiratory duration highly variable) at relatively constant duration of expiration (**Figures 5C** and **6A**). This prolongation of inspiration after vagotomy increased with the degree of pontine suppression (reducing the weights of excitatory synaptic inputs to pontine neurons) (**Figure 6A**) and accompanied by a suppression or full elimination of post-I activity and reduced amplitude of integrated PN (**Figure 5C**). Both these features are typical for apneusis (see Cohen, 1979; Wang et al., 1993; Jodkowski et al., 1994; Morrison et al., 1994; Fung and St. John, 1995; St. John, 1998). The durations of inspiration and expiration after vagotomy at different degrees of pontine suppression were the following: $T_I = 0.437 \pm 0.143$ s with $T_E = 0.433 \pm 0.030$ s at 25% suppression; $T_I = 0.885 \pm 0.339$ s with $T_E = 0.417 \pm 0.004$ s at 75% suppression; and $T_I = 571 \pm 0.310$ s with $T_E = 0.431 \pm 0.003$ s at 100% suppression.

The results of our simulations reflecting changes in T_I and T_E following different combinations of vagotomy with pontine suppression at different degrees are shown together in **Figure 6A**. Our general conclusions made from these simulations are the following. (1) A suppression of pontine activity with the intact pulmonary feedback leads to a moderate prolongation of inspiration, slight shortening of expiration, and an increase in variability of T_E (with 100% pontine suppression). (2) The simulated vagotomy (with the intact pontine-medullary interactions) causes a moderate prolongation of inspiration with an increase in variability of T_I and a strong prolongation of expiration. (3) Combination of both perturbations does not produce visible effects on T_E, but leads to a significant prolongation of inspiration (increasing with the degree of pontine suppression), increasing of T_I variability,

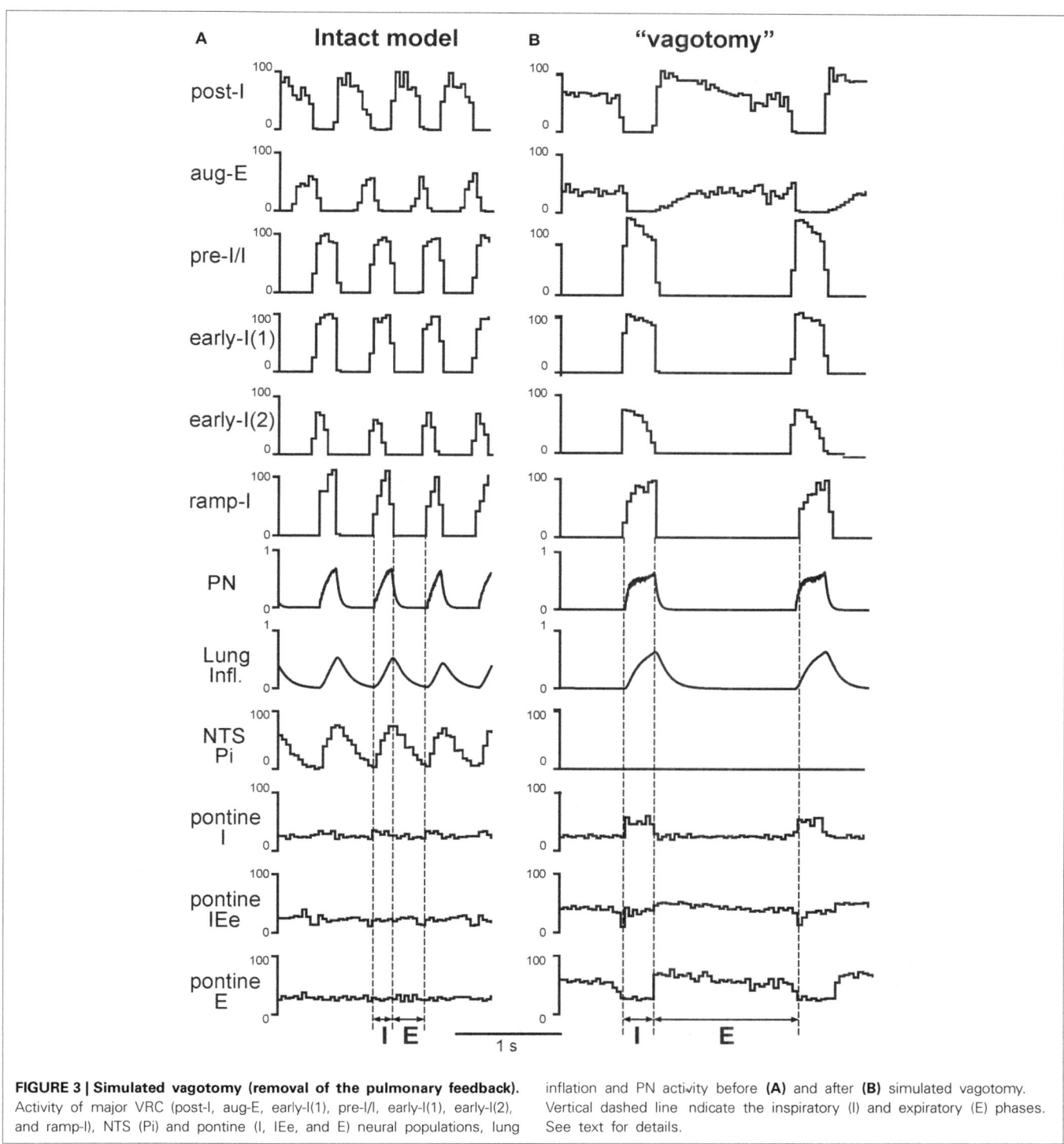

FIGURE 3 | Simulated vagotomy (removal of the pulmonary feedback). Activity of major VRC (post-I, aug-E, early-I(1), pre-I/I, early-I(1), early-I(2), and ramp-I), NTS (Pi) and pontine (I, IEe, and E) neural populations, lung inflation and PN activity before **(A)** and after **(B)** simulated vagotomy. Vertical dashed line ndicate the inspiratory (I) and expiratory (E) phases. See text for details.

and other typical characteristics of apneusis (suppressed post-I activity and reduced PN amplitude).

COMPARISON WITH EXPERIMENTAL DATA

To test our model, we performed simulation with 25%, 75%, and 100% suppression of the pontine control loop before and after simulated vagotomy (removal of the pulmonary feedback).

The resultant changes in T_I and T_E are shown in **Figure 6A**. To compare these simulation results with the related experimental data, we built similar diagrams from the early study of Connelly et al. (1992), which examined spontaneously breathing in Wistar rats during the administration of NMDA blocker MK-801 before and after vagotomy (**Figure 6B**). In this study, the experiments on Wistar rats (in contrast to the Sprague-Dawley strain) did not end

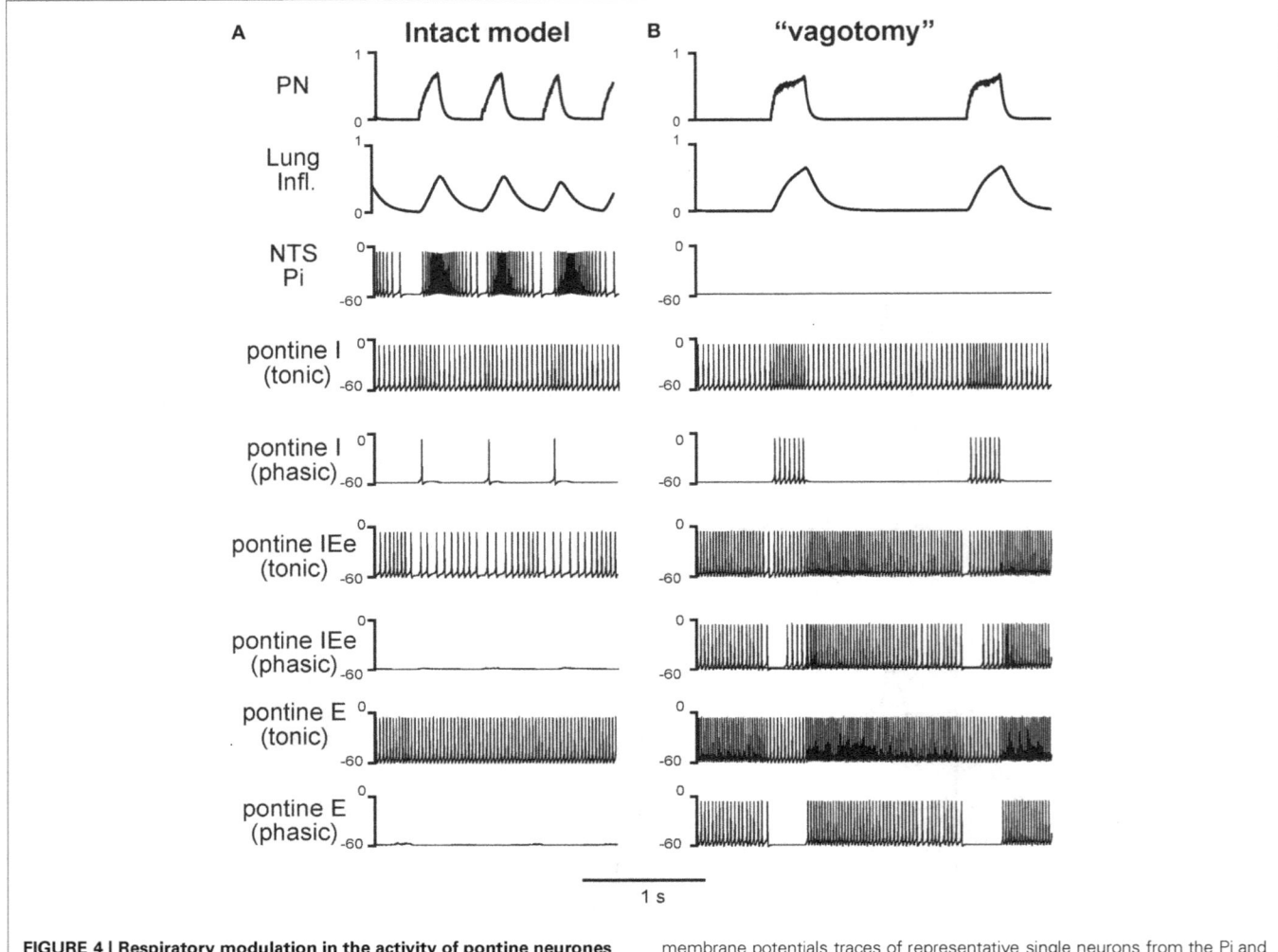

FIGURE 4 | Respiratory modulation in the activity of pontine neurones before (A) and after (B) simulated vagotomy. The changes of phrenic activity (PN) and the lung inflation are shown at the top. Below these graphs, membrane potentials traces of representative single neurons from the Pi and pontine populations (tonic and phasic subpopulations) are shown. See text for details.

with apneusis, due to (in our opinion) an insufficient suppression of the pontine feedback by the performed MK-801 injections. Nevertheless, the effects of vagotomy and MK-801 administration on T_I and T_E before and after vagotomy reported in Connelly et al. study are qualitatively similar to our simulations with 25% suppression of pontine feedback (see **Figures 6A,B**). Specifically, the 25% pontine suppression in our simulations and the administration of MK-801 in Connelly et al. experiments result in an increase of T_I and slight reduction of T_E before vagotomy and in a significant prolongation of inspiration after vagotomy. In addition, vagotomy alone without other perturbations in both cases results in an increase of T_I and significant prolongation of T_E (see **Figures 6A,B**). Moreover, the changes in the respiratory frequency and the shape and amplitude of integrated phrenic activity after vagotomy and/or pontine suppression in our model are similar to that in the experimental studies with MK-801 administration (**Figure 7**). The other comparison of our simulations was made with the experimental study of Monteau et al. (1990) performed in anaesthetized vagotomized rats by

using MK-801 administration, which results are summarized in **Figure 6C**. This study did demonstrate that MK-801 application after vagotomy produced switching from a normal breathing pattern to the typical apneusis. The relationships between T_I and T_E in our simulation after vagotomy and their changes following 100% pontine suppression (apneusis) are similar to these in the Monteau et al. study (see **Figures 6A,C**).

DISCUSSION

The results of our simulations promote the concept that both pulmonary and pontine feedback loops contribute to the control of the respiratory pattern and, specifically, the durations of inspiration (T_I) and expiration (T_E). Furthermore, our modeling results are consistent with the previous suggestion of specific interactions between these feedback loops, in particular that the PSR afferents involved in the pulmonary control of T_I and T_E attenuate the gain of the pontine control of these phase durations (via the presynaptic inhibition of excitatory inputs from medullary to pontine populations) (Feldman and Gautier, 1976;

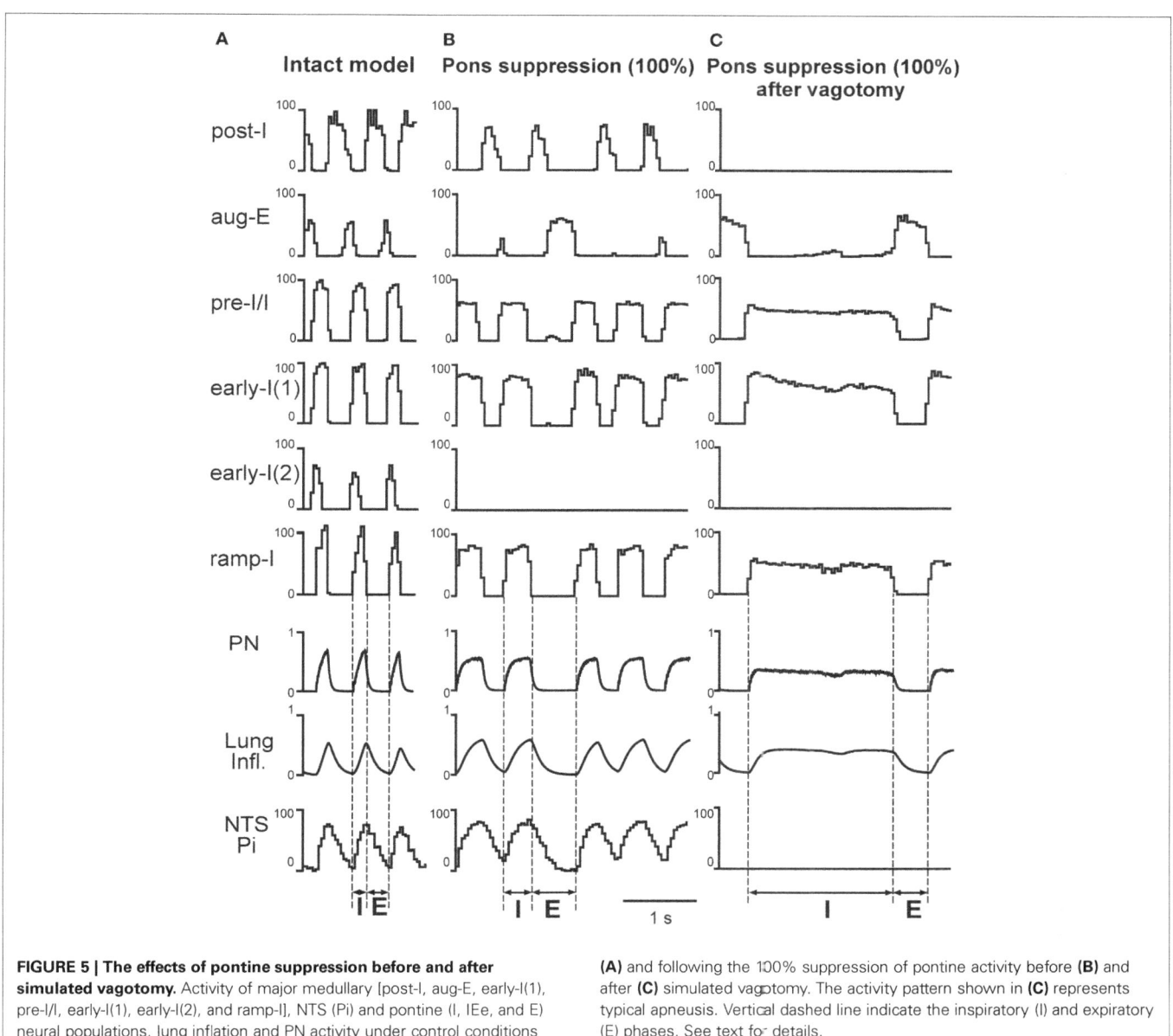

FIGURE 5 | The effects of pontine suppression before and after simulated vagotomy. Activity of major medullary [post-I, aug-E, early-I(1), pre-I/I, early-I(1), early-I(2), and ramp-I], NTS (Pi) and pontine (I, IEe, and E) neural populations, lung inflation and PN activity under control conditions (A) and following the 100% suppression of pontine activity before (B) and after (C) simulated vagotomy. The activity pattern shown in (C) represents typical apneusis. Vertical dashed line indicate the inspiratory (I) and expiratory (E) phases. See text for details.

Feldman et al., 1976; Cohen and Feldman, 1977; Cohen, 1979; Mörschel and Dutschmann, 2009). Nevertheless, according to our simulations, pontine activity still plays a role in the control of inspiration and expiration even when the pulmonary feedback is intact, although the gain of this pontine control is significantly reduced by the presynaptic inhibition. This presynaptic inhibition is expected to suppress the respiratory modulation in the activity of pontine neurons expressing either tonic or phasic firing patterns (Feldman and Gautier, 1976; Feldman et al., 1976; Cohen and Feldman, 1977; Cohen, 1979; St. John, 1987, 1998; Shaw et al., 1989; Dick et al., 1994, 2008; Song et al., 2006; Segers et al., 2008), which is reproduced by our model (**Figure 4**). Also, the model offers a plausible mechanistic explanation for the previous experimental findings that injection of NMDA antagonists in the dorsolateral pons (specifically in the Kölliker-Fuse area) leads to

a prolongation of inspiration and to apneusis in the case of a lack of pulmonary feedback (Foutz et al., 1989; Connelly et al., 1992; Pierrefiche et al., 1992, 1998; Fung et al., 1994; Ling et al., 1994; Bianchi et al., 1995; Borday et al., 1998; St. John, 1998).

In contrast to previous suggestions and models (Okazaki et al., 2002; Cohen and Shaw, 2004; Rybak et al., 2004; Dutschmann and Herbert, 2006; Mörschel and Dutschmann, 2009; Dutschmann and Dick, 2012), the mechanisms of action of the two feedbacks considered in the current model are not exactly symmetric. Excitatory inputs from both these feedbacks (from PSRs via the NTS's Pe cells, and from the pontine I, IEe, and E populations) activate the ramp-I, pre-I/I, post-Ie, and post-I medullary populations (see **Figure 1B**). The majority of these excitatory connections are the ones activating the inhibitory post-I population that controls the inspiratory off-switching, i.e., the timing

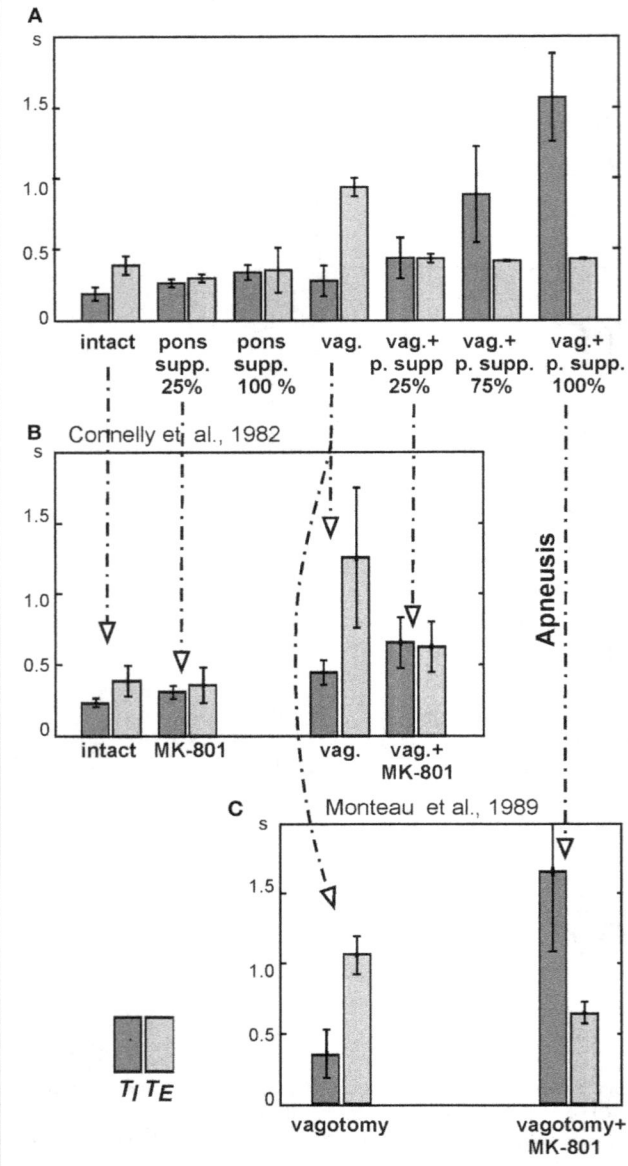

FIGURE 6 | Changes in the durations of inspiration (T_I) and expiration (T_E) following pontine suppression and/or vagotomy. (A) Changes in T_I and T_E following the simulated pontine suppression at different degrees (25%, 75%, and 100%) before and after (vag. +) vagotomy. **(B)** Changes in T_I and T_E in the study of Connelly et al. (1992): diagrams are built for spontaneously breathing Wistar rats under control conditions and after administration of NMDA blocker MK-801 before and after vagotomy. **(C)** Changes in T_I and T_E in the study of Monteau et al. (1990) performed in anaesthetized vagotomized rats using MK-801 administration.

the pontine neurons (**Figure 1B**). The organization of inhibitory inputs of these feedbacks to the medullary populations in the model is different. While the pulmonary feedback inhibits the aug-E population (via PSRs and Pi cells) causing a complex effect on the respiratory pattern, the pontine IEi population inhibits the early-I(1) population hence promoting expiration, which is clearly seen after vagotomy (**Figure 1B**).

It is important to mention that the current model of the medullary core respiratory circuits in the VRC (including the BötC, pre-BötC, and rVRG) used in our model was derived from the model of Smith et al. (2007) without significant changes. Starting with that first publication, this basic model (with necessary additions) was able to reproduce multiple experimental results, including the characteristic changes of the respiratory pattern following a series of pontine and medullary transections and effect of riluzole (persistent sodium current blocker) on the intact and sequentially reduced *in situ* preparation (Rybak et al., 2007; Smith et al., 2007), the emergence of the additional late-expiratory oscillations in the RTN/parafacial respiratory group (RTN/pFRG) during hypercapnia and interactions between the BötC/pre-BötC and RTN/pFRG oscillators (Abdala et al., 2009; Molkov et al., 2010), the effects of baroreceptor stimulation and the respiratory-sympathetic coupling including this following the intermittent hypoxia (Baekey et al., 2010; Molkov et al., 2011; Rybak et al., 2012), etc. The extended model described here was also able to reproduce the above behaviors, including the biologically plausible changes of membrane potentials and firing patterns of different respiratory neurons (**Figure 2B**). The ability of the extended model to reproduce the experimentally observed effects of the two feedback loops provides an additional support for the model of the core respiratory circuits used in all these previous models.

The exact mechanisms of pontine control of breathing are not well-understood and the pontine-medullary connections incorporated in the model are currently speculative. However, the general importance of the pons in the control of the respiratory pattern is well-recognized (see Dutschmann and Dick, 2012, for review). Studies utilizing the classic neurophysiological approaches of lesioning, stimulating and recording neurons have established that the lateral pons influences not only phase duration, phrenic amplitude, and response to afferent stimulation, but also the dynamic changes in respiratory pattern associated with persistent stimuli. For instance, blocking neural activity in the dorsolateral pons not only prolongs inspiration but also blocks the adaptation to vagal stimulation (Siniaia et al., 2000), and the shortening of expiration associated with repeated lung inflation (Dutschmann et al., 2009). Thus, the pons is not only intimately involved in the initial response to various stimuli, but also in the complex processes of accommodation and habituation. In the cardiovascular control system, parabrachial stimulation attenuates the NTS response to carotid sinus nerve stimulation by inhibition of NTS neurons receiving these inputs (Felder and Mifflin, 1988).

With normally operating pontine-medullary interactions, the simulated vagotomy results in a prolongation of inspiration and significant increase of the expiratory duration

of inspiratory phase termination and T_I, and those activating the excitatory pre-I/I population which, in a balance with the inputs to post-I, control the onset of inspiration (and T_E). However the effect of these excitatory inputs from the two feedbacks on the medullary circuitry is not identical and depends on the particular synaptic weights and the activity pattern of the inhibitory NTS's Pi cells providing presynaptic inhibition of medullary inputs to

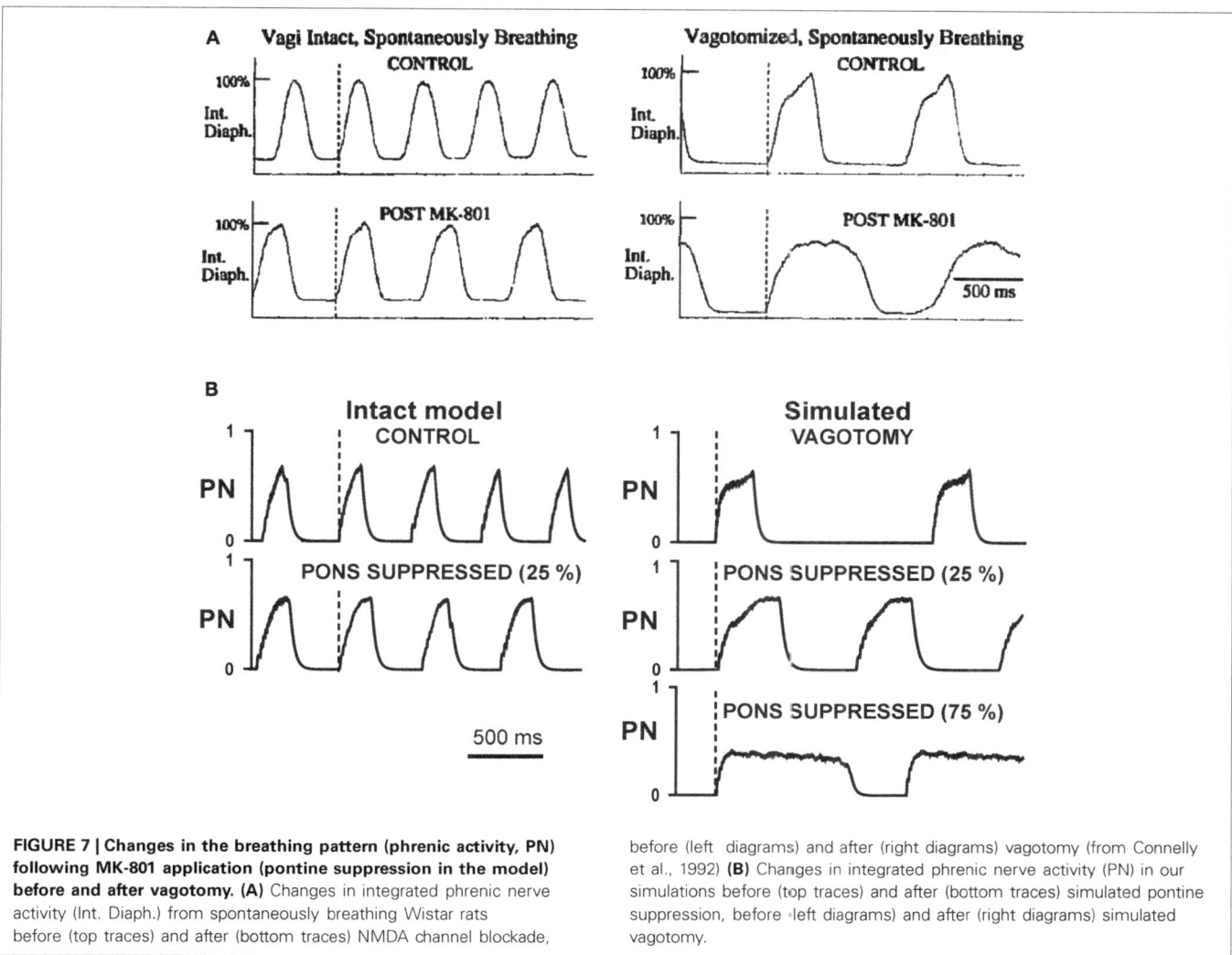

FIGURE 7 | Changes in the breathing pattern (phrenic activity, PN) following MK-801 application (pontine suppression in the model) before and after vagotomy. (A) Changes in integrated phrenic nerve activity (Int. Diaph.) from spontaneously breathing Wistar rats before (top traces) and after (bottom traces) NMDA channel blockade, before (left diagrams) and after (right diagrams) vagotomy (from Connelly et al., 1992) **(B)** Changes in integrated phrenic nerve activity (PN) in our simulations before (top traces) and after (bottom traces) simulated pontine suppression, before (left diagrams) and after (right diagrams) simulated vagotomy.

(**Figures 3B** and **6A**). However, despite these changes, the breathing pattern after vagotomy remains similar to that in eupnea (**Figure 3**). This maintenance of the eupneic breathing pattern occurs because the control performed by the pulmonary loop is now partly mimicked by the pontine loop, whose gain is increasing after vagotomy, as the latter removes the presynaptic inhibition of medullary inputs to pontine neurons (**Figure 1B**). Our model suggests that the pulmonary feedback yet performs the major function in the control of respiratory phase transitions and phase durations, and that a removal of this control loop places the full responsibility for this control on the pontine feedback loop.

The complementary role of the pontine and pulmonary feedbacks in control of phase duration (especially T_I) in our model is consistent with the classical interpretation of their function in respiratory control (see Dutschmann and Dick, 2012, for review). In particular, a premature termination of inspiration and switching to expiration can be elicited by stimulation of either the rostral pons or the pulmonary afferents (Bertrand and Hugelin, 1971; Cohen, 1979; Oku and Dick, 1992; Wang et al., 1993; St. John, 1998; Haji et al., 1999; Okazaki et al., 2002; Rybak et al., 2004;

Dutschmann and Herbert, 2006). This observation was explained by their common excitatory input on the post-inspiratory neurons in the medullary VRC which are critically involved in this phase transition (Okazaki et al., 2002; Rybak et al., 2004; Dutschmann and Herbert, 2006; Mörschel and Dutschmann, 2009).

Alternatively, our results suggest that the pontine-medullary feedback does not simply function as an "internal pulmonary feedback," performing a redundant function and compensating for the potential loss of vagal input. The specific increase in the variability of T_E with the suppression pontine activity and the significant prolongation of T_E after vagotomy (**Figure 6A**) indicate that the pontine and pulmonary feedbacks differ in the control of T_E. Indeed, our modeling results show that these control loops may complement each other in differential control of phase duration and breathing pattern variability. For example, an increase of T_E variability with pontine suppression, as seen in **Figures 5B** and **6A**, may be the case during various breathing disorders, such as sleep apnea or ventilator weaning (Tobin et al., 2012). In this connection, the stability of

T_E can be critically important and is primarily being controlled by the pons. Moreover, the Kölliker-Fuse area of the dorsolateral pons was explicitly identified to contribute to breathing disorders in a mouse model for a neurodevelopmental disease called Rett-syndrome (Stettner et al., 2007; Abdala et al., 2010).

Consistent with the many earlier and recent experimental data from cats and rats (Lumsden, 1923; Cohen, 1979; Wang et al., 1993; Jodkowski et al., 1994; Morrison et al., 1994; St. John, 1998), our simulations show that a strong pontine suppression (e.g., 75%) or its removal after vagotomy leads to apneusis, characterized by a significant increase of inspiratory duration and its variability (**Figures 5C** and **6A**). The other specific characteristics of apneusis are a lack of post-inspiratory activity and a reduction of phrenic amplitude during inspiration (Cohen, 1979; Wang et al., 1993; Jodkowski et al., 1994; Morrison et al., 1994; Fung

and St. John, 1995; St. John, 1998), which were reproduced in our simulations (**Figure 5C**).

Our understanding of interactions between individual components of complex systems is often insufficient to explain emergent properties of these systems. The present study elucidates the important role of two major feedback loops and interactions between them in regulation of the respiratory rate and breathing pattern allowing the brainstem respiratory network to maintain system's homeostasis and adjust breathing to various metabolic and physiologic demands.

ACKNOWLEDGMENTS

This study was supported by the National Institutes of Health: grants R33 HL087377, R33 HL087379, R01 NS057815, and R01 NS069220.

REFERENCES

Abdala, A. P., Dutschmann, M., Bissonnette, J. M., and Paton, J. F. (2010). Correction of respiratory disorders in a mouse model of Rett syndrome. *Proc. Natl. Acad. Sci. U.S.A.* 107, 18208–18213.

Abdala, A. P., Rybak, I. A., Smith, J. C., and Paton, J. F. (2009). Abdominal expiratory activity in the rat brainstem-spinal cord *in situ*: patterns, origins and implications for respiratory rhythm generation. *J. Physiol.* 587, 3539–3559.

Anders, K., Ohndorf, W., Dermietzel, R., and Richter, D. W. (1993). Synapses between slowly adapting lung stretch receptor afferents and inspiratory beta-neurons in the nucleus of the solitary tract of cats: a light and electron microscopic analysis. *J. Comp. Neurol.* 335, 163–172.

Averill, D. B., Cameron, W. E., and Berger, A. J. (1984). Monosynaptic excitation of dorsal medullary respiratory neurons by slowly adapting pulmonary stretch receptors. *J. Neurophysiol.* 52, 771–785.

Backman, S. B., Anders, C., Ballantyne, D., Rohrig, N., Camerer, H., Mifflin, S., et al. (1984). Evidence for a monosynaptic connection between slowly adapting pulmonary stretch receptor afferents and inspiratory beta neurones. *Pflugers Arch.* 402, 129–136.

Baekey, D. M., Molkov, Y. I., Paton, J. F., Rybak, I. A., and Dick, T. E. (2010). Effect of baroreceptor stimulation on the respiratory pattern: insights into respiratory-sympathetic interactions. *Respir. Physiol. Neurobiol.* 174, 135–145.

Bajic, J., Zuperku, E. J., and Hopp, F. A. (1989). Processing of pulmonary afferent input patterns by respiratory I-beta neurons. *Am. J. Physiol.* 256, R379–R393.

Berger, A. J., and Dick, T. E. (1987). Connectivity of slowly adapting pulmonary stretch receptors with dorsal medullary respiratory neurons. *J. Neurophysiol.* 58, 1259–1274.

Bertrand, F., and Hugelin, A. (1971). Respiratory synchronizing function of nucleus parabrachialis medialis: pneumotaxic mechanisms. *J. Neurophysiol.* 34, 189–207.

Bianchi, A. L., Denavit-Saubie, M., and Champagnat, J. (1995). Central control of breathing in mammals: neuronal circuitry, membrane properties, and neurotransmitters. *Physiol. Rev.* 75, 1–45.

Bianchi, A. L., and St. John, W. M. (1982). Medullary axonal projections of respiratory neurons of pontile pneumotaxic center. *Respir. Physiol.* 48, 357–373.

Blitz, D. M., and Nusbaum, M. P. (2008). State-dependent presynaptic inhibition regulates central pattern generator feedback to descending inputs. *J. Neurosci.* 28, 9564–9574.

Borday, V., Foutz, A. S., Nordholm, L., and Denavit-Saubie, M. (1998). Respiratory effects of glutamate receptor antagonists in neonate and adult mammals. *Eur. J. Pharmacol.* 348, 235–246.

Buchanan, J. T., and Einum, J. F. (2008). The spinobulbar system in lamprey. *Brain. Res. Rev.* 57, 37–45.

Chamberlin, N. L., and Saper, C. B. (1994). Topographic organization of respiratory responses to glutamate microstimulation of the parabrachial nucleus in the rat. *J. Neurosci.* 14, 6500–6510.

Chamberlin, N. L., and Saper, C. B. (1998). A brainstem network mediating apneic reflexes in the rat. *J. Neurosci.* 18, 6048–6056.

Cohen, M. I. (1979). Neurogenesis of respiratory rhythm in the mammal. *Physiol. Rev.* 59, 1105–1173.

Cohen, M. I., and Feldman, J. L. (1977). Models of respiratory phase-switching. *Fed. Proc.* 36, 2367–2374.

Cohen, M. I., Huang, W. X., Barnhardt, R., and See, W. R. (1993). Timing of medullary late-inspiratory neuron discharges: vagal afferent effects indicate possible off-switch function. *J. Neurophysiol.* 69, 1784–1787.

Cohen, M. I., and Shaw, C. F. (2004). Role in the inspiratory off-switch of vagal inputs to rostral pontine inspiratory-modulated neurons. *Respir. Physiol. Neurobiol.* 143, 127–140.

Connelly, C. A., Otto-Smith, M. R., and Feldman, J. L. (1992). Blockade of NMDA receptor-channels by MK-801 alters breathing in adult rats. *Brain Res.* 596, 99–110.

Côté, M.-P., and Gossard, J.-P. (2003). Task-dependent presynaptic inhibition. *J. Neurosci.* 23, 1886–1893.

Dick, T. E., Bellingham, M. C., and Richter, D. W. (1994). Pontine respiratory neurons in anesthetized cats. *Brain Res.* 636, 259–269.

Dick, T. E., Shannon, R., Lindsey, B. G., Nuding, S. C., Segers, L. S., Baekey, D. M., et al. (2008). Pontine respiratory-modulated activity before and after vagotomy in decerebrate cats. *J. Physiol.* 586, 4265–4282.

Dubuc, R., and Grillner, S. (1989). The role of spinal cord inputs in modulating the activity of reticulospinal neurons during fictive locomotion in the lamprey. *Brain Res.* 483, 196–200.

Dutschmann, M., and Dick, T. E. (2012). Pontine mechanisms of respiratory control. *Compr. Physiol.* 2443–2469.

Dutschmann, M., and Herbert, H. (2006). The Kolliker-Fuse nucleus gates the postinspiratory phase of the respiratory cycle to control inspiratory off-switch and upper airway resistance in rat. *Eur. J. Neurosci.* 24, 1071–1084.

Dutschmann, M., Morschel, M., Rybak, I. A., and Dick, T. E. (2009). Learning to breathe: control of the inspiratory-expiratory phase transition shifts from sensory- to central-dominated during postnatal development in rats. *J. Physiol.* 587, 4931–4948.

Elsen, F. P., and Ramirez, J. M. (1998). Calcium currents of rhythmic neurons recorded in the isolated respiratory network of neonatal mice. *J. Neurosci.* 18, 10652–10662.

Ezure, K. (1990). Synaptic connections between medullary respiratory neurons and considerations on the genesis of respiratory rhythm. *Prog. Neurobiol.* 35, 429–450.

Ezure, K., Otake, K., Lipski, J., and She, R. B. (1991). Efferent projections of pulmonary rapidly adapting receptor relay neurons in the cat. *Brain Res.* 564, 268–278.

Ezure, K., and Tanaka, I. (1996). Pump neurons of the nucleus of the solitary tract project widely to the medulla. *Neurosci. Lett.* 215, 123–126.

Ezure, K., and Tanaka, I. (1997). Convergence of central respiratory and locomotor rhythms onto single neurons of the lateral reticular nucleus. *Exp. Brain Res.* 113, 230–242.

Ezure, K., and Tanaka, I. (2004). GABA, in some cases together with glycine, is used as the inhibitory transmitter by pump cells in the Hering-Breuer reflex pathway of the rat. *Neuroscience* 127, 409–417.

Ezure, K., and Tanaka, I. (2006). Distribution and medullary projection of respiratory neurons in the dorsolateral pons of the rat. *Neuroscience* 141, 1011–1023.

Ezure, K., Tanaka, I., and Miyazaki, M. (1998). Inspiratory inhibition of pulmonary rapidly adapting receptor relay neurons in the rat. *Neurosci. Lett.* 258, 49–52.

Ezure, K., Tanaka, I., and Saito, Y. (2003). Brainstem and spinal projections of augmenting expiratory neurons in the rat. *Neurosci. Res.* 45, 41–51.

Felder, R. B., and Mifflin, S. W. (1988). Modulation of carotid sinus afferent input to nucleus tractus solitarius by parabrachial nucleus stimulation. *Circ. Res.* 63, 35–49.

Feldman, J. L., Cohen, M. I., and Wolotsky, P. (1976). Powerful inhibition of pontine respiratory neurons by pulmonary afferent activity. *Brain Res.* 104, 341–346.

Feldman, J. L., and Gautier, H. (1976). Interaction of pulmonary afferents and pneumotaxic center in control of respiratory pattern in cats. *J. Neurophysiol.* 39, 31–44.

Foutz, A. S., Champagnat, J., and Denavit-Saubie, M. (1989). Involvement of N-methyl-D-aspartate (NMDA) receptors in respiratory rhythmogenesis. *Brain Res.* 500, 199–208.

Frermann, D., Keller, B. U., and Richter, D. W. (1999). Calcium oscillations in rhythmically active respiratory neurones in the brain stem of the mouse. *J. Physiol.* 515, 119–131.

Fung, M. L., and St. John, W. M. (1994a). Electrical stimulation of pneumotaxic center: activation of fibers and neurons. *Respir. Physiol.* 96, 71–82.

Fung, M. L., and St. John, W. M. (1994b). Neuronal activities underlying inspiratory termination by pneumotaxic mechanisms. *Respir. Physiol.* 98, 267–281.

Fung, M. L., and St. John, W. M. (1994c). Separation of multiple functions in ventilatory control of pneumotaxic mechanisms. *Respir. Physiol.* 96, 83–98.

Fung, M. L., and St. John, W. M. (1995). The functional expression of a pontine pneumotaxic centre in neonatal rats. *J. Physiol.* 489(Pt 2), 579–591.

Fung, M. L., Wang, W., and St. John, W. M. (1994). Involvement of pontile NMDA receptors in inspiratory termination in rat. *Respir. Physiol.* 96, 177–188.

Gaytan, S. P., Calero, F., Nunez-Abades, P. A., Morillo, A. M., and Pasaro, R. (1997). Pontomedullary efferent projections of the ventral

respiratory neuronal subsets of the rat. *Brain Res. Bull.* 42, 323–334.

Haji, A., Okazaki, M., and Takeda, R. (1999). Synaptic interactions between respiratory neurons during inspiratory on-switching evoked by vagal stimulation in decerebrate cats. *Neurosci. Res.* 35, 85–93.

Harris, M. B., and Milsom, W. K. (2003). Apneusis follows disruption of NMDA-type glutamate receptors in vagotomized ground squirrels. *Respir. Physiol. Neurobiol.* 134, 191–207.

Hayashi, F., Coles, S. K., and McCrimmon, D. R. (1996). Respiratory neurons mediating the Breuer-Hering reflex prolongation of expiration in rat. *J. Neurosci.* 16, 6526–6536.

Jiang, C., and Lipski, J. (1990). Extensive monosynaptic inhibition of ventral respiratory group neurons by augmenting neurons in the Botzinger complex in the cat. *Exp. Brain Res.* 81, 639–648.

Jodkowski, J. S., Coles, S. K., and Dick, T. E. (1994). A 'pneumotaxic centre' in rats. *Neurosci. Lett.* 172, 67–72.

Jodkowski, J. S., Coles, S. K., and Dick, T. E. (1997). Prolongation in expiration evoked from ventrolateral pons of adult rats. *J. Appl. Physiol.* 82, 377–381.

Koshiya, N., and Smith, J. C. (1999). Neuronal pacemaker for breathing visualized *in vitro*. *Nature* 400, 360–363.

Kubin, L., Alheid, G. F., Zuperku, E. J., McCrimmon, D. R. (2006). Central pathways of pulmonary and lower airway vagal afferents. *J. Appl. Physiol.* 101, 618–627.

Ling, L., Karius, D. R., and Speck, D. F. (1994). Role of N-methyl-D-aspartate receptors in the pontine pneumotaxic mechanism in the cat. *J. Appl. Physiol.* 76, 1138–1143.

Loewy, A. D., and Spyer, K. M. (1990). *Central Regulation of Autonomic Functions*. New York, NY: Oxford University Press.

Lumsden, T. (1923). Observations on the respiratory centres in the cat. *J. Physiol.* 57, 153–160.

McCrimmon, D. R., Speck, D. F., and Feldman, J. L. (1987). Role of the ventrolateral region of the nucleus of the tractus solitarius in processing respiratory afferent input from vagus and superior laryngeal nerves. *Exp. Brain Res.* 67, 449–459.

Ménard, A., Leblond, H., and Gossard, J.-P. (2002). Sensory integration in presynaptic inhibitory pathways during fictive locomotion in the cat. *J. Neurophysiol.* 88, 163–171.

Molkov, Y. I., Abdala, A. P., Bacak, B. J., Smith, J. C., Paton, J. F., and

Rybak, I. A. (2010). Late-expiratory activity: emergence and interactions with the respiratory CPG. *J. Neurophysiol.* 104, 2713–2729.

Molkov, Y. I., Zoccal, D. B., Moraes, D. J., Paton, J. F., Machado, B. H., and Rybak, I. A. (2011). Intermittent hypoxia-induced sensitization of central chemoreceptors contributes to sympathetic nerve activity during late expiration in rats. *J. Neurophysiol.* 105 3080–3091.

Monteau, R., Gauthier, P., Rega, P., and Hilaire, G. (1990). Effects of N-methyl-D-aspartate (NMDA) antagonist MK-801 on breathing pattern in rats. *Neurosci. Lett.* 109, 134–139.

Morrison, S. F., Cravo, S. L., and Wilfehrt, H. M. (1994). Pontine lesions produce apneusis in the rat. *Brain Res.* 652, 83–86.

Mörschel, M., and Dutschmann, M. (2009). Pontine respiratory activity involved in inspiratory/expiratory phase transition. *Philos. Trans. R. Soc. B Biol. Sci.* 364, 2517–2526.

Nunez-Abades, P. A., Morillo, A. M., and Pasaro, R. (1993). Brainstem connections of the rat ventral respiratory subgroups: afferent projections. *J. Auton. Nerv. Syst.* 42, 99–118.

Nushbaum, M. P., El Manira, A., Cossard, J.-P., and Rossignol, S. (1997). "Presynaptic mechanisms during rhythmic activity in vertebrates and invertebrates," in *Neurons, Networks, and Motor Behavior*, eds P. S. G. Stein, S. Grillner, A. I. Selverston, and D. G. Stuart (Cambridge, MA: MIT Press), 237–253.

Okazaki, M., Takeda, R., Yamazaki, H., and Haji, A. (2002). Synaptic mechanisms of inspiratory off-switching evoked by pontine pneumotaxic stimulation in cats. *Neurosci. Res.* 44, 101–110.

Oku, Y., and Dick, T. E. (1992). Phase resetting of the respiratory cycle before and after unilateral pontine lesion in cat. *J. Appl. Physiol.* 72, 721–730.

Pierrefiche, O., Foutz, A. S., Champagnat, J., and Denavit-Saubie, M. (1992). The bulbar network of respiratory neurons during apneusis induced by a blockade of NMDA receptors. *Exp. Brain Res.* 89, 623–639.

Pierrefiche, O., Haji, A., Bischoff, A., and Richter, D. W. (1999). Calcium currents in respiratory neurons of the cat *in vivo*. *Pflugers Arch.* 438, 817–826.

Pierrefiche, O., Haji, A., Foutz, A. S., Takeda, R., Champagnat, J., and Denavit-Saubie, M. (1998).

Synaptic potentials in respiratory neurones during evoked phase switching after NMDA receptor blockade in the cat. *J. Physiol.* 508(Pt 2), 549–559.

Rekling, J. C., and Feldman, J. L. (1998). PreBotzinger complex and pacemaker neurons: hypothesized site and kernel for respiratory rhythm generation. *Annu. Rev. Physiol.* 60, 385–405.

Richter, D. W. (1996). "Neural regulation of respiration: rhythmogenesis and afferent control," in *Comprehensive Human Physiology*, eds R. Greger and U. Windhorst (Berlin: Springer-Verlag), 2079–2095.

Richter, D. W., and Spyer, K. M. (2001). Studying rhythmogenesis of breathing: comparison of *in vivo* and *in vitro* models. *Trends Neurosci.* 24, 464–472.

Rubin, J. E., Shevtsova, N. A., Ermentrout, G. B., Smith, J. C., and Rybak, I. A. (2009). Multiple rhythmic states in a model of the respiratory central pattern generator. *J. Neurophysiol.* 101, 2146–2165.

Rybak, I. A., Abdala, A. P., Markin, S. N., Paton, J. F., and Smith, J. C. (2007). Spatial organization and state-dependent mechanisms for respiratory rhythm and pattern generation. *Prog. Brain Res.* 165, 201–220.

Rybak, I. A., Molkov, Y. I., Paton, J. F., Abdala, A. P., and Zoccal, D. B. (2012). "Modeling the autonomic nervous system," in *Primer on the Autonomic Nervous System*, eds D. Robertson, I. Biaggioni, P. A. Burnstock, P. A. Lowe, and J. F. Paton (Oxford: Academic Press), 681–687.

Rybak, I. A., O'Connor, R., Ross, A., Shevtsova, N. A., Nuding, S. C., Segers, L. S., et al. (2008). Reconfiguration of the pontomedullary respiratory network: a computational modeling study with coordinated *in vivo* experiments. *J. Neurophysiol.* 100, 1770–1799.

Rybak, I. A., Paton, J. F. R., and Schwaber, J. S. (1997). Modeling neural mechanisms for genesis of respiratory rhythm and pattern: I. Models of respiratory neurons. *J. Neurophysiol.* 77, 1994–2006.

Rybak, I. A., Ptak, K., Shevtsova, N. A., and McCrimmon, D. R. (2003). Sodium currents in neurons from the rostroventrolateral medulla of the rat. *J. Neurophysiol.* 90, 1635–1642.

Rybak, I. A., Shevtsova, N. A., Paton, J. F., Dick, T. E., St. John, W. M., Mörschel, M., et al. (2004).

Modeling the ponto-medullary respiratory network. *Respir. Physiol. Neurobiol.* 143, 307–319.

Segers, L. S., Nuding, S. C., Dick, T. E., Shannon, R., Baekey, D. M., Solomon, I. C., et al. (2008). Functional connectivity in the pontomedullary respiratory network. *J. Neurophysiol.* 100, 1749–1769.

Shaw, C. F., Cohen, M. I., and Barnhardt, R. (1989). Inspiratory-modulated neurons of the rostrolateral pons: effects of pulmonary afferent input. *Brain Res.* 485, 179–184.

Siniaia, M. S., Young, D. L., and Poon, C. S. (2000). Habituation and desensitization of the Hering-Breuer reflex in rat. *J. Physiol.* 523(Pt 2), 479–491.

Smith, J. C., Abdala, A. P., Koizumi, H., Rybak, I. A., and Paton, J. F. (2007). Spatial and functional architecture of the mammalian brain stem respiratory network: a hierarchy of three oscillatory mechanisms. *J. Neurophysiol.* 98, 3370–3387.

Smith, J. C., Abdala, A. P., Rybak, I. A., and Paton, J. F. (2009). Structural and functional architecture of respiratory networks in the mammalian brainstem. *Philos. Trans. R. Soc. B Biol. Sci.* 364, 2577–2587.

Smith, J. C., Ellenberger, H. H., Ballanyi, K., Richter, D. W., and Feldman, J. L. (1991). Pre-Botzinger complex: a brainstem region that may generate respiratory rhythm in mammals. *Science* 254, 726–729.

Song, G., Yu, Y., and Poon, C. S. (2006). Cytoarchitecture of pneumotaxic integration of respiratory and nonrespiratory information in the rat. *J. Neurosci.* 26, 300–310.

St. John, W. M. (1987). Influence of pulmonary inflations on discharge of pontile respiratory neurons. *J. Appl. Physiol.* 63, 2231–2239.

St. John, W. M. (1998). Neurogenesis of patterns of automatic ventilatory activity. *Prog. Neurobiol.* 56, 97–117.

Stettner, G. M., Huppke, P., Brendel, C., Richter, D. W., Gartner, J., and Dutschmann, M. (2007). Breathing dysfunctions associated with impaired control of postinspiratory activity in Mecp2-/y knockout mice. *J. Physiol.* 579, 863–876.

Tian, G. F., Peever, J. H., and Duffin, J. (1999). Botzinger-complex, bulbospinal expiratory neurones monosynaptically inhibit ventral-group respiratory neurones in the decerebrate rat. *Exp. Brain Res.* 124, 173–180.

Tobin, M. J., Laghi, F., and Jubran, A. (2012). Ventilatory failure, ventilator support, and ventilator weaning. *Compr. Physiol.* 2, 2871–2921.

Wang, W., Brandle, M., and Zucker, I. H. (1993). Influence of vagotomy on the baroreflex sensitivity in anesthetized dogs with experimental heart failure. *Am. J. Physiol.* 265, H1310–H1317.

Zheng, Y., Riche, D., Rekling, J. C., Foutz, A. S., and Denavit-Saubie, M. (1998). Brainstem neurons projecting to the rostral ventral respiratory group (VRG) in the medulla oblongata of the rat revealed by co-application of NMDA and biocytin. *Brain Res.* 782, 113–125.

APPENDIX

SINGLE NEURON MODEL

All neurons were modeled in the Hodgkin-Huxley style as single-compartment models:

$$C \cdot \frac{dV}{dt} = -I_{Na} - I_{NaP} - I_K - I_{CaL} - I_{K,Ca} - I_L - I_{SynE} - I_{SynI},$$
(A1)

where V is the membrane potential, C is the membrane capacitance, and t is time. The terms in the right part of this equation represent ionic currents: I_{Na}—fast sodium (with maximal conductance $\bar{g}_{Na}$); I_{NaP}—persistent (slow inactivating) sodium (with maximal conductance $\bar{g}_{NaP}$); I_K—delayed rectifier potassium (with maximal conductance $\bar{g}_K$); I_{CaL}—high-voltage activated calcium (with maximal conductance $\bar{g}_{CaL}$); $I_{K,Ca}$—calcium-dependent potassium (with maximal conductance $\bar{g}_{K,Ca}$), I_L—leakage (with constant conductance g_L); I_{SynE} (with conductance g_{SynE}) and I_{SynI} (with conductance g_{SynI})—excitatory and inhibitory synaptic currents, respectively.

Currents are described as follows:

$$I_{Na} = \bar{g}_{Na} \cdot m_{Na}^3 \cdot h_{Na} \cdot (V - E_{Na});$$

$$I_{NaP} = \bar{g}_{NaP} \cdot m_{NaP} \cdot h_{NaP} \cdot (V - E_{Na});$$

$$I_K = \bar{g}_K \cdot m_K^4 \cdot (V - E_K);$$

$$I_{CaL} = \bar{g}_{CaL} \cdot m_{CaL} \cdot h_{CaL} \cdot (V - E_{Ca});$$

$$I_{K,Ca} = \bar{g}_{K,Ca} \cdot m_{K,Ca}^2 \cdot (V - E_K);$$
(A2)

$$I_L = g_L \cdot (V - E_L);$$

$$I_{SynE} = g_{SynE} \cdot (V - E_{SynE});$$

$$I_{SynI} = g_{SynI} \cdot (V - E_{SynI}),$$

where E_{Na}, E_K, E_{Ca}, E_L, E_{SynE}, and E_{SynI} are the reversal potentials for the corresponding channels.

Variables m_i and h_i with indexes indicating ionic currents represent, respectively, the activation and inactivation variables of the corresponding ionic channels. Kinetics of activation and inactivation variables is described as follows:

$$\tau_{mi}(V) \cdot \frac{d}{dt} m_i = m_{\infty i}(V) - m_i;$$

$$\tau_{hi}(V) \cdot \frac{d}{dt} h_i = h_{\infty i}(V) - h_i.$$
(A3)

The expressions for steady state activation and inactivation variables and time constants are shown in **Table A1**. The value of maximal conductances for all neuron types are shown in **Table A2**.

The kinetics of intracellular calcium concentration Ca is described as follows (Rybak et al., 1997):

$$\frac{d}{dt} Ca = -k_{Ca} \cdot I_{CaL} \cdot (1 - P_B) + (Ca_0 - Ca)/\tau_{Ca},$$
(A4)

where the first term constitutes influx (with the coefficient k_{Ca}) and buffering (with the probability P_B), and the second term

Table A1 | Steady state activation and inactivation variables and time constants for different ionic channels.

Ionic channels	$m_\infty(V)$, V in mV; $\tau_m V$), ms; $h_\infty(V)$, V in mV; $\tau_h(V)$, ms
Fast sodium Na	$m_{\infty Na} = 1/(1 + \exp(-(V + 43.8)/6));$ $\tau_{mNa} = \tau_{mNa\,max}/\cosh((V + 43.8)/14),\ \tau_{mNa\,max} = 0.252;$ $h_{\infty Na} = 1/(1 + \exp((V + 67.5)/10.8));$ $\tau_{hNa} = \tau_{hNa\,max}/\cosh((V + 67.5)/12.8),\ \tau_{hNa\,max} = 8.456$
Persistent sodium NaP	$m_{\infty NaP} = 1/(1 + \exp(-(V + 47.1)/3.1));$ $\tau_{mNaP} = \tau_{mNaP\,max}/\cosh((V + 47.1)/6.2),\ \tau_{mNaP\,max} = 1;$ $h_{\infty NaP} = 1/(1 + \exp((V + 60)/9));$ $\tau_{hNaP} = \tau_{hNaP\,max}/\cosh(V + 60)/9),\ \tau_{hNaP\,max} = 5000$
Delayed rectifier potassium K	$\alpha_{\infty K} = 0.01 \cdot (V + 44)/(1 - \exp(-(V + 44)/5));$ $\beta_{\infty K} = 0.17 \cdot \exp(-(V + 49)/40));$ $m_{\infty K} = \alpha_{\infty K}/(\alpha_{\infty K} + \beta_{\infty K}).$ $\tau_{mK} = \tau_{mK\,max}/(\alpha_{\infty K} + \beta_{\infty K}),\ \tau_{mK\,max} = 1$
High-voltage activated calcium Ca$_L$	$m_{\infty CaL} = 1/(1 + \exp(-(V + 27.4)/5.7));$ $\tau_{mCaL} = 0.5;$ $h_{\infty CaL} = (1 + \exp((V + 52.4)/5.2));$ $\tau_{hCaL} = 18$
Calcium-dependent potassium K(Ca^{2+})	$\alpha_{\infty K,Ca} = 1.25 \cdot 10^8 \cdot [Ca]_i^2,\ \beta_{\infty K,Ca} = 2.5;$ $m_{\infty K,Ca} = \alpha_{\infty K,Ca}/(\alpha_{\infty K,Ca} + \beta_{\infty K,Ca}).$ $\tau_{mk,Ca} = \tau_{mK,Ca\,max} \cdot 1000/(\alpha_{\infty K,Ca} + \beta_{\infty K,Ca}),$ $\tau_{mk\,max} = 0.7 - 1.0$

Table A2 | Maximal conductances of ionic channels in different neuron types.

Neuron type	$\bar{g}_{Na}$, nS	$\bar{g}_{NaP}$, nS	$\bar{g}_K$, nS	$\bar{g}_{CaL}$, nS	$\bar{g}_{K,Ca}$, nS	g_L, nS
pre-I	170	5.0	180			2.5
post-I, post-Ie	400		250	0.1	6.0	6.0
aug-E	400		250	0.1	3.0	6.0
early-I(1)	400		250	0.1	3.5	6.0
early-I(2)	400		250	0.1	11.0	6.0
All others	400		250			6.0

describes pump kinetics with resting level of calcium concentration Ca_0 and time constant τ_{Ca}.

$$P_B = B/(Ca + B + K),$$
(A5)

where B is the total buffer concentration and K is the rate parameter.

The calcium reversal potential is considered a variable and is a function of Ca:

$$E_{Ca} = 13.27 \cdot \ln(4/Ca) \text{ (at rest } Ca = Ca_0$$

$$= 5 \times 10^{-5} \text{ mM and } E_{Ca} = 150 \text{ mV}).$$
(A6)

The excitatory (g_{SynE}) and inhibitory synaptic (g_{SynI}) conductances are equal to zero at rest and may be activated (opened) by the excitatory or inhibitory inputs respectively:

$$g_{SynEi}(t) = \bar{g}_E \cdot F_i^{presyn} \cdot \sum_j S\{w_{ji}\} \cdot \sum_{t_{kj} < t} \exp\left(-\left(t - t_{kj}\right)/\tau_{SynE}\right)$$

$$+ \bar{g}_{Ed} \cdot \sum_m S\{w_{dmi}\} \cdot d_{mi};$$

$$g_{SynIi}(t) = \bar{g}_I \cdot \sum_j S\{-w_{ji}\} \cdot \sum_{t_{kj} < t} \exp\left(-\left(t - t_{kj}\right)/\tau_{SynI}\right)$$

$$+ \bar{g}_{Id} \cdot \sum_m S\{-w_{dmi}\} \cdot d_{mi}, \tag{A7}$$

where the function $S\{x\} = x$, if $x \geq 0$, and 0 if $x < 0$. In Equations (A7), each of the excitatory and inhibitory synaptic conductances has two terms. The first term describes the integrated effect of inputs from other neurons in the network (excitatory or inhibitory). The second term describes the integrated effect of inputs from external drives d_{mi}. Each spike arriving to neuron i from neuron j at time t_{kj} increases the excitatory synaptic conductance by $\bar{g}_E \cdot w_{ji}$ if the synaptic weight $w_{ji} > 0$, or increases the inhibitory synaptic conductance by $-\bar{g}_I \cdot w_{ji}$ if the synaptic weight $w_{ji} < 0$. $\bar{g}_E$ and $\bar{g}_I$ are the parameters defining an increase in the excitatory or inhibitory synaptic conductance, respectively, produced by one arriving spike at $|w_{ji}| = 1$. τ_{SynE} and τ_{SynE} are the decay time constants for the excitatory and inhibitory conductances respectively. In the second terms of Equation (A7), $\bar{g}_{Ed}$ and $\bar{g}_{Id}$ are the parameters defining the increase in the excitatory or inhibitory synaptic conductance, respectively, produced by external input drive $d_{mi} = 1$ with a synaptic weight of $|w_{dmi}| = 1$. All drives were set to 1.

Presynaptic inhibition is simulated as an attenuator of excitatory synapses by means of a factor $F^{presyn} \leq 1$. This factor is calculated according to the following equation:

$$F_i^{presyn} = \left(1 + \sum_j S\left\{-w_{ji}^p\right\} \cdot \sum_{t_{kj} < t} \exp\left(-\left(t - t_{kj}\right)/\tau_{SynI}\right)\right)^{-1}, \tag{A8}$$

where $w_{ji}^p \leq 0$ is the weight of presynaptic inhibitory connection that synapse i receives from neuron j. If a synapse i does not receive any presynaptic inhibition, then $w_{ji}^p = 0$ for and hence for this synapse $F_i^{presyn} = 1$.

The relative weights of synaptic connections (w_{ji}, w_{ji}^p, and w_{dmi}) are shown in **Table A3**.

The following neuronal and synaptic parameters were used:

$$C = 36\,\text{pF}; E_{Na} = 55\,\text{mV}; E_K = -94\,\text{mV}; E_{SynE} = -10\,\text{mV};$$

$$E_{SynI} = E_{Cl} = -75\,\text{mV};$$

$$\bar{g}_E = \bar{g}_I = \bar{g}_{Ed} = \bar{g}_{Id} = 1.0\,\text{nS}; \tau_{SynE} = 5\,\text{ms}; \tau_{SynI} = 15\,\text{ms};$$

$$Ca_0 = 5 \times 10^{-5}\,\text{mM}; k_{Ca} = 2 \times 10^{-5}\,\text{mM/C}; \tau_{Ca} = 250\,\text{ms},$$

$$B = 0.030\,\text{mM}; K = 0.001\,\text{mM}.$$

Table A3 | Weights of synaptic connections in the network.

Target population (location)	Excitatory drive (weight of synaptic input from this drive) or source population (from single neuron)
ramp-I (rVRG)	drive(Pons) (0.7); post-I (−1.0); aug-E(−0.15); pre-I /I (0.06); early-I(2) (−0.2); pontine I (0.2); Pe (0.115)
early-I(2) (rVRG)	drive(Pons) (2); post-I (−0.5); Pi (−0.15)
pre-I/I (pre-BötC)	drive(Pons) (0.03); drive(Raphe) (0.3); drive(RTN) (0.2); post-I (−0.1625); aug-E (−0.0275); pre-I /I (0.03); pontine I (0.2); Pe (0.025)
early-I(1) (pre-BötC)	drive(Pons) (0.75); drive(RTN) (2.03); post-I (−0.4); aug-E (−0.2); pre-I /I (0.04); pontine IEi (−0.15)
aug-E (BötC)	drive(Pons) (0.6); drive(RTN) (1.25); post-I (−0.09); early-I(1) (−0.135); Pi (−0.075)
post-I and post-Ie (BötC)	drive(Pons) (0.5); aug-E (−0.025); early-I(1) (−0.15); pontine IEe (0.35); pontine E (0.075); Pe (0.275)
pontine I (Pons)	drive(Pons) (0.25) (only to tonic subpopulation); ramp-I (0.025); Pi (−0.5^p)
pontine IEe and IEi (Pons)	drive(Pons) (0.2) (only to tonic subpopulations); ramp-I (0.03); post-Ie (0.05); Pi (−0.5^p)
pontine E (Pons)	drive(Pons) (0.3) (only to tonic subpopulations); post-Ie (0.05); Pi (−5.0^p)
Pe and Pi (NTS)	PSRs (1.0)
Phrenic Nerve (PN)	ramp-I (0.065)
Lungs	PN (1.2)
PSRs	Lungs (3.0)

Values in brackets represent relative weights of synaptic inputs from the corresponding source populations;
^{p}presynaptic inhibition.

MODELING NEURAL POPULATIONS

Each functional type of neuron in the model was represented by a population of 50 neurons. Connections between the populations were established so that, if a population A was assigned to receive an excitatory or inhibitory input from a population B or external drive D, then each neuron of population A received the corresponding excitatory or inhibitory synaptic input from each neuron of population B or from drive D, respectively. The pontine I, IEi, IEe, and E population represent an exception: only half of each population (the tonic subpopulation) receives tonic drive (see in the section "Pontine Feedback Loop"). To provide heterogeneity of neurons within neural populations, the value of E_L was randomly assigned from normal distributions using average value ± SD. Leakage reversal potential for all neurons (except for the pre-I ones) was $E_L = -60 \pm 1.2$ mV; for pre-I neurons $E_L = -68 \pm 1.36$ mV.

MODELING OF LUNGS, PN, AND PSR

The phrenic motoneuron population and phrenic nerve (PN) were not modeled. Integrated activity of the ramp-I population were considered as PN motor output. An increase in lung volume (lung inflation) V was modeled as a low-pass filter of PN activity:

$$\tau_V \cdot \frac{dV}{dt} = -V + w_{PN \to V} \cdot PN, \tag{A9}$$

where $\tau_V = 100$ ms is a lung time constant. The PSR output was considered proportional to the lung inflation V.

13

Closed-loop, multichannel experimentation using the open-source NeuroRighter electrophysiology platform

Jonathan P. Newman[1], Riley Zeller-Townson[1], Ming-Fai Fong[1,2], Sharanya Arcot Desai[1,3,4], Robert E. Gross[3,4,5] and Steve M. Potter[1]*

[1] Laboratory for Neuroengineering, Department of Biomedical Engineering, Georgia Institute of Technology and Emory University School of Medicine, Atlanta, GA, USA
[2] Department of Physiology, Emory University School of Medicine, Atlanta, GA, USA
[3] Department of Neurosurgery, Emory University School of Medicine, Atlanta, GA, USA
[4] Department of Neurology, Emory University School of Medicine, Atlanta, GA, USA
[5] Department of Biomedical Engineering, Georgia Institute of Technology and Emory University School of Medicine, Atlanta, GA, USA

Edited by:
Eberhard E. Fetz, University of Washington, USA

Reviewed by:
Yang Dan, University of California, Berkeley, USA
Stavros Zanos, University of Washington, USA

*Correspondence:
Steve M. Potter, Laboratory for Neuroengineering, Department of Biomedical Engineering, The Georgia Institute of Technology, 313 Ferst Drive, Atlanta, GA 30332, USA.
e-mail: steve.potter@bme.gatech.edu

Single neuron feedback control techniques, such as voltage clamp and dynamic clamp, have enabled numerous advances in our understanding of ion channels, electrochemical signaling, and neural dynamics. Although commercially available multichannel recording and stimulation systems are commonly used for studying neural processing at the network level, they provide little native support for real-time feedback. We developed the open-source NeuroRighter multichannel electrophysiology hardware and software platform for closed-loop multichannel control with a focus on accessibility and low cost. NeuroRighter allows 64 channels of stimulation and recording for around US $10,000, along with the ability to integrate with other software and hardware. Here, we present substantial enhancements to the NeuroRighter platform, including a redesigned desktop application, a new stimulation subsystem allowing arbitrary stimulation patterns, low-latency data servers for accessing data streams, and a new application programming interface (API) for creating closed-loop protocols that can be inserted into NeuroRighter as plugin programs. This greatly simplifies the design of sophisticated real-time experiments without sacrificing the power and speed of a compiled programming language. Here we present a detailed description of NeuroRighter as a stand-alone application, its plugin API, and an extensive set of case studies that highlight the system's abilities for conducting closed-loop, multichannel interfacing experiments.

Keywords: closed-loop, multichannel, real-time, multi-electrode, micro-electrode array, electrophysiology, open-source, network

1. INTRODUCTION

Multi-electrode neural interfacing systems, such as planar electrode arrays, silicon probes, and microwire arrays are commonly used to record spatially distributed neural activity *in vitro* and *in vivo*. Advances in nanoscale fabrication techniques have continued to push channel counts and electrode resolution (Du et al., 2011; Fiscella et al., 2012; Robinson et al., 2012), allowing for increasingly detailed measurements of network activity states. Because multi-electrode neural interfaces provide many parallel measurements, they can be used to rapidly estimate ensemble features of network activity (e.g., the population firing rate or network-level synchronization). This makes them well suited for real-time applications.

However, most commercial software interfaces for controlling multichannel hardware lack flexible support for real-time, bi-directional communication with neural tissue. Additionally, commercial software is often hard to integrate into complex multi-component experimental configurations. As a result, multichannel hardware has not been incorporated into closed-loop interfacing schemes to the degree of single-cell recording systems, such as voltage and dynamic clamp (Cole, 1949; Marmont, 1949; Hamill et al., 1981; Prinz et al., 2004; Arsiero et al., 2007; Kispersky et al., 2011). There are some exceptions to this trend (Jackson et al., 2006b; Azin and Guggenmos, 2011; Zanos et al., 2011). These systems are typically limited to low channel counts and/or low recording resolution in order to achieve embedded real-time processing at the recording site using a microcontroller or DSP. This approach has clear advantages for experiments on freely moving animals, but is limited in terms of input and output bandwidth, processing power to enable complex experimental protocols, and ease of programming. Neuroscience research would benefit from a multichannel acquisition platform that (1) enables bi-directional interaction with neuronal networks, (2) is practical for everyday use, (3) is straightforwardly extensible for complex closed-loop protocols, (4) works with a variety multi-electrode interfaces, (5) provides large channel counts and high recording resolution, and (6) is low cost. This type of system would be particularly applicable to three areas of neuroscience research:

- Feedback Control of Network Variables: Neuronal networks are complex systems with many recurrently interacting components. This often results in ambiguity in cause and effect relationships between network variables (Rich and Wenner, 2007; Turrigiano, 2011). Feedback control can be used to parse variables of neural activation that are causally linked (Cole, 1949). Feedback control of network-level variables (e.g., population firing rate, neuronal synchronization, or neurotransmission levels) can potentially clarify their causal relationships (Wagenaar et al., 2005; Wallach et al., 2011).

- Artificial Embodiment: Dissociated neural cultures, slice preparations, and anesthetized or paralyzed animals allow stable electrophysiological access but cannot engage in natural behaviors with their environment. By artificially embodying reduced neuronal preparations using a virtual environment or a robot, experimental access is maintained while neural tissue is engaged in complex behaviors (Reger et al., 2000; DeMarse et al., 2001; Ahrens et al., 2012).

- Clinical Applications: Responsive (Morrell, 2011) or predictive (Mormann et al., 2007) application of neural therapies have the potential to improve the efficacy and safety of treatments that are currently used in open-loop. Examples include brain stimulation and local drug perfusion techniques that are used to treat movement disorders, clinical depression, chronic pain, and epilepsy. Additionally, electrical stimuli delivered to one region of motor cortex in response to spiking activity in another motor area has been shown to facilitate a functional reorganization of motor output, indicating a potential role for activity-dependent stimulation in rehabilitation therapy (Jackson et al., 2006a).

Here, we present substantial improvements to NeuroRighter, an open-source, multichannel neural interfacing platform which we designed specifically to enable bi-directional, real-time communication with neuronal networks (Rolston et al., 2009a, 2010). In the first half of the paper, we provide a description of NeuroRighter's capabilities, including an application programming interface (API) that facilitates the creation of custom real-time experiment protocols. In the second half of the paper, we demonstrate these features with a variety of case studies. Each case-study highlights a different aspect of NeuroRighter's abilities in the areas of network-level feedback control, artificial embodiment, and closed-loop control of aberrant activity states in freely moving animals.

2. THE NEURORIGHTER MULTICHANNEL ELECTROPHYSIOLOGY PLATFORM

NeuroRighter is an open-source, low-cost multichannel electrophysiology system designed for bi-directional neural interfacing (Rolston et al., 2009a, 2010). A complete system, including all necessary electronics and a host computer, can be assembled for less than $10,000 USD. The NeuroRighter software is free. Extensive documentation on the construction and usage of a NeuroRighter system is available online[1]. NeuroRighter's source code, the API reference, and demonstration closed-loop protocol code, are available from the NeuroRighter code repository[2]. Questions on NeuroRighter assembly and usage can be submitted to the NeuroRighter-Users forum[3]. Tutorials on API usage are provided in sections 1 and 2 of the Supplementary Material.

2.1. HARDWARE

Here we provide a summary of NeuroRighter's hardware building blocks. Hardware components can be used with neural interfaces designed for applications both *in vivo* and *in vitro*. Printed circuit board (PCB) performance specifications are provided in (Rolston et al., 2009a) and layouts are available online. A complete NeuroRighter system meets or exceeds the performance of commercial alternatives in terms of noise levels, stimulation channel count, stimulation recovery times, and flexibility (Rolston et al., 2009a). NeuroRighter's PCBs are designed to be modular: electrode interfacing and stimulation PCBs have identical footprints and use vertical headers to route power between boards. This allows interfacing PCBs to be stacked on top of one another for increased channel counts and the use of a single DC power supply (or set of batteries) for all hardware.

2.1.1. ADC/DAC boards

NeuroRighter uses National Instruments (NI; National Instruments Corp, Austin, TX, USA) data acquisition hardware driven with NI's hardware control library, DAQmx. NI PCI-6259, PCIe-6259, PCIe-6353, and PCIe-6363 16-bit, 1 M sample/sec data acquisition cards are currently supported. Each card supports 32 analog inputs (AI), 4 analog outputs (AO), and 48 I/O-configurable digital channels. NI SCB-68 screw-terminal connector boxes are used to interface each data acquisition card with external hardware. Up to 3 cards can be used in a single NeuroRighter system to meet channel count requirements.

2.1.2. Multichannel amplifier interfacing boards

NeuroRighter provides two types of PCB to interface the NI data acquisition cards with multi-electrode amplifier systems. For *in vivo* applications, a 16-channel filter module provides 1.6X signal buffering, anti-aliasing filtering (−3 dB point at 8.8 KHz), DC offset subtraction (−3 dB point at 1 Hz), and regulated power to the headstage. Up to four of these modules can be stacked together in order to meet channel count requirements. For *in vitro* applications, a 68 channel conversion board provides power and signal routing for planar electrode array amplifier systems, e.g., Multichannel Systems' 60 channel amplifiers (Multichannel Systems, Reutlingen, Germany), which have a manufacturer settable pass-band. Both boards interface with the SCB-68 connector boxes using 34-channel ribbon cables, wired as signal/ground pairs to reduce capacitive crosstalk between adjacent lines during stimulation.

2.1.3. Electrical micro-stimulation hardware

NeuroRighter includes all-channel (up to 64 electrodes) stimulation capabilities for both *in vivo* and *in vitro* systems. This system is based upon the circuits presented in (Wagenaar and Potter, 2004; Wagenaar et al., 2004) and includes two separate PCBs: (1) a voltage- or current-controlled signal generation PCB, and (2) a

---

[1] https://sites.google.com/site/neurorighter/
[2] http://code.google.com/p/neurorighter/

[3] http://groups.google.com/group/neurorighter-users

signal multiplexing and isolation PCB to select different electrodes for stimulation and isolate recording electrodes from stimulation cables between stimulus pulses.

(1) *Signal generation board.* The signal generation PCB is identical for all applications. This board provides both voltage controlled or constant current stimulation modes. It stacks into the amplifier interfacing board(s) and therefore does not require an additional power source. Aside from stimulus generation, this PCB can be used to perform electrode impedance measurements, which are useful for diagnosing the health of micro-electrodes and their insulated leads, and for electroplating (Desai et al., 2010). Only one signal generation PCB is required for up to 64 electrodes.

(2) *Signal multiplexing boards.* Stimulus multiplexing and isolation occurs at PCBs that piggyback directly on electrode pre-amplifiers. These PCBs are located close to the initial stages of electrode amplification so that the recording amplifier can be isolated from long electrical leads, which reduces capacitive pickup. Because recording amplifiers (e.g., headstages *in vivo* or multichannel amplifiers *in vitro*) come in many shapes and sizes, the design of the multiplexer PCBs is application dependent. For *in vivo* applications, we have designed multiplexer systems that use an 18-pin Omnetics Nano connector, which interfaces with headstages from Triangle Biosystems (Durham, NC), Tucker-Davis Technologies (Alachua, FL), and Neurolinc Corporation (New York, NY), among others (Rolston et al., 2009a). This board employs a single 1-of-16 multiplexer. For *in vitro* applications, four separate multiplexing modules, each of which houses two 1-of-8 multiplexers, plug directly into exposed $0.1''$ pitch sockets of a 60 channel Multichannel Systems amplifier (Wagenaar and Potter, 2004). The creation of custom multiplexer boards or adapters for other systems is straightforward due to the simplicity of these PCBs (they generally consist of a single multiplexer integrated circuit).

2.1.4. Generic I/O

NeuroRighter provides 4 analog output channels and 32 bits of programmable digital I/O for controlling or recording digital signals from laboratory equipment. An auxiliary set of up to 32 analog input channels and 32 bits of digital I/O can also be used. Channel counts of generic I/O in a NeuroRighter system depend on the number of data acquisition cards in the user's system, and the amount of analog input channels reserved for the electrodes.

NeuroRighter's hardware serves as an adaptable interface between multi-electrode sensors and data acquisition cards for recording and microstimulation. There are many other options for routing signals to and from the acquisition cards. Therefore, except for the acquisition cards themselves, the hardware we present here is not required to make use of NeuroRighter's software.

2.2. SOFTWARE

The NeuroRighter software application was written in C# (pronounced "C-Sharp"). C# is a modern, general purpose,

object-oriented programming language. The software is free and its source code is maintained on a publicly accessible repository[4]. For standard installations, NeuroRighter is distributed as an installation package for 32- or 64-bit Windows operating systems (Microsoft Corp., Redmond, WA). NeuroRighter installations contain two software components:

1. A stand-alone multichannel recording and stimulation application. This includes a graphical user interface (GUI) for data visualization, hardware configuration, data filtering, spike detection and sorting, all-channel stimulation, stimulus artifact rejection, and data recording (section 2.2.1).
2. An application programming interface (API) that allows NeuroRighter to be used as a real-time hardware interface and data server for user-coded protocols (section 2.2.2).

2.2.1. The NeuroRighter application

As a stand-alone application, NeuroRighter can be used for high-quality multichannel recordings (16-bit resolution, 31 k Samples/sec/channel) and all-channel stimulation protocols. NeuroRighter's graphical interface is organized into tabbed pages, each of which encapsulates a particular group of functions or visualization tools (**Figure 1**). In the following section, we discuss the main functional aspects of the stand-alone NeuroRighter application.

2.2.1.1. Main interface. The main NeuroRighter interface (**Figure 1C**) is an access point for all of the application's functionality. It facilitates user manipulation of hardware settings, online filter settings, data visualization windows, stimulation tools, and other features, which are discussed below. Additionally, some recording settings can be manipulated within the main interface itself:

Online acquisition settings. Many filter settings can be adjusted during data collection. This allows the user to fine tune acquisition settings while gaining visual feedback of the effect on incoming data streams. Bandpass, spike detection, and spike sorting parameters can be adjusted during a recording.

Data visualization. Data visualization tools in NeuroRighter use the Microsoft XNA game development framework. This ensures that online visualization does not consume CPU cycles by offloading plotting routines to a supported graphics card. Visualization tools are provided for single-unit activity, local field potentials (LFP), multiunit activity (MUA), electroencephalograph (EEG) traces, and auxiliary analog input streams. Additionally, overlay plots are used to display sorted spike waveforms for each channel (**Figure 1C**).

File saving. Data streams selected by the user are written to disk with a unique file extension that designates their type. These binary files can be read with MATLAB (Mathworks, Natick, MA) functions included with NeuroRighter installations.

---

[4]http://code.google.com/p/neurorighter/

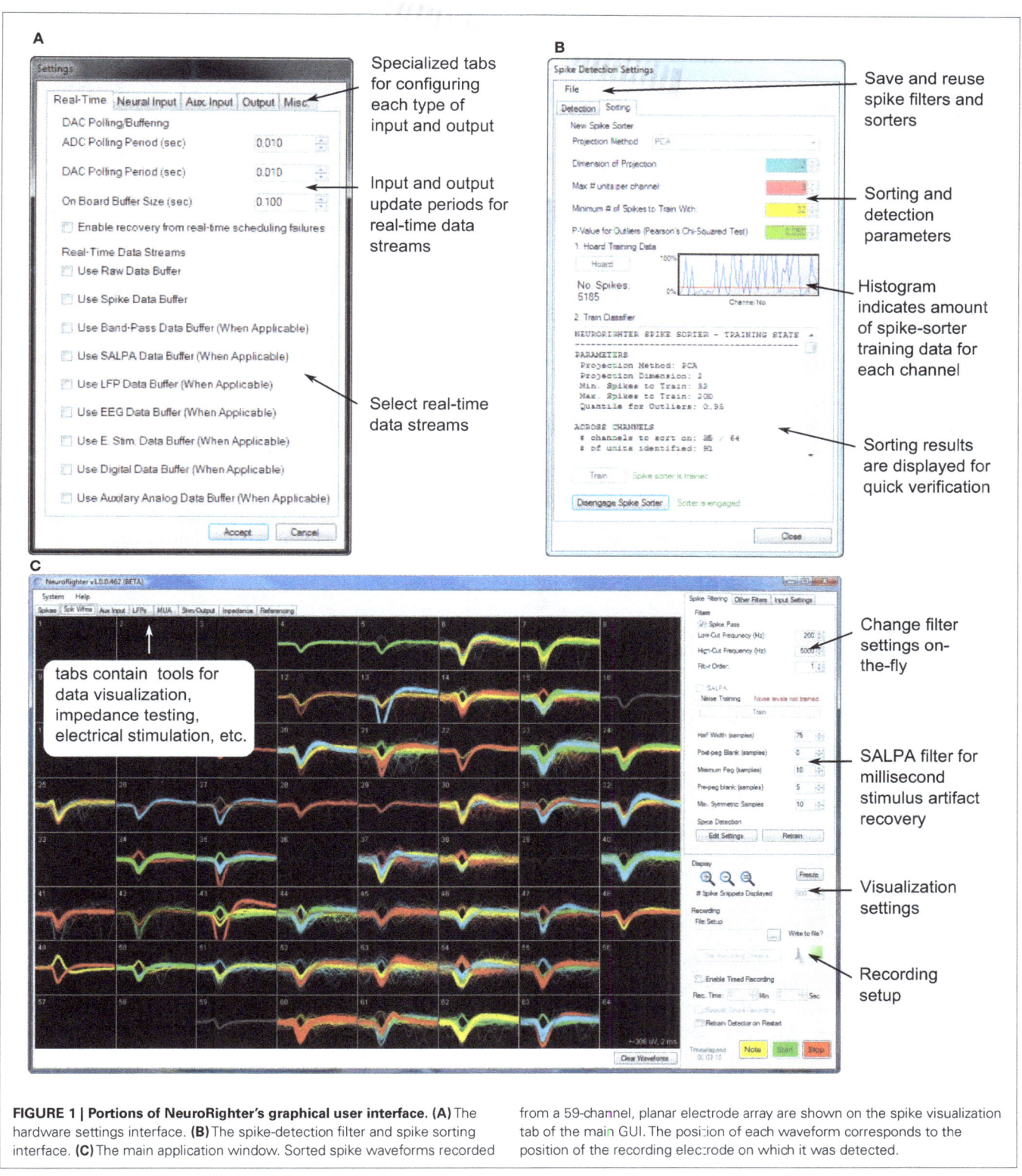

FIGURE 1 | Portions of NeuroRighter's graphical user interface. (A) The hardware settings interface. **(B)** The spike-detection filter and spike sorting interface. **(C)** The main application window. Sorted spike waveforms recorded from a 59-channel, planar electrode array are shown on the spike visualization tab of the main GUI. The position of each waveform corresponds to the position of the recording electrode on which it was detected.

2.2.1.2. Hardware configuration. Correctly specifying mixed digital and analog signal routing, clock synchronization, and trigger synchronization on a multi-board data acquisition system can be complicated. NeuroRighter simplifies this process using a graphical hardware settings interface (**Figure 1A**). Here, the user specifies the types of signals carried by the NI acquisition cards in his or her system, amplifier gain settings, auxiliary input and output channels, options for electrode impedance measurement, signal referencing, and real-time data streaming options. Upon closing the settings dialog, NeuroRighter performs the required signal routing and clock synchronization. All NI cards are synchronized to a single clock oscillator using an NI real-time system integration bus (RTSI, **Figure 3**).

2.2.1.3. *Time-series filtering.*

Incoming data from the A/D converters are passed through a cascade of digital filters to produce different neural data streams. First, channel voltages are passed through several linear filters to extract frequency bands for single-unit activity ($\simeq$200–5000 Hz) and LFP ($\simeq$1–500 Hz). MUA, which reflects the firing rate of neurons within the vicinity of the recording electrode, is extracted by rectifying and then low pass filtering the single-unit activity data stream (Supèr and Roelfsema, 2005).

In addition to traditional filtering methods, NeuroRighter provides several specialized filtering options. Common-mode noise sources such as AC mains pickup or movement artifacts in freely moving animals can corrupt neural recordings. NeuroRighter allows the mean or median of all recording electrodes (with appropriate scaling) to be subtracted from individual electrode voltage streams to combat common-mode interference (Rolston et al., 2009b). This is an effective method for reducing non-periodic common-mode interference, such as movement artifacts, where template subtraction methods are inappropriate. Finally, NeuroRighter includes an implementation of the SALPA filter (Wagenaar and Potter, 2002), which subtracts locally fit cubic splines from electrode traces following the application of a stimulus pulse. This removes the capacitive artifacts from non-saturated recording channels and allows online action potential detection within 2 ms after a stimulus pulse.

Sampling rates for different data streams can be set independently. Filter settings (pass-band and filter order) can be modified during data acquisition (**Figure 1C**). Raw data, as well as the result of each filtering stage, yield separate data streams (**Table 1**).

2.2.1.4. *Spike filtering.*

Spike filtering in NeuroRighter is a three-step process: (1) detection, (2) validation, and (3) sorting. NeuroRighter detects spikes using a threshold criterion that compares individual voltage samples to the estimated RMS voltage on the corresponding electrode. Upon threshold crossing, a peak-aligned voltage "snippet" is extracted from the raw voltage stream. Each snippet is validated using a series of *ad hoc* criteria based upon waveform slope, width, and peak-to-peak amplitude. Finally, spikes can be sorted online using an automated Gaussian mixture modeling algorithm. Details of the spike detection and sorting algorithms used by NeuroRighter are provided in section 3 in the Supplementary Material.

The spike detection/sorting configuration is controlled through a child GUI (**Figure 1B**). All relevant spike detection, validation, and sorting parameters are under user control and are manipulated using the spike detection GUI. Because spike-detection settings are changed using a secondary GUI, the effects of parameter changes can be simultaneously monitored on the visualization tabs in the main interface while data collection occurs. A complete list of these parameters is shown in Table S1 in the Supplementary Material. Spike filters, including trained spike sorters, can be saved and reused.

2.2.1.5. *Stimulation.*

NeuroRighter provides several options for delivering complex stimulus patterns to neural tissue either manually through the NeuroRighter application or using scripted protocols. Simple, periodic stimulation protocols, consisting of single or double phase, square, current- or voltage-controlled pulses on any electrode, can be performed directly from the main GUI. Stimuli can be triggered "on demand" in response to a mouse click or by using hardware-timed, periodic sequence of triggers.

Scripted protocols can be used to deliver complex, potentially non-periodic stimulus patterns and to access general purpose analog and digital output lines. Neurorighter uses a double-buffered output engine, called `StimSrv` (**Table 2**), to produce arbitrary, hardware-timed stimulation, analog-output, or digital output signals (**Table 1**, bottom). `StimSrv` can be accessed on-the-fly using NeuroRighter's API (section 2.2.2) or with user-written scripts. The schematic in **Figure 2A** demonstrates how `StimSrv` delivers uninterrupted output. First, a block of the NI cards' memory is reserved and divided into two sections, each of which comprises a single output buffer. At a given instant, one buffer is reserved for sample generation and one is available for writing. When the all samples in the read buffer are exhausted, the buffers switch roles, allowing seamless delivery of constantly varying output signals. This allows the delivery of complex, aperiodic stimulation patterns and the orchestration of experimental apparatuses using analog and digital output lines. All output is clock-synchronized to input data streams, allowing *a priori* specification of stimulus delivery times, relative to the start of the experiment, with single-sample precision. Stimulation scripts can be created with a set of MATLAB functions that are included with NeuroRighter installations (see section 1 in the Supplementary Material).

Figure 2B demonstrates the use of a scripted stimulation protocol to deliver spatio-temporal patterns of electrical stimuli. One-second trials of spatially uniform, and temporally Poisson random stimulus pulses were delivered to a dissociated cortical network. Each trial consisted of either a new, random stimulus realization or a single repeated realization. Each type of stimulus sequence was interleaved with no delay between adjacent trials. **Figure 2Bi** shows stimulus raster plots for 100 trials each stimulus type, with a gray-scale indicating the stimulus trial. For repeated stimuli, individual trials cannot be seen since the recording and stimulation subsystems are clock-synchronized and every repeated stimulus sequence occupies the same set of samples relative to the start of a trial. **Figure 2Bii** shows spiking patterns in response to random and repeated stimuli for 4 units across trials. The delivery of repeated stimuli to the network results in extremely reproducible spiking patterns, and non-repeated, random stimuli probe the variability of population spiking response. This type of stimulus protocol is commonly used to estimate the mutual information between a stimulation process and the population spiking response (Strong et al., 1998; Yu et al., 2010).

2.2.2. *NeuroRighter's application programming interface*

NeuroRighter installations include an API that facilitates the creation of real-time protocols. The API comprises a set of tools for interacting with NeuroRighter's input and output streams. Protocols written using the API are externally compiled libraries that can "plug in" to the NeuroRighter application in order to impart

Table 1 | Overview of NeuroRighter's input and output streams.

Input	Source	Server (DataSrv)	Buffer type	Max. channel count
	Raw electrodes	RawElectrodeSrv	Circular double[][]	64
	SALPA Filter	SalpaSrv	Circular double[][]	64
	Spike-band filter	SpikeBandSrv	Circular double[][]	64
	Spike filter	SpikeSrv	List <SpikeEvent>	64 or No. units
	LFP filter	LFPSrv	Circular double[][]	64
	EEG filter	EEGSrv	Circular double[][]	64
	MUA filter	MUASrv	Circular double[][]	64
	Electrical stimuli	ElecStimuliSrv	List <SpikeEvent>	64
	Auxiliary analog	AuxAnalogSrv	Circular double[][]	32
	Auxiliary digital	AuxDigitalSrv	List <DigitalEvent>	32 bits
Output	**Source**	**Server (StimSrv)**	**Buffer type**	**Max. channel count**
	Electrical stimuli	StimOut	List <StimulusEvent>	64
	Analog output	AnalogOut	List <AnalogEvent>	4
	Digital output	DigitalOut	List <DigitalEvent>	32 bits

Each stream is accessed using a dedicated server that includes functions for reading from, or writing to, its data buffer.

Table 2 | Packages included with NeuroRighter's Plugin API.

Package	Component	Description
Server	DataSrv	Contains input server objects (**Table 1**, top)
	StimSrv	Contains output server objects (**Table 1**, bottom)
Datatypes	MultiChannelBuffer	Circular buffer for time series data
	SpikeEvent	Spike event type (time, channel, waveform, unit)
	DigitalEvent	Digital event type (time, 32-bit port state)
	StimulusEvent	Stimulus event type (time, channel, waveform)
	AuxEvent	Auxiliary voltage event (time, channel, voltage)
NeuroRighterTask	NRTask	Abstract class for real-time NeuroRighter interfacing
Log	Logger	Used for debugging real-time protocols

real-time and closed-loop functionality. The software packages included with the API are shown in **Table 2**. Each package contains different set of tools for interacting with NeuroRighter's data streams. Here we discuss the contents and usage of each of these tools. Additionally, a detailed API reference is available online[5].

2.2.2.1. *NeuroRighterTask.* User-defined protocols employ the NeuroRighter application as a real-time data server. These protocols are inherited from a base component called `NRTask`, which belongs to the NeuroRighterTask package. Closed-loop protocols created with the plugin API are derived from `NRTask` (see section 2 in the Supplementary Material for details). Three functions included in `NRTask` can then be accessed to impart real-time functionality.

1. `NRTask.Setup()`: This function is called when the base `NRTask` component is instantiated. It allows one-time setup operations to take place, such as the declaration of variables,

allocation of internal buffers, file streaming setup, GUI initialization, etc.

2. `NRTask.Loop()`: This function is executed periodically by a hardware-timed clock. Execution periods of 1 to 150 ms are allowed and can be set from the Hardware Settings GUI in the main application (**Figure 1A**). To achieve closed-loop functionality, code within the `Loop` function should access other components of the API, most importantly components from the Server and DataTypes packages (**Table 2**). These packages provide access to incoming neural data streams and output buffers and can be used to form a bi-directional interface with neural tissue. Output can be sent from within the `Loop` function using the StimSrv package (**Table 2**) or through natively supported communication interfaces such as TCP/IP ports, serial ports, or USB communication.

3. `NRTask.Cleanup()`: This function is called a single time when the protocol is stopped from the NeuroRighter GUI. It allows the deconstruction of GUIs, the closure of file streams that may have been created during the execution of the plugin, and other cleanup routines.

[5]https://potterlab.gatech.edu/main/neurorighter-api-ref/

```
A
/// StimSrv-based plugin
using NeuroRighter.NeuroRighterTask;
using NeuroRighter.DataTypes;
using NeuroRighter.DatSrv;
using NeuroRighter.StimSrv;
namespace Example
{
  public class MyTask : NRTask
  {
 // Called once at plugin start
    protected override void Setup(){
    }
    // Called by output buffer
    protected override void Loop(){
      data = NRDataSrv.SpikeSrv.Read();
      if (myUnit member of data)
      {
        NRStimSrv.Write();
      }
    }
    // Called upon plugin termination
    protected override void Cleanup(){
    }
  }
}
```

```
B
/// NewData-based plugin
using NeuroRighter.NeuroRighterTask;
using NeuroRighter.DataTypes;
using NeuroRighter.DatSrv;

namespace Example
{
  public class MyTask : NRTask
  {
    // Called once at plugin start
    protected override void Setup(){
      SpikeSrv.NewData += NewData_Hander();
    }
    // Called on NewData event
    private void NewData_Hander(){
      if(myUnit member of data)
      {
        NI Card sends output;
      }
    }
    // Called upon plugin termination
    protected override void Cleanup(){
    }
  }
}
```

LISTING 1 | Code structure for two types of real-time plugin implemented with the API. (A) Pseudocode for a StimSrv-based real-time plugin.
(B) Pseudocode for real-time plugin triggered by NewData events.

Listing 1A and **1B** provide pseudocode for a two real-time plug-ins that both respond to a spike produced by a particular detected unit. A real-time protocol written using the API will follow the structure of one of these code skeletons, regardless of its complexity. First, the user references the required packages from the API. Next, the plugin is designated to be a child of NRTask, which provides the protocol with automatic access to NeuroRighter's data servers. Finally, the Setup(), Loop(), and Cleanup() functions are overridden (**Listing 1A**), or a NewData event is sub-scribed to (**Listing 1B**), to impart real-time functionality. After it is compiled (either using Visual Studio or Mono[6]), the plugin can be executed through NeuroRighter's GUI. Plugin protocols exe-cuted through NeuroRighter operate on a high-priority thread to decrease closed-loop response latency. The diagram shown in **Figure 3** shows the interaction between a plugin created using the API, the NeuroRighter executable, and hardware. Functional

examples of plugin protocols are provided in section 5 of the Supplementary Material.

2.2.2.2.   Server. Components derived from NRTask have auto-matic access to NeuroRighter's input and output servers, which belong to the Server package. There are two banks of data servers: (1) DataSrv, which can be used to read NeuroRighter's input streams (**Table 1**, top) and (2) StimSrv, which can be used to write to output streams (**Table 1**, bottom). DataSrv and StimSrv objects encapsulate isolated data servers, each of which handles a particular data stream. Each server includes methods for reading the hardware clock, reading from and writing to its own data buffer, and accessing stream metadata. Because input and output servers are simultaneously accessible from within a user-defined NRTask, sending output signals (e.g., stimuli) contingent on recorded input is straightforward. The user can select which data streams are sent to DataSrv or available for writing on StimSrv using the Hardware Settings GUI (**Figure 1A**).

---

[6]http://www.mono-project.com/Main_Page

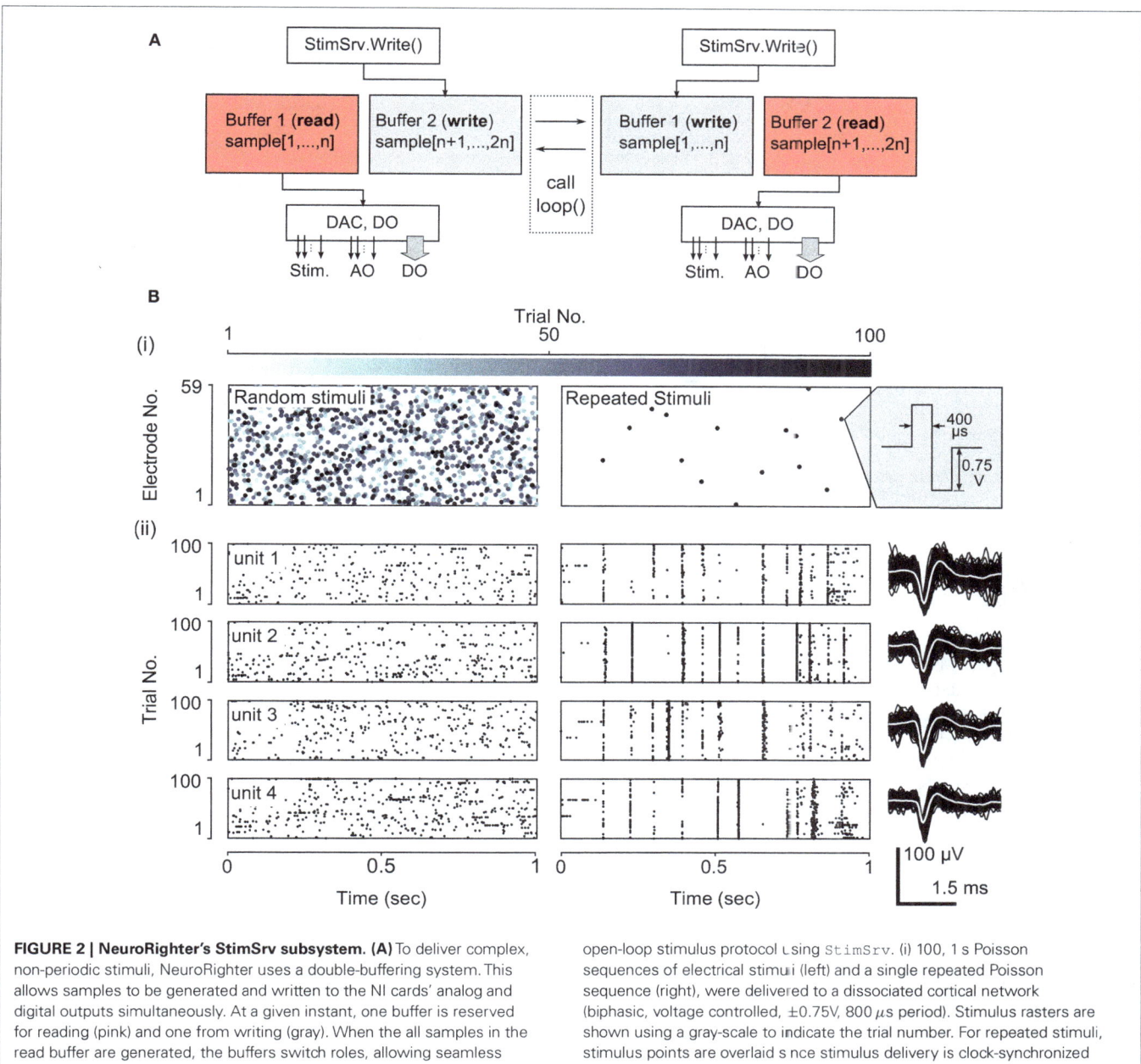

FIGURE 2 | NeuroRighter's StimSrv subsystem. (A) To deliver complex, non-periodic stimuli, NeuroRighter uses a double-buffering system. This allows samples to be generated and written to the NI cards' analog and digital outputs simultaneously. At a given instant, one buffer is reserved for reading (pink) and one from writing (gray). When the all samples in the read buffer are generated, the buffers switch roles, allowing seamless delivery of constantly varying stimulus patterns and generic analog and digital signals. When using `StimSrv` for closed-loop protocols, the `loop()` function is called at the instant of a buffer switch. **(B)** Example open-loop stimulus protocol using `StimSrv`. (i) 100, 1 s Poisson sequences of electrical stimuli (left) and a single repeated Poisson sequence (right), were delivered to a dissociated cortical network (biphasic, voltage controlled, ±0.75V, 800 μs period). Stimulus rasters are shown using a gray-scale to indicate the trial number. For repeated stimuli, stimulus points are overlaid since stimulus delivery is clock-synchronized with the acquisition subsystem. (ii) Rastergrams of 4 units are shown below each stimulus raster, across trials. Example waveforms for each of the 4 units are shown to the right.

A final important feature of each data server within `DataSrv` is a `NewData` event. A `NewData` event is fired for a given stream each time it receives new data for the A/D card or a digital filter. Functions within a plugin can subscribe to these events so that feedback processing only occurs when new data is acquired. This reduces computational overhead and the latency of the closed-loop response. Plugins that use `NewData` events to generate feedback are not required to include a `Loop()` function or to use `StimSrv` to send output signals. Instead, standard calls to the National Instrument driver library (DAQmx) can be used to access the NI cards' directly. Alternatively, output can be generated using natively supported external communication protocols (USB, TCP/IP, UDP, serial, etc.). **Listing II. B.2(b)** provides pseudocode for a real-time protocol analogous to **Listing II.B.2(a)**, but using the `NewData` event to trigger a response. This type of plugin provides a lower response latencies but is less capable of producing complex, precisely timed output signals. A functional example of a `NewData`-based plugin is provided in section 5.2 in the Supplementary Material.

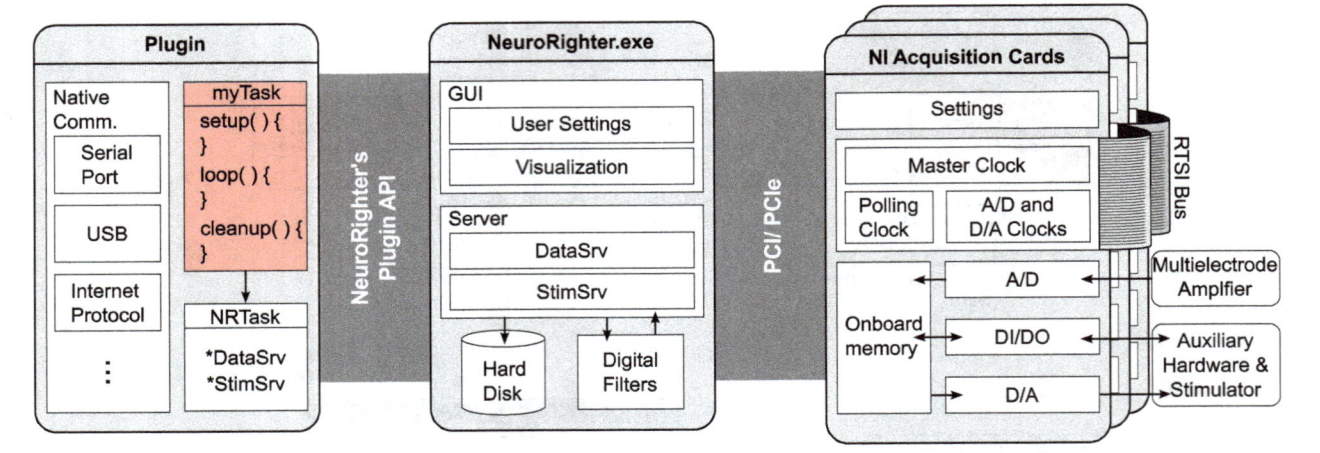

FIGURE 3 | Conceptual schematic of NeuroRighter's hardware and software elements. NeuroRighter serves as a high-level interface between hardware and custom user-written protocols (pink box). NeuroRighter simplifies hardware level programming by using datatypes and methods that are specialized for multichannel neural recording and stimulation. This facilitates the creation of low-latency, closed-loop protocols. Neural signals and secondary data streams are fed into the NI cards' analog and digital inputs where they are digitalized and stored temporarily in on-board memory. NeuroRighter periodically transfers data from the acquisition cards' FIFO memory to RAM using direct memory access. Data is then pushed to NeuroRighter's `DataSrv` server object. `DataSrv` serves data to NeuroRighter's visualization tools, filtering algorithms, and externally compiled plugins. The plugin API provides functions for safe interaction with `DataSrv` so that custom operations can be performed on incoming data streams. User-written plugins can interact with any of the computer's native communication ports, or write data back to `StimSrv` in order to control external hardware as a function of recorded neural signals.

2.2.2.3.   Datatypes. NeuroRighter's input and output servers operate on high-level data types that encapsulate different forms of multichannel input and output data. These include multichannel buffers for continuous data streams (such as raw electrode voltages or LFP recordings) and discrete event types (such a detected spikes or stimulation events). Extensive documentation on each of these data types is provided in the API reference.

2.2.2.4.   Log. The Log package provides accesses to a data logging tool that operates within the NeuroRighter executable, but can be invoked from a user protocol. This tool can be used to write information to a log file using a separate, low-priority thread. This is useful in the development of real-time protocols because core NeuroRighter operations (such as the timing of hardware reads, writes, and other triggers) are logged to this file as well, providing context for messages written from the plugin.

3.   CASE STUDIES

NeuroRighter's abilities for orchestrating closed-loop experiments are best demonstrated through example. Here we present five case studies in which protocols created with the API were used to measure NeuroRighter's closed-loop reaction-time, clamp network firing levels in dissociated cultured cortical networks, react to seizures in freely moving animals with multi-electrode electrical stimulation, and control robots serving as artificial embodiments. Experimental methods, and plugin examples are provided in the section 4 in the Supplementary Material. The plugin code used in these case studies is available for download on NeuroRighter's code repository. [7]. Additionally, we provide all code used

in the reaction-time case study in section 5 in the Supplementary Material.

3.1.   LOW-LATENCY CONTROL OF REAL-TIME HARDWARE

Rapid response times are critical for maintaining a tight feedback loop in which features of incoming data streams (e.g., spikes, EEG, temperature, or animal motion) are used to trigger or adjust the delivery of stimuli. To benchmark the response speed of protocols written using the API, we wrote a protocol that generated output signals in response to recorded action potentials. We picked two sorted units from a dissociated neural culture to serve as triggers for hardware activation. When one of these units fired, it triggered the output of a digital word encoding the identity of the detect unit. These signals serve as a generic stand-in for a stimulation pattern or any other hardware control signal that might be used in a feedback control scheme. Output signals were then recorded using NeuroRighter's digital input port. The delay between action potential detection and signal generation could then be measured using the same sample clock. A diagram of the experimental protocol is shown in **Figure 4A**. We wrote protocols to test three hardware options for generating the required digital output:

1. StimSrv: Buffered manipulation of the NI cards using NeuroRighter's native stimulation server (**Figure 2** and **Listing II.B.2(a)**).
2. NewData: Unbuffered manipulation of the NI cards whenever new data enters NeuroRighter's spike server (**Listing II.B.2(b)**).
3. Arduino: An Arduino ATmega2560-based microcontroller board[8] communicating via serial port (RS-232).

---

[7] http://code.google.com/p/neurorighter/source/browse/NR-ClosedLoop-Examples/

[8] http://www.arduino.cc/

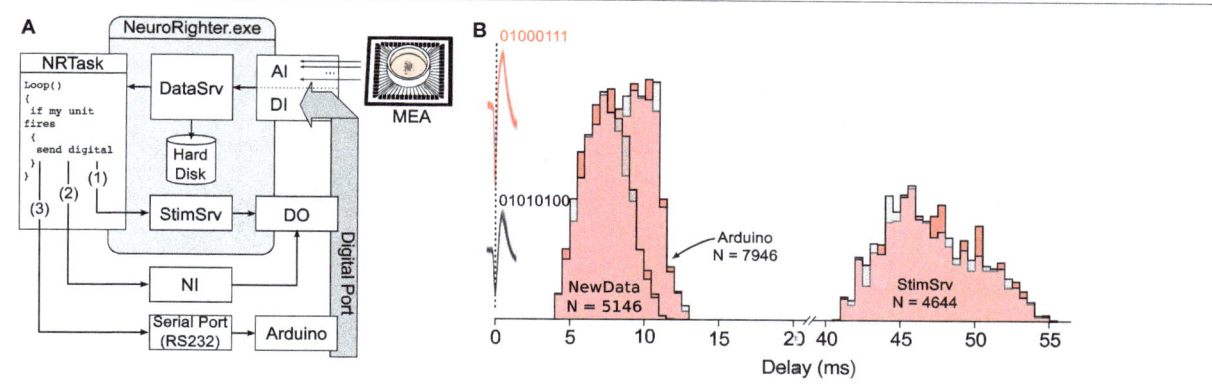

FIGURE 4 | Estimated loop times for bi-directional communication using different hardware configurations. (A) Schematic of experiment used to test reaction delays for different real-time hardware options. Spikes detected and sorted from 59-channel planar electrode array were passed to the real-time plugin. The plugin determined if a spike originated from one of two units of interest. In the case that a spike was produced by one of the two units, the plugin triggered the generation of a digital word encoding the detected unit using either StimSrv, unbuffered digital output triggered by a NewData event, or an Arduino board. Digital signals were then, recorded though NeuroRighter's digital input port. **(B)** Normalized histogram of time delays from spikes produced by the two units of interest (action potential waveforms are shown in pink and gray and occur at 0 ms) to the recorded digital signals produced by the plugin to encode the units (01000111 or 01010100). Delay histograms are shown for each unit (pink and gray) and the three different hardware options. N is the number of spikes recorded for each hardware option.

The response latency, calculated from the time of an action potential peak to the corresponding change in the digital port was calculated for each hardware option (**Figure 4**). Mean response latencies were 46.9 ± 3.1 ms for rb StimSrv, 7.1 ± 1.5 ms for NewData, and 9.2 ± 1.3 ms for the Arduino board. Latencies where measured while NeuroRighter performed bandpass filtering, spike detection, spike sorting, data streaming, and data saving for 64 electrode inputs, each sampled at 25 kHz. Experiments were conducted on a desktop computer using an Intel Core i7 processor (Santa Clara, California, USA.) and running running 64-bit Windows Vista.

The differences in reaction latency for different hardware options are a result of both the method used to communicate with the hardware and the how the input sent from NeuroRighter is interpreted and transformed into a physical output signal. The differences in response times for NewData and Arduino are largely attributable to the different communication protocols and command interpretation by the client device. For instance the Arduino used a RS-232 serial interface where as NewData communicates with the NI cards via PCIe. StimSrv's long latency in comparison to other options is a result of its double buffering system, which requires a relatively long time period between updates to the NI D/A's output buffer. While StimSrv is slow in comparison to the NewData and microcontroller options, it provides an interface that is easier to use and allows the uninterrupted delivery of arbitrary complex signal outputs. On the other hand, the Arduino and NewData methods can only respond by generating finite-sample or periodic control signals. We have found that StimSrv is fast enough for most of our closed-loop requirements. For this reason, we used StimSrv to generate physical outputs for the remainder of the case studies. However, as demonstrated above, the API's modularity allows the use of faster hardware options with little change in coding complexity.

3.2. MULTICHANNEL POPULATION FIRING CLAMP

The population firing rate is a building block of the neural code. The ability to precisely control population firing in the face of experimental perturbations can be used to understand its role in network function. To demonstrate NeuroRighter's ability to control the network firing rate, we implemented the feedback controller presented in Wagenaar et al. (2005) to control the firing activity in dissociated cortical cultures grown on 59-channel micro-electrode arrays. This algorithm adjusts the stimulation amplitude of voltage controlled, biphasic pulses on 10 electrodes to desynchronize population firing and force the network firing rate to track target values. The control law is given by

$$v_k[t + \Delta T] = v_k[t] - \alpha v_k[t] \left(\frac{\langle f_u[t] \rangle}{f^*} - 1 \right), \quad (1)$$

where v_k is the stimulation voltage on electrode k, $\langle f_u[t] \rangle$ is the average firing rate across sorted units detected with the 59 electrode array extending over a 2 s window into the past, f^* is the target firing rate, ΔT is the update period of the feedback loop (as defined within NeuroRighter's Hardware Settings GUI), and α defines the time constant of the feedback controller as

$$\tau_{FB} = \Delta T / \alpha. \quad (2)$$

We used $\Delta T = 10$ ms and $\alpha = 0.002$ so that $\tau_{FB} = 5$ s. Electrodes were stimulated at a 10 Hz aggregate frequency (1 Hz per electrode for 10 electrodes) in a random, repeating sequence. Additionally, individual electrode voltages were multiplied by a tuning factor that was inversely proportional to the number of spikes that occurred within 30 ms following a stimulus pulse on that electrode, as described in Wagenaar et al. (2005). This factor equalizes each electrode's ability to evoke a spiking response, and is critical for achieving the desynchronizing effect of the controller on population activity.

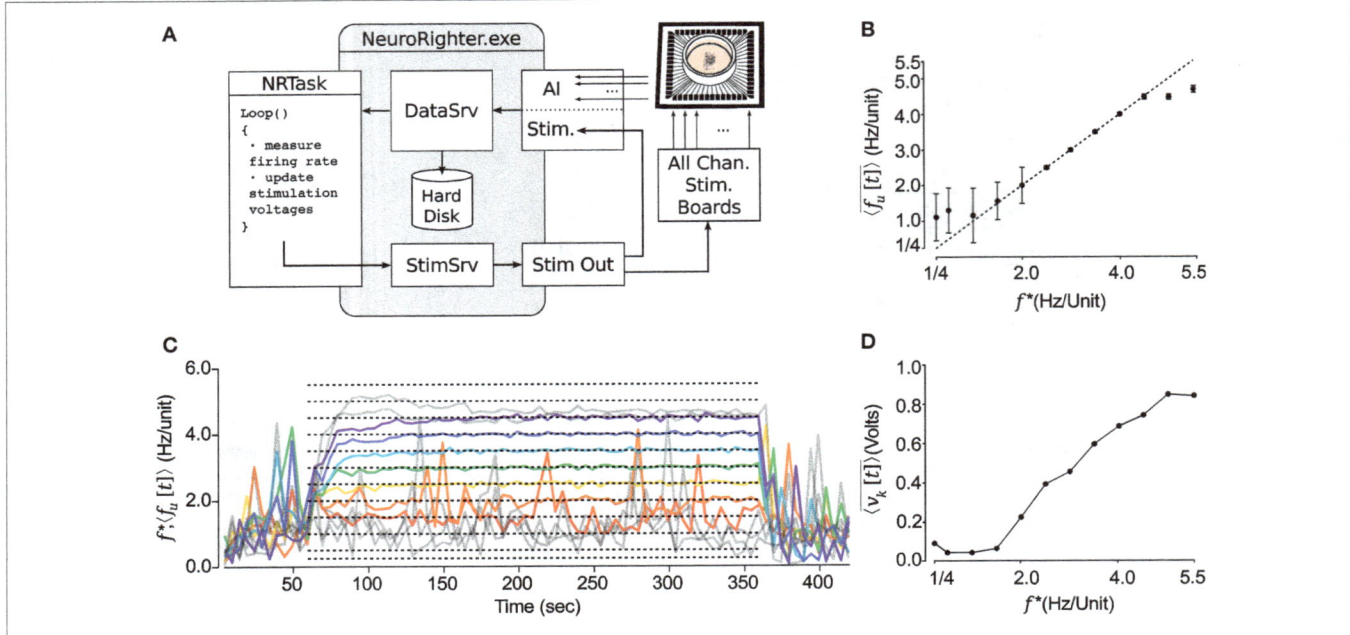

FIGURE 5 | NeuroRighter can be used to clamp population firing rates *in vitro* using closed-loop electrical stimulation. (A) Schematic of the multi-electrode population firing clamp. **(B)** Step tracking performance is shown for a range of target firing rates, f^* (dotted lines). The average neuronal firing rate across detected units, $\langle f_u[t] \rangle$ (colored lines), is shown for each step in f^*. Tracking failures are colored gray. **(C)** Time averaged neuronal firing rate for the last 2.5 min of each 5 min protocol compared to the reference signal, f^*. The dotted line is identity. **(D)** The mean control voltage across the stimulating electrodes over the final 2.5 min of each step protocol at different values of f^*.

We used the controller to clamp network firing at target rates for 5 min epochs. These results are shown in **Figure 5**. The controller was able to achieve target rates within the range of $f^* = 1.5$–4.5 Hz/Unit. An animation of neural activity before and during firing-rate clamping is provided in the Supplementary Material.

The monotonically increasing relationship between the mean stimulation voltage $\overline{\langle v_k[t] \rangle}$, and target firing rate f^* (**Figure 5D**) might indicate that knowledge of the stimulation voltage versus firing rate relationship is sufficient to design an open-loop controller capable of holding network firing rates. To test this, we clamped firing at $f^* = 3.0$ Hz/Unit over 10 min epochs for 15 trials. Five minutes into each 10 min protocol, we stopped updating stimulation voltages on the ten stimulating electrodes, but continued multi-electrode stimulation in open-loop mode (**Figure 6**). Although the desired mean firing rate was achieved fairly consistently, the open-loop control scheme could not react to the rapid changes in excitability that are typical of cultured cortical networks (Wagenaar et al., 2006b). This variability is reflected in the large range of control signals required to track the target rate over the first 5 min of each trial. As a result the RMS error of $\langle f_u[t] \rangle$ about f^* increased by a factor of 5.1 for open-loop compared to closed-loop epochs. The variance of firing during open-loop stimulation is comparable to that of spontaneous (non-evoked) firing behavior that was recorded before the controller was switched on (**Figure 6**, top).

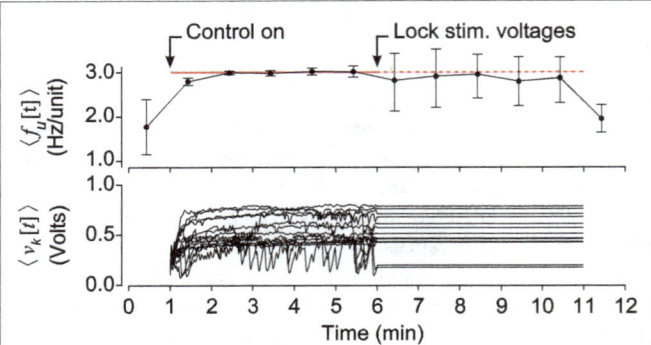

FIGURE 6 | Closed-loop stimulation is required to robustly clamp population firing. (Top) The average neuronal firing rate over 1 min periods across 15 trials. Half-way through a multichannel population clamp protocol, real-time voltage updates stop and microstimulation is applied in open-loop. Error bars are ± standard deviation. (Bottom) The mean electrode stimulation voltage across 10 stimulating electrodes, for each of the 15 trials.

3.3. LONG-TERM POPULATION FIRING CLAMP WITH SYNAPTIC DECOUPLING

3.3.1. Experiment 1

In vitro neural preparations allow continuous experimental access to neural tissue over very long time scales (Potter and DeMarse,

2001), and therefore serve as important models for understanding slowly occurring developmental processes (Turrigiano et al., 1998; Minerbi et al., 2009; Gal et al., 2010). To demonstrate that NeuroRighter is capable of stable closed-loop neural interfacing over long time scales, we used the multi-electrode feedback controller used in section 3.2 for 6 h epochs. This protocol started with a 1 h recording of spontaneous activity. Then, the controller was engaged to clamp population firing to $f^* = 3.0\,Hz/Unit$ for 6 h. Following the clamping protocol, spontaneous network activity was recorded for an additional hour.

Figure 7A shows the resulting multichannel stimulation signal (**Figure 7Ai**), neuronal firing rate in relation to f^* (**Figure 7Aii**), individual unit firing rates (**Figure 7Aiii**), and zoomed rastergrams before, during, and after multi-electrode stimulation was applied (**Figure 7Aiv**). The controller achieved the $f^* = 3.0\,Hz/Unit$ tracking over the duration of the 6 h protocol. Additionally, network activity was desynchronized through most of the control epoch, but occasionally the controller allowed bouts of synchronized network activity (Wagenaar et al., 2006b).

3.3.2. Experiment 2

Spiking and neurotransmission have a strong reciprocal influence on one another, making their individual effects on network development difficult to quantify (Turrigiano, 2011). For instance, N-methyl-D-aspartate (NMDA)-ergic neurotransmission plays a large role in sustained network recruitment (Nakanishi and Kukita, 1998). For this reason, long-term changes in the state of *in vitro* networks following the application synaptic blockers (e.g., changes in firing rate, spiking patterns, or synaptic-strength) is difficult to attribute directly to effects on neurotransmission because of secondary, confounding effects on network activity levels. However, the closed-loop population clamp provides a solution to this problem. A firing rate controller has the potential to compensate for changes in network excitability induced by the application of a drug, removing its confounding effect on network activity.

To test this, we used the multichannel population clamp during the bath application of d(−)-2-amino-5-phosphonopentanoic acid (AP5), a competitive antagonist of NMDA receptor. This protocol proceeded identically to experiment 1 except that at 1-h following the start of closed-loop stimulation, NeuroRighter triggered the perfusion of $50\,\mu m$ AP5 into the culturing medium using a syringe pump and a custom, gas-permeable perfusion lid (Potter and DeMarse, 2001; Figure S5 in the Supplementary Material). Four hours after AP5 was applied, NeuroRighter triggered the pump a second time to perform a series of washes with normal culturing medium that removed AP5 from the bath.

Time-series results of this protocol are shown in **Figure 7B**. The contents of these plots are analogous to **Figure 7A** but have arrows to indicate when AP5 was added to, and removed from, the culturing chamber. The controller was able to successfully compensate for changes in network excitability caused by the addition of AP5. Changes in network dynamics were reflected in the control signal, which became smoother in the presence of the AP5 (**Figure 7Bi**).

3.3.3. Comparing Experiments 1 and 2

Figure 7C shows the average, pair-wise firing rate correlation functions (Tchumatchenko et al., 2010) for 30 randomly selected units

from experiment 1 (black lines) and experiment 2 (red lines). **Figures 7Ci,iii** show the correlation functions of spontaneous network activity before and after the controller was engaged, respectively. **Figure 7Cii** shows correlation functions for epochs during the clamping phase (which included the AP5 treatment for experiment 2). The periodicity of this correlation function follows the 10 Hz aggregate stimulation frequency during the clamping period.

Intriguingly, although the pair-wise spiking correlations for experiments 1 and 2 were very similar for epochs of spontaneous activity before and during multichannel stimulation (**Figures 7Ci,ii**), they were remarkably different once the stimulator was turned off (**Figure 7Ciii**). When AP5 was not present during the clamping phase (experiment 1), the firing correlation between units appeared to be enhanced following multichannel stimulation. In contrast, pair-wise correlations were almost non-existent following the a population clamp in which AP5 was present (experiment 2). Because the firing statistics (firing rate and correlation structure) during the 6-h clamping period were nearly identical for the both experiments 1 and 2, this effect on the correlation structure of network activity can not be due to effects on firing activity, but required blocking NMDAergic transmission. Without the closed-loop controller in place, AP5 would have affected network activity levels, obfuscating the mechanism of AP5's effect.

This case study demonstrates the ability of the closed-loop controller to quickly adapt to drug-induced changes in network excitability, to decouple network variables that are normally causally intertwined, and to operate robustly over many hours. Additionally, this case study demonstrates NeuroRighter's ability control peripheral equipment aside from electrical stimulators.

3.4. REAL-TIME SEIZURE INTERVENTION IN FREELY MOVING RATS

Aside from *in vitro* recording hardware, NeuroRighter can interface with many different types of neural probes, including those designed to record from and stimulate freely moving animals. To demonstrate this, we performed electrical micro-stimulation in response to paroxysmal activity of hippocampal recordings taken from a rat with induced temporal lobe epilepsy. Many studies have shown potentially therapeutic effects of electrical stimulation on epileptic brain tissue, which could serve as an alternative to pharmacological or surgical treatment methods. For instance, electrical stimulation triggered by characteristic field potential abnormalities can potentially abrogate seizures and lead to a decreased frequency of behavioral symptoms (Mormann et al., 2007; Morrell, 2011; Nelson et al., 2011).

We used the plugin API to create a closed-loop protocol that could detect temporal lobe seizures in freely moving rats and react with multi-electrode stimulation (**Figure 8A**). This control scheme is similar to that of the NeuroPace responsive neurostimulation system (Sun et al., 2008) (NeuroPace Inc., Moutain View, CA, USA), with the exception that we used multi-micro-electrode stimulation instead of driving a single macroelectrode.

Rats were rendered epileptic using focal injections of tetanus toxin into the right-dorsal hippocampus (Hawkins and Mellanby, 1987; see section 4C in the Supplementary Material). LFPs were recorded from CA1 and CA3 regions of the hippocampus using

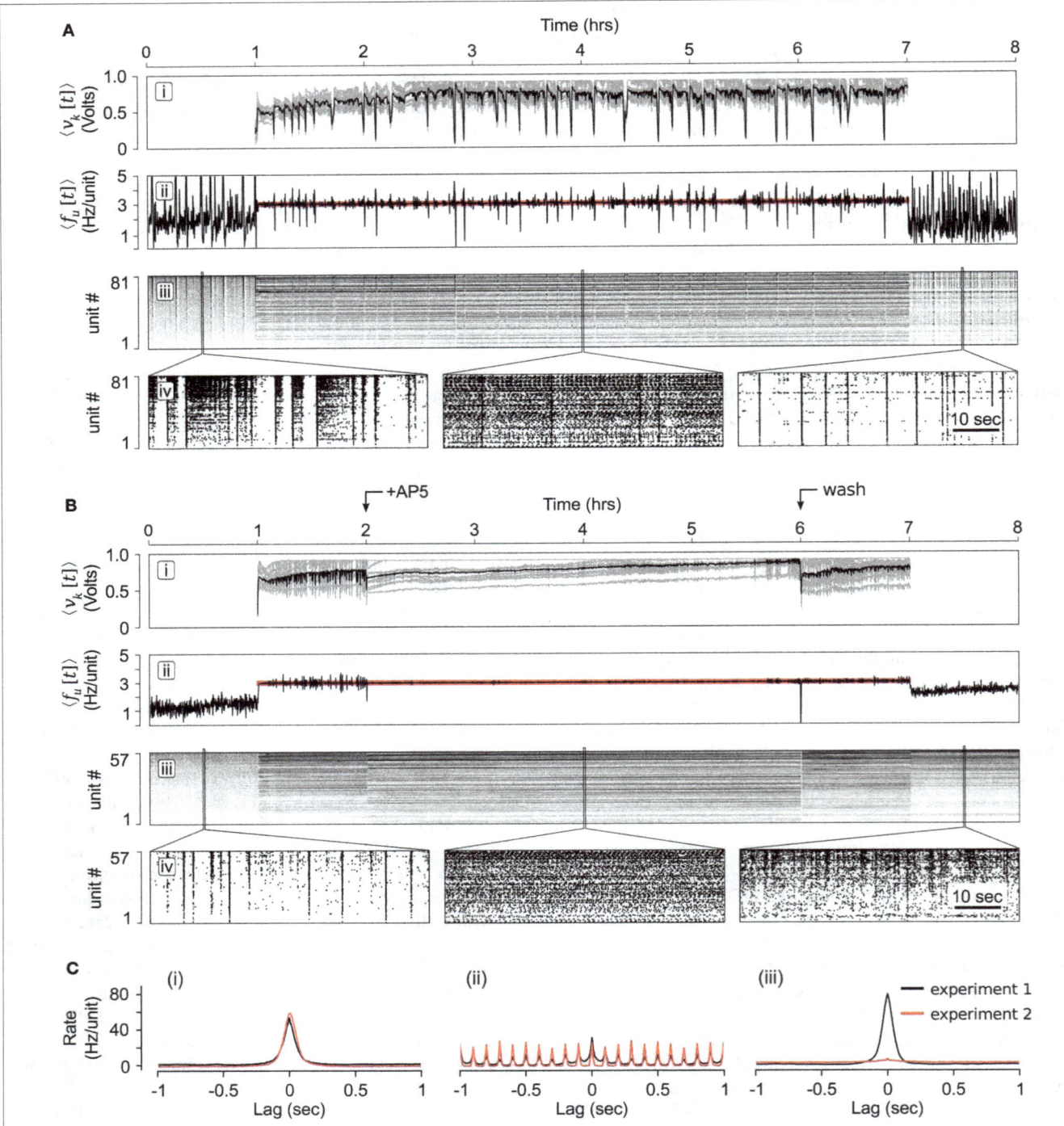

FIGURE 7 | Long-term population clamp. (A) (i) The mean stimulation voltage (black) and individual electrode stimulation voltages (gray) over the course of the 6-h clamping protocol. (ii) The neuronal firing rate (black) compared to the target rate (red line). (iii) Individual unit firing rates, sorted in order of increasing rate during the 1 h period prior to the start of closed-loop control. (iv) Zoomed rastergrams showing short time scale network spiking before, during and after the controller was engaged. **(B)** Same as **(A)** except that AP5 was added 1 h after the start of the closed-loop controller and removed 4 h later. This is indicated by the arrows at the top of the figure. **(C)**

Average pair-wise correlation functions between units for experiments with and without AP5 application (red and black lines, respectively). Cross-correlations were created from spiking data (i) during spontaneous activity before the closed-loop controller was engaged, (ii) half-way through the closed-loop-control period, and (iii) during spontaneous network activity following closed-loop control. The data used to create the correlation functions is centered about locations used to create the rastergrams shown in **(A**iv) and **(B**iv). To create the correlation functions, unit firing rates were calculated using 10 ms time bins.

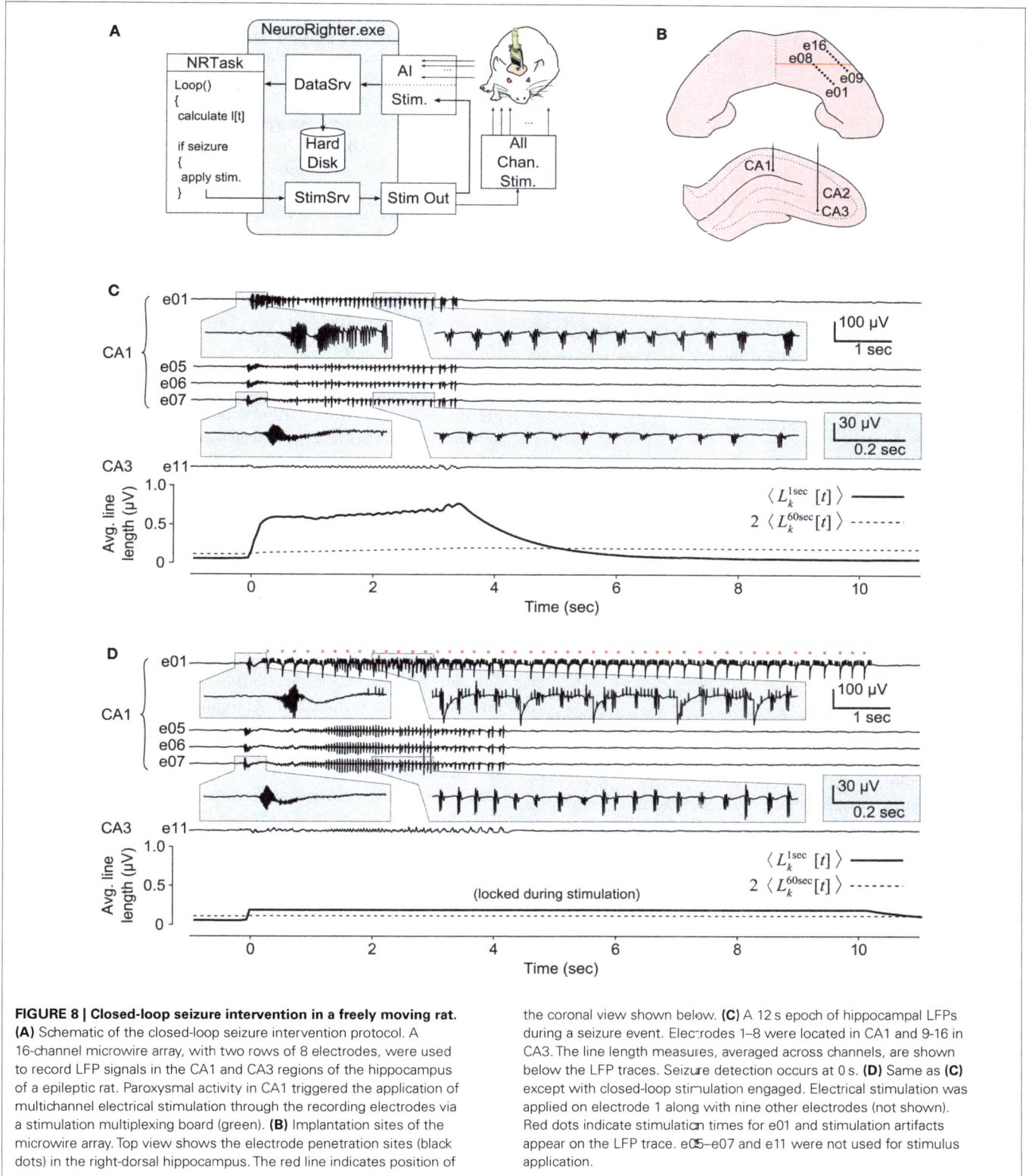

FIGURE 8 | Closed-loop seizure intervention in a freely moving rat.
(A) Schematic of the closed-loop seizure intervention protocol. A
16-channel microwire array, with two rows of 8 electrodes, were used
to record LFP signals in the CA1 and CA3 regions of the hippocampus
of a epileptic rat. Paroxysmal activity in CA1 triggered the application of
multichannel electrical stimulation through the recording electrodes via
a stimulation multiplexing board (green). **(B)** Implantation sites of the
microwire array. Top view shows the electrode penetration sites (black
dots) in the right-dorsal hippocampus. The red line indicates position of
the coronal view shown below. **(C)** A 12 s epoch of hippocampal LFPs
during a seizure event. Electrodes 1–8 were located in CA1 and 9-16 in
CA3. The line length measures, averaged across channels, are shown
below the LFP traces. Seizure detection occurs at 0 s. **(D)** Same as **(C)**
except with closed-loop stimulation engaged. Electrical stimulation was
applied on electrode 1 along with nine other electrodes (not shown).
Red dots indicate stimulation times for e01 and stimulation artifacts
appear on the LFP trace. e05–e07 and e11 were not used for stimulus
application.

a chronically implanted 16-channel microwire array (Tucker-Davis Technologies, Alachua, FL; **Figure 8B**). The microwire array consisted of two rows of electrodes, with 8 electrodes per row.

Multi-electrode stimulation was triggered in response to detected seizures while the rat moved around its cage. To accomplish this, a "line length" measure on each LFP channel, which has been shown to be effective for threshold based seizure detection, was calculated online (Esteller et al., 2001). A line length increment for a single LFP channel is defined as absolute difference between successive samples of the LFP,

$$l_k[t] = |x_k[t] - x_k[t - T_s]| \qquad (3)$$

where $x_k[t]$ is the LFP value on the kth channel at time t, and T_s is the LFP sampling period of 500 μs. $l_k[t]$ was passed through a first order averaging filter,

$$L_k^{\tau_{filt}}[t + T_s] = l_k[t] + \exp\left(\frac{-T_s}{\tau_{filt}}\right) \cdot (L_k^{\tau_{filt}}[t] - l_k[t]) \qquad (4)$$

where τ_{filt} is the filter time constant. For each recording channel, we calculated $L_k^{\tau_{filt}}[t + T_s]$ using two values of τ_{filt}, 1 and 60 s, which resulted in short and long time averages that could be compared to detect rapidly occurring trends in $l_k[t]$. Specifically, seizures were defined as events for which the criterion

$$L_k^{1sec}[t] > 2 \cdot L_k^{60sec}[t] \qquad (5)$$

was met on at least 4 of the 16 recordings channels. Upon seizure detection, 10 randomly chosen electrodes were stimulated sequentially at 45 Hz (aggregate frequency) for 10 s using biphasic, 1 V, 400 μs per phase, square waves. **Figures 8C,D** shows seizure events without and with closed-loop stimulation engaged. During stimulus application, $L_k^{\alpha}[t]$ values were frozen to prevent stimulation artifacts from affecting the line length averages.

There was no easily discernible effect of microstimulation on seizure duration or intensity during this pilot experiment. However, this proof of concept demonstrates the API's utility in experiments conducted on freely moving animals and to modulate aberrant neural activity states. These features are useful for testing stimulation algorithms that do not just react to a seizure occurrence, but *predict* oncoming seizures ahead of time in order to apply a preventative action, which has proven a difficult goal to achieve (Mormann et al., 2007).

3.5. SILENT BARRAGE AND ROBOTIC EMBODIMENT
The complexity of neural systems often necessitates intricate experimental protocols for proper investigation. To meet this requirement, the plugin API can be used to integrate NeuroRighter with complicated configurations external hardware and software. Working in collaboration with the SymbioticA group at the University of Western Australia, we used NeuroRighter for intercontinental neural control of a robotic system. This project was part of an art-science collaboration called Silent Barrage (Zeller-Townson et al., 2011), in which a dissociated cortical culture in Atlanta, Georgia, USA, was embodied with a remote array of robotic drawing machines situated in an interactive art gallery[9]. This system is an extension of the MEART project (Bakkum et al., 2007).

Figure 9A shows an illustration of the Silent Barrage system. Using the plugin API, a protocol was written to communicate

between NeuroRighter and a custom web server running on the same computer. The web server in turn communicated with a client computer controlling a robotic body consisting of 32 independent robots. Each robot had a rotating actuator capable of climbing up and down a vertical column (**Figure 9C**). Columns were arranged in a grid that reflected the electrode layout of the MEA (**Figures 9A,B**). The height of each rotating actuator at a given moment was determined by the instantaneous firing rate detected on two adjacent electrodes from the 59-channel MEA. As the actuators traveled up and down, they periodically marked their positions on the vertical poles using an ink pen. Over time, this resulted in a visual record of spatiotemporal activity of the culture inscribed on each column (**Figure 9C**).

Silent Barrage was exhibited in the United States (New York), Spain (Madrid), Brazil (Sao Paolo), Ireland (Dublin), and China (Beijing). Visitors to the exhibitions were encouraged to mingle amongst the robotic embodiment and they were observed using overhead cameras (**Figures 9A,B**). The resulting video feed was processed on site to extract features of audience movement (Horn and Schunck, 1981) and these data were streamed back to NeuroRighter's web server in Atlanta. Audience movement measures were then used to adjust stimulation patterns delivered through NeuroRighter's all-channel stimulator. The relationship between incoming video data and electrical stimulation varied from exhibit to exhibit, from simple single-electrode rate coding schemes to more complex multi-electrode schemes where artificial neural networks were used to deliver certain stimulus pattern based upon learned features of incoming video data. Electrical stimulation modulated the activity state of the culture's firing patterns, thus closing the loop around the dissociated culture, robotic body, and audience members separated by thousands of kilometers. While on exhibit in the National Art Museum of China, Silent Barrage was perhaps the Earth's largest behaving "organism."

4. DISCUSSION
Closed-loop electrophysiology systems are powerful tools for neuroscience research because they can be used to parse recurrent systems into independently manipulable components. Voltage clamp techniques use feedback control to separate membrane potential from the recurrent influence of voltage-dependent ionic conductances (Marmont, 1949). Seminal experiments using voltage clamp have fostered our understanding of ion channels, neuronal excitability, and synaptic transmission. More recently, dynamic clamp has been used to deliver artificial transmembrane or synaptic conductances into living neurons (Prinz et al., 2004; Kispersky et al., 2011). Using these approaches, feedback control transforms dynamic features of *individual neurons* into controlled experimental variables. Similarly, closed-loop multichannel systems like NeuroRighter can transform features of *neural networks* into controlled experimental variables (Arsiero et al., 2007). NeuroRighter is a powerful tool for controlling network variables, improving upon currently available systems in terms of cost, usability, accessibility, extensibility, and hardware standardization (Wagenaar et al., 2006a; Stirman et al., 2011; Wallach et al., 2011; Ahrens et al., 2012). We have this demonstrated NeuroRighter's power in conducting basic and translational neuroscience research through a variety of case studies.

---

[9]http://silentbarrage.com/

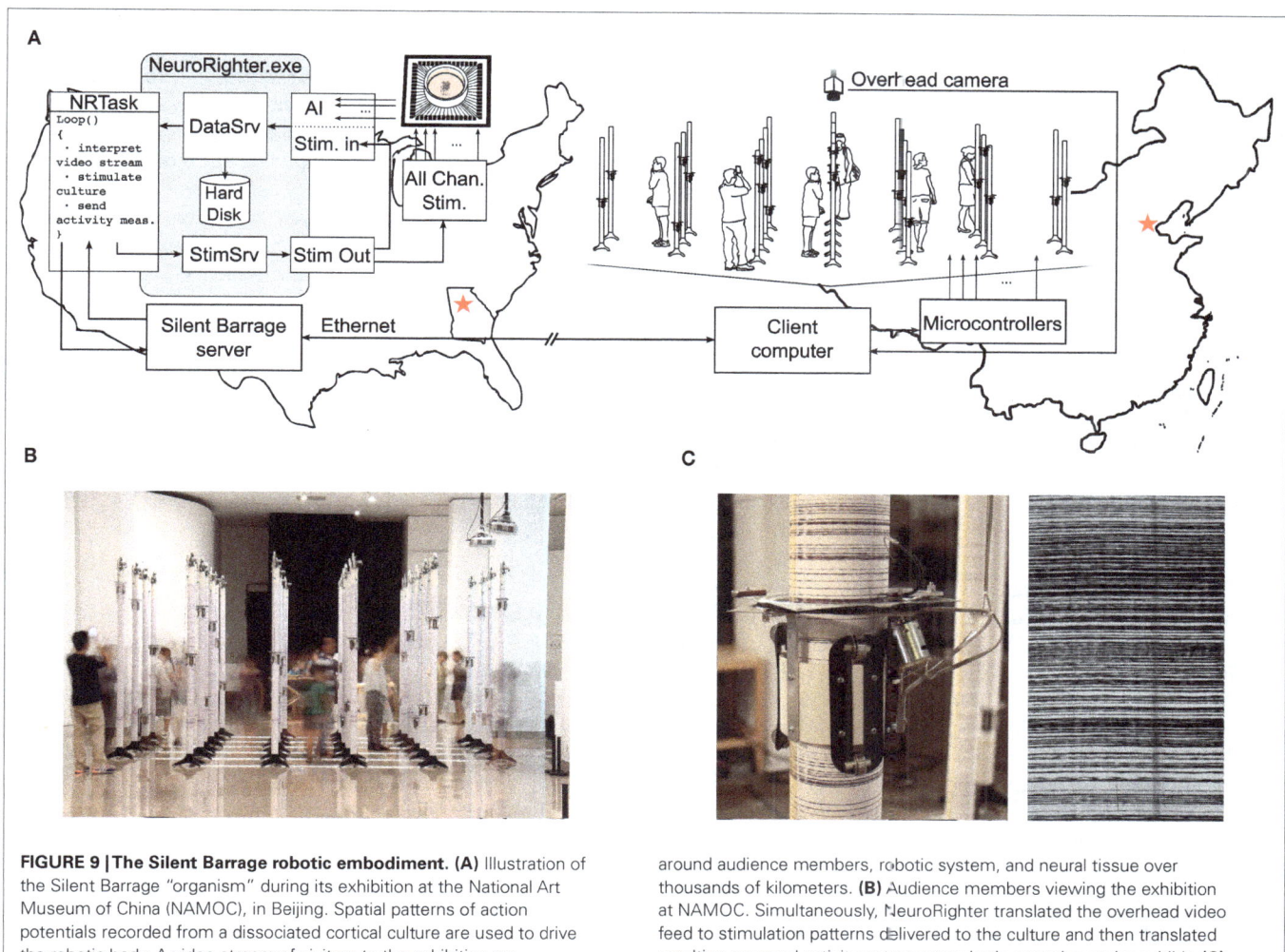

FIGURE 9 | The Silent Barrage robotic embodiment. (A) Illustration of the Silent Barrage "organism" during its exhibition at the National Art Museum of China (NAMOC), in Beijing. Spatial patterns of action potentials recorded from a dissociated cortical culture are used to drive the robotic body. A video stream of visitors to the exhibition are interpreted by NeuroRighter's plugin protocol and used to control multichannel electrical stimulation though the MEA, closing the loop around audience members, robotic system, and neural tissue over thousands of kilometers. **(B)** Audience members viewing the exhibition at NAMOC. Simultaneously, NeuroRighter translated the overhead video feed to stimulation patterns delivered to the culture and then translated resulting neuronal activity patterns to robotic actuation at the exhibit. **(C)** Photograph of an individual robot and the traces it produced during the NAMOC exhibition.

Altered gene expression, synaptic input, or environmental conditions can induce changes in spiking activity, which in turn trigger activity-dependent processes. Because of this, it becomes difficult to distinguish the role these factors play in shaping network dynamics and neural plasticity independent of firing rate. Closed-loop multichannel feedback systems provide an opportunity to render the population firing rate a controlled experimental variable and enable study of cellular and network processes as a function of a defined activity state. We used Neurorighter to clamp the firing rate of a living neural network to user-defined setpoints over both short and long timescales (Sections 3.2, 3.3). Further, we were able to control population firing rate during prolonged application of the NMDA receptor antagonist, AP5 (Section 3.3). Our controller compensated for the loss of NMDA-mediated excitation and maintained network spiking at the target firing rate. Therefore, the effects of AP5 could be deduced through comparison with a control culture that underwent an identical clamping protocol but with intact synaptic transmission. In most studies that use long-term drug application, the individual roles of spiking and

excitatory neurotransmission on plasticity are ambiguous (Turrigiano, 2011). By using a real-time multichannel feedback system, we have begun to unravel the independent effects of spiking and NMDAergic transmission on network behavior. This approach could also be used to more directly study the effects of altered genetic or environmental factors on network activity.

In addition to better controlled experimental variables, real-time feedback can be used to improve the relevance of experiments using reduced neural preparations in studies of behavior. Implicit to animal behavior is the interplay between motor output and sensory perception (e.g., head movement affects the visual input stream and vice-versa). While reduced neural preparations or immobilized animals provide excellent experimental accessibility, their major weakness is that they do not preserve a functional sensory-motor loop. We have demonstrated that Neurorighter is well-equipped for performing closed-loop experiments that restore the sensory-motor loop by interfacing living neural networks with artificial bodies (Section 3.5). The advantages of this approach over traditional open-loop techniques are twofold. First, neural systems can engage in "motor" behaviors without sacrificing delicate optical (Ahrens et al., 2012) or electrophysiological (Harvey et al., 2009) access due to actual motion. Secondly, the experimenter has complete control over the mapping between a recorded neural signal and its resulting "motor" effect (DeMarse et al., 2001; Ahrens et al., 2012). For example, Ahrens et al. (2012) recently examined optomotor adaptation in paralyzed larval zebrafish by embedding them in a virtual environment. Visual stimuli in the virtual environment provided a perception of motion, and induced fictive motor-nerve activity. Recorded motor-nerve activity was used to drive motion of the virtual environment. Changes in sensory-motor feedback gain could be achieved by adjusting the efficacy by which fictive motor patterns propelled the fish through its virtual world. All the while, full brain activity was recorded through single-cell resolution imaging, which would be nearly impossible to achieve in a freely moving animal. This study highlights how closed-loop interfaces between artificial bodies or environments and a living neural system allows excellent experimental access during behaviors requiring an intact sensory-motor loop.

Aside from basic research, closed-loop multichannel electrophysiology has possible medical applications. Predictive application of drugs or electrical stimulation has the potential to increase the efficacy and safety of treatments for various neurological disorders (Mormann et al., 2007; Rosin et al., 2011) and improve neural rehabilitation procedures (Jackson et al., 2006a). For example, a reliable seizure prediction algorithm would open the possibility for targeted interventions that abort seizures before they occur. Mormann et al. (2007) provide an extensive comparison of different methods for seizure prediction. Unfortunately, the clinical applicability of these algorithms remains quite pessimistic and future studies will require a high-throughput validation system to test robustness of seizure prediction algorithms under a variety of circumstances. We have demonstrated that NeuroRighter can be used for this purpose (Section 3.4). The stimulation algorithm we used is very similar to a method called responsive neurostimulation (NeuroPace Inc., Mountain View, CA, USA) that recently showed very promising results in a large, double-blind, pivotal clinical trial (Morrell, 2011). This form of closed-loop seizure modulation is not truly predictive as it was triggered on the occurrence of "unequivocal seizure onset" (Litt and Echauz, 2002). However, the API provides a means for easy reconfiguration in order to test alternative, predictive methods to abort seizures before they begin, using multichannel electrical stimulation or the local application of an anti-convulsive drug. Additionally, a plugin could be reconfigured for closed-loop modulation

of other pathological neuronal activities or to facilitate motor rehabilitation (Jackson et al., 2006a).

Tools that enable closed-loop interaction with neural tissue at the network level have great potential to advance experimental neuroscience. Historically, open-source projects have been extremely good at adapting equipment and code designed for a singular purpose to other uses. For this reason, we envision a large role for open-source software and open-access hardware communities in the development of technologies for closed-loop eletrophysiology systems. Rapid improvements in microprocessor performance, embedded computer systems, on-chip multichannel signal processing, and A/D conversion technology must be matched by projects that can expose their powerful features for researchers with little or no background in embedded systems or computer science. NeuroRighter is one of several open-source hardware/software projects that are enabling more labs to carry out sophisticated electrophysiology with less money and more experimental flexibility[10].

ACKNOWLEDGMENTS

This work was supported by NSF COPN grant 1238097 and NIH grant 1R01NS079757-01, NSF GRFP Fellowship 08-593 to Jonathan P Newman, NSF GRFP Fellowship 09-603 to Ming-fai Fong, and NSF IGERT Fellowship DGE-0333411 to Jonathan P Newman and Ming-fai Fong. Sharanya Arcot Desai was supported by a Faculty for the Future fellowship, provided by the Schlumberger Foundation. We thank Guy Ben-Ary, Phil Gamblen, Peter Gee, Stephen Bobic, and Douglas Swehla for their contributions to the Silent Barrage robotic embodiment project. We thank J. T. Shoemaker for performing tissue harvests. We thank Ted French for his work creating the gas-permeable perfusion caps for delivery of AP5. Finally, we gratefully acknowledge all those who have contributed to NeuroRighter's hardware forums and supplied bug reports to the NeuroRighter code repository. Jon Erickson and Neal Laxpati have been especially helpful in this regard.

---

http://www.its.caltech.edu/~daw/meabench/
http://code.google.com/p/arte-ephys/
http://open-ephys.com/
http://www.backyardbrains.com/Home.aspx

REFERENCES

Ahrens, M. B., Li, J. M., Orger, M. B., Robson, D. N., Schier, A. F., Engert, F., et al. (2012). Brain-wide neuronal dynamics during motor adaptation in zebrafish. *Nature* 485, 471–477.

Arsiero, M., Lüscher, H. R., and Giugliano, M. (2007). Real-time closed-loop electrophysiology: towards new frontiers in in vitro investigations in the neurosciences. *Arch. Ital. Biol.* 145, 193–209.

Azin, M., and Guggenmos, D. J. (2011). A battery-powered activity-dependent intracortical microstimulation IC for brain-machine-brain interface. *IEEE J. Solid-State Circuits* 46, 731–745.

Bakkum, D. J., Gamblen, P. M., Ben-Ary, G., Chao, Z. C., and Potter, S. M. (2007). MEART: The Semi-Living Artist. *Front. Neurorob.* 1:5. doi:10.3389/neuro.12.005.2007

Cole, K. S. (1949). Dynamic electrical characteristics of the squid axon membrane. *Annu. Rev. Physiol.* 3, 253–258.

DeMarse, T. B., Wagenaar, D. A., Blau, A. W., and Potter, S. M. (2001). The neurally controlled animat: biological brains acting with simulated bodies. *Auton. Robots* 11, 305–310.

Desai, S. A., Rolston, J. D., Guo, L., and Potter, S. M. (2010). Improving impedance of implantable microwire multi-electrode arrays by ultrasonic electroplating of durable platinum black. *Front. Neuroeng.* 3:5. doi:10.3389/fneng.2010.00005

Du, J., Blanche, T. J., Harrison, R. R., Lester, H., and Masmanidis, S. C. (2011). Multiplexed, high density electrophysiology with nanofabricated neural probes. *PLoS ONE* 6:e26204. doi:10.1371/journal.pone.0026204

Esteller, R., Echauz, J., and Tcheng, T. (2001). Line length: an efficient feature for seizure onset detection. *Conf. Proc. IEEE Eng. Med. Biol. Soc.* 2, 1707–1710.

Fiscella, M., Farrow, K., Jones, I. L., Jäckel, D., Müller, J., Frey, U., et al. (2012). Recording from defined populations of retinal ganglion cells using a high-density CMOS-integrated microelectrode array with real-time switchable electrode selection. *J. Neurosci. Methods* 211, 103–113.

Gal, A., Eytan, D., Wallach, A., Sandler, M., Schiller, J., and Marom, S. (2010). Dynamics of excitability over extended timescales in cultured cortical neurons. *J. Neurosci.* 30, 16332–16342.

Hamill, O. P., Marty, A., Neher, E., and Sakmann, B. (1981). Improved patch-clamp techniques for high-resolution current recording from cells and cell-free membrane patches. *Pflugers Arch.* 391, 85–100.

Harvey, C. D., Collman, F., Dombeck, D. A., and Tank, D. W. (2009). Intracellular dynamics of hippocampal place cells during virtual navigation. *Nature* 461, 941–946.

Hawkins, C. A., and Mellanby, J. H. (1987). Limbic epilepsy induced by tetanus toxin: A longitudinal electroencephalographic study. *Epilepsia* 28, 431–444.

Horn, B. K. P., and Schunck, B. G. (1981). Determining optical flow. *Artif. Intell.* 17, 185–203.

Jackson, A., Mavoori, J., and Fetz, E. E. (2006a). Long-term motor cortex plasticity induced by an electronic neural implant. *Nature* 444, 56–60.

Jackson, A., Moritz, C. T., Mavoori, J., Lucas, T. H., and Fetz, E. E. (2006b). The Neurochip BCI: towards a neural prosthesis for upper limb function. *IEEE Trans. Neural Syst. Rehabil. Eng.* 14, 187–190.

Kispersky, T. J., Economo, M. N., Randeria, P., and White, J. A. (2011). GenNet: a platform for hybrid network experiments. *Front. Neuroinform.* 5:11. doi:10.3389/fninf.2011.00011

Litt, B., and Echauz, J. (2002). Prediction of epileptic seizures. *Lancet Neurol.* 1, 22–30.

Marmont, G. (1949). Studies on the axon membrane. *J. Cell. Comp. Physiol.* 34, 351–381.

Minerbi, A., Kahana, R., Goldfeld, L., Kaufman, M., Marom, S., and Ziv, N. E. (2009). Long-term relationships between synaptic tenacity, synaptic remodeling, and network activity. *PLoS Biol.* 7:e1000136. doi:10.1371/journal.pbio.1000136

Mormann, F., Andrzejak, R. G., Elger, C. E., and Lehnertz, K. (2007). Seizure prediction: the long and winding road. *Brain* 130, 314–333.

Morrell, M. J. (2011). Responsive cortical stimulation for the treatment of medically intractable partial epilepsy. *Neurology* 77, 1295–1304.

Nakanishi, K., and Kukita, F. (1998). Functional synapses in synchronized bursting of neocortical neurons in culture. *Brain Res.* 795, 137–146.

Nelson, T. S., Suhr, C. L., Freestone, D. R., Lai, A., Halliday, A. J., Mclean, K. J., et al. (2011). Closed-loop seizure control with very high frequency electrical stimulation at seizure onset in the Gaers model of absence epilepsy. *Int. J. Neural Syst.* 21, 163.

Potter, S. M., and DeMarse, T. B. (2001). A new approach to neural cell culture for long-term studies. *J. Neurosci. Methods* 110, 17–24.

Prinz, A. A., Abbott, L. F., and Marder, E. (2004). The dynamic clamp comes of age. *Trends Neurosci.* 27, 218–224.

Reger, B. D., Fleming, K. M., Sanguineti, V., and Alford, S. (2000). Connecting brains to robots: an artificial body for studying the computational properties of neural tissues. *Artif. Life* 324, 307–324.

Rich, M. M., and Wenner, P. (2007). Sensing and expressing homeostatic synaptic plasticity. *Trends Neurosci.* 30, 119–125.

Robinson, J. T., Jorgolli, M., Shalek, A. K., Yoon, M.-H., Gertner, R. S., and Park, H. (2012). Vertical nanowire electrode arrays as a scalable platform for intracellular interfacing to neuronal circuits. *Nat. Nanotechnol.* 7, 180–184.

Rolston, J. D., Gross, R. E., and Potter, S. M. (2009a). A low-cost multielectrode system for data acquisition enabling real-time closed-loop processing with rapid recovery from stimulation artifacts. *Front. Neuroeng.* 2:12. doi:10.3389/neuro.16.012.2009

Rolston, J. D., Gross, R. E., and Potter, S. M. (2009b). Common median referencing for improved action potential detection with multielectrode arrays. *Conf. Proc. IEEE Eng. Med. Biol. Soc.* 2009, 1604–1607.

Rolston, J. D., Gross, R. E., and Potter, S. M. (2010). Closed-loop, open-source electrophysiology. *Front. Neurosci.* 4:31. doi:10.3389/fnins.2010.00031

Rosin, B., Slovik, M., Mitelman, R., Rivlin-Etzion, M., Haber, S. N., Israel, Z., et al. (2011). Closed-loop deep brain stimulation is superior in ameliorating parkinsonism. *Neuron* 72, 370–384.

Stirman, J. N., Crane, M. M., Husson, S. J., Wabnig, S., Schultheis, C., Gottschalk, A., et al. (2011). Real-time multimodal optical control of neurons and muscles in freely behaving Caenorhabditis elegans. *Nat. Methods* 8, 153–158.

Strong, S. P., Koberle, R., de Ruyter Van Steveninck, R. R., and Bialek, W. (1998). Entropy and information in neural spike trains. *Phys. Rev. Lett.* 80, 197–200.

Sun, F. T., Morrell, M. J., and Wharen, R. E. (2008). Responsive cortical stimulation for the treatment of epilepsy. *Neurotherapeutics* 5, 68–74.

Supèr, H., and Roelfsema, P. R. (2005). Chronic multiunit recordings in behaving animals: advantages and limitations. *Prog. Brain Res.* 147, 263–282.

Tchumatchenko, T., Geisel, T., Volgushev, M., and Wolf, F. (2010). Signatures of synchrony in pairwise count correlations. *Front. Comput. Neurosci.* 4:1. doi:10.3389/neuro.10.001.2010

Turrigiano, G. (2011). Too many cooks? Intrinsic and synaptic homeostatic mechanisms in cortical circuit refinement. *Annu. Rev. Neurosci.* 34, 89–103.

Turrigiano, G. G., Leslie, K. R., Desai, N. S., Rutherford, L. C., and Nelson, S. B. (1998). Activity-dependent scaling of quantal amplitude in neocortical neurons. *Nature* 391, 892–896.

Wagenaar, D. A., Madhavan, R., Pine, J., and Potter, S. M. (2005). Controlling bursting in cortical cultures with closed-loop multi-electrode stimulation. *J. Neurosci.* 25, 680–688

Wagenaar, D. A., Pine, J., and Potter, S. M. (2004). Effective parameters for stimulation of dissociated cultures using multi-electrode arrays. *J. Neurosci. Methods* 138, 27–37.

Wagenaar, D. A., Pine, J., and Potter, S. M. (2006a). An extremely rich repertoire of bursting patterns during the development of cortical cultures. *BMC Neurosci.* 7:11. doi:10.1186/1471-2202-7-11

Wagenaar, D., DeMarse, T. B., and Potter, S. M. (2006b). "MEABench: a toolset for multi-electrode data acquisition and on-line analysis," in *International IEEE EMBS Conference on Neural Engineering*, Washington, 518–521.

Wagenaar, D. A., and Potter, S. M. (2002). Real-time multi-channel stimulus artifact suppression by local curve fitting. *J. Neurosci. Methods* 120, 113–120.

Wagenaar, D. A., and Potter, S. M. (2004). A versatile all-channel stimulator for electrode arrays, with real-time control. *J. Neural. Eng.* 1, 39–45.

Wallach, A., Eytan, D., Gal, A., Zrenner, C., and Marom, S. (2011). Neuronal response clamp. *Front. Neuroeng.* 4:3. doi:10.3389/fneng.2011.00003

Yu, Y., Crumiller, M., Knight, B., and Kaplan, E. (2010). Estimating the amount of information carried by a neuronal population. *Front. Comput. Neurosci.* 4:10. doi:10.3389/fncom.2010.00010

Zanos, S., Richardson, A. G., Shupe, L., Miles, F. P., and Fetz, E. E. (2011). The Neurochip-2: an autonomous head-fixed computer for recording and stimulating in freely behaving monkeys. *IEEE Trans. Neural Syst. Rehabil. Eng.* 19, 427–435.

Zeller-Townson, R., Ben-Ary, G., and Gamblen, P. (2011). "Silent barrage: interactive neurobiological art," in *The Proceedings of the 8th ACM Conference on Creativity and Cognition*, Atlanta, 407–408.

14

A neurochemical closed-loop controller for deep brain stimulation: toward individualized smart neuromodulation therapies

Peter J. Grahn[1], Grant W. Mallory[2], Obaid U. Khurram[1], B. Michael Berry[1], Jan T. Hachmann[2], Allan J. Bieber[2,3], Kevin E. Bennet[2,4], Hoon-Ki Min[2,5], Su-Youne Chang[2], Kendall H. Lee[2,5] and J. L. Lujan[2,5]*

[1] Mayo Clinic College of Medicine, Mayo Clinic, Rochester, MN, USA
[2] Department of Neurologic Surgery, Mayo Clinic, Rochester, MN, USA
[3] Department of Neurology, Mayo Clinic, Rochester, MN, USA
[4] Division of Engineering, Mayo Clinic, Rochester, MN, USA
[5] Department of Physiology and Biomedical Engineering, Mayo Clinic, Rochester, MN, USA

Edited by:
Mitsuhiro Hayashibe, University of Montpellier, France

Reviewed by:
Matthew Johnson, University of Minnesota, USA
Christian J. Hartmann, Heinrich Heine University Duesseldorf, Germany

*Correspondence:
J. L. Lujan, Departments of Neurologic Surgery and Physiology and Biomedical Engineering, Mayo Clinic, 200 First Street SW, Rochester, MN 55905, USA
e-mail: lujan.luis@mayo.edu

Current strategies for optimizing deep brain stimulation (DBS) therapy involve multiple postoperative visits. During each visit, stimulation parameters are adjusted until desired therapeutic effects are achieved and adverse effects are minimized. However, the efficacy of these therapeutic parameters may decline with time due at least in part to disease progression, interactions between the host environment and the electrode, and lead migration. As such, development of closed-loop control systems that can respond to changing neurochemical environments, tailoring DBS therapy to individual patients, is paramount for improving the therapeutic efficacy of DBS. Evidence obtained using electrophysiology and imaging techniques in both animals and humans suggests that DBS works by modulating neural network activity. Recently, animal studies have shown that stimulation-evoked changes in neurotransmitter release that mirror normal physiology are associated with the therapeutic benefits of DBS. Therefore, to fully understand the neurophysiology of DBS and optimize its efficacy, it may be necessary to look beyond conventional electrophysiological analyses and characterize the neurochemical effects of therapeutic and non-therapeutic stimulation. By combining electrochemical monitoring and mathematical modeling techniques, we can potentially replace the trial-and-error process used in clinical programming with deterministic approaches that help attain optimal and stable neurochemical profiles. In this manuscript, we summarize the current understanding of electrophysiological and electrochemical processing for control of neuromodulation therapies. Additionally, we describe a proof-of-principle closed-loop controller that characterizes DBS-evoked dopamine changes to adjust stimulation parameters in a rodent model of DBS. The work described herein represents the initial steps toward achieving a "smart" neuroprosthetic system for treatment of neurologic and psychiatric disorders.

Keywords: deep brain stimulation (DBS), feedback control systems, local field potentials (LFP), fast scan cyclic voltammetry (FSCV), machine learning, individualized medicine

INTRODUCTION

Neurologic and psychiatric disorders can be characterized by motor, behavioral, cognitive, affective, or perceptual traits that affect how individuals move, feel, think, and behave (Benabid et al., 2005; Nemeroff, 2007; Williams and Okun, 2013). These disorders affect over 94 million people in the United States alone with health-care related costs exceeding $648 billion (Logothetis, 2003b; Benabid et al., 2005; Speert et al., 2012; Williams and Okun, 2013). Although most individuals suffering from neurologic and psychiatric disorders are successfully treated with a combination of medications and therapy, up to 30% of patients are unable to respond to standard therapeutic interventions

(Olanow et al., 2000; Benabid et al., 2005; Hamani et al., 2006; Nemeroff, 2007; Williams and Okun, 2013). For these treatment-resistant patients, high-frequency electrical stimulation of subcortical brain structures, known as deep brain stimulation (DBS), presents a highly successful therapeutic alternative (Benabid et al., 2005; Williams and Okun, 2013). DBS is FDA-approved for the treatment of Parkinson's disease (PD) and essential tremor (ET) (Benabid et al., 1987, 1991; Burchiel et al., 1999; Koller et al., 2001; Obeso and Guridi, 2001; Simuni et al., 2002; Rehncrona et al., 2003; Germano et al., 2004; Rodriguez-Oroz, 2004; Blomstedt and Hariz, 2010; Moro et al., 2010; Weiss et al., 2013). Additionally, DBS has received humanitarian device exemptions for dystonia and obsessive-compulsive disorder, and there are multiple studies underway for the treatment of other neurologic and psychiatric disorders (Benabid et al., 1987, 1991; Burchiel et al., 1999; Obeso and Guridi, 2001; Simuni et al., 2002; Velasco et al., 2005; Lim et al., 2007; Mueller et al., 2008; Blomstedt and Hariz, 2010; Denys et al., 2010; Fisher et al., 2010; Ramasubbu et al., 2013).

Brain stimulation has been an important tool in the field of neurosurgery pioneered by Spiegel and Wycis (Blomstedt and Hariz, 2010). Intra-operative electrical stimulation of neural tissue has been used since the early days of human stereotaxis to identify surgical targets (Gildenberg, 2003, 2005). Application of brain stimulation in modern-day neurosurgery was revolutionized by Benabid and colleagues, who used high frequency stimulation (typically 100–130 Hz) delivered directly into specific brain regions to mimic the effects of surgical lesions without performing any tissue resection (Benabid et al., 1987, 1991; Blomstedt and Hariz, 2010). DBS achieves therapeutic benefits by delivering electrical currents to specific anatomical targets within the brain via multi-contact electrodes connected to implanted pulse generators. In DBS therapy, a balance between maximal clinical improvement and minimal stimulation-induced side effects is typically achieved by adjusting active electrode contacts, stimulus frequency, amplitude, and pulse duration.

Clinical DBS programming is an iterative process in which stimulation parameters are adjusted in order to maximize therapeutic benefits while minimizing side effects (Morishita et al., 2013) Although many DBS patients require minimal stimulation adjustment following surgery, many more require several months of regular parameter adjustments before optimal therapeutic results can be achieved (Okun et al., 2005; Bronstein et al., 2011; Kluger et al., 2011). However, sustaining these therapeutic benefits requires subsequent adjustment of stimulation parameters every few months (Mayberg et al., 2000, 2005; Deuschl et al., 2006; Moro et al., 2006; Frankemolle et al., 2010; Mure et al., 2011). Therefore, existing clinical programming and stimulation paradigms are poorly suited to cope with the dynamic and comorbid nature of most neurologic disorders. This, in turn, highlights the need for dynamic feedback systems that can continually and automatically adjust stimulation parameters in response to changes within the environment of the brain.

THERAPEUTIC STIMULATION PARADIGMS

The therapeutic success of DBS depends not only on accurate surgical targeting and electrode implantation, but also on the ability to optimize stimulation parameters to maximize therapeutic benefits while minimizing side effects. Clinical strategies for therapeutic DBS programming require multiple post-operative visits during which experienced clinicians perform clinical evaluations and corresponding device programming. In each visit, a series of inputs (active contacts, stimulus amplitude, pulse width, and frequency) are adjusted in an attempt to minimize adverse effects while maximizing clinical benefits. Although this strategy has provided significant patient benefit, the results are far from optimal. First, this open loop strategy relies on the subjective experiences of both the patient and clinician, without providing objective feedback to support parameter optimization. Second, the therapeutic response observed in this acute setting

does not guarantee sustained therapeutic effects. Disease progression, environmental factors, and behaviorally induced changes in network activity can all render therapeutic stimulation ineffective, requiring additional programming sessions (Obeso and Guridi, 2001; Hunka et al., 2005; Kupsch et al., 2011). Third, the procedure is costly and time consuming. As such, only a fraction of the stimulation parameter space can be practically explored during each session. Fourth, DBS device programming can differ according to the target chosen, the orientation of the electrode relative to the target, the disorder being treated, and the symptoms being treated for a given disorder (Velasco et al., 2007; Ricchi et al., 2012; Min et al., 2013; Miocinovic et al., 2013). Additionally, the timing of programming as well as the waiting time between adjustments can influence when different therapeutic responses can be observed, and these responses also vary between disorders (e.g., Tremor is nearly immediate, whereas depression could take several weeks to observe the effect of a disorder) (Velasco et al., 2007; Ricchi et al., 2012; Min et al., 2013; Miocinovic et al., 2013). Therefore, it is necessary to implement DBS control strategies that can adjust stimulation parameters in real-time according to quantifiable and objective neurochemical, physiological, and behavioral changes while reducing the frequency of clinical interventions. However, before such control strategies can be implemented, it is necessary to improve the understanding of the cellular mechanisms responsible for the network effects of DBS.

The cellular response of single neurons to extracellular electrical fields has been well characterized over short time scales (Smith and Grace, 1992; Benazzouz et al., 2000; Hashimoto et al., 2003; Maurice et al., 2003; Kita et al., 2005; Miocinovic et al., 2006). It is known that excitation of efferent axons or fibers of passage near the site of stimulation results in network changes in neurotransmission and electrical activity (Grill et al., 2004; McIntyre et al., 2004a,b; Johnson et al., 2008; McIntyre and Hahn, 2010; Shah et al., 2010). Furthermore, functional and metabolic imaging studies have shown that successful treatment of neurologic and psychiatric disorders is associated with metabolic normalization in proximal and distal regions of the brain (Mayberg et al., 2000, 2005; Mure et al., 2011). The precise relationships between therapeutic improvement and changes in metabolic patterns remain unknown. As such, current research efforts focus on the use electrophysiology and electrochemistry to elucidate the network effects of DBS (Bledsoe et al., 2009; Lee et al., 2011; Vitek et al., 2012).

REAL-TIME MONITORING OF NEURAL ACTIVITY

Signaling within the brain occurs both electrically and chemically. Technological advances in neural activity monitoring have enabled real-time investigation of cellular and molecular dynamics using electrophysiological and neurochemical probes. While the most used technique involves electrophysiological monitoring of extra-cellular neuronal activity (Smith and Grace, 1992; Benazzouz et al., 2000; Hashimoto et al., 2003; Maurice et al., 2003; Johnson et al., 2005; Kita et al., 2005; Miocinovic et al., 2006) recent advances in electrode technology allow *in vivo* monitoring of synaptic neurotransmitter activity (Roham et al., 2007; van Gompel et al., 2010).

Electrophysiological analysis has been widely used to study stimulation-evoked changes in brain activity, such as increased pallidal (Hashimoto et al., 2003; Kita et al., 2005; Miocinovic et al., 2006) and nigral activity (Smith and Grace, 1992; Benazzouz et al., 2000; Maurice et al., 2003) during subthalamic nucleus (STN) DBS. This has been accomplished by recording single neuron activity (single unit recordings), activity from local groups of neurons (multi unit activity, local field potentials), and distributed signals representing global brain activity [electrocorticograms (ECoGs), electroencephalograms (EEGs)]. Alternatively, neurochemical analysis techniques such as microdialysis, amperometry, and voltammetry, can detect local changes in neurotransmitter concentration evoked by internal and external mechanical, electrical, and chemical stimuli (Dale et al., 2005; Wightman, 2006). Neurochemical recordings have been used to monitor *in vivo* release of analytes such as oxygen, dopamine, adenosine, serotonin, and glutamate in small and large animal models of DBS (Agnesi et al., 2009; Bledsoe et al., 2009; Chang et al., 2009; Kimble et al., 2009; Griessenauer et al., 2010; Shon et al., 2010a,b).

SINGLE-UNIT RECORDINGS

Single unit recordings capture the activity of distinct neurons *in vivo* by placing a high-impedance microelectrode within the extracellular space surrounding the cell body. These electrodes, having surface areas under $2 \times 10\text{-}5\,\text{cm}^2$ (Loffler, 2012), record extracellular potentials representative of intracellular action potentials from neurons adjacent to the electrode tip. The high spatial and temporal resolution provided by single unit recordings allows for precise measurements of neuronal spikes (Buzsáki et al., 2012). However, activity from single units can be difficult to isolate due to crosstalk from neighboring cells (Bai and Wise, 2001). Additionally, single unit recordings can be biased toward activity from larger (e.g., pyramidal) cells (Buzsáki et al., 1983). Furthermore, electrode migration, immune responses (e.g., glial scarring), and disruption of surrounding neural tissue interfere with signal quality and limit reliable single unit activity to acute recording conditions (Carter and Houk, 1993; Polikov et al., 2005).

MULTI-UNIT RECORDINGS

Multi unit recordings capture fast spiking activity from groups of neurons using high-impedance microelectrode arrays. Similar to single unit recordings, this technique provides good spatial and temporal resolution reflecting synaptic events occurring at high frequencies (>800 Hz) (Logothetis, 2003a,b; Mattia et al., 2010). Unfortunately, multi-unit recording arrays suffer from stiff form factors that result in shear-induced inflammation of the surrounding tissue (Cheung, 2007). Furthermore, recording can only occur from the tips of the electrodes, limiting recording selectivity (Maynard et al., 1997).

LOCAL FIELD POTENTIALS

Local field potential (LFP) analysis is an electrophysiological technique for detecting changes in brain activity that offers great potential for understanding the network effects of DBS (Tsang et al., 2012; Priori et al., 2013). This technique is capable of recording chronic electrical activity directly from single

and multiple neural units using micro and macro electrodes implanted within the nucleus of interest (Bronte-Stewart et al., 2009; Giannicola et al., 2012). LFPs are typically used to record low-frequency changes in activity across groups of neurons within a volume of interest (Andersen et al., 2004; Buzsáki et al., 2012; Rosa et al., 2012). These activity changes reflect a weighted average of integrative processes and associations between cells that can be detected over longer distances through extracellular space (Logothetis, 2003a,b; Bronte-Stewart et al., 2009). Unfortunately, the longer recording range of LFP techniques is associated with decreased spatial resolution. Despite this limitation, LFP recordings can be performed in real-time using the same DBS electrode, which eliminates the need for additional electrode penetrations (Rossi et al., 2007). Therefore, local field potentials present a good starting point for establishing closed-loop neurostimulation control systems (Rosin et al., 2011; Santaniello et al., 2011; Berényi et al., 2012; Little et al., 2013).

GLOBAL FIELD POTENTIALS

Analysis of global brain activity can be used to identify both spontaneous and event-related responses from large groups of neurons. Whole-brain electrophysiological brain activity (i.e., global field potentials) is typically measured using far-field sensors located on the scalp (EEG) or directly on the brain surface (ECoG). These global field potentials can be used to identify information regarding high-level sensory processing, perception, and locomotor activity (Issa and Wang, 2013). For example, EEG signals with low spatial resolution can be recorded non-invasively by non-surgically attaching recording electrodes to the scalp. Alternatively, ECoG signals offer increased spatial resolution, but recording electrodes must be surgically attached at the cortical surface (Buzsáki et al., 2012). Despite the advantages of global field potentials, these signals do not provide insight into activity changes within specific subcortical structures. As such, a system that combines activity analysis within cortical (e.g., EcOG) and subcortical (e.g., LFP) networks should provide a better depiction of network dynamics which, in turn, will be required to develop optimal closed-loop stimulation paradigms (Rosa et al., 2012).

NEUROCHEMICAL RECORDINGS

Neurochemical sensing allows real-time characterization of neural activity with high spatial resolution and signal specificity (Lee et al., 2004). Microdialysis, amperometry, and voltammetry are three widely used techniques for neurochemical monitoring (Blaha and Phillips, 1996).

Microdialysis is a technique for sampling different analytes and determining their concentration in extracellular fluid (Chefer et al., 2009). This technique offers excellent specificity, selectivity, and sensitivity for quantifying neurotransmitter release in a laboratory setting (Watson et al., 2006). However, it suffers from limited temporal resolution (Smolders et al., 1997; Khan et al., 1999). Therefore, microdialysis is not suitable for real-time clinical application in closed-loop systems.

Amperometry is an alternative technique for measuring analytes in the extracellular space. Amperometric recordings involve the application of a fixed electric potential through a carbon fiber microelectrode (CFM) placed in close proximity to the target

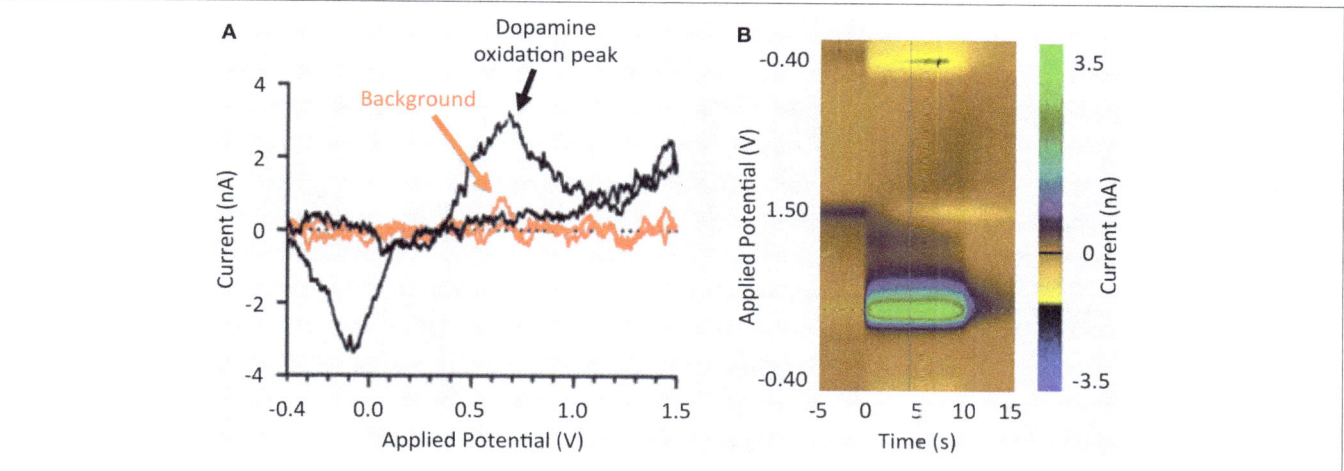

FIGURE 1 | Stimulation-evoked dopamine responses. (A) Dopamine redox reactions at the tip of a carbon fiber microelectrode during fast scan cyclic voltammetry. As the potential applied to the electrode increases from −0.4 to 0.0 V, extracellular dopamine is reduced (reduction peak at −3.5 nA). As the applied potential is further increased from 0.0 to 1.0 V, dopamine is oxidized (oxidation peak at 3.5 nA). Measured current background is shown in red. **(B)** Pseudo-color representation of dopamine oxidation current at +0.6 V at DBS onset (100 Hz, 2 ms, 300 μA .

cells (Gale et al., 2013; Tye et al., 2013). These CFM are coated with specific enzymes known to react with non-electrolytic analytes of interest, resulting in electroactive products that can be electrically measured (Oldenziel et al., 2004). This allows continuous monitoring of changes in electrical currents within the surrounding extracellular fluid. The detected changes in current are caused by oxidative reactions between the applied potential and analyte molecules within the extracellular space (van Gompel et al., 2010). The downfall of this technique is the high complexity associated with chronic *in vivo* measurements, which require continuous enzyme delivery to detect the breakdown products of the neurotransmitter of interest (Jacobs et al., 2010).

Analogous to amperometry, voltammetry provides real-time high-resolution analyte measurements (Blaha et al., 1990). Specifically, fast scan cyclic voltammetry (FSCV) is a voltammetry technique in which a linearly varying potential is applied to a carbon fiber electrode, allowing for oxidation and reduction of surrounding electroactive molecules to take place (Robinson et al., 2003; Lee et al., 2007). The magnitudes of the analyte oxidation and reduction current peaks are directly proportional to the concentration of analyte oxidized and reduced at the electrode surface (Atcherley et al., 2013). Furthermore, the resulting electrical current vs. applied potential relationships (**Figure 1**) provide a chemical signature (i.e., voltammogram) that allows identification of specific neurotransmitters or other electroactive analytes (Robinson et al., 2003). FSCV detection of analytes is limited to electroactive molecules such as dopamine, adenosine, and oxygen (van Gompel et al., 2010). Furthermore, the lifetime of CFM is limited to a few months (Kim et al., under review), restricting clinical application of FSCV detection methods to intraoperative approaches.

SMART DBS CONTROL
Clinical DBS systems follow an open-loop paradigm. That is, stimulation parameters are pre-programmed into the DBS device and held constant until the next programming session, regardless of the internal state of the system or environmental factors (Foltynie and Hariz, 2010). In contrast, closed-loop DBS systems rely on sensor feedback to monitor the environment and internal state of the system in order to adjust stimulation parameters accordingly (Abbott, 2006; Fagg et al., 2007). That is, stimulation parameters (e.g., stimulation frequency, stimulus amplitude, etc.) are automatically adjusted to maintain specific therapeutic outputs such as tremor suppression in the presence of disturbances, environmental perturbations, and internal network changes (**Figure 2**). To date, development of closed-loop neuroprosthetic devices has largely focused on using electrophysiological activity as feedback signals (Avestruz et al., 2008; Skarpaas and Morrell, 2009; Rosin et al., 2011; Basu et al., 2013; Grant and Lowery, 2013). Neurochemical-based feedback, however, offers the prospect of finer control of stimulation-induced effects, as it allows activity monitoring from individual types of neurons by virtue of their neurotransmitters. The ability to use neurochemical feedback to control DBS has been demonstrated by characterizing glutamate release using mathematical models linking electrical stimulation to glutamate release in a rat model of DBS (Behrend et al., 2009). Thus, chemical sensing presents a unique opportunity for developing closed-loop smart neurocontrol systems that are optimized for specific disorders and targets, and which can account for intra- and inter-patient variability.

NEUROCHEMISTRY OF DBS
Studies using small and large animal models suggest that therapeutic DBS coincides with changes in neurotransmitter release (Lee et al., 2004; Shon et al., 2010a,b). It has been established that dopaminergic cell loss in the substantia nigra leads to striatal dopamine deficiency and movement abnormalities in PD patients (MacDonald et al., 2013). It has also been shown that therapeutic STN DBS for treatment of PD decreases the need for exogenous levodopa (Moro et al., 1999; Molinuevo et al.,

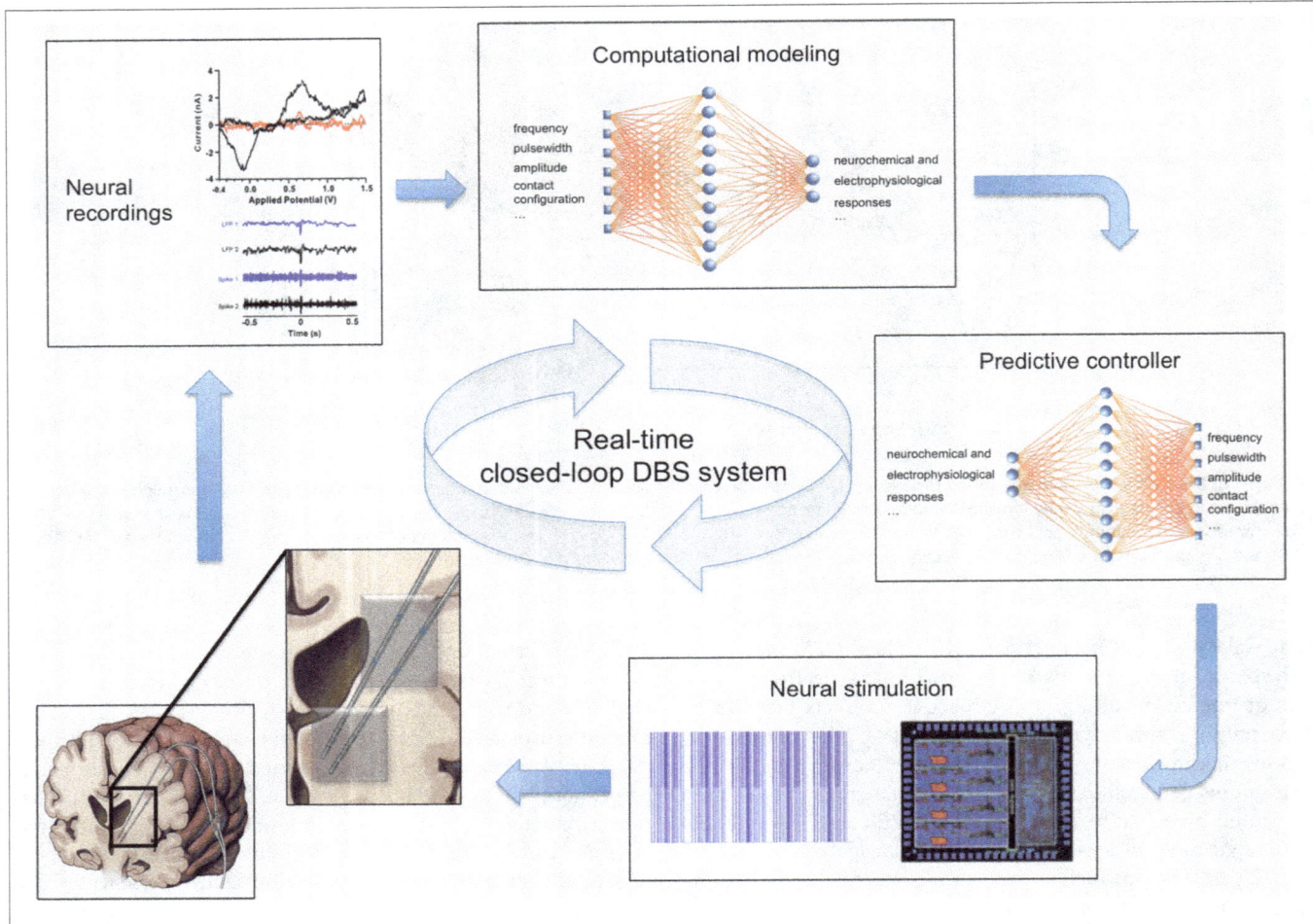

FIGURE 2 | Real-time closed-loop deep brain stimulation system.
Clockwise from bottom left: (1) Schematic of the human brain with two electrodes (inset) for simultaneous stimulation (gray contacts) and recording of neural activity (blue contacts). (2) Example voltammogram, local field potentials, and single unit activity signals representing recorded neurochemical and electrophysiological neural activity. (3) Computational

model of neurochemical and electrophysiological dynamics allows generation and optimization of data beyond the time constraints imposed by experimental conditions. (4) Smart controller uses existing neural activity to predict stimulation parameters required to achieve therapeutic neuromodulation. (5) Predicted stimulation parameters are applied to the brain using an implanted neurostimulation system.

2000) and has been hypothesized to increase striatal dopamine release (Lee et al., 2009). Complementing findings in electrophysiological and neurochemical sensing studies have shown that STN DBS evokes dopamine release in the striatum of parkinsonian rats (Blaha and Phillips, 1996; Lee et al., 2006). Similarly, stimulation-evoked adenosine release has been recorded intraoperatively in the ventral intermediate nucleus of the thalamus in human patients undergoing DBS for treatment of ET (Chang et al., 2012). However, the specific relationship between DBS and neurochemical activity changes remains unknown. Therefore, understanding the relationships between stimulation parameters and neurotransmitter concentration levels is paramount for developing closed-loop DBS control strategies.

In the following paragraphs, we describe a proof-of-principle approach to closed-loop DBS that automatically adjusts stimulation parameters in order to sustain stable dopamine levels in a rodent model of DBS. The paradigm proposed herein uses FSCV to quantify striatal dopamine release evoked by medial forebrain

bundle (MFB) DBS. Additionally, this paradigm relies on nonlinear regression, computational modeling, and constrained optimization techniques to parameterize stimulation-evoked dopamine responses. The inverse dynamics of stimulation-evoked dopaminergic responses are modeled using artificial neural networks (ANN), which also predict stimulation parameters required for sustaining target dopaminergic concentration levels. The performance of this closed-loop paradigm was evaluated by comparing target dopaminergic responses to *in vivo* dopaminergic responses achieved using ANN-predicted stimulation parameters (**Figure 4**). While focused on DBS of ascending dopaminergic fibers in the MFB for evoking dopamine release in the rat striatum (Agnesi et al., 2009), this closed-loop paradigm is applicable to a variety of analytes, targets, and neurologic disorders.

EXPERIMENTAL PARADIGM

To quantify the dynamics of stimulation-evoked dopamine release, recording FSCV CFM and bipolar DBS macroelectrodes were implanted into the striatum and MFB, respectively, in four anesthetized rats. All animal procedures were performed according to the guidelines of the Mayo Clinic Institutional Animal Care and Use Committee (IACUC). Animals were kept on a standard 12 h light-dark cycle with access to food and water *ad libitum* in conventional housing in accordance with National Institutes of Health (NIH) and US Department of Agriculture guidelines.

Animals were anesthetized and the head was fixed in a Kopf stereotactic frame (David Kopf Instruments, California) for electrode targeting. Following brain exposure, one bipolar stimulating electrode, one FSCV recording electrode, and one silver-chloride reference electrode was inserted into the left MFB, striatum, and contralateral cortex, respectively. Recording electrodes were allowed to stabilize within the tissue environment for 20 min. Finally, the electrodes were connected to a wireless stimulator and neurotransmitter sensor for real-time detection of stimulation-evoked dopamine release (Kimble et al., 2009; Chang et al., 2013).

Following electrode implantation, a comprehensive range of stimulation parameters (**Table 1**) was used to determine the magnitudes and temporal patterns of stimulation-evoked dopamine release. Stimulation was divided into 65 20-s bins. Each bin corresponded to one combination of stimulation parameters delivered through the active electrode contact. Each stimulation bin was followed by a stabilization and washout period of 180 s.

STIMULATION-EVOKED NEUROCHEMICAL MONITORING

Stimulation-evoked dopamine measurements were obtained by changing the CFM potential from a resting potential of −0.4–1.3 V and back, at a rate of 400 V/s. This triangular waveform was repeated at a frequency of 10 Hz (Chang et al., 2012). The CFM was held at the resting potential between scans. We converted the measured oxidation and reduction current peaks to dopamine concentration using post-operative *in vitro* flow injection analysis calibration of each CFM (Griessenauer et al., 2010). Our preliminary results showed that as MFB DBS amplitude increases, extracellular dopamine levels within the striatum also increase (**Figure 3A**). A similar response is also observed as pulse duration is increased from 0.1 to 2.0 ms (**Figure 3B**). Changes in frequency, however, give rise to a different dopaminergic response. Maximum response was observed at 100 Hz, followed by a decrease in dopamine oxidation currents at higher frequencies (**Figure 3C**).

Table 1 | Stimulation parameters.

Frequency (Hz)	Amplitude (μA)	Pulse width (ms)	Duration (s)
60	100–450	2.0	2
100	100–450	2.0	2
20–200	250	2.0	2
20–200	350	2.0	2
60	300	2.0	2
100	300	0.1–2.0	2
60	300	2.0	0.5–8

NEUROCHEMICAL RESPONSE MODELING

Implementation of neurochemically-driven closed-loop DBS control strategies requires characterization of the relationship between electrical stimulation and neurochemical responses. To characterize this relationship, stimulation-evoked FSCV dopamine signals were low pass filtered (5th-order Butterworth filter, 100 Hz cutoff frequency) to remove signal noise. Additionally, the responses to individual stimuli were characterized using a combination of 7th-degree polynomial and 2nd-order exponential mathematical models. The mathematical model parameters (eight for the polynomial fit and four for the exponential fit) and corresponding stimuli were presented to a double-layer feedforward ANN with sigmoidal and linear transfer functions (Lujan and Crago, 2009). The hidden layer contained 150-hidden neurons. The inputs to the ANN consisted on the stimulation frequency, pulsewidth, and stimulus amplitude, while system outputs corresponded to the 12 model parameters. Initial weights and biases were selected at random for 10 different initial conditions. Ten corresponding ANNs were trained on 80% of the data (selected at random) using the Levenberg-Marquardt algorithm. The trained ANN with the lowest generalization error, calculated using the remaining 20% of data, was selected as a system model. The resulting system model, when combined with constrained optimization for minimization of stimulation energy, can identify and eliminate mathematical redundancies for the optimal design of the closed-loop controller (Lujan and Crago, 2009).

STIMULATION PREDICTION

In order to provide optimal stimulation, a predictive model that characterizes the inverse relationship between stimulation parameters and dopamine levels was created. Similarly to the system model, the predictive model was created using a double-layer ANN with 600 hidden neurons, as well as sigmoidal and linear transfer functions (Lujan and Crago, 2009). The inputs to the predictive model corresponded to the sets of 12 model parameters, while the outputs corresponded to the three stimulation parameters. This inverse model was then used to predict the stimulation parameters required to sustain specific extracellular dopamine levels within the striatum, thus allowing for feedback control. This was followed by stimulation of the MFB using the predicted parameters, and simultaneous recording of extracellular dopamine levels. Root mean squared (RMS) errors between experimentally measured and desired stimulation-evoked dopamine responses were used to determine controller efficacy. Least-squares regression analysis of the dependencies of actual dopamine levels on target levels was used in an effort to identify systematic (e.g., slope, offset) sources of error (Lujan and Crago, 2009).

CLOSED-LOOP CONTROL

Our preliminary results in four anesthetized rats suggest that mathematical models can be used to describe the relationships between stimulation-evoked extracellular dopamine responses and DBS parameters ($R^2 = 0.8$). Furthermore, these results show that adjusting stimulation parameter intensity can modulate dopamine concentration, and that we can use ANN to

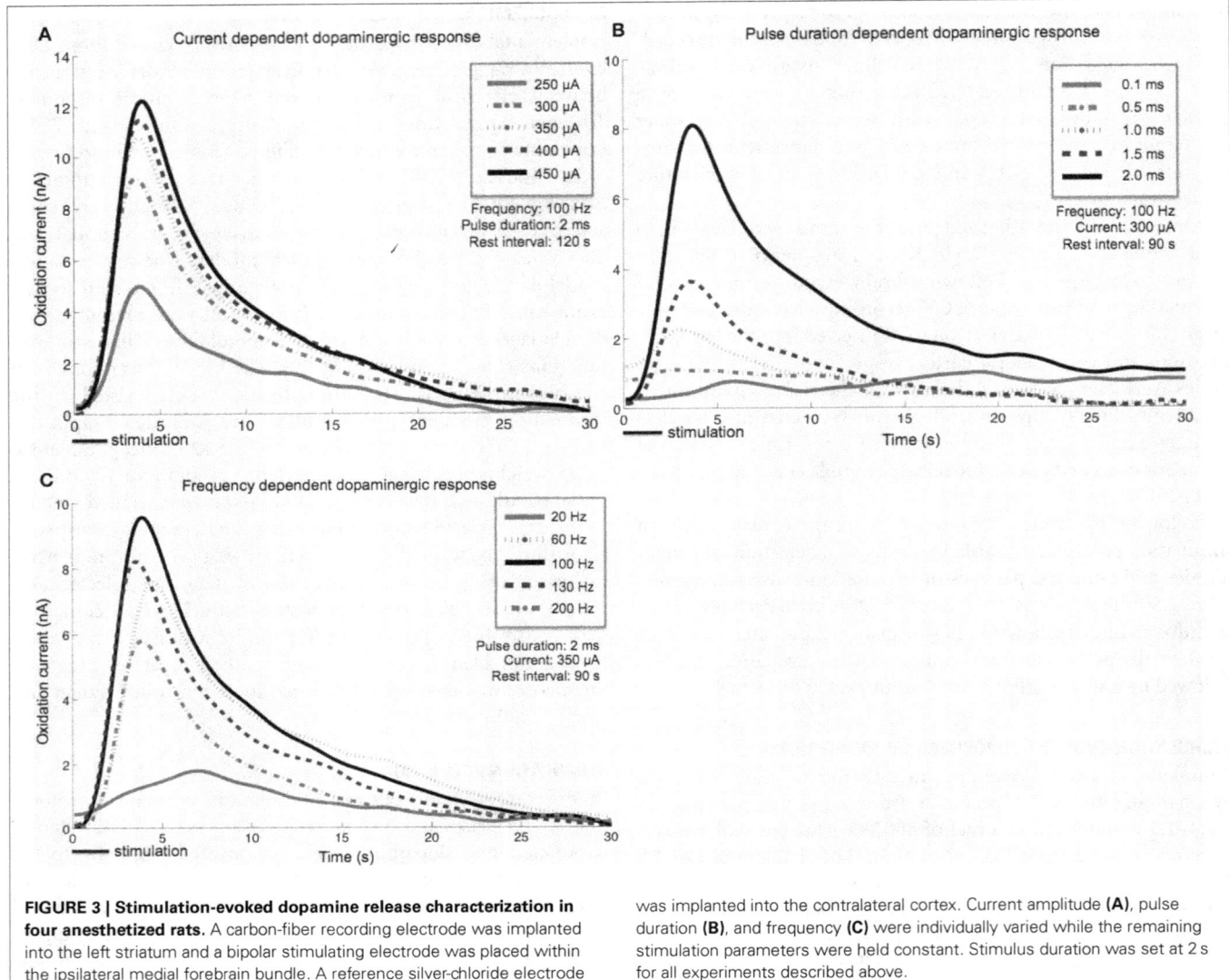

FIGURE 3 | Stimulation-evoked dopamine release characterization in four anesthetized rats. A carbon-fiber recording electrode was implanted into the left striatum and a bipolar stimulating electrode was placed within the ipsilateral medial forebrain bundle. A reference silver-chloride electrode was implanted into the contralateral cortex. Current amplitude **(A)**, pulse duration **(B)**, and frequency **(C)** were individually varied while the remaining stimulation parameters were held constant. Stimulus duration was set at 2 s for all experiments described above.

dynamically predict stimulation parameters required to adjust stimulation-evoked dopamine levels (**Figure 4**). However, to further understand the network effects of DBS and optimize the therapeutic efficacy of stimulation, it may be necessary to combine electrophysiological (e.g., LFP, ECoG) and neurochemical feedback signals.

DISCUSSION

Frequent adjustment of stimulation settings has been shown to improve the efficacy of DBS therapy (Rosin et al., 2011), which highlights the nature of the changing brain environment. Thus, a smart, automated system capable of dynamically adjusting stimulation parameters in response to a changing environment becomes critical for improving the therapeutic efficacy of DBS therapy. The proof-of-principle closed-loop DBS system proposed above offers the potential for maintaining therapeutic responses during disease progression. By taking advantage of mathematical models, the paradigm presented here can potentially replace the trial-and-error process currently used in clinical

programming with deterministic approaches, thereby achieving optimal therapeutic outcomes while minimizing the number of clinical interventions. In turn, this will ultimately reduce required hospital visits and associated healthcare costs (Fraix et al., 2006).

Before automated adjustment of stimulation parameters can be clinically implemented, however, several key clinical questions need to be investigated. Specifically, the relationship between neurotransmitter levels and symptoms of neurologic disease needs further elucidation. For example, there is indirect evidence to suggest that dopamine depletion plays a role in the symptoms of PD and that dopaminergic medications have a therapeutic response. However, precise concentration changes that occur with symptom exacerbation and amelioration are unknown. Additionally, multiple neurotransmitters may play a critical role in the disease (Fitzgerald, 2014). Thus, optimal neurotransmitters and optimal recording locations should be identified for each disorder. Future work should be directed toward validating closed-loop algorithms, correlating neurotransmitter release to clinical benefit in a large animal disease model of Parkinsonism or ET.

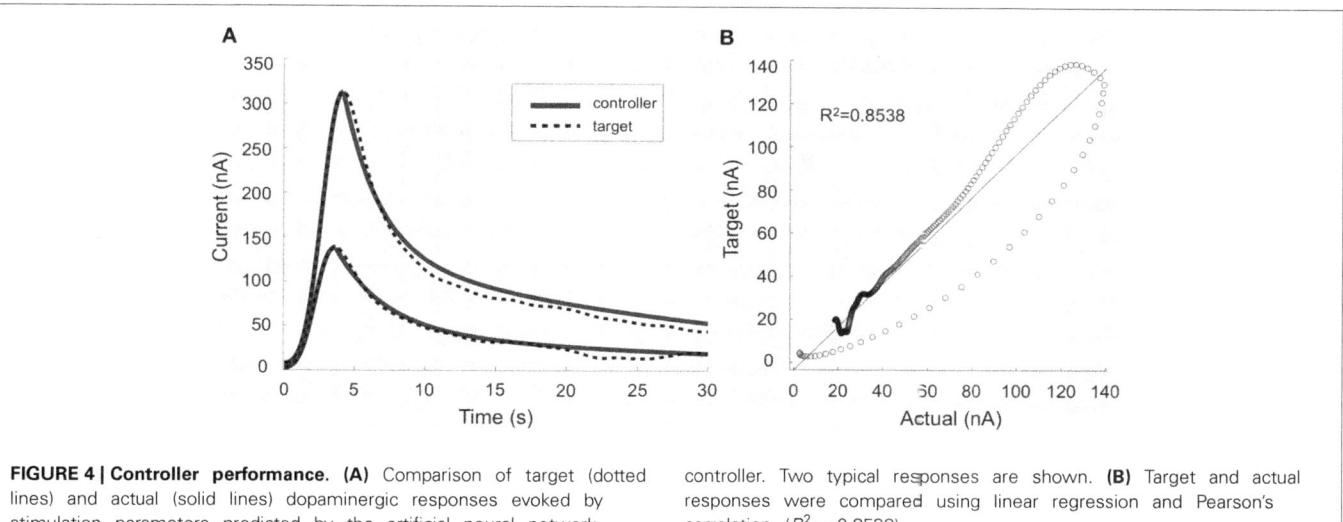

FIGURE 4 | Controller performance. (A) Comparison of target (dotted lines) and actual (solid lines) dopaminergic responses evoked by stimulation parameters predicted by the artificial neural network controller. Two typical responses are shown. **(B)** Target and actual responses were compared using linear regression and Pearson's correlation ($R^2 = 0.8538$).

Similarly, an important technical barrier that needs to be addressed is that chronic recordings are not possible using current electrode technology. CFMs are subject to electrode fouling due to the charge imbalance of the waveforms required for FSCV. Efforts are underway to develop electrochemical-sensing techniques capable of extending electrode longevity by renewing the electrochemically active surface following adsorption of chemical species (Takmakov et al., 2010). Additionally, it has been reported that diamond coating may potentially prolong the life of recording electrodes (Roham et al., 2007). Once these technologies have been developed, they will need to undergo extensive safety and efficacy testing and validation in pathological animal models before advancing to clinical trials.

CONCLUSIONS

Conventional neuromodulation systems have been successful at achieving therapeutic outcomes in patients with neurologic and psychiatric disorders. However, limitations in existing technology make ensuring optimal benefits a difficult and expensive endeavor. Correlation of multi-modal electrophysiological and neurochemical recordings may provide new insight into the cellular and molecular mechanisms of therapeutic neuromodulation. Therefore, development of smart DBS controllers that rely on the relationships between neurochemical and electrophysiological recordings with the clinical effects of DBS offers the potential of replacing the trial-and-error process used in clinical programming with a deterministic approach. Furthermore, the versatility and adaptability of such controllers will allow expansion of the clinical indications that can be treated with DBS while tailoring its application to individual patients and symptoms. In turn, these will likely improve clinical outcomes, reduce the time and frequency of patient visits, and lower overall health care costs.

ACKNOWLEDGMENTS

This work is supported by The Grainger Foundation, NIH grants R01 NS084975 (J. L. Lujan) and R01 NS070872 (Kendall H. Lee). The authors thank Brian Paek, James Baek, and Megan Settel for their assistance with FSCV electrode manufacture and animal surgery.

REFERENCES

Abbott, A. (2006). Neuroprosthetics: in search of the sixth sense. *Nature* 442, 125–127. doi: 10.1038/442125a

Agnesi, F., Tye, S. J., Bledsoe, J. M., Griessenauer, C. J., Kimble, C. J., Sieck, G. C., et al. (2009). Wireless Instantaneous Neurotransmitter Concentration System–based amperometric detection of dopamine, adenosine, and glutamate for intraoperative neurochemical monitoring. *J. Neurosurg.* 111, 701–711. doi: 10.3171/2009.3.JNS0990

Andersen, R. A., Musallam, S., and Pesaran, B. (2004). Selecting the signals for a brain–machine interface. *Curr. Opin. Neurobiol.* 14, 720–726. doi: 10.1016/j.

conb.2004.10.005

Atcherley, C. W., Laude, N. D., Parent, K. L., and Heien, M. L. (2013). Fastscan controlled-adsorption voltammetry for the quantification of absolute concentrations and adsorption dynamics. *Langmuir* 29, 14885–14892. doi: 10.1021/la402686s

Avestruz, A.-T., Santa, W., Carlson, D., Jensen, R., Stanslaski, S., Helfenstine, A., et al. (2008). A 5 uW/Channel spectral analysis IC for chronic bidirectional brain-machine interfaces. *IEEE J. Solid-State Circuits* 43, 3006–3024. doi: 10.1109/JSSC.2008.2006460

Bai, Q., and Wise, K. D. (2001). Single-unit neural recording with active microelectrode arrays. *IEEE Trans. Biomed. Eng.* 48, 911–920.

doi: 10.1109/10.936367

Basu, I., Graupe, D., Tuninetti, D., Shukla, P., Slavin, K. V., Metman, L. V., et al. (2013). Pathological tremor prediction using surface electromyogram and acceleration: potential use in ON-OFF demand driven deep brain stimulator design. *J. Neural Eng.* 10:036019. doi: 10.1088/1741-2560/10/3/036019

Behrend, C. E., Cassim, S. M., and Pallone, M. J. (2009). Toward feed- back controlled deep brain stimulation: dynamics of glutamate release in the subthalamic nucleus in rats. *J. Neurosci. Methods* 180, 278–289. doi: 10.1016/j.jneumeth.2009.04.001

Benabid, A.-L., Chabardès, S., and Seigneuret, E. (2005). Deep-

brain stimulation in Parkinson's disease: long-term efficacy and safety What happened this year? *Curr. Opin. Neurol.* 18, 623–630. doi: 10.1097/01.wco.0000186839.53807.93

Benabid, A.-L., Pollak, P., Gervason, C., Hoffmann, D., Gao, D. M., Hommel, M., et al. (1991). Long-term suppression of tremor by chronic stimulation of the ventral intermediate thalamic nucleus. *Lancet* 337, 403–406. doi: 10.1016/01406736(91)91175-T

Benabid, A.-L., Pollak, P., Louveau, A., Henry, S., and de Rougemont, J. (1987). Combined (thalamotomy and stimulation) stereotactic surgery of the VIM thalamic nucleus for bilateral Parkinson disease. *Appl. Neurophysiol.* 50,

344–346.

Benazzouz, A., Gao, D. M., Ni, Z. G., Piallat, B., Bouali-Benazzouz, R., and Benabid, A.-L. (2000). Effect of high-frequency stimulation of the subthalamic nucleus on the neuronal activities of the substantia nigra pars reticulata and ventrolateral nucleus of the thalamus in the rat. *Neuroscience* 99, 289–295. doi: 10.1016/S0306-4522(00)00199-8

Berényi, A., Belluscio, M., Mao, D., and Buzsáki, G. (2012). Closed-loop control of epilepsy by transcranial electrical stimulation. *Science* 337, 735–737. doi: 10.1126/science.1223154

Blaha, C. D., Coury, A., Fibiger, H. C., and Phillips, A. G. (1990). Effects of neurotensin on dopamine release and metabolism in the rat striatum and nucleus accumbens: cross-validation using *in vivo* voltammetry and microdialysis. *Neuroscience* 34, 699–705. doi: 10.1016/0306-4522(90)90176-5

Blaha, C. D., and Phillips, A. G. (1996). A critical assessment of electrochemical procedures applied to the measurement of dopamine and its metabolites during drug-induced and species-typical behaviours. *Behav. Pharmacol.* 7, 675–708. doi: 10.1097/00008877-199611000-00014

Bledsoe, J. M., Kimble, C. J., Covey, D. P., Blaha, C. D., Agnesi, F., Mohseni, P., et al. (2009). Development of the wireless instantaneous neurotransmitter concentration system for intraoperative neurochemical monitoring using fast-scan cyclic voltammetry. *J. Neurosurg.* 111, 712–723. doi: 10.3171/2009.3.JNS081348

Blomstedt, P., and Hariz, M. I. (2010). Deep brain stimulation for movement disorders before DBS for movement disorders. *Parkinsonism Relat. Disord.* 16, 429–433. doi: 10.1016/j.parkreldis.2010.04.005

Bronstein, J. M., Tagliati, M., Alterman, R. L., Lozano, A. M., Volkmann, J., Stefani, A., et al. (2011). Deep brain stimulation for Parkinson disease: an expert consensus and review of key issues. *Arch. Neurol.* 68, 165. doi: 10.1001/archneurol.2010.260

Bronte-Stewart, H., Barberini, C., Koop, M. M., Hill, B. C., Henderson, J. M., and Wingeier, B. (2009). The STN beta-band profile in Parkinson's disease is stationary and shows prolonged attenuation after deep brain stimulation. *Exp. Neurol.* 215, 20–28. doi: 10.1016/j.expneurol.2008.09.008

Burchiel, K. J., Anderson, V. C., Favre, J., and Hammerstad, J. P. (1999).

Comparison of pallidal and subthalamic nucleus deep brain stimulation for advanced Parkinson's disease: results of a randomized, blinded pilot study. *Neurosurgery* 45, 1375–1382. discussion: 1382–1384.

Buzsáki, G., Anastassiou, C. A., and Koch, C. (2012). The origin of extracellular fields and currents—EEG, ECoG, LFP and spikes. *Nat. Rev. Neurosci.* 13, 407–420. doi: 10.1038/nrn3241

Buzsáki, G., Leung, L. W., and Vanderwolf, C. H. (1983). Cellular bases of hippocampal EEG in the behaving rat. *Brain Res.* 287, 139–171. doi: 10.1016/01650173(83)90037-1

Carter, R. R., and Houk, J. C. (1993). Multiple single-unit recordings from the CNS using thin-film electrode arrays. *IEEE Trans. Rehab. Eng.* 1, 175–184. doi: 10.1109/86.279266

Chang, S.-Y., Kim, I., Marsh, M. P., Jang, D. P., Hwang, S.-C., van Gompel, J. J., et al. (2012). Wireless fast-scan cyclic voltammetry to monitor adenosine in patients with essential tremor during deep brain stimulation. *Mayo Clin. Proc.* 87, 760–765. doi: 10.1016/j.mayocp.2012.05.006

Chang, S.-Y., Kimble, C. J., Kim, I., Paek, S. B., Kressin, K. R., Boesche, J. B., et al. (2013). Development of the mayo investigational neuromodulation control system: toward a closed-loop electrochemical feedback system for deep brain stimulation. *J. Neurosurg.* 119, 1556–1565. doi: 10.3171/2013.8.JNS122142

Chang, S. Y., Shon, Y. M., and Agnesi, F. (2009). "Microthalamotomy effect during deep brain stimulation: potential involvement of adenosine and glutam," in *31st Annual International Conference of the IEEE EMBS* (Minneapolis, MN).

Chefer, V. I., Thompson, A. C., Zapata, A., and Shippenberg, T. S. (2009). Overview of brain microdialysis. *Curr. Protoc. Neurosci.* 47, 1–28. doi: 10.1002/0471142301.ns0701s47

Cheung, K. C. (2007). Implantable microscale neural interfaces. *Biomed. Microdevices* 9, 923–938. doi: 10.1007/s10544-006-9045-z

Dale, N., Hatz, S., Tian, F., and Llaudet, E. (2005). Listening to the brain: microelectrode biosensors for neurochemicals. *Trends Biotechnol.* 23, 420–428. doi: 10.1016/j.tibtech.2005.05.010

Denys, D., Mantione, M., Figee, M., van den Munckhof, P., Koerselman, F., Westenberg, H., et al. (2010). Deep brain

stimulation of the nucleus accumbens for treatment-refractory obsessive-compulsive disorderobsessive-compulsive disorder. *Arch. Gen. Psychiatry* 67, 1061–1068. doi: 10.1001/archgenpsychiatry.2010.122

Deuschl, G., Herzog, J., Kleiner-Fisman, G., Kubu, C., Lozano, A. M., Lyons, K. E., et al. (2006). Deep brain stimulation: postoperative issues. *Mov. Disord.* 21, S219–S237. doi: 10.1002/mds.20957

Fagg, A. H., Hatsopoulos, N. G., de Lafuente, V., Moxon, K. A., Nemati, S., Rebesco, J. M., et al. (2007). Biomimetic brain machine interfaces for the control of movement. *J. Neurosci.* 27, 11842–11846. doi: 10.1523/JNEUROSCI.351607.2007

Fisher, R., Salanova, V., Witt, T., Worth, R., Henry, T., Gross, R., et al. (2010). Electrical stimulation of the anterior nucleus of thalamus for treatment of refractory epilepsy. *Epilepsia* 51, 899–908. doi: 10.1111/j.1528-1167.2010.02536.x

Fitzgerald, P. J. (2014). Is elevated norepinephrine an etiological factor in some cases of Parkinson's disease? *Med. Hypotheses* 82, 462–469. doi: 10.1016/j.mehy.2014.01.026

Foltynie, T., and Hariz, M. I. (2010). Surgical management of Parkinson's disease. *Expert Rev. Neurother.* 10, 903–914. doi: 10.1586/ern.10.68

Fraix, V., Houeto, J.-L., Lagrange, C., Le Pen, C., Krystkowiak, P., Guehl, D., et al. (2006). Clinical and economic results of bilateral subthalamic nucleus stimulation in Parkinson's disease. *J. Neurol. Neurosurg. Psychiatry* 77, 443–449. doi: 10.1136/jnnp.2005.077677

Frankemolle, A. M. M., Wu, J., Noecker, A. M., Voelcker-Rehage, C., Ho, J. C., Vitek, J. L., et al. (2010). Reversing cognitive-motor impairments in Parkinson's disease patients using a computational modelling approach to deep brain stimulation programming. *Brain* 133, 746–761. doi: 10.1093/brain/awp315

Gale, J. T., Lee, K. H., Amirnovin, R., Roberts, D. W., Williams, Z. M., Blaha, C. D., et al. (2013). Electrical stimulation-evoked dopamine release in the primate striatum. *Stereotact. Funct. Neurosurg.* 91, 355–363. doi: 10.1159/000351523

Germano, I. M., Gracies, J.-M., Weisz, D. J., Tse, W., Koller, W. C., and Olanow, C. W. (2004). Unilateral stimulation of the subthalamic nucleus in Parkinson disease:

a double-blind 12-month evaluation study. *J. Neurosurg.* 101, 36–42. doi: 10.3171/jns.2004.101.1.0036

Giannicola, G., Rosa, M., Servello, D., Menghetti, C., Carrabba, G., Pacchetti, C., Zangaglia, R., Cogiamanian, F., Scelzo, E., Marceglia, S., et al. (2012). Subthalamic local field potentials after seven-year deep brain stimulation in Parkinson's disease. *Experimental Neurology* 237, 312–317. doi: 10.1016/j.expneurol.2012.06.012

Gildenberg, P. L. (2003). History repeats itself. *Stereotact Funct Neurosurg* 80, 61–75. doi: 10.1159/000075162

Gildenberg, P. L. (2005). Evolution of neuromodulation. *Stereotact Funct Neurosurg* 83, 71–79. doi: 10.1159/000086865

Grant, P. F., and Lowery, M. M. (2013). Simulation of cortico-basal ganglia oscillations and their suppression by closed loop deep brain stimulation. *IEEE Trans. Neural Syst. Rehabil. Eng.* 21, 584–594. doi: 10.1109/TNSRE.2012.2202403

Griessenauer, C. J., Chang, S.-Y., Tye, S. J., Kimble, C. J., Bennet, K. E., Garris, P. A., et al. (2010). Wireless instantaneous neurotransmitter concentration system: electrochemical monitoring of serotonin using fast-scan cyclic voltammetry-a proof-of-principle study. *J. Neurosurg.* 113, 656–665. doi: 10.3171/2010.3.JNS091627

Grill, W. M., Snyder, A. N., and Miocinovic, S. (2004). Deep brain stimulation creates an informational lesion of the stimulated nucleus. *Neuroreport* 15, 1137–1140. doi: 10.1097/00001756-200405190-00011

Hamani, C., Neimat, J., and Lozano, A. M. (2006). Deep brain stimulation for the treatment of Parkinson's disease. *J. Neural Transm. Suppl.* 70, 393–399. doi: 10.1007/978-3-211-45295-0_59

Hashimoto, T., Elder, C. M., Okun, M. S., Patrick, S. K., and Vitek, J. L. (2003). Stimulation of the subthalamic nucleus changes the firing pattern of pallidal neurons. *J. Neurosci.* 23, 1916–1923.

Hunka, K., Suchowersky, O., Wood, S., Derwent, L., and Kiss, Z. H. T. (2005). Nursing time to program and assess deep brain stimulators in movement disorder patients. *J. Neurosci. Nurs.* 37, 204–210. doi: 10.1097/01376517-20050800000006

Issa, E. B., and Wang, X. (2013). Increased neural correlations in primate auditory cortex during slow-wave sleep. *J. Neurophysiol.* 109, 2732–2738. doi: 10.1152/jn.00695.2012

Jacobs, C. B., Peairs, M. J., and Venton, B. J. (2010). Review: carbon nanotube based electrochemical sensors for biomolecules. *Anal. Chim. Acta.* 662, 105–127. doi: 10.1016/j.aca.2010.01.009

Johnson, M., Franklin, R., Scott, K. A., Brown, R., and Kipke, D. (2005). Neural probes for concurrent detection of neurochemical and electrophysiological signals *in vivo. Conf. Proc. IEEE Eng. Med. Biol. Soc.* 7, 7325–7328. doi: 10.1109/IEMBS.2005.1616203

Johnson, M. D., Miocinovic, S., McIntyre, C. C., and Vitek, J. L. (2008). Mechanisms and targets of deep brain stimulation in movement disorders. *Neurotherapeutics* 5, 294–308. doi: 10.1016/j.nurt.2008.01.010

Khan, G. M., Smolders, I., Lindekens, H., Manil, J., Ebinger, G., and Michotte, Y. (1999). Effects of diazepam on extracellular brain neurotransmitters in pilocarpine-induced seizures in rats. *Eur. J. Pharmacol.* 373, 153–161. doi: 10.1016/S0014-2999(99)00209-5

Kimble, C. J., Johnson, D. M., Winter, B., Whitlock, S. V., Kressin, K. R., Horne, A. E., et al. (2009). "Wireless Instantaneous Neurotransmitter Concentration Sensing System (WINCS) for intraoperative neurochemical monitoring," in *31st Annual International Conference of the IEEE EMBS*, 1–4. Available online at: http://ieeexplore.ieee.org/xpls/abs_all.jsp?arnumber=5332773

Kita, H., Tachibana, Y., Nambu, A., and Chiken, S. (2005). Balance of monosynaptic excitatory and disynaptic inhibitory responses of the globus pallidus induced after stimulation of the subthalamic nucleus in the monkey. *J. Neurosci.* 25, 8611–8619. doi: 10.1523/JNEUROSCI.1719-05.2005

Kluger, B. M., Foote, K. D., Jacobson, C. E., and Okun, M. S. (2011). Lessons learned from a large single center cohort of patients referred for DBS management. *Parkinsonism Relat. Disord.* 17, 236–239. doi: 10.1016/j.parkreldis.2010.05.003

Koller, W. C., Lyons, K. E., Wilkinson, S. B., and Pahwa, R. (2001). Efficacy of unilateral deep brain stimulation of the vim nucleus of the thalamus for essential head tremor. *Mov. Disord.* 14, 847–850. doi: 0.1002/15318257(199909)14:5%3C847::AID-MDS1021%3E3.0.CO;2-G

Kupsch, A., Tagliati, M., Vidailhet, M., Aziz, T., Krack, P., Moro, E., et al. (2011). Early postoperative management of DBS in dystonia: programming, response to stimulation, adverse events, medication changes, evaluations, and troubleshooting. *Mov. Disord.* 26(Suppl. 1), S37–S53. doi: 10.1002/mds.23624

Lee, K. H., Blaha, C. D., Garris, P. A., Mohseni, P., Horne, A. E., Bennet, K. E., et al. (2009). Evolution of deep brain stimulation: human electrometer and smart devices supporting the next generation of therapy. *Neuromodulation* 12, 85–103. doi: 10.1111/j.1525-1403.2009.00199.x

Lee, K. H., Blaha, C. D., Harris, B. T., Cooper, S., Hitti, F. L., Leiter, J. C., et al. (2006). Dopamine efflux in the rat striatum evoked by electrical stimulation of the subthalamic nucleus: potential mechanism of action in Parkinson's disease. *Eur. J. Neurosci.* 23, 1005–1014. doi: 10.1111/j.1460-9568.2006.04638.x

Lee, K. H., Chang, S.-Y., Jang, D. P., Kim, I., Goerss, S., van Gompel, J., et al. (2011). Emerging techniques for elucidating mechanism of action of deep brain stimulation. *Conf. Proc. IEEE Eng. Med. Biol. Soc.* 2011, 677–680. doi: 10.1109/IEMBS.2011.6090152

Lee, K. H., Chang, S.-Y., Roberts, D. W., and Kim, U. (2004). Neurotransmitter release from high-frequency stimulation of the subthalamic nucleus. *J. Neurosurg.* 101, 511–517. doi: 10.3171/jns.2004.101.3.0511

Lee, K. H., Kristic, K., van Hoff, R., Hitti, F. L., Blaha, C., Harris, B., et al. (2007). High-frequency stimulation of the subthalamic nucleus increases glutamate in the subthalamic nucleus of rats as demonstrated by *in vivo* enzyme-linked glutamate sensor. *Brain Res.* 1162, 121–129. doi: 10.1016/j.brainres.2007.06.021

Lim, S.-N., Lee, S.-T., Tsai, Y.-T., Chen, I.-A., Tu, P.-H., Chen, J.-L., et al. (2007). Electrical stimulation of the anterior nucleus of the thalamus for intractable epilepsy: a long-term follow-up study. *Epilepsia* 48, 342–347. doi: 10.1111/j.1528-1167.2006.00898.x

Little, S., Pogosyan, A., Neal, S., Zavala, B., Zrinzo, L., Hariz, M., et al. (2013). Adaptive deep brain stimulation in advanced Parkinson disease. *Ann. Neurol.* 74, 449–457. doi: 10.1002/ana.23951

Loffler, S. (2012). *Towards Closed Loop Deep Brain Stimulation: An Integrated Approach for Neural Recording and Microstimulation.* 1–235.

Logothetis, N. K. (2003a). MR imaging in the non-human primate: studies of function and of dynamic connectivity. *Curr. Opin. Neurobiol.* 13, 630–642. doi: 10.1016/j.conb.2003.09.017

Logothetis, N. K. (2003b). The underpinnings of the BOLD functional magnetic resonance imaging signal. *J. Neurosci.* 23, 3963–3971.

Lujan, J. L., and Crago, P. E. (2009). Automated optimal coordination of multipleDOF neuromuscular actions in feedforward neuroprostheses. *IEEE Trans. Biomed. Eng.* 56, 179–187. doi: 10.1109/TBME.2008.2002159

MacDonald, A. A., Monchi, O., Seergobin, K. N., Ganjavi, H., Tamjeedi, R., and MacDonald, P. A. (2013). Parkinson's disease duration determines effect of dopaminergic therapy on ventral striatum function. *Mov. Disord.* 28, 153–160. doi: 10.1002/mds.25152

Mattia, M., Ferraina, S., and del Giudice, P. (2010). Dissociated multi-unit activity and local field potentials: a theory inspired analysis of a motor decision task. *Neuroimage* 52, 812–823. doi: 10.1016/j.neuroimage.2010.01.063

Maurice, N., Thierry, A.-M., Glowinski, J., and Deniau, J.-M. (2003). Spontaneous and evoked activity of substantia nigra pars reticulata neurons during high-frequency stimulation of the subthalamic nucleus. *J. Neurosci.* 23, 9929–9936.

Mayberg, H. S., Brannan, S. K., Tekell, J. L., Silva, J. A., Mahurin, R. K., McGinnis, S., et al. (2000). Regional metabolic effects of fluoxetine in major depression: serial changes and relationship to clinical response. *Biol. Psychiatry* 48, 830–843. doi: 10.1016/S0006-3223(00)01036-2

Mayberg, H. S., Lozano, A. M., Voon, V., McNeely, H. E., Seminowicz, D., Hamani, C., et al. (2005). Deep brain stimulation for treatment-resistant depression. *Neuron* 45, 651–660. doi: 10.1016/j.neuron.2005.02.014

Maynard, E. M., Nordhausen, C. T., and Normann, R. A. (1997). The Utah intracortical Electrode Array: a recording structure for potential brain-computer interfaces. *Electroencephalogr. Clin. Neurophysiol.* 102, 228–239. doi: 10.1016/S0013-4694(96)95176-0

McIntyre, C. C., and Hahn, P. J. (2010). Network perspectives on the mechanisms of deep brain stimulation. *Neurobiol. Dis.* 38, 329–337. doi: 10.1016/j.nbd.2009.09.022

McIntyre, C. C., Savasta, M., Kerkerian-Le Goff, L., and Vitek, J. L. (2004a). Uncovering the mechanism(s) of action of deep brain stimulation: activation, inhibition, or both. *Clin. Neurophysiol.* 115, 1239–1248. doi: 10.1016/j.clinph.2003.12.024

McIntyre, C. C., Savasta, M., Walter, B. L., and Vitek, J. L. (2004b). How does deep brain stimulation work? Present understanding and future questions. *J. Clin. Neurophysiol.* 21, 40–50. doi: 10.1097/00004691-200401000-00006

Min, B., Guoming, L., and Jian, Z. (2013). Treatment of mesial temporal lobe epilepsy with amygdalohippocampal stimulation: a case series and review of the literature. *Exp. Ther. Med.* 5, 1264–1268. doi: 10.3892/etm.2013.968

Miocinovic, S., Parent, M., Butson, C. R., Hahn, P. J., Russo, G. S., Vitek, J. L., et al. (2006). Computational analysis of subthalamic nucleus and lenticular fasciculus activation during therapeutic deep brain stimulation. *J. Neurophysiol.* 96, 1569–1580. doi: 10.1152/jn.00305.2006

Miocinovic, S., Somayajula, S., Chitnis, S., and Vitek, J. L. (2013). History, applications, and mechanisms of deep brain stimulation. *JAMA Neurol.* 70, 163–171. doi: 10.1001/2013.jamaneurol.45

Molinuevo, J. L., Valldeoriola, F., Tolosa, E., Rumia, J., Valls-Sole, J., Roldan, H., et al. (2000). Levodopa withdrawal after bilateral subthalamic nucleus stimulation in advanced Parkinson disease. *Arch. Neurol.* 57, 983–988. doi: 10.1001/archneur.57.7.983

Morishita, T., Fayad, S. M., Goodman, W. K., Foote, K. D., Chen, D., Peace, A., et al. (2013). Surgical neuroanatomy and programming in deep brain stimulation for obsessive compulsive disorder. *Neuromodulation.* doi: 10.1111/ner.12141. [Epub ahead of print].

Moro, E., Lozano, A. M., Pollak, P., Agid, Y., Rehncrona, S., Volkmann, J., et al. (2010). Long-term results of a multicenter study on subthalamic and pallidal stimulation in Parkinson's disease. *Mov. Disord.* 25, 578–586. doi: 10.1002/mds.22735

Moro, E., Poon, Y.-Y. W., Lozano, A. M., Saint-Cyr, J. A., and Lang, A. (2006). Subthalamic nucleus stimulation: improvements in outcome with reprogramming. *Arch. Neurol.* 63, 1266–1272. doi: 10.1001/archneur.63. 9.1266

Moro, E., Scerrati, M., Romito, L. M., Roselli, R., Tonali, P., and Albanese, A. (1999). Chronic subthalamic nucleus stimulation reduces medication requirements in Parkinson's disease. *Neurology* 53, 85–90. doi: 10.1212/WNL.53.1.85

Mueller, J., Skogseid, I. M., and Benecke, R. (2008). Pallidal deep brain stimulation improves quality of life in segmental and generalized dystonia: results from a prospective, randomized sham-controlled trial. *Mov. Disord.* 23, 131–134. doi: 10.1002/mds.21783

Mure, H., Hirano, S., Tang, C. C., Isaias, I. U., Antonini, A., Ma, Y., et al. (2011). Parkinson's disease tremor-related metabolic network: characterization, progression, and treatment effects. *Neuroimage* 54, 1244–1253. doi: 10.1016/j.neuroimage.2010.09.028

Nemeroff, C. B. (2007). The burden of severe depression: a review of diagnostic challenges and treatment alternatives. *J. Psychiatr. Res.* 41, 189–206. doi: 10.1016/j.jpsychires.2006.05.008

Obeso, J. A., and Guridi, J. (2001). Deep-brain stimulation of the subthalamic nucleus or the pars interna of the globus pallidus in Parkinson's Disease. *N. Engl. J. Med.* 345, 956–963. doi: 10.1056/NEJMoa000827

Okun, M. S., Tagliati, M., Pourfar, M., Fernandez, H. H., Rodriguez, R. L., Alterman, R. L., et al. (2005). Management of referred deep brain stimulation failuresa retrospective analysis from 2 movement disorders centers. *Arch. Neurol.* 62, 1250–1255. doi: 10.1001/archneur.62.8.noc40425

Olanow, W., Schapira, A. H., and Rascol, O. (2000). Continuous dopaminereceptor stimulation in early Parkinson's disease. *Trends Neurosci.* 23, S117–S126. doi: 10.1016/S1471-1931(00)00030-6

Oldenziel, W. H., Beukema, W., and Westerink, B. H. C. (2004). Improving the reproducibility of hydrogel-coated glutamate microsensors by using an automated dipcoater. *J. Neurosci. Methods* 140, 117–126. doi: 10.1016/j.jneumeth.2004.04.038

Polikov, V. S., Tresco, P. A., and Reichert, W. M. (2005). Response of brain tissue to chronically implanted neural electrodes. *J. Neurosci. Methods* 148, 1–18. doi: 10.1016/j.jneumeth.2005.08.015

Priori, A., Foffani, G., Rossi, L., and Marceglia, S. (2013). Experimental neurology. *Exp. Neurol.* 245, 77–86. doi: 10.1016/j.expneurol.2012.09.013

Ramasubbu, R., Anderson, S., Haffenden, A., Chavda, S., and

Kiss, Z. H. (2013). Double-blind optimization of subcallosal cingulate deep brain stimulation for treatment-resistant depression: a pilot study. *J. Psychiatry Neurosci.* 38, 325–332. doi: 10.1503/jpn.120160

Rehncrona, S., Johnels, B., and Widner, H. (2003). Long-term efficacy of thalamic deep brain stimulation for tremor: double-blind assessments. *Mov. Disord.* 18, 163–170. doi: 10.1002/mds.10309

Ricchi, V., Zibetti, M., Angrisano, S., Merola, A., Arduino, N., Artusi, C. A., et al. (2012). Transient effects of 80 Hz stimulation on gait in STN DBS treated PD patients: a 15 months follow-up study. *Brain Stimul.* 5, 388–392. doi: 10.1016/j.brs.2011.07.001

Robinson, D. L., Venton, B. J., Heien, M. L. A. V., and Wightman, R. M. (2003). Detecting subsecond dopamine release with fast-scan cyclic voltammetry *in vivo*. *Clin. Chem.* 49, 1763–1773. doi: 10.1373/49.10.1763

Rodriguez-Oroz, M. C. (2004). Efficacy of deep brain stimulation of the subthalamic nucleus in Parkinson's disease 4 years after surgery: double blind and open label evaluation. *J. Neurol. Neurosurg. Psychiatry* 75, 1382–1385. doi: 10.1136/jnnp.2003.031294

Roham, M., Halpern, J. M., Martin, H. B., Chiel, H. J., and Mohseni, P. (2007). "Diamond microelectrodes and CMOS microelectronics for wireless transmission of fast-scan cyclic voltammetry," in *Engineering in Medicine and Biology Society, 2007. EMBS 2007. 29th Annual International Conference of the IEEE*, 6044–6047. doi: 10.1109/IEMBS.2007.4353726

Rosa, M., Giannicola, G., Marceglia, S., Fumagalli, M., Barbieri, S., and Priori, A. (2012). "Neurophysiology of deep brain stimulation: emerging horizons in neuromodulation—new frontiers in brain and spine stimulation," in *International Review of Neurobiology*, Vol. 107 (Philadelphia, PA), 23–55. doi: 10.1016/B978-0-12-404706-8.00004-8

Rosin, B., Slovik, M., Mitelman, R., Rivlin-Etzion, M., Haber, S. N., Israel, Z., et al. (2011). Closed-loop deep brain stimulationis superior in ameliorating parkinsonism. *Neuron* 72, 370–384. doi: 10.1016/j.neuron.2011.08.023

Rossi, L., Foffani, G., Marceglia, S., Bracchi, F., Barbieri, S., and Priori, A. (2007). An electronic

device for artefact suppression in human local field potential recordings during deep brain stimulation. *J. Neural Eng.* 4, 96–106. doi: 10.1088/1741-2560/4/2/010

Santaniello, S., Fiengo, G., Glielmo, L., and Grill, W. M. (2011). Closed-loop control of deep brain stimulation: a simulation study. *IEEE Trans. Neural Syst. Rehabil. Eng.* 19, 15–24. doi: 10.1109/TNSRE.2010.2081377

Shah, R. S., Chang, S.-Y., Min, H.-K., Cho, Z.-H., Blaha, C. D., and Lee, K. H. (2010). Deep brain stimulation: technology at the cutting edge. *J. Clin. Neurol.* 6, 167–182. doi: 10.3988/jcn.2010.6.4.167

Shon, Y.-M., Chang, S.-Y., Tye, S. J., Kimble, C. J., Bennet, K. E., Blaha, C. D., et al. (2010a). Comonitoring of adenosine and dopamine using the wireless instantaneous neurotransmitter concentration system: proof of principle. *J. Neurosurg.* 112, 539–548. doi: 10.3171/2009.7.JNS09787

Shon, Y.-M., Lee, K. H., Goerss, S. J., Kim, I. Y., Kimble, C., van Gompel, J. J., et al. (2010b). High frequency stimulation of the subthalamic nucleus evokes striatal dopamine release in a large animal model of human DBS neurosurgery. *Neurosci. Lett.* 475, 136–140. doi: 10.1016/j.neulet.2010.03.060

Simuni, T., Jaggi, J. L., Mulholland, H., Hurtig, H. I., Colcher, A., Siderowf, A. D., et al. (2002). Bilateral stimulation of the subthalamic nucleus in patients with Parkinson disease: a study of efficacy and safety. *J. Neurosurg.* 96, 666–672. doi: 10.3171/jns.2002.96.4.0666

Skarpaas, T. L., and Morrell, M. J. (2009). Intracranial stimulation therapy for epilepsy. *Neurotherapeutics* 6, 238–243. doi: 10.1016/j.nurt.2009.01.022

Smith, I. D., and Grace, A. A. (1992). Role of the subthalamic nucleus in the regulation of nigral dopamine neuron activity. *Synapse* 12, 287–303. doi: 10.1002/syn.890120406

Smolders, I., van Belle, K., Ebinger, G., and Michotte, Y. (1997). Hippocampal and cerebellar extracellular amino acids during pilocarpine-induced seizures in freely moving rats. *Eur. J. Pharmacol.* 319, 21–29. doi: 10.1016/S00142999(96)00830-8

Speert, D., Bentsen, T., and Fenichel, M. (eds.). (2012). *Brain Facts*. 7th Edn. Washington, DC: Society for Neuroscience.

Takmakov, P., Zachek, M. K., Keithley, R. B., Walsh, P. L., Donley, C., McCarty, G. S., et al. (2010). Carbon microelectrodes with a renewable surface. *Anal. Chem.* 82, 2020–2028. doi: 10.1021/ac902753x

Tsang, E. W., Hamani, C., Moro, E., Mazzella, F., Saha, U., Lozano, A. M., et al. (2012). Subthalamic deep brain stimulation at individualized frequencies for Parkinson disease. *Neurology* 78, 1930–1938. doi: 10.1212/WNL.0b013e3182 59e183

Tye, S. J., Miller, A. D., and Blaha, C. D. (2013). Ventral tegmental ionotropic glutamate receptor stimulation of nucleus accumbens tonic dopamine efflux blunts hindbrain-evoked phasic neurotransmission: implications for dopamine dysregulation disorders. *Neuroscience* 252, 337–345. doi: 10.1016/j.neuroscience.2013.08.010

van Gompel, J. J., Chang, S.-Y., Goerss, S. J., Kim, I. Y., Kimble, C., Bennet, K. E., et al. (2010). Development of intraoperative electrochemical detection: wireless instantaneous neurochemical concentration sensor for deep brain stimulation feedback. *Neurosurg. Focus* 29, E6. doi: 10.3171/2010.5.FOCUS10110

Velasco, F., Carrillo-Ruiz, J. D., Brito, F., Velasco, M., Velasco, A. L., Marquez, I., et al. (2005). Double-blind, randomized controlled pilot study of bilateral cerebellar stimulation for treatment of intractable motor seizures. *Epilepsia* 46, 1071–1081 doi: 10.1111/j.1528-1167.2005.70504.x

Velasco, F., Velasco, A. L., Velasco, M., Jiménez, F., Carrillo-Ruiz, J. D., and Castro, G. (2007). Deep brain stimulation for treatment of the epilepsies: the centromedian thalamic target. *Acta Neurochir. Suppl.* 97, 337–342. doi: 10.1007/978-3-211-33081-4_38

Vitek, J. L., Zhang, J., Hashimoto, T., Russo, G. S., and Baker, K. B. (2012). External pallidal stimulation improves parkinsonian motor signs and modulates neuronal activity throughout the basal ganglia thalamic network. *Exp. Neurol.* 233, 581–586. doi: 10.1016/j.expneurol.2011.09.031

Watson, C. J., Venton, B. J., and Kennedy, R. T. (2006). *In vivo* measurements of neurotransmitters by microdialysis sampling. *Anal. Chem.* 78, 1391–1399. doi: 10.1021/ac0693722

Weiss, D., Walach, M., Meisner, C., Fritz, M., Scholten, M., Breit, S., et al. (2013). Nigral stimulation for resistant axial motor impairment

A neurochemical closed-loop controller for deep brain stimulation: toward individualized smart neuromodulation...

205

in Parkinson's disease? A randomized controlled trial. *Brain* 136, 2098–2108. doi: 10.1093/brain/awt122

Wightman, R. M. (2006). Detection technologies. Probing cellular chemistry in biological systems with microelectrodes. *Science* 311, 1570–1574. doi: 10.1126/science.1120027

Williams, N. R., and Okun, M. S. (2013). Deep brain stimulation (DBS) at the interface of neurology and psychiatry. *J. Clin. Invest.* 123, 4546–4556. doi: 10.1172/JCI68341

15

Assisted closed-loop optimization of SSVEP-BCI efficiency

Jacobo Fernandez-Vargas, Hanns U. Pfaff, Francisco B. Rodríguez and Pablo Varona*

Grupo de Neurocomputación Biológica, Departamento de Ingeniería Informática, Escuela Politécnica Superior, Universidad Autónoma de Madrid, Madrid, Spain

Edited by:
Steve M. Potter, Georgia Institute of Technology, USA

Reviewed by:
Attila Szücs, Balaton Limnological Research Institute HAS, Hungary
Pablo F. Diez, Universidad Nacional de San Juan, Argentina

*Correspondence:
Pablo Varona, Grupo de Neurocomputación Biológica, Departamento de Ingeniería Informática, Universidad Autónoma de Madrid, Calle Francisco Tomás y Valiente, 11, 28049 Madrid, Spain.
e-mail: pablo.varona@uam.es

We designed a novel *assisted closed-loop optimization protocol* to improve the efficiency of brain-computer interfaces (BCI) based on steady state visually evoked potentials (SSVEP). In traditional paradigms, the control over the BCI-performance completely depends on the subjects' ability to learn from the given feedback cues. By contrast, in the proposed protocol *both* the subject and the machine share information and control over the BCI goal. Generally, the innovative *assistance* consists in the delivery of online information together with the online adaptation of BCI stimuli properties. In our case, this adaptive optimization process is realized by (1) a *closed-loop search* for the best set of *SSVEP* flicker frequencies and (2) feedback of actual *SSVEP* magnitudes to both the subject and the machine. These closed-loop interactions between subject and machine are evaluated in *real-time* by continuous measurement of their efficiencies, which are used as online criteria to adapt the BCI control parameters. The proposed protocol aims to compensate for variability in possibly unknown subjects' state and trait dimensions. In a study with $N = 18$ subjects, we found significant evidence that our protocol *outperformed* classic SSVEP-BCI control paradigms. Evidence is presented that it takes indeed into account interindividual variabilities: e.g., under the new protocol, baseline resting state EEG measures predict subjects' BCI performances. This paper illustrates the promising potential of *assisted closed-loop* protocols in BCI systems. Probably their applicability might be expanded to innovative uses, e.g., as possible new diagnostic/therapeutic tools for clinical contexts and as new paradigms for basic research.

Keywords: brain-computer interface, brain-machine interface, activity-dependent stimulation, resting state EEG, resting state network, individual alpha frequency, BCI illiteracy, BCI performance predictor

INTRODUCTION

The use of closed-loop interaction with biological nervous systems for observation and control purposes goes back to the beginnings of electrophysiology in the 1940s when the *voltage clamp* technique was developed (Marmont, 1949; Cole, 1955). Later on, the *dynamic clamp* technology to implement artificial membrane or synaptic conductances (Robinson and Kawai, 1993; Sharp et al., 1993) has produced many examples of successful closed-loop interactions with neural systems at the cellular and circuit levels (for reviews see Prinz et al., 2004; Goaillard and Marder, 2006; Destexhe and Bal, 2009; Economo et al., 2010).

We recently proposed a generalization of the dynamic clamp concept in electrophysiology and animal ethology to design closed-loop interactions with biological nervous systems beyond electrical stimulation and recording. In particular, we investigated in our previous work goal-driven real-time closed-loop interactions with drug microinjectors, mechanical stimulation devices and video event driven stimulators (Muniz et al., 2008, 2011; Chamorro et al., 2009, 2012). These examples illustrate that modern activity-dependent stimulation protocols can reveal dynamics otherwise hidden under traditional stimulation techniques, provide control of regular and pathological states, induce learning processes, bridge between distinct levels of analysis and lead to a further automation of experiments. In this paper, we propose

the same assisted closed-loop approach described in our previous work to optimize the efficiency of steady state visually evoked potentials (SSVEP) based brain-computer interfaces (BCI) which might have a large impact for applied uses, such as computer control and biomedical or prosthetic uses, but also as novel paradigms for basic research. Generally, the innovative assistance consists in the delivery of online information with regard to the control over the given BCI goal both to the human subject and to the system, together with the online adaptation of BCI stimuli properties.

BCIs use measures of brain activity, typically real-time human EEG recordings, usually in order to interact with devices such as virtual keyboards, etc. (for recent reviews see e.g., Birbaumer, 2006; Van Gerven et al., 2009; Nicolas-Alonso and Gomez-Gil, 2012). Among the most successful BCIs are those which rely on SSVEPs, a type of event related potentials (ERPs) generated by the nervous system in response to repetitive visual stimulation (flicker) by linear superposition of transient visually evoked potentials (VEPs) (Capilla et al., 2011) up to 90 Hz (Herrmann, 2001): apart from smaller responses in higher harmonic frequencies, the brain mainly generates electrical activity at just the same fundamental frequency as its visual system is exposed to the visual flicker frequency. SSVEPs are frequently used in basic and applied research because of their relatively large magnitudes which lead to superior signal-to-noise ratios (SNRs) and make them relatively stable against artifacts as compared to other ERPs (Vialatte et al., 2010).

SSVEP-BCIs make use of the physiological property that SSVEP magnitudes can be modulated by visual-spatial selective attention (e.g., Morgan et al., 1996). Thus, SSVEP based BCIs employ multiple visual stimuli (e.g., LEDs or regions on a screen) flickering at different frequencies. Apart from these intraindividual state changes due to attention, SSVEP magnitudes further depend both on extrinsic variables as the spatial and temporal frequencies of the stimulus, and on other intrinsic intra- and interindividual dimensions of the subjects themselves (Ding et al., 2006; Lopez-Gordo et al., 2011). The optimal spatial frequency of a structured stimulus is related to individual traits such as visual acuity or age (Vialatte et al., 2010). There is also a significant difference in the magnitude of SSVEPs between flicker stimulation of the center (fovea centralis) vs. the periphery of the visual field. Environmental conditions (e.g., screen brightness and frequency, distance to the screen, etc.) also influence the performance of the BCI. Although determined by multiple factors, SSVEP magnitudes are modulated by the subjects' states of attention. Hence, online monitoring of SSVEP magnitudes elicited by arrays of multiple flickering light sources allows BCI systems to detect to which flicker source the subject is attending to at a given moment. Taken altogether, these aspects call for automated mechanisms to optimize parameters of the stimuli and of the BCI control, aiming toward flexible adaptiveness to specific individual and contextual situations of SSVEP-BCI use.

Commonly, SSVEP-BCIs use only one prefixed set of flicker frequencies, but nonetheless there are studies employing two different prefixed sets (e.g., Volosyak et al., 2009, 2011) which lead to remarkably different results. Those findings imply that BCI efficiency may crucially depend on flicker frequency selection. Following this idea, we created an assisted closed-loop adaptive algorithm to search for the best frequencies for each subject and for each particular time point/situation of use. The adaptive

and informative nature of this novel online approach aims to improve the BCI efficiency as compared to traditional paradigms (see **Figure 1**). Firstly, this optimization process is realized by performing a real-time closed-loop search for the best set of frequencies to achieve the given BCI goal. The number of stimuli and their effectiveness with regard to the BCI goal modulate this real-time search strategy. The closed-loop search is evaluated in real-time by a continuous measurement of the actual BCI efficiency (see section "Efficiency Measures"), which is used as an online criterion to select the BCI control parameters. Secondly, the SSVEP online recording is processed, on the one hand, to an online auditory feedback to inform the subject and, on the other, is used to inform the system to select the best flicker frequencies. This shared information constitutes the assisted part of the closed-loop. The proposed protocol aims to address the problems which arise from different hardware configurations, subjects' intra- and inter-individual variabilities, e.g., in neuropsychological dimensions of executive functioning (see e.g., Funahashi, 2001) etc., and other sources of variability in experimental settings and intrinsic dimensions.

The paper is organized as follows: in section "Materials and Methods" the new assisted closed-loop system is described; in section "Results" analyses and correlates efficiency as compared with traditional BCI paradigms are presented; finally, in "Discussion" section we discuss about the generalization and applicability of the proposed novel protocol.

MATERIALS AND METHODS
PARTICIPANTS

A convenience non-probability sample of $N = 18$ healthy subjects from our department was used applying the exclusion criteria self-reported chronic medication/substance intake and neurological diseases as e.g., epilepsy. Our sample consisted of 6 females and 12 males with age $Mdn = 26.00$ years (25th percentile = 23.00, 75th = 35.75), range = 18–59. Subjects had a normal or

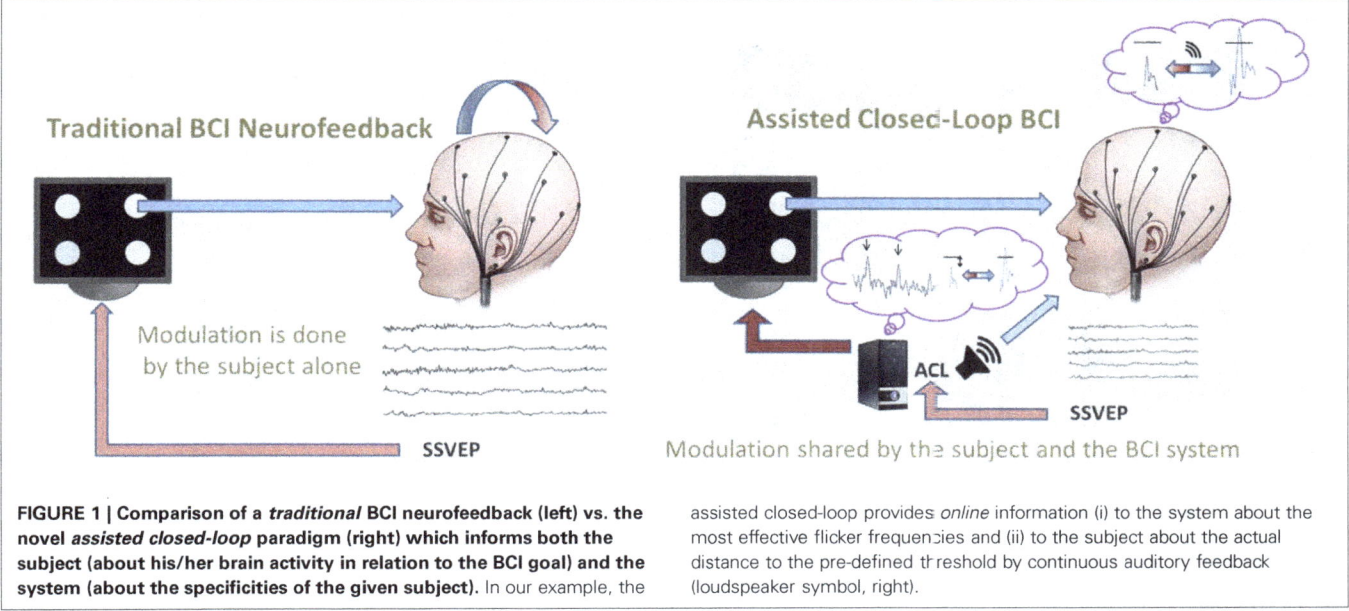

FIGURE 1 | Comparison of a *traditional* BCI neurofeedback (left) vs. the novel *assisted closed-loop* paradigm (right) which informs both the subject (about his/her brain activity in relation to the BCI goal) and the system (about the specificities of the given subject). In our example, the assisted closed-loop provides *online* information (i) to the system about the most effective flicker frequencies and (ii) to the subject about the actual distance to the pre-defined threshold by continuous auditory feedback (loudspeaker symbol, right).

corrected-to-normal vision and were right-handed. Permission of the ethics committee of Autonomous University of Madrid was obtained; all subjects participated voluntarily in the sense of an *informed consent* without receiving any incentives. Participants were informed that they could leave the experiments at any time without giving any explication.

SSVEP BCI SYSTEM

Stimulation device

We constructed a stimulation panel with four white color LEDs (manufacturer *Seoul Semiconductor, white lamp LED LW500AM,* Ø 5 mm, viewing angle 100°), using a 100 Ω series resistor to the digital +5V output of the acquisition board (see below) which results in a luminous intensity output $I_V \approx 700$ mcd for each LED.

On a black background panel, each LED was mounted into a reflector with Ø40 mm diffuser cap carrying an outstanding non-transparent cylindrical black screen of 45 mm length; the spatial organization is illustrated in **Figure 2**. Below each white flicker light source we placed a green color standard signaling LED to instruct the subject where to look during the BCI task. The distance of the LED stimulation panel to the subject was kept ~60 cm, resulting in a visual angle of ~3.8° for every light source.

BCI task

The BCI task consisted in subjects trying to follow a prefixed sequence of 16 steps by focusing their vision onto a specific flickering white light source out of the four possible ones at each step, as continuously indicated by the smaller green signaling LEDs below. This sequence was identical for all subjects. A brief beep sound confirmed the indicated flickering light source as correctly detected.

STIMULATION

We compared the BCI efficiency under three conditions of flicker frequency selection: (i) by the assisted closed-loop (*ACL*)

protocol, (ii) by a standard protocol with stimulation frequencies *prefixed* at 27, 28, 29, and 30 Hz (because 1 Hz distances are commonly employed in SSVEP-BCIs e.g., Herrmann, 2001; Diez et al., 2011; Volosyak et al., 2011), and (iii) by a protocol which used a selection of *top* frequencies for each subject (see section "ACL Algorithm"). In order to compensate for possible presentation order effects, the order of (i), (ii), y (iii) was permutated over the subjects.

Figure 3 shows the timeline of the experiment. The first phase of the experiment consisted in the measurement of the individual EEG *baseline* and the *frequency scanning phase* to select a set of flicker stimulation frequencies for each subject (the number of frequencies in this set is specific for each participant—see below). The second phase is the BCI phase with its three conditions (i), (ii), and (iii) mentioned above.

SIGNAL ACQUISITION AND PREPROCESSING

The signal acquisition and preprocessing steps are summarized in **Figure 4**. The EEG signal was recorded at 1024 Hz with eight sintered Ag/AgCl electrodes mounted into a "*Aegis Array*" stretch lycra cap (*Sands Research Inc.*, Texas/USA) using a "*BRAINBOX® EEG-1166*" 64 channel EEG amplifier (*Braintronics B.V,* Almere/Netherlands) with in-house software written in *C*. Vertical and horizontal EOG was recorded bipolarly by an in-house battery driven analog amplifier following a circuitry of Usakli and Gurkan (2010) with sintered Ag/AgCl electrodes fixed by adhesive rings above/below the left eye vs. at left/right *epicanthus* connected to a data acquisition board (*NI-PCI-6251, National Instruments*) at 1024 Hz. The eight standard 10–20 positions were FPz, F3, Fz, F4, Cz, Pz, POz, and Oz (Jasper, 1958). For *online* SSVEP detection as BCI input only POz and Oz were used, while for later *offline* studies the signals from *all* eight mentioned electrodes were analyzed. The EEG reference electrode was placed at nose tip, EOG ground electrode at *glabella* and impedances were kept <10 kΩ.

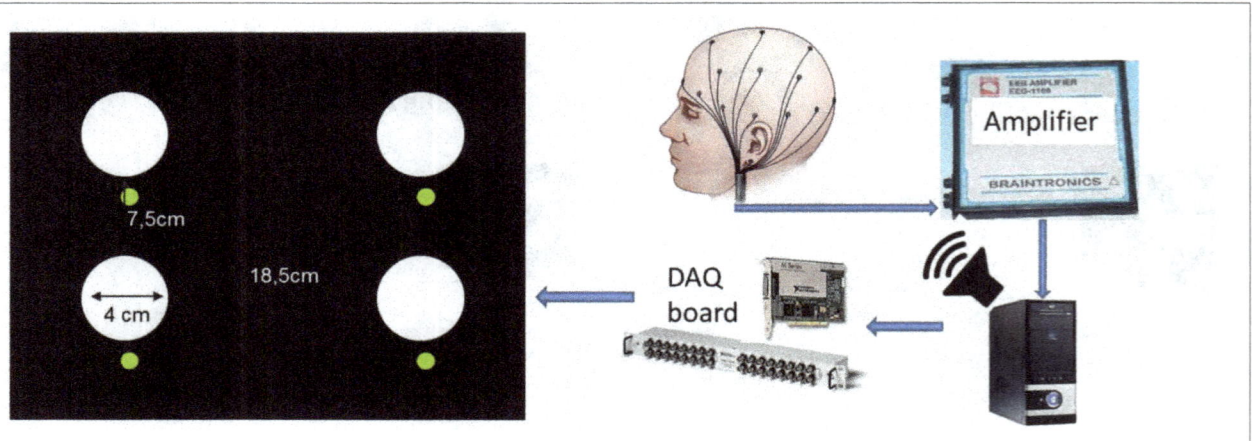

FIGURE 2 | Diagram of the *BCI flicker stimulation setup* (left) and the signal acquisition/stimulation system. The flickering frequency was controlled by a software driving the digital output of a National Instruments data acquisition (DAQ) board (model *NI-PCI-6251*) directly connected to the white colored LEDs, generating 0/+5V *off* vs. *on* signals according to the desired flicker frequency. We verified the intended flicker frequency for each light source independently by a photodiode connected to a digital oscilloscope. Luminous intensity output is $I_V \approx 700$ mcd for each white LED. Smaller green color standard signaling LEDs were placed below to instruct subjects where to look during the BCI task.

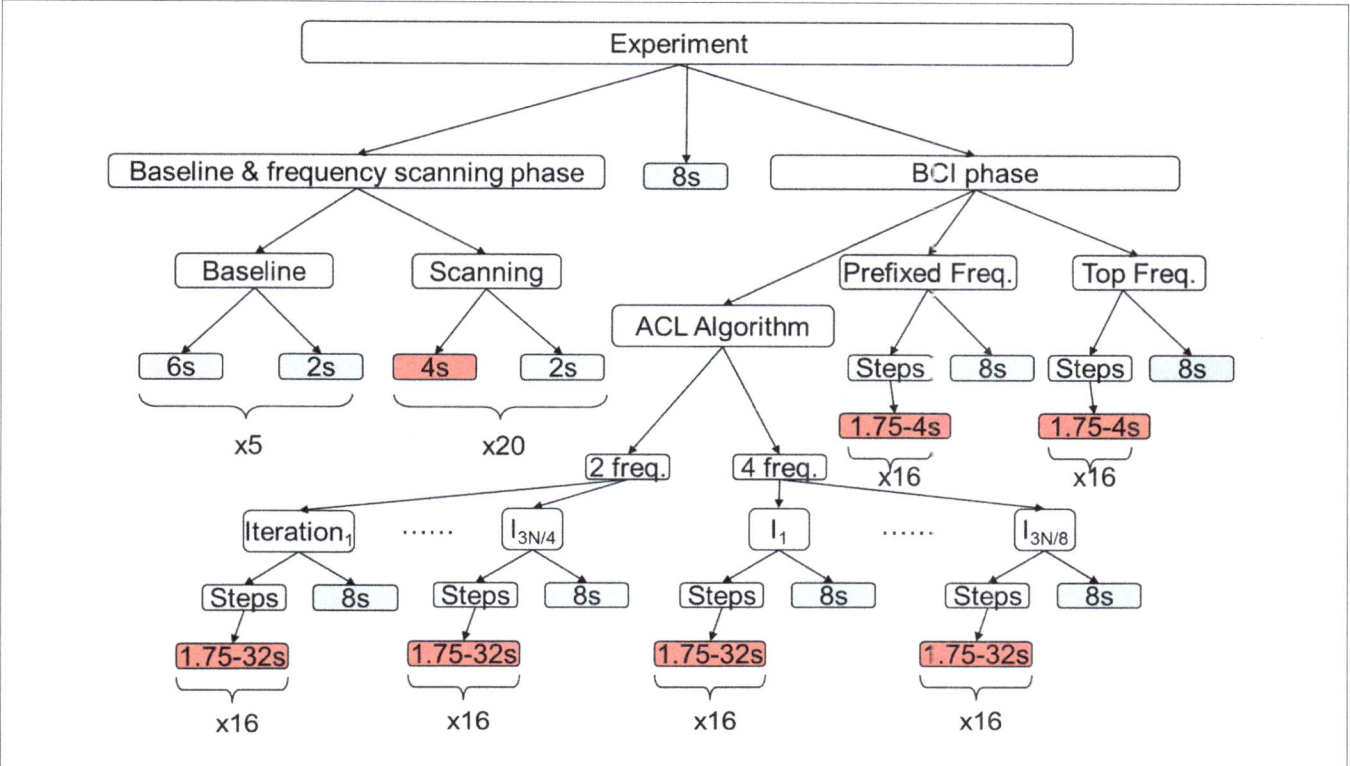

FIGURE 3 | Timeline of the experiment. In the first phase individual EEG *baseline* activity is measured and in the following *frequency scanning phase* those frequencies electing largest SSVEP magnitudes are selected for each subject individually, while those below a predefined threshold are excluded (*Top Freq.*). Later, these values are used in the BCI phase. Under the *prefixed frequency* condition, always the same frequency set of 27, 28, 29, and 30 Hz is used for stimulation. *Red* boxes indicate stimulation, *blue* resting periods and *gray* baseline recording; in each box durations are reported.

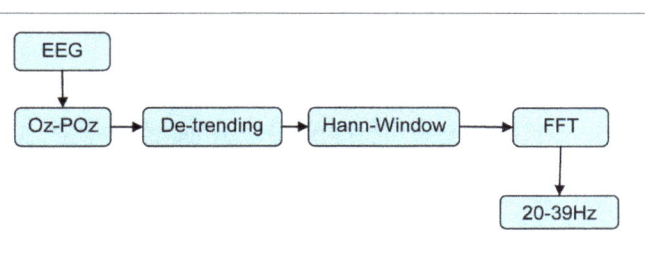

FIGURE 4 | Signal chain of acquisition and *online* preprocessing. Input signals are the *time domain* EEG signals at electrodes Oz and POz sampled at 1024 Hz which finally result in normalized SSVEP spectral power densities S_f for each of the 20 stimulation frequencies *f* using as transformation to *frequency domain* the Fast Fourier Transform (FFT).

To improve SSVEP detection, we used the online computed difference signal between Oz and POz as bipolar montage as the only input signal to our BCI system. This reduces both EOG/EMG artifacts and EEG activity not related to the visual cortex because this montage implements a simple and computationally inexpensive *spatial high pass filter* (see **Figure 5**). Thus, the *SNR* for the SSVEP detection is increased as compared to unipolar montages (Diez et al., 2010). In a time window of 2 s, this difference signal was then linearly detrended, treated by a *Hann*-window and then converted into *frequency domain* by Fast Fourier Transform

(FFT) with a window length of 2048 sample points. The chosen *Hann-window function* has a quite narrow main lobe, which determines a good frequency resolution, and reasonable side lobe suppression (Harris, 1978). Those FFT coefficients meeting the exact flicker frequencies were used, one single coefficient for each flicker frequency. Thus, 20 real numbers were obtained and squared to represent the *power spectral densities* (PSDs) in the flicker range 20–39 Hz (see **Figure 4**). This procedure was developed following Diez et al. (2011). The described analysis was continuously repeated as *sliding windows* with a displacement of 250 ms, resulting in 87.5% overlapping. With all four LEDs emitting steady light, magnitudes of baseline EEG activities B_f were measured over 30 s at each future flicker stimulation frequency, determined as M_{PSD} by the described procedure (5 sets of 6s with 2 s resting periods in-between, see **Figure 3** *Baseline*). Subjects were instructed to use only the resting periods in-between for eye blinks/relaxation and otherwise maintain their eyes quietly open, trying to avoid jaw and tongue movements to reduce EOG/EMG artifacts.

For the *frequency scanning phase* of the experiment an identical measurement procedure was used, but with time windows for flicker stimulation of 4 s in each frequency *f* of the 20–39 Hz range resulting in magnitudes of SSVEPs as response, R_f. Each stimulation epoch is followed by a 2 s resting period. In the *BCI phase* of the experiment, the same procedure is used for the

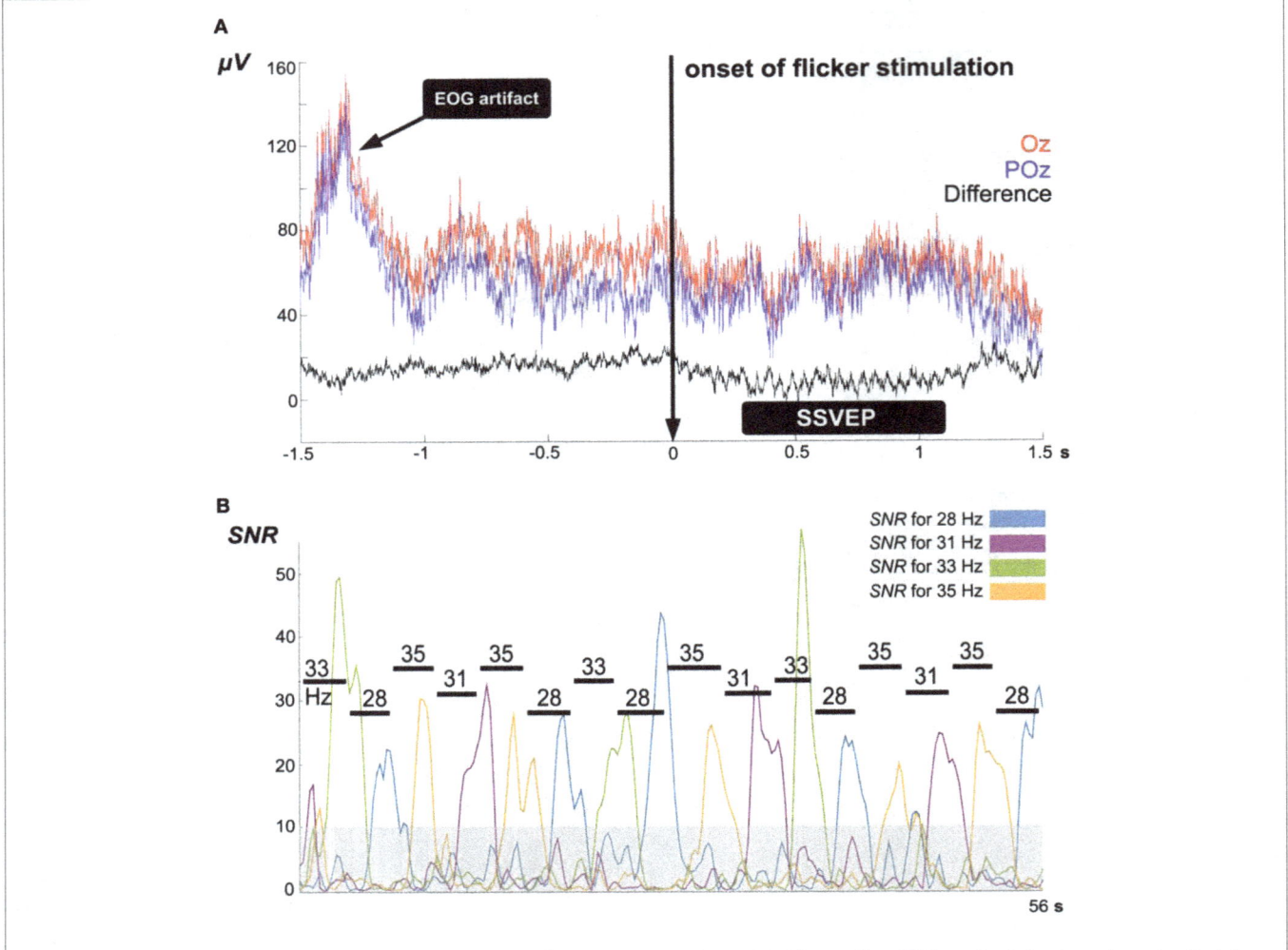

FIGURE 5 | (A) Example of EEG *time domain* signals during 3 s before and after 21 Hz flicker stimulation at electrodes Oz (red) and POz (blue). Using their difference signal (black) as BCI input, in the sense of a *bipolar montage,* remarkably reduces common DC offsets, EOG/EMG artifacts and EEG contributions other than due to the visual cortex: the difference signal offers a simple *spatial high-pass filter.* **(B)** Example of signal-to-noise ratios S_f during a single iteration of the algorithm ACL using four different flicker frequencies. The gray shadowed area represents the *noise floor* with dimensionless value 10; this level was defined as SSVEP detection threshold for all subjects. Horizontal lines indicate the detection duration of each target frequency at each *step.*

selected stimulation frequencies in a single measurement window of 2 s.

SSVEP PSD magnitudes were normalized to EEG baseline activity in a given frequency f as dimensionless *signal-to-noise ratios:*

$$S_f = R_f / B_f \qquad (1)$$

In order to minimize fatigue, we tried to keep the baseline and frequency scanning phase as short as possible, 40 s in total for the baseline and 160 s for frequency scanning.

ACL ALGORITHM
Selection of the top frequencies for each subject
A closed-loop approach is used to select the set of the four *top* stimulation frequencies by compatibility for each subject and in the given experimental context. As a first step, the specified range is scanned which results in a-priori score for each of them.

Stimulation frequencies are defined as valid if their S_f exceeds a prefixed threshold (set to 10) any time during the ongoing flicker stimulation. For N valid frequencies, the frequency corresponding to the largest S_f gets an initial score of $s_1(0) = N$, the second to best $s_2(0) = N - 1$, etc. The frequency corresponding to the lowest S_f gets a score of $s_N(0) = 1$. Finally, the four best scores define the selection of the four *top* stimulation frequencies.

First closed-loop in the ACL-algorithm: iterative selection of the most compatible frequencies
The previous procedure provides initial scores for each frequency $s_1(0), s_2(0), \ldots, s_N(0)$ which depend on subjects' intra- and interindividual *state* and *trait* dimensions and on the extrinsic conditions in which the BCI is used. The selection of the four stimulation frequencies is then further optimized in an iterative approach attending to their compatibility. Thus, as the next step, we calculate the following compatibility measure between all

possible pairs of frequencies x and y taking into account a measure of their distance and their scores:

$$c_{xy}(t) = \alpha \cdot \left(s_x(t) + s_y(t)\right) + \beta \cdot d_{xy} \tag{2}$$

Here t represents the iteration number. We assigned the following weights to the distance and the scores: $\alpha = 1.5$ and $\beta = 1$, respectively, where d_{xy} is a measure of the distance between the frequencies which we define below. The values for α and β were set empirically based on several trials. Because four frequencies are used simultaneously in our specific BCI implementation, the most compatible four frequencies have to be selected out of N valid frequencies, determined by the protocol described above: the first step is to identify pairs of frequencies with optimal compatibility ("2 freq." search in the ACL branch in **Figure 2**). This search consists of $3N/4$ iterations (see below), each of them divided into 16 steps with a resting period at its end. The ACL departs from the scores calculated in the scanning procedure $s_1(0), s_2(0),\dots, s_N(0)$: they are modified in the successive iterations to search for the best compatibility.

In each iteration, the subject has to follow a sequence of flicker light sources by focusing upon them, as continuously indicated by the location of the green light. The flicker frequencies are chosen by selecting $max_{xy}(c_{xy})$ at the end of the iteration. To update the scores, we take into account both the success rate and the time as:

$$s_x(t) = s_x(t-1) \cdot \left(\delta \cdot SR - \gamma \cdot T\right) \tag{3}$$

where SR is the success rate (correct SSVEP detections over 16, the number of possible detections) and δ and γ are parameters of the ACL algorithm which were set to $\delta = 1.2$ and $\gamma = 0.02$. T is the duration of the detection in seconds. The values for δ and γ were chosen based upon the range of SR and T and several simulations.

In this first part of the algorithm, the distance between two specific frequencies f_x and f_y for Equation (2) is calculated as:

$$d_{xy} = |f_x - f_y| \tag{4}$$

Each $c_{xy}(t)$ is updated by the new scores after each iteration. Once this procedure has run $p = \lfloor 3N/4 \rfloor$ times, the highest $c_{xy}(p)$ is selected and a new set is created with the union of both frequencies. Now, the next highest $c_{x'y'}(p)$ disjoint from the previous set is chosen and a new set is constructed. This is repeated $\lfloor N/2 \rfloor$ times because this is the total number of possible disjoint pairs. It is ensured that each set is disjoint from all others. $p = \lfloor 3N/4 \rfloor$ is chosen to test $\lfloor 3N/2 \rfloor$ frequencies, so that the best frequencies are tested more than once. It is important to note that the duration of the frequency tests has to be restricted.

Afterwards, the second part of the algorithm is performed, the selection of four frequencies. The same procedure as in the first part is employed, but instead of single frequencies, sets of two frequencies are used. The values of $s_{x'}(p + 1)$ of each set are adjusted according to the values $c_{xy}(p)$, where $x' = x \cup y$. In this way, the set with the highest value gets $s_{1'}(p + 1) = \lfloor N/2 \rfloor$, the second best $s_{2'}(p + 1) = \lfloor N/2 \rfloor - 1$ and so on. The last one gets $s_{\lfloor N/2 \rfloor'}(p + 1) = 1$. From this point of the algorithm on, these sets are indivisible.

Using the same procedure performed with two frequencies, the process is repeated with four of them. The compatibility and the score actualization rules are still the same. The only difference is the distance measure for Equation (2) calculated as:

$$d_{xy} = \frac{\sum_{i=1}^{2k} \sum_{j=1}^{2k} |f_i - f_j|}{2k \cdot (2k - 1)} \tag{5}$$

where k is the number of frequencies of each set (in this case 2), and f_i and f_j are the individual frequencies taken from the union of the sets x and y. Note that here x and y refer to sets of two frequencies while in Equation (4) x and y referred to individual frequencies. This distance expresses the arithmetic mean of all possible pairs in the set resulting from the union of the initial sets x and y. Note that for $k = 1$, this distance measure is exactly the same distance (Equation 4) as used in the first part of the algorithm. In this second part $\lfloor 3N/8 \rfloor$ iterations are performed, which is $N/2$ (the number of disjoint sets) times 3/4 (see above).

Second closed-loop in the ACL-algorithm: online auditory feedback of SSVEP magnitudes

In order to offer additional dynamic information to the subject related to his/her brain activity beyond the SSVEP detection confirmation cue, we provide a continuous online auditory feedback during the trials which represents the distance between the actual state and the pre-defined goal. The feedback signal consists of a 20 possible sinusoids with a range between 100 and 575 Hz which are updated every 0.25 s. The represented distance measure is defined as the difference between the EEG-SSVEP *signal to noise ratio* for the target frequency (S_f^{target}) and the threshold. Once S_f^{target} has reached this threshold level, the auditory feedback is muted. Previously, subjects are instructed that their goal is to raise the pitch of the sinusoids as high as possible, and that after possible success their further goal would be trying to keep the sounds muted for 1.75 s; after this silence, the program automatically proceeds to the trial's next step. This kind of continuous auditory feedback aims to help subjects to learn to gain control *in their particular way* over SSVEP magnitudes by attracting their attentional resources to these voluntary attempts to increase self-regulation of their resonating brain states.

Concluding, there are two assisted closed loops in our system: the first one operates over the stimulation frequency set with the aim to directly improve the ITRs of each subject. This closed-loop informs the system about subject and environment specificities. The second one informs the subject about his/her brain activity in relation to the use of the interface and helps him/her to do so faster and more accurately. This closed loop works several times for each step of a trial.

SSVEP DETECTION

In order to reduce the experiment's complexity in terms of a reductionistic paradigm, we choose a simple SSVEP detection strategy in our study. During the *top* and *prefixed* frequency stimulation, the S_f^{target} value is calculated every 0.25 s. If this value exceeds the threshold for 1.75 consecutive seconds, then this SSVEP is defined as "detected." The threshold value was set to

10 which reflects the observed noise flow (see **Figure 5**). To avoid longer waiting periods when the subject is unable to exceed the threshold, a time limit of 4 s is used, after which that step is considered as fault.

During the ACL, to favor SSVEP detection in case that the subject exceeds the threshold and more time than the 1.75 s is needed to be classified as "detected," there is a small modification in this protocol to allow adaptive time extensions. When S_f^{target} exceeds the threshold in a given 0.25 s time step, the time limit is increased for another 0.25 s.

EFFICIENCY MEASURES

After each iteration of the algorithm, both the success rate and time needed are saved. For the *prefixed* and *top* frequencies, *standard Information Transfer Rate* (ITR) is calculated:

$$\text{ITR}(SR,\ t) = \big(\log_2(N) + SR \cdot \log_2(SR) + (1 - SR) \cdot$$
$$\log_2((1 - SR)/(N - 1))\big) \cdot Norm/t \quad (6)$$

where N is the number of targets ($N = 4$ in our case). The value SR represents the success rate and t is the time taken in minutes. *Norm* is a normalization value set to 960 (60 s times 16 steps in each iteration). Note that if $SR \leq 1/N$, then $\text{ITR}(SR, t) = 0$.

In contrast to the conditions *prefixed* and *top*, ITR is measured *several* times during the ACL. Thus, for further a-posteriori analyses these ITR distributions have to be represented by descriptive statistics: for condition *ACL* therefore M and Mdn of success rates and needed times are used to calculate ITR_{Mean} and ITR_{Median}, completed by maximum ITR (ITR_{Max}).

CONVERGENCE MEASURE

For a-posteriori analyses, a *convergence measure* for the algorithm in terms of the stimulus frequency exploration was defined: the duration of the 2 freq. search of the algorithm is divided into two parts. For each part, the numbers of explored frequencies are determined and divided by the maximal number of possible frequencies which could be explored (twice the number of iterations). The decrease comparing this measure in the second part vs. in the first part is a sign for how much the frequency exploration is converging. As can be seen in **Table 1**, the number of iterations varies over the subjects. The convergence measure is not reported for the first part because in our sample all subjects had the same maximal value 1, i.e., all possible frequencies were explored. We will use this measure to discuss how the ACL algorithm seems to adapt to subjects' interindividual differences.

STUDY DESIGN

A three conditions (*ACL, top, prefixed*) balanced *within*-subjects design with three times full permutation of presentation order (ABC, ACB, BAC, BCA, CAB, CBA) and with random assignment of subjects, resulting in $N = 18$ was employed.

BASELINE RESTING STATE EEG MEASURES AS POSSIBLE INTERINDIVIDUAL CORRELATES OF ITR PERFORMANCES

Aiming to investigate possible correlations between baseline resting state EEG measures and the variables of the experiment,

the 30 s baseline EEG (see **Figure 3**) at all eight electrodes reported above were manually cleaned from artifacts with the result of $M = 20.02$ s, $SD = 5.54$ artifact free epochs. Under *MATLAB 7.11.0.584 win64*, EEG signals were preprocessed in a first step by linear detrending followed by a 8th order *Butterworth* 1.5–70 Hz band pass filter and finally by a 8th order *Butterworth* 45–55 Hz notch filter against 50 Hz power line electromagnetic interferences. Then, preprocessed EEG signals were converted into *frequency domain* by a sliding windows FFT transform of 2 s window length (2048 sample points) with 3.906 ms displacement (4 sample points, which correspond to a 256 Hz sample frequency in the resulting frequency domain signals), after linear detrending and treatment by a *Hann*-window function. Obtained FFT coefficients were squared to obtain the power spectrum and then normalized by dividing by 2048 sample points. In order to obtain *absolute PSDs* for the defined EEG frequencies bands of interest, corresponding coefficients were summed: *thetaLow* (3.5–6.5 Hz), *thetaHigh* (6.5–7.5 Hz); *alphaLow* (7.5–9 Hz), *alphaHigh* (9–12.5 Hz); *betaLow* (12.5–18 Hz), *betaMid* (18–24 Hz), *betaHigh* (18–30 Hz); *totalSpectrum* (0.5–70 Hz). In a first step, those absolute frequency domain *PSDs* signals were normalized dividing every sample point by the corresponding one of *totalSpectrum* which resulted in dimensionless ratios. These ratios indicate for every 256 time points per second the *relative* energy contribution of the frequency band of interest to the EEG total energy at this particular moment. In a last step, in order to represent EEG baseline resting state activities in the analyzed artifact free epochs by one single value for every frequency band, means of these normalized signals were computed over all corresponding time points. Thus, finally we obtained the desired baseline resting state EEG measures as *relative mean PSDs* for further correlational analyses, single values for every frequency band over all subjects.

Another measure of interindividual EEG variability is the resting state *individual alpha frequency* (IAF), because it has been found to be remarkably stable *within* subjects, but relatively variable *between* subjects (Kondacs and Szabó, 1999). In order to determine IAF in our experiment, coefficients of PSDs corresponding to the frequency band 8–13 Hz at *Oz* were normalized by *totalSpectrum* PSDs and averaged over all sliding windows in the artifact free baseline resting state epochs. In this averaged and normalized power spectrum the *alpha* frequency with the highest PSD was manually measured and defined as IAF (*peak frequency method*).

STATISTICAL ANALYSES

All statistical analyses were computed using SPSS 17.0 and STATISTICA 6.0. Previously, *Shapiro–Wilk* tests were calculated to check each of the three conditions for normal distribution in the underlying populations. If one or more conditions showed significant departures from normality, *non-parametric* tests were preferred for further analyses: a *Friedman* test was performed as an *omnibus* test to investigate whether the *central tendencies* of one or more conditions differed significantly from the rest. In case of such a significant result, *post hoc pairwise comparisons* were performed in order to find out what conditions exactly differed significantly from each other, based upon comparison of *mean*

Table 1 | Data of the $N = 18$ subjects under the three experimental conditions.

No. of subject	SR Pre	SR Top	SR Mean ACL	SR Mdn ACL	SR Max ACL	ITR Pre	ITR Top	ITR Mean ACL	ITR Mdn ACL	ITR Max ACL	Age	SNR SSVEPs in scanning phase	Convergence measure N trials	Convergence measure 2nd half
1	0.31	0.88	0.77	0.78	0.88	**0.24**	**21.19**	**15.01**	**15.34**	**21.57**	23	15.20	13	0.5
2	0.56	0.63	0.57	0.5	0.75	**5.65**	**7.34**	**5.03**	**3.06**	**11.7**	23	15.89	11	0.4
3	0.75	0.38	0.80	0.88	0.94	**11.88**	**0.82**	**15.25**	**19.48**	**26.33**	27	14.44	14	0.57
4	0.81	0.94	0.95	0.97	1	**17.89**	**27.29**	**26.62**	**29.21**	**34.9**	33	31.38	15	0.71
5	0.75	0.56	0.68	0.59	0.69	**16.9**	**7.09**	**12.08**	**8.42**	**12.98**	24	8.02	15	0.36
6	0.06	0.25	0.35	0.25	0.63	**0**	**0**	**0.56**	**0**	**6.98**	25	8.08	9	0.5
7	0.81	0.69	0.85	0.81	1	**19.32**	**11.68**	**21.18**	**18.58**	**36.92**	59	23.76	12	0.92
8	0	0.44	0.59	0.59	0.75	**0**	**1.88**	**5.12**	**5.12**	**10.56**	18	8.03	5	0.5
9	0.63	0.44	0.69	0.69	0.75	**6.76**	**1.79**	**9.17**	**9.17**	**12.47**	52	8.68	4	1
10	0.75	0.75	0.83	0.84	0.94	**16.53**	**16.18**	**21.16**	**22.31**	**30.02**	23	59.20	14	1
11	0.56	0.81	0.88	0.88	1	**5.35**	**18.23**	**21.84**	**22.16**	**31.47**	50	37.70	14	0.64
12	0.19	0.25	0.56	0.69	0.69	**0**	**0**	**4.67**	**9.42**	**9.73**	24	6.35	6	0.33
13	0.69	0.81	0.81	0.81	0.94	**10.07**	**19.32**	**18.06**	**18.06**	**28.32**	34	8.43	8	0.87
14	0.69	0.75	0.66	0.69	0.75	**12.7**	**16.53**	**11.13**	**12.7**	**16.18**	27	48.58	14	0.93
15	0.31	0.31	0.58	0.56	0.69	**0.21**	**0.22**	**5.4**	**4.96**	**9.57**	45	12.01	14	0.43
16	0.18	0.5	0.63	0.56	0.94	**0**	**3.43**	**6.34**	**4.42**	**21.14**	20	16.35	9	0.38
17	0	0	0.34	0.34	0.38	**0**	**0**	**0.42**	**0.42**	**0.76**	22	14.15	11	0.6
18	0.5	0.69	0.76	0.75	0.81	**3.43**	**12.98**	**15.43**	**14.63**	**18.58**	32	30.03	13	0.67
Shapiro–Wilk's W	0.883	0.961	0.947	0.952	0.896	0.850	0.886	0.950	0.960	0.956	0.832	0.819	0.876	0.909
p	0.030	0.631	0.385	0.460	0.049	0.008	0.034	0.420	0.594	0.520	0.005	0.003	0.022	0.082
Mdn	**0.56**	**0.60**	**0.69**	**0.69**	**0.78**	5.5	7.22	**11.61**	**11.06**	**17.33**	**26.00**	**14.82**	**12.50**	**0.59**
Percentile 25	0.19	0.36	0.58	0.56	0.69	0.00	0.67	5.10	4.83	10.35	23.00	8.34	8.75	0.42
Percentile 75	0.75	0.77	0.82	0.82	0.94	13.66	16.96	18.84	18.81	28.75	36.75	30.37	14.00	0.88

Note: Information transfer rates (ITRs) in bits/min as measures of individual BCI performances under the different experimental conditions and all Mdn values are highlighted in bold for further analyses.

N trials refers to the number of iterations in the first part of ACL (using two flicker LEDs).

Convergence measure first half is not reported in the table because all subjects had the same value 1.

SNR SSVEPs in Scanning phase are means over all used 20 flicker frequencies.

rank differences using as significance criteria the *critical rank differences* proposed by the more progressive approach of Conover (1980) vs. the more conservative of Schaich and Hamerle (1984).

In order to quantify the *effect sizes* of those *post hoc* pairwise comparisons which resulted in significant differences, we used the probability of superiority of dependent scores, PS_{dep}, recommended by Grissom and Kim (2012) and developed in Grissom (1994). It expresses the probability that in a randomly sampled matched pair the value from the condition containing the higher scores is indeed larger than that from the one containing lower scores. PS_{dep} is calculated by dividing the number of *positive* differences between the condition *containing the higher scores* minus the condition *containing the lower scores* by the total number of matched pairs. For classifying PS_{dep} into small, middle and large effect sizes based upon the standards of Cohen (1988), the *cut-off* values reported by Grissom (1994) are used: *small* 0.56, *medium* 0.64, and *large* 0.71. The same author offers a table to directly convert PS into equivalent *Cohen's Δ*. Thus, as effect size measures both PS_{dep} and *Cohen's Δ* are reported with standards *small* $\Delta = 0.20$, *medium* $\Delta = 0.50$ and *large* $\Delta = 0.80$ (Cohen, 1988).

In order to check whether significant differences over all six possible permutations of the presentation order might be found, a *mixed-design repeated measures ANOVA* was computed with *stimulation condition* as repeated *within*-subjects factor with three levels (i) ACL algorithm represented as ITR_{Median}, (ii) prefixed and (iii) top and *presentation order* as *between*-subjects factor with the six possible permutations as levels (ABC, ACB, BAC etc.). Previously, *Levene's* tests were performed in order to check for homogeneities of error variance. Moreover, the assumption of *sphericity* of the covariance matrix was verified previously by a *Mauchly's sphericity test* in order to assure that the F ratios match an F distribution. If there was a significant departure from sphericity, *Greenhouse-Geisser* estimates were used to correct degrees of freedom which results in fractions instead of usual integers. Although data may not follow a normal distribution, *ANOVA* has been demonstrated to be relatively robust against moderate deviations from normality (see e.g., Khan and Rayner, 2003). Univariate analyses were used to examine whether there is a significant *between*-subjects main effect of *presentation order* and further if there is a significant *interaction* effect between *presentation order* × *stimulation condition*. Analyses were repeated representing condition (i) ACL algorithm also as ITR_{Mean} vs. ITR_{Max}.

For the investigation of linear correlational relationships, *Spearman's rank order correlation coefficient Rho* was additionally used apart from the common *Pearson product-moment correlation coefficient r* due to its relative robustness firstly against outliers, but also against other than linear, but still monotonic relationships and against departures from normality or homoscedasticity. Whenever relevant influence of outliers was suspected, *Spearman's rank correlation coefficient Rho* was preferred.

A-priori *statistical test power* analyses with the program G*Power 3 (Faul et al., 2007) show that *Pearson* correlation significance tests in the employed sample size of $N = 18$ and with standard significance level $\alpha = 0.05$ have test powers $(1 - \beta) \geq 0.80$ as recommend by Cohen (1988), when they have effect sizes in the underlying population $\rho \geq 0.60$, as compared to $H_0 : \rho = 0.00$. For $\rho = 0.50$ test power is $(1 - \beta) \geq 0.60$, for $\rho = 0.40$ $(1 - \beta) = 0.40$ and for $\rho = 0.30$ $(1 - \beta) \approx 0.20$. Thus, although the employed sample size $N = 18$ is relatively small, hypothesis testing of *Pearson* correlations with full recommended strictness is definitely possible at the level of assumed large effect sizes.

RESULTS

Table 1 reports the data for all $N = 18$ subjects under the three experimental conditions, representing (i) *ACL algorithm* as ITR_{Mean}, ITR_{Median} and ITR_{Max}. Inferential statistical hypotheses testing that (i) outperformed the other two flicker stimulation conditions is reported below.

Figure 6 shows the SSVEP frequency-response curves in our experiments. For all subjects, the 20 flicker frequencies in the scanning phase were presented in the same order: 23, 37, 30, 31, 36, 22, 29, 33, 39, 24, 35, 21, 25, 27, 32, 34, 28, 20, 26, and 38 Hz. Sequential randomness of this order is confirmed with $Z = -0.230$ and $p_{exact} = 0.828$ (*Wald–Wolfowitz* runs test after *Mdn* split dichotomization). Our findings that in the 20–39 Hz range, lower flicker frequencies *over all subjects* (**Figure 6A**) evoke higher SSVEP magnitudes are in line with other studies which reported a global maximum SSVEP amplitude around 10 Hz with additional local maxima around 20, 40, and 80 Hz (Regan, 1989; Herrmann, 2001; Bayram et al., 2011). In our sample, we found that SSVEP frequency-response curves differed remarkably *between subjects* (**Figure 6B**) probably due to trait and state variabilities which justifies that they are determined in our experiment in the scanning phase for every subject *individually*.

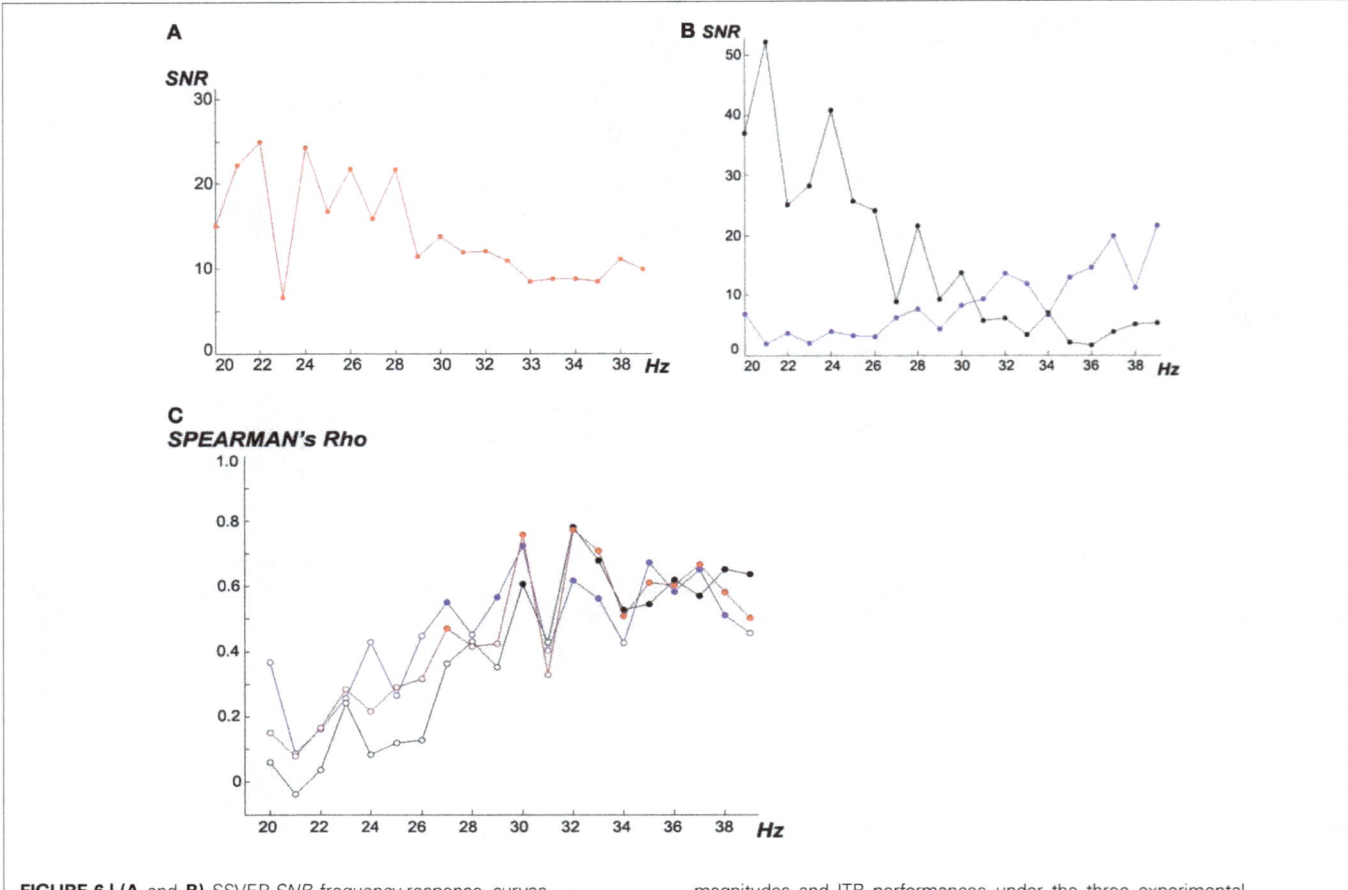

FIGURE 6 | (A and **B)** SSVEP-*SNR* frequency-response curves. **(A)** *Mdn*s over all $N = 18$ subjects, **(B)** example of two subjects with opposed frequency-response curves (black # subject 16, blue #9). **(C)** Frequency-dependent interindividual association between SSVEP-*SNR*

magnitudes and ITR performances under the three experimental conditions, computed as *Spearman's* rank order correlations: (i) *ACL algorithm* (red), (ii) *top* (blue) and (iii) *prefixed* (black), filled circles represent significant $p < 0.05$.

Analyzing **Figure 6C**, higher frequencies ≥ 30 Hz lead to higher correlations; no relevant differences can be seen comparing the three experimental conditions. Interestingly, following e.g., Zschocke and Hansen (2012), 30 Hz is the upper boundary of *beta* activity observable in scalp EEGs by conventional amplifiers.

SIGNIFICANT AND LARGE IMPROVEMENT OF SSVEP-BCI EFFICIENCY BY THE NOVEL ACL ALGORITHM

Analyzing the differences in the *central tendencies* between the three experimental conditions (i) *ACL algorithm* (ii) *prefixed* (iii) *top* we represented condition (i) based upon three different descriptive statistics, (a) ITR_{Mean}, (b) ITR_{Median}, (d) ITR_{Max} (see section "Materials and Methods" and **Table 1**). Applying non-parametric inferential statistics we found a very significant and very large superiority of condition (i) *ACL algorithm* over the other two (ii) and (iii) which is independent of its three types of representation (a), (b), and (c), while there is no significant difference between (ii) and (iii). The used statistical methods and measures for the following results are found in section "Statistical Analyses."

(a) A *Friedman* omnibus test comparing the ITRs between the three experimental conditions (i) *ACL algorithm* **represented as ITR_{Mean}**, (ii) *prefixed* and (iii) *top* shows a significant overall difference with $\chi^2(2) = 10.116$, $p = 0.006$.

Post-hoc pairwise comparisons based upon *critical mean rank differences* 0.82 (Schaich and Hamerle, 1984) vs. 0.58 (Conover, 1980) indicate that ITRs are significantly higher in (i) *ACL algorithm* as compared to (ii) *prefixed* (*mean rank difference* = 1.03, very large effect size $PS_{dep} = 0.83$, $\Delta = 1.37$) and also as compared to (iii) *top* (*mean rank difference* = 0.64, large effect size $PS_{dep} = 0.72$, $\Delta = 0.83$). Comparison of (ii) *prefixed* with (iii) *top* results in a non-significant difference (*mean rank difference* = 0.39).

(b) A *Friedman* omnibus test comparing the ITRs between the three experimental conditions (i) *ACL algorithm* **represented as ITR_{Median}**, (ii) *prefixed* and (iii) *top* shows a significant overall difference with $\chi^2(2) = 9.262$, $p = 0.01$.

Post-hoc pairwise comparisons based upon *critical mean rank differences* 0.82 (Schaich and Hamerle, 1984) vs. 0.57 (Conover, 1980) indicate that ITRs are significantly higher in (i) *ACL algorithm* as compared to (ii) *prefixed* (*mean rank difference* = 0.94, very large effect size $PS_{dep} = 0.81$, $\Delta = 1.25$) and also as compared to (iii) *top* (*mean rank difference* = 0.64, very large effect size $PS_{dep} = 0.76$, $\Delta = 1.21$) applying the less conservative criterion of (Conover, 1980). Comparison of (ii) *prefixed* with (iii) *top* results in a non-significant difference (*mean rank difference* = 0.31).

(c) A *Friedman* omnibus test comparing the ITRs between the three experimental conditions (i) *ACL algorithm* **represented as ITR_{Max}**, (ii) *prefixed* and (iii) *top* shows a significant overall difference with $\chi^2(2) = 22.986$, $p = 0.00001$.

Post-hoc pairwise comparisons based upon *critical mean rank differences* 0.82 (Schaich and Hamerle, 1984) vs. 0.41 (Conover, 1980) indicate that ITRs are significantly higher in (i) *ACL algorithm* as compared to (ii) *prefixed* (*mean rank difference* = 1.47, extremely large effect size $PS_{dep} = 0.94$,

$\Delta = 2.25$) and also as compared to (iii) *top* (*mean rank difference* = 1.19, extremely large effect size $PS_{dep} = 0.94$, $\Delta = 2.25$). Comparison of (ii) *prefixed* with (iii) *top* results in a non-significant difference (*mean rank difference* = 0.28).

THE ACL ALGORITHM SEEMS TO ADAPT TO SUBJECTS' INTERINDIVIDUAL DIFFERENCES

N_{Trials} in condition (i) *ACL algorithm* using two flicker LEDs (see **Table 1**) is deterministically given by 3/4 of the total number of the SSVEP-*SNR* responses under the 20 flicker frequencies in the scanning phase of the experiment which had exceeded the defined threshold value of 10 (*suitable* frequencies), see *ACL Algorithm* of section "Materials and Methods." Thus, in order to make the investigation of possible interindividual associations between the SSVEP-*SNR* magnitudes with the convergence measure second half (see section "Materials and Methods") relatively independent from N_{Trials}, all subjects with $N_{Trials} <$ 25th percentile ($8.75 \approx 9$) were excluded, # subject 6, 8, 9, 12, 13, and 16. The resulting rest of $N = 12$ subjects showed a relatively small variability with range of N_{Trials} between 11 and 15. The measure SSVEP-*SNR* mean magnitudes in the scanning phase of the experiment (a) over all flicker frequencies from 20 to 39 Hz was split into two measures, one for (b) *lower* frequencies from 20 to 29 Hz and the other for (c) *higher* frequencies from 30 to 39 Hz. In this subsample, convergence measure second half shows large and highly significant correlations with (a) of $r = 0.839$, $p = 0.001$, with (b) of $r = 0.843$, $p = 0.001$ and with (c) of $r = 0.763$, $p = 0.004$. Checking these relationships against the remaining variability of N_{Trials} and age as controlled third variables in *partial correlation* analyses, indeed no changes are observed; those found relationships can be considered as linearly independent from N_{Trials} and age. Hence, these findings show that the convergence of the *ACL* algorithm highly depends on the subjects' *trait* ability to generate higher SSVEP-*SNR* magnitudes, with no relevant differences observed between *lower* vs. *higher* flicker frequencies: focusing on a subsample with a more or less constant number of *suitable* frequencies, the ACL algorithm explored the more distinct frequencies in those subjects who displayed the *larger* SSVEP-*SNR* magnitudes in the scanning phase of the experiment.

In conclusion, these findings imply that the ACL algorithm shows a distinct exploration behavior for different subjects and thus indeed is able to adapt to subjects' interindividual differences. Whether this adaptation is the *cause* for the ACL algorithm's outperformance of (ii) *top* and (iii) *prefixed* cannot be examined in depth with the employed experimental design and has to be investigated in further studies.

BASELINE RESTING STATE EEG MEASURES AS CORRELATES OF INTERINDIVIDUAL DIFFERENCES

Searching for significant and relevant associations between interindividual variabilities of ITR performances under the three experimental conditions vs. of baseline resting state EEG relative mean PSDs in all computed frequency bands at all eight used electrodes, effects were only found in *thetaHigh* (6.5–7.5 Hz) and *betaMid* (18–24 Hz). In all the other bands nothing could be observed.

Whereas *Pearson* correlations showed no relationships between the resting state relative mean *thetaHigh* PSDs at *Oz* vs. ITRs in conditions (iii) *prefixed* ($r = 0.034$, $p = 0.894$) and (ii) *top* ($r = 0.196$, $p = 0.436$), a significant positive correlation with condition (i) *ACL algorithm* was found ($r = 0.467$, $p = 0.048$) representing the performance as ITR$_{Median}$. Searching for similar relationships in the other seven used electrodes, no associations were observed; these effects exclusively occur at *Oz* in our sample. Following the effects size classifications of Cohen (1988), this correlation is to be considered as *moderate*. *Partial correlation* analyses confirmed that this correlation is linearly independent against age and all means of SSVEP-*SNRs* in the previous scanning phase of the experiment over (a) *all* 20 flicker frequencies, (b) also over the *lower* frequencies 20–29 Hz and (c) also over the *higher* frequencies 30–39 Hz.

At least in the examined sample, interindividual variability in relative mean *thetaHigh PSD* at *Oz* seems to differentiate between *ACL algorithm* and the other two conditions: the larger the observed relative mean PSDs among subjects in the baseline resting state are, the better will be their later SSVEP-BCI performance exclusively under the use of *ACL algorithm*.

At first sight, analyzing baseline resting state relative mean *betaMid* PSDs, an exclusive relationship with only the ITRs in condition (iii) *top* was found for *F3* ($r = 0.484$, $p = 0.042$), although its neighbor electrodes also showed relationships not very far away from significance, probably due to small sample

size: *F4* with $r = 0.425$, $p = 0.117$ and *Fz* with $r = 0.410$, $p = 0.091$. All the other used electrodes showed no associations. After further graphic inspection of relevant scatterplots and *Box-Whisker-Plots*, a possible negative relationship between baseline resting state relative mean *betaMid* PSDs at *Oz* and ITR$_{Mean}$ in condition (i) *ACL algorithm* was suspected, hidden by outliers. *Box-Whisker-Plots* suggested case 15 and 11 as outliers, so for further analysis *Mahalanobis distances* were computed in a linear regression analysis with the ITRs$_{Mean}$ of condition (i) *ACL algorithm* as criterion variable and baseline resting state relative mean *betaMid* PSDs at *Oz* as predictor variable. The inspection of *Mahalanobis distances* and the scatterplot (see **Figure 7**) suggest that subject 15 and 11 might be considered as outliers. Excluding them changes the correlation from $r = -0.262$, $p = 0.294$ to significant $r = -0.530$, $p = 0.042$. *Partial correlation* analyses confirmed that this correlation is linearly independent against age and all means of SSVEP-*SNRs* in the previous scanning phase of the experiment (a), (b), and (c) mentioned above.

Interestingly, excluding case 15 and 11, baseline resting state relative mean PSDs *betaMid* vs. *thetaHigh* both at *Oz* show an almost significant correlation over the subjects with $r = -0.482$ and $p = 0.059$, probably due to the small sample size, which is stable against the third variables age and all SSVEP-*SNRs* in the previous scanning phase of the experiment (a), (b), and (c), mentioned above.

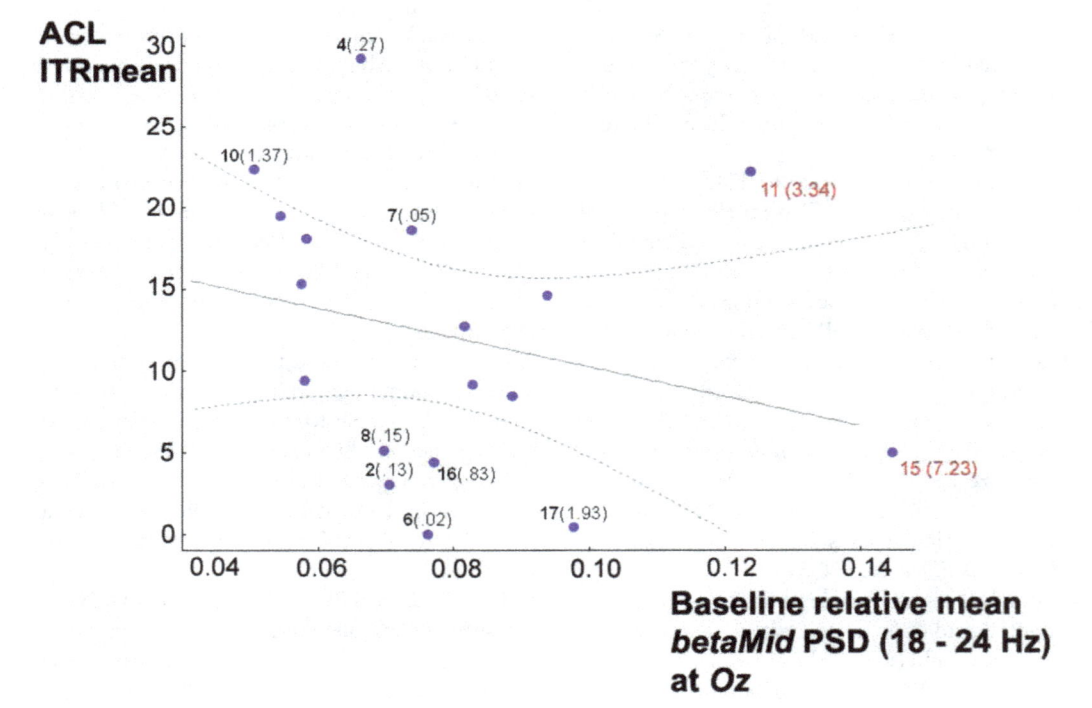

FIGURE 7 | Scatterplot of baseline resting state relative mean *betaMid* PSDs at *Oz* vs. ITR$_{Mean}$ in condition (i) *ACL* algorithm, 95% confidence regression bands as dotted lines, subject numbers in bold, *Mahalanobis distances* in brackets calculated in a linear regression analysis with the ITR$_{Mean}$ as criterion variables and relative mean *betaMid* PSDs as predictor variables. Subject 15 and 11 (in red) might be considered as outliers (see text). Excluding them changes the *Pearson* correlation from $r = -0.262$, $p = 0.294$ to significant $r = -0.510$, $p = 0.043$.

In conclusion, baseline resting state relative mean *betaMid* PSDs seem to predict ITR performances under (i) *ACL algorithm* vs. (iii) *top* in an opposed fashion depending on the electrodes: the *lower* baseline resting state relative mean *betaMid* PSDs are at Oz, the *higher* will be the ITRs under condition (i); and the *higher* baseline resting state relative mean *betaMid* PSDs are at frontal electrodes (*F3, Fz, F4*) the *higher* will be the ITRs under condition (iii). In addition to these findings in *betaMid*, the higher the baseline resting state relative mean *thetaHigh* PSDs at Oz are, the higher will be the ITRs exclusively under condition (i).

Returning to the above described subsample of $N = 12$ obtained by exclusion of all subjects with $N_{Trials} <$ 25th percentile ($8.75 \approx 9$), an interesting observation was found: IAF shows differentiating relationships with ITR performances: a significant correlation of $r = 0.577, p = 0.0496$ was only found with ITRs under (i) *ACL algorithm* (see scatterplot **Figure 8**), but neither under (ii) *top* with $r = 0.394, p = 0.205$ nor under (iii) *prefixed* $r = 0.283, p = 0.373$. The higher subjects' IAF are in the subsample, the better will be their ITR performance exclusively under the ACL algorithm. *Partial correlation* analyses confirmed that this association is linearly independent against age. Repeating this analysis for the entire sample of $N = 18$ *no* significant correlations between individual alpha frequency (IAF) and ITR performances under the three experimental conditions become apparent (i) with $r = 0.282, p = 0.257$, (ii) $r = 0.198, p = 0.432$ and (iii) $r = 0.243, p = 0.332$. These findings imply that subjects with *low* ITRs in all three conditions might represent another population as compared to the rest. Further studies may try to replicate these findings and identify dimensions which discriminate between these possible two different populations. Moreover, these findings could be relevant for the understanding

of the so-called *BCI illiteracy* phenomenon (Blankertz et al., 2010; Vidaurre and Blankertz, 2010; Volosyak et al., 2011), see section "Discussion."

Inspired by the findings of Koch et al. (2008) who found correlations of IAF with both magnitudes of *visually evoked potentials* (VEPs) and also with cortical oxygenation measured by *near-infrared spectroscopy* (NIRS), *Spearman* rank order correlations were computed between IAF and means of SSVEP-*SNR* magnitudes in the scanning phase of the experiment (a) over *all* 20 used flicker frequencies 20–39 Hz, (b) over the *lower* frequencies 20–29 Hz and (c) over the *higher* frequencies 30–39 Hz in the described subsample of $N = 12$. Although not fully reaching significance level, probably due to the relatively small sample size, an interesting pattern was found: IAF vs. (a) with $rho = 0.561, p = 0.058$, IAF vs. (b) with $rho = 0.183, p = 0.568$ and IAF vs. (c) $rho = 0.557, p = 0.060$. Although not fully significant, probably due to the small sample size, interindividual differences in SSVEP-*SNR* magnitudes under the employed *higher* flicker frequencies seem to show a tendency of positive association to higher IAFs while this relationship might not exist for the stimulation with the *lower* frequencies (or if so, it may presumably be lower). These findings motivated the re-analysis of the found relationship in **Figure 8** by *partial correlations* whether it would be linearly independent against SSVEP-*SNR* magnitudes in the scanning phase of the experiment (a), (b) and (c) as described above. While (a) and (b) showed no relevant influence on this relationship, controlling for (c) resulted in a reduction from former *Pearson* $r = 0.577, p = 0.0496$ to $r = 0.396, p = 0.228$. Hence, these findings imply that IAF and (c) the magnitude of SSVEP responses to only the employed *higher* flicker frequencies share remarkably amounts of common interindividual variability while explaining variability of ITR_{Mean} under the ACL algorithm.

EFFECTS OF THE PERMUTATION OF PRESENTATION ORDER

Investigating possible effects of the permutation of presentation order, a *mixed-design repeated measures ANOVA* was computed with *stimulation condition* as repeated *within*-subjects factor with three levels (i) ACL algorithm represented as ITR_{Median}, (ii) prefixed and (iii) top and *presentation order* as *between*-subjects factor with the six possible permutations as levels (ABC, ACB, BAC etc.). *Levene's* tests showed homogeneities of error variances. There was no significant *between*-subjects main effect of *presentation order* with $F_{(5, 18)} = 2.26, p = 0.115, \eta_p^2 = 0.485$. Because *Mauchly's sphericity* test indicated a significant departure from the assumption of *sphericity* with $\chi^2(2) = 6.54, p = 0.038$, *Greenhouse-Geisser* estimates were used to correct degrees of freedom ($\varepsilon = 0.691$). There was no significant *interaction* between *presentation order* × *stimulation condition* with $F_{(10, 18)} = 0.67, p = 0.738, \eta_p^2 = 0.219$. *ANOVA* analyses were repeated also for condition (i) ACL algorithm represented as ITR_{Mean} and ITR_{Max} which resulted in similar findings. In conclusion, neither significant main effects nor significant interactions could be found over all six possible permutations of presentation order. Hence, the found effects in the *central tendencies* reported above with regard to all ITR performances can be considered as independent from possible presentation order effects.

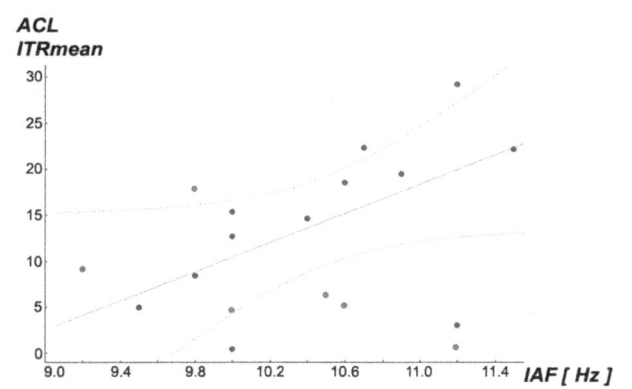

FIGURE 8 | Scatterplot of individual alpha frequency (IAF) vs. ITR$_{Mean}$ under condition (i) *ACL algorithm* (best-fit regression line for $N = 12$ as continuous line, 95% confidence regression bands as dotted lines). A significant *Pearson* correlation with $r = 0.577, p = 0.0496$ was found in the remaining subsample of $N = 12$ (blue points), removing subjects with $N_{Trials} <$ 25th percentile ($8.75 \approx 9$) (red points), while over the entire sample of $N = 18$ the correlation is hidden with $r = 0.282, p = 0.257$ (all points). This relationship seems to exist exclusively for condition (i) *ACL algorithm*: the higher subjects' IAF are in this subsample, the better will be their ITR$_{Mean}$ performance exclusively under (i). *Partial correlation* analyses confirmed that this association is linearly independent against age.

DISCUSSION

Although electrophysiology-based closed-loop interactions with biological nervous systems have been used since the 1940s, modern computers and online software control techniques allow a wide variety of novel activity dependent protocols in neuroscience research and related applications. Current BCI bring up a number of problems related to relatively long previous training times and still relatively low efficiencies (ITRs). This calls for novel techniques which can also address context and subject specificities, e.g., adaptive detection of SSVEPs (e.g., Krauledat et al., 2008).

In this paper we described an *assisted closed-loop protocol* which enhances BCI efficiency, as compared to classic BCI protocols, by providing both the subject and the system with online information which helps them to reach the BCI goal in their interaction. We used a reductionistic paradigm to constrain the inherent complexity of closed-loop exploration: four simultaneous frequencies, a basic SSVEP detection strategy and a relatively simple task to be accomplished by the user. More complex BCI systems might further benefit from the described approach. Our paradigm calls for many possible improvements, ranging from advanced SSVEP detection algorithms, stimuli which inform the user more effectively, up to a more adaptive online control of the interface itself by measuring and exploring additional dimensions (multimodality).

The literature on SSVEP-BCIs does not report general recommendations for the selection of the properties of the visual stimuli (Wu et al., 2008; Zhu et al., 2010), although it is known that the SSVEP magnitudes depend on extrinsic and intrinsic dimensions (Ding et al., 2006; Lopez-Gordo et al., 2011). Our study shows that a closed-loop subject-specific selection of the stimulation frequencies together with the closed-loop auditory feedback lead to increased BCI ITR performance which outperformed the employed control conditions.

Although *assisted closed-loop protocols* seem to enhance BCI efficiency, their use is limited by the additional time needed for the exploration process. In the protocol discussed in this paper, the average time to perform the experiment was around half an hour, flicker frequency selection took most of this time. Due to time restrictions, the parameter space can never be explored completely, so BCI efficiency improvement might remain suboptimal. Thus, there is some unknown *trade-off* between improvement and time needed, which should be explored in further studies. Furthermore, the question how replicable the found flicker frequencies are in the same subjects over multiple follow-up time points could be explored. Probably, observing this stability over time (e.g., *test-retest reliability*) may help to discover important trait vs. state dimensions related to variability of BCI performance. Another limitation due to the SSVEP physiology is that the time window for the auditory feedback is relatively short, so subjects have to establish control over the BCI goal in the range of a few seconds. This implies possible interactions with subjects' traits and states related to cognitive *processing speed* and dimensions of learning abilities.

ACL algorithms offer new possibilities as compared to traditional open-loop paradigms, but require additional decisions and new perspectives for their design and analysis, e.g., with regard to online measurement of actual states and performance, parameter search responding to the particular dynamic behavior of the system, properties of the feedback stimuli, *actuation laws*, etc. However, our findings imply that this additional effort can improve BCI efficiency and contribute to reveal dynamics of the nervous system which would remain hidden under traditional paradigms. Because our analyses showed that EEG resting state measures can predict assisted closed-loop SSVEP-BCI performance, our novel approach seems to flexibly adapt/interact with interindividual cerebral variability. Although found in the context of a *sensory motor rhythms* (SMRs) based BCI, other recent work also demonstrated that EEG resting state measures can be relevant predictors of BCI performance (Blankertz et al., 2010). In this emerging field, it could be fruitful to identify possible EEG resting state measures which can differentiate/predict between BCI performances based on biosignals originating from distinct physiological mechanisms: SSVEPs, P300, SMRs, *slow cortical potentials* (SCPs), *electrocorticogram* (ECoG), *magnetoencephalography* (MEG), NIRS or *blood-oxygen-level-dependent* (BOLD). Apart from these biosignals reflecting *brain* activity, *peripheral* psychophysiological measures have been investigated in the context of BCIs, especially as performance predictors, such as *parasympathic/vagal* parameters of resting state *heart rate variability* (HRV) (Kaufmann et al., 2011).

Our proposed approach of new adaptive-interactive paradigms might offer innovative ways how to address the problem of the so-called *BCI illiteracy*, i.e., the incapacity of some subjects to achieve control of BCIs (Blankertz et al., 2010; Vidaurre and Blankertz, 2010; Volosyak et al., 2011). It might be fruitful to explore the possible different impact of ACL algorithms in BCIs based on the mentioned distinct physiological mechanisms, especially with regard to their specific BCI illiteracies.

As mentioned in section "Baseline Resting State EEG Measures as Possible Interindividual Correlates of ITR Performances," the IAF is a measure of *interindividual* EEG variability because it is remarkably stable *within* subjects, but relatively variable *between* subjects (Kondacs and Szabó, 1999). IAF seems to be highly heritable, e.g., Posthuma et al. (2001) found in a study comparing mono- vs. dizygotic twins, analyzing a large representative sample of healthy Dutch adults ($N = 688$), that 71–83% of total IAF variance could be ascribed to genetic variances. Thus, IAF may be considered as an *endophenotype* following the definition of Gottesman and Gould (2003). Klimesch (1997) found in a sample of age matched subjects that the IAF of good working memory performers is about 1 Hz higher vs. that of bad performers. Jin et al. (2006) found that IAF is positively correlated with conflict reaction time. Severity of *Alzheimer's* disease is positively related to the extent of typical IAF slowing in this pathology (Rodriguez et al., 1999). On the neurophysiological level, Steriade et al. (1990) reported that IAF depends on membrane properties of the thalamic neurons which project to the cortex, implying thalamo-cortical feedback loops as one of the important generators of alpha activity (Lopes da Silva, 1991). Mayer et al. (2007) successfully modeled the synchronization of locally coupled bistable thalamic oscillators as controlled by the influence of corticothalamic projections, probably responsible for widespread spindle oscillations in the thalamus. Given these findings, IAF might be understood as a positive correlate of thalamo-cortical information processing speed. With regard of possible correlations of IAF with SSVEP magnitudes, Koch et al. (2008) found interesting correlations of IAF with both magnitudes of VEPs and cortical oxygenation measured by NIRS. Concluding, IAF seems to open new insights into the understanding of the neural circuits underlying BCI performance and thus should be considered as a promising predictor for further studies.

In this study, only eight EEG electrodes were used to investigate EEG resting state measures as performance predictors, but further works might use more electrodes of the 10–20 system to allow a-posteriori offline analyses of *scalp maps* and the use of *source localization* techniques, e.g., *LORETA* (for a review see Grech et al., 2008). Findings of research concerning the cerebral *resting-state networks* call for further studies which use simultaneous EEG/fMRI recordings (for reviews see e.g., Fox and Raichle,

2007; Van den Heuvel and Hulshoff-Pol, 2010; for typical studies see e.g., Damoiseaux et al., 2006; Van den Heuvel et al., 2009; Yuan et al., 2012).

Opening the scope to other uses, the demonstrated advantage of our adaptive-interactive BCI protocol can be expanded conceptually, e.g., to innovative applications such as diagnostic/therapeutic tools in clinical contexts: exploring the subject-specific dynamical trajectory of machine-subject interaction could extract information which otherwise would remain undiscovered. Thus, far beyond an engineering focus, the proposed approach might be employed as a new paradigm for basic neuroscientific and biomedical research.

ACKNOWLEDGMENTS

We thank Víctor Bonilla for technical help. This work was supported by UAM CEMU 2012-004, MINECO TIN2012-30883 and TIN-2010-19607.

REFERENCES

Bayram, A., Bayraktaroglu, Z., Karahan, E., Erdogan, B., Bilgic, B., Ozker, M., et al. (2011). Simultaneous EEG/fMRI analysis of the resonance phenomena in steady-state visual evoked responses. *Clin. EEG Neurosci.* 42, 98–106.

Birbaumer, N. (2006). Breaking the silence: brain-computer interfaces (BCI) for communication and motor control. *Psychophysiology* 43, 517–532.

Blankertz, B., Sannelli, C., Halder, S., Hammer, E. M., Kübler, A., Müller, K.-R., et al. (2010). Neurophysiological predictor of SMR-based BCI performance. *Neuroimage* 51, 1303–1309.

Capilla, A., Pazo-Alvarez, P., Darriba, A., Campo, P., and Gross, J. (2011). Steady-state visual evoked potentials can be explained by temporal superposition of transient event-related responses. *PLoS ONE* 6:e14543. doi: 10.1371/journal.pone.0014543

Chamorro, P., Levi, R., Rodriguez, F. B., Pinto, R. D., and Varona, P. (2009). Real-time activity-dependent drug microinjection. *BMC Neuroscience* 10:P296. doi: 10.1186/1471-2202-10-S1-P296

Chamorro, P., Muñiz, C., Levi, R., Arroyo, D., Rodríguez, F. B., and Varona, P. (2012). Generalization of the dynamic clamp concept in neurophysiology and behavior. *PLoS ONE* 7:e40887. doi: 10.1371/journal.pone.0040887

Cohen, J. (1988). *Statistical Power Analysis for the Behavioral Sciences.* 2nd Edn. Hillsdale, NJ: Erlbaum.

Cole, K. S. (1955). "Ions, potentials and the nerve impulse," in *Electrochemistry in Biology and Medicine,* ed T. Shedlovsky (New York, NY: Wiley), 121–140.

Conover, W. J. (1980). *Practical Nonparametric Statistics.* 2nd Edn. New York, NY: John Wiley and Sons.

Damoiseaux, J. S., Rombouts, S. A. R. B., Barkhof, F., Scheltens, P., Stam, C. J., Smith, S. M., et al. (2006). Consistent resting-state networks across healthy subjects. *Proc. Natl. Acad. Sci. U.S.A.* 103, 13848–13853.

Destexhe, A., and Bal, T. (eds.). (2009). *Dynamic-Clamp: From Principles to Applications.* New York, NY: Springer.

Diez, P. F., Mut, V., Laciar, E., and Avila, E. (2010). A comparison of monopolar and bipolar EEG recordings for SSVEP detection. *Conf. Proc. IEEE Eng. Med. Biol. Soc.* 2010, 5803–5806.

Diez, P. F., Mut, V. A., Avila-Perona, E. M., and Laciar-Leber, E. (2011). Asynchronous BCI control using high-frequency SSVEP. *J. Neuroeng. Rehabil.* 8:39. doi: 10.1186/1743-0003-8-39

Ding, J., Sperling, G., and Srinivasan, R. (2006). Attentional modulation of SSVEP power depends on the network tagged by the flicker frequency. *Cereb. Cortex* 16, 1016–1029.

Economo, M. N., Fernandez, F. R., and White, J. A. (2010). Dynamic clamp: alteration of response properties and creation of virtual realities in neurophysiology. *J. Neurosci.* 30, 2407–2413.

Faul, F., Erdfelder, E., Lang, A.-G., and Buchner, A. (2007). G*Power 3: a flexible statistical power analysis program for the social, behavioral, and biomedical sciences. *Behav. Res. Methods* 39, 175–191.

Fox, M. D., and Raichle, M. E. (2007). Spontaneous fluctuations in brain activity observed with functional magnetic resonance imaging. *Nat. Rev. Neurosci.* 8, 700–711.

Funahashi, S. (2001). Neuronal mechanisms of executive control by the prefrontal cortex. *Neurosci. Res.* 39, 147–165.

Goaillard, J.-M., and Marder, E. (2006). Dynamic clamp analyses of cardiac, endocrine, and neural function. *Physiology (Bethesda)* 21, 197–207.

Gottesman, I. I., and Gould T. D. (2003). The endophenotype concept in psychiatry: etymology and strategic intentions. *Am. J. Psychiatry* 160, 636–645.

Grech, R., Cassar, T., Muscat, J., Camilleri, K. P., Fabri, S. G., Zervakis, M., et al. (2008). Review on solving the inverse problem in EEG source analysis. *J. Neuroeng. Rehabil.* 5:25. doi: 10.1186/1743-0003-5-25

Grissom, R. J. (1994). Probability of the superior outcome of one treatment over another. *J. Appl. Psychol.* 79, 314–316.

Grissom, R. J., and Kim, J. J. (2012). *Effect Sizes for Research: Univariate and Multivariate Applications.* 2nd Edn. New York, NY: Routledge.

Harris, F. J. (1978). On the use of windows for harmonic analysis with the discrete Fourier transform. *Proc. IEEE* 66, 51–83.

Herrmann, C. S. (2001). Human EEG responses to 1-100 Hz flicker: resonance phenomena in visual cortex and their potential correlation to cognitive phenomena. *Exp. Brain Res.* 137, 346–353.

Jasper, H. H. (1958). The ten-twenty electrode system of the International

Federation. *Electroencephalogr. Clin. Neurophysiol.* 10, 370–375.

Jin, Y., O'Halloran, J. P., Plon, L., Sandman, C. A., and Potkin, S. G. (2006). Alpha EEG predicts visual reaction time. *Int. J. Neurosci.* 116, 1035–1044.

Kaufmann, T., Vögele, C., Sütterlin, S., Lukito, S., and Kübler, A. (2011). Effects of resting heart rate variability on performance in the P300 brain-computer interface. *Int. J. Psychophysiol.* 83, 336–341.

Khan, A., and Rayner, G. D. (2003). Robustness to non-normality of common tests for the many-sample location problem. *J. Appl. Math. Decis. Sci.* 7, 187–206.

Klimesch, W. (1997). EEG-alpha rhythms and memory processes. *Int. J. Psychophysiol.* 26, 319–340.

Koch, S. P., Koendgen, S., Bourayou, R., Steinbrink, J., and Obrig, H. (2008). Individual alpha-frequency correlates with amplitude of visual evoked potential and hemodynamic response. *Neuroimage* 41, 233–242.

Kondacs, A., and Szabó, M. (1999). Long-term intra-individual variability of the background EEG in normals. *Clin. Neurophysiol.* 110, 1708–1716.

Krauledat, M., Tangermann, M., Blankertz, B., and Müller, K.-R. (2008). Towards zero training for brain-computer interfacing. *PLoS ONE* 3:e2967. doi: 10.1371/journal.pone.0002967

Lopes da Silva, F. (1991). Neural mechanisms underlying brain waves: from neural membranes to networks. *Electroencephalogr. Clin. Neurophysiol.* 79, 81–93.

Lopez-Gordo, M. A., Prieto, A., Pelayo, F., and Morillas, C. (2011). Customized stimulation enhances performance of independent binary SSVEP-BCIs. *Clin. Neurophysiol.* 122, 128–133.

Marmont, G. (1949). Studies on the axon membrane; a new method. *J. Cell. Physiol.* 34, 351–382.

Mayer, J., Schuster, H. G., Claussen, J. C., and Mölle, M. (2007). Corticothalamic projections control synchronization in locally coupled bistable thalamic oscillators. *Phys. Rev. Lett.* 99, 068102.

Morgan, S. T., Hansen, J. C., and Hillyard, S. A. (1996). Selective attention to stimulus location modulates the steady-state visual evoked potential. *Proc. Natl. Acad. Sci. U.S.A.* 93, 4770–4774.

Muniz, C., Forlim, C. G., Guariento, R. T., Pinto, R., Rodriguez, F., and Varona, P. (2011). Online video tracking for activity-dependent stimulation in neuroethology. *BMC Neuroscience* 12:P358. doi: 10.1186/1471-2202-12-S1-P358

Muniz, C., Levi, R., Benkrid, M., Rodriguez, F. B., and Varona, P. (2008). Real-time control of stepper motors for mechano-sensory stimulation. *J. Neurosci. Methods* 172, 105–111.

Nicolas-Alonso, L. F., and Gomez-Gil, J. (2012). Brain computer interfaces, a review. *Sensors* 12, 1211–1279.

Posthuma, D., Neale, M. C., Boomsma, D. I., and De Geus, E. J. (2001). Are smarter brains running faster? Heritability of alpha peak frequency, IQ, and their interrelation. *Behav. Genet.* 31, 567–579.

Prinz, A. A., Abbott, L. F., and Marder, E. (2004). The dynamic clamp comes of age. *Trends Neurosci.* 27, 218.

Regan, D. (1989). *Human Electrophysiology: Evoked Potentials and Evoked Magnetic Fields in Science and Medicine*. New York, NY: Elsevier.

Robinson, H. P., and Kawai, N. (1993). Injection of digitally synthesized synaptic conductance transients to measure the integrative properties of neurons. *J. Neurosci. Methods* 49, 157.

Rodriguez, G., Copello, F., Vitali, P., Perego, G., and Nobili, F. (1999). EEG spectral profile to stage Alzheimer's disease. *Clin. Neurophysiol.* 110, 1831–1837.

Schaich, E., and Hamerle, A. (1984). *Verteilungsfreie Statistische Prüfverfahren*. Berlin: Springer.

Sharp, A. A., O'Neil, M. B., Abbott, L. F., and Marder, E. (1993). Dynamic clamp: computer-generated conductances in real neurons. *J. Neurophysiol.* 69, 992–995.

Steriade, M., Gloor, P., Llinás, R. R., Lopes de Silva, F. H., and Mesulam, M. M. (1990). Report of IFCN Committee on Basic Mechanisms. Basic mechanisms of cerebral rhythmic activities. *Electroencephalogr. Clin. Neurophysiol.* 76, 481–508.

Usakli, A. B., and Gurkan, S. (2010). Design of a novel efficient human-computer interface: an electrooculagram based virtual keyboard. *IEEE Trans. Instrum. Meas.* 59, 2099–2108.

Van den Heuvel, M. P., and Hulshoff-Pol, H. E. (2010). Exploring the brain network: a review on resting-state fMRI functional connectivity. *Eur. Neuropsychopharmacol.* 20, 519–534.

Van den Heuvel, M. P., Mandl, R. C. W., Kahn, R. S., and Hulshoff Pol, H. E. (2009). Functionally linked resting-state networks reflect the underlying structural connectivity architecture of the human brain. *Hum. Brain Mapp.* 30, 3127–3141.

Van Gerven, M., Farquhar, J., Schaefer, R., Vlek, R., Geuze, J., Nijholt, A., et al. (2009). The brain-computer interface cycle. *J. Neural Eng.* 6:41001. doi: 10.1088/1741-2560/6/4/041001

Vialatte, F.-B., Maurice, M., Dauwels, J., and Cichocki, A. (2010). Steady-state visually evoked potentials: focus on essential paradigms and future perspectives. *Prog. Neurobiol.* 90, 418–438.

Vidaurre, C., and Blankertz, B. (2010). Towards a cure for BCI illiteracy. *Brain Topogr.* 23, 194–198.

Volosyak, I., Cecotti, H., and Gräser, A. (2009). "Impact of frequency selection on LCD screens for SSVEP based brain-computer interfaces," in *Proceedings of the 4th International IEEE/EMBS Conference on Neural Engineering NER 09* (Antalya, Turkey), 706–713.

Volosyak, I., Valbuena, D., Luth, T., Malechka, T., and Gräser, A. (2011). BCI demographics II: how many (and what kinds of) people can use a high-frequency SSVEP BCI? *IEEE Trans. Neural Syst. Rehabil. Eng.* 19, 232–239.

Wu, Z., Lai, Y., Xia, Y., Wu, D., and Yao, D. (2008). Stimulator selection in SSVEP-based BCI. *Med. Eng. Phys.* 30, 1079–1088.

Yuan, H., Zotev, V., Phillips, R., Drevets, W. C., and Bodurka, J. (2012). Spatiotemporal dynamics of the brain at rest—exploring EEG microstates as electrophysiological signatures of BOLD resting state networks. *Neuroimage* 60, 2062–2072.

Zhu, D., Bieger, J., Garcia Molina, G., and Aarts, R. M. (2010). A survey of stimulation methods used in SSVEP-based BCIs. *Comput. Intell. Neurosci.* 2010:702357. doi: 10.1155/2010/702357

Zschocke, S., and Hansen, H.-C. (eds.). (2012). *Klinische Elektroenzephalographie*. Berlin/Heidelberg: Springer.

16

Developing an EEG-based on-line closed-loop lapse detection and mitigation system

Yu-Te Wang[1,2], Kuan-Chih Huang[3], Chun-Shu Wei[2,4], Teng-Yi Huang[3], Li-Wei Ko[5], Chin-Teng Lin[3], Chung-Kuan Cheng[1,6] and Tzyy-Ping Jung[2,4,6]*

[1] Department of Computer Science and Engineering, Jacobs School of Engineering, University of California San Diego, La Jolla, CA, USA
[2] Swartz Center for Computational Neuroscience, Institute for Neural Computation, University of California San Diego, La Jolla, CA, USA
[3] Department of Electrical Engineering, National Chiao-Tung University, Hsinchu, Taiwan
[4] Department of Bioengineering, Jacobs School of Engineering, University of California San Diego, La Jolla, CA, USA
[5] Department of Biological Science and Technology, National Chiao-Tung University, Hsinchu, Taiwan
[6] Center for Advanced Neurological Engineering, Institute of Engineering in Medicine, University of California San Diego, La Jolla, CA, USA

Edited by:
Thorsten O. Zander, Technical
University of Berlin, Germany

Reviewed by:
Klas Ihme, German Aerospace
Center, Germany
Johanna Wagner, Graz University of
Technology, Austria

*Correspondence:
Tzyy-Ping Jung, Swartz Center for
Computational Neuroscience,
Institute for Neural Computation,
University of California San Diego,
La Jolla, CA 92092, USA
e-mail: jung@sccn.ucsd.edu

In America, 60% of adults reported that they have driven a motor vehicle while feeling drowsy, and at least 15–20% of fatal car accidents are fatigue-related. This study translates previous laboratory-oriented neurophysiological research to design, develop, and test an On-line Closed-loop Lapse Detection and Mitigation (OCLDM) System featuring a mobile wireless dry-sensor EEG headgear and a cell-phone based real-time EEG processing platform. Eleven subjects participated in an event-related lane-keeping task, in which they were instructed to manipulate a randomly deviated, fixed-speed cruising car on a 4-lane highway. This was simulated in a 1st person view with an 8-screen and 8-projector immersive virtual-reality environment. When the subjects experienced lapses or failed to respond to events during the experiment, auditory warning was delivered to rectify the performance decrements. However, the arousing auditory signals were not always effective. The EEG spectra exhibited statistically significant differences between effective and ineffective arousing signals, suggesting that EEG spectra could be used as a countermeasure of the efficacy of arousing signals. In this on-line pilot study, the proposed OCLDM System was able to continuously detect EEG signatures of fatigue, deliver arousing warning to subjects suffering momentary cognitive lapses, and assess the efficacy of the warning in near real-time to rectify cognitive lapses. The on-line testing results of the OCLDM System validated the efficacy of the arousing signals in improving subjects' response times to the subsequent lane-departure events. This study may lead to a practical on-line lapse detection and mitigation system in real-world environments.

Keywords: electroencephalogram (EEG), drowsiness, fatigue, driving, smartphone, cell-phone, brain computer interface (BCI)

INTRODUCTION

Fatigue-related performance decrements such as lapses in attention and slowed reaction time could lead to catastrophic incidents in occupations ranging from ship navigators to airplane pilots, railroad engineers, truck and auto drivers, and nuclear plant monitors. Fatigue (or drowsiness) "concerns the inability or disinclination to continue an activity, generally because the activity has been going on for too long," defined by European Transport Safety Council (Croo et al., 2001). Sixty percent of American adults reported that they have been driving a motor vehicle when feeling drowsy (National Sleep Foundation, 2005). Furthermore, studies have concluded that at least 15–20% of fatal car accidents are fatigue-related (The Royal Society for the Prevention of Accidents, 2001; Connor et al., 2002; National Highway Traffic Safety Administration, 2003). Therefore, an earlier detection of driving fatigue is a crucial issue for preventing catastrophic incidents.

In order to detect the driving fatigue, several approaches have been proposed in scientific literature. (1) Computer vision-based systems (Bergasa et al., 2006; D'Orazio et al., 2007; Golz et al., 2010). Bergasa et al. (2006) used a real-time image-acquisition system to monitor drivers' visual behaviors that revealed a drivers' alertness level. Six parameters: percentage of eye closure, eye closure duration, blink frequency, nodding frequency, face position, and fixed gaze were included in a fuzzy classifier for identifying a driver's vigilance level. D'Orazio et al. (2007) proposed a neural classifier to recognize the eye activities from images without being constrained to head rotation or partially occluded eyes. (2) Driving behavior counter-measurements (Lin et al., 2009, 2010a, 2013). Lin et al. (2009) performed an event-related, lane-keeping driving task in an immersive virtual-reality environment. Subjects were asked to steer the stimulated car back to the middle of the cruising lane once they perceived the randomized lane-departure events. The results showed that the reaction time (RT), defined as the time interval between the onset of the simulated car deviation and the user response, could be improved by providing arousing auditory warning to the subjects combating with fatigue.

A Brain Computer Interface (BCI) translates neural activities into control signals to provide a direct communication pathway between the human brain and an external device (Wolpaw et al., 2002). Broadly speaking, BCIs can be grouped into three categories: active, passive and reactive BCIs (Zander and Kothe, 2011). Electroencephalogram (EEG)-based passive BCIs measure brain electrical activities from the scalp and enrich a human–machine interaction with implicit information on the actual user state without conscious effort from the user (Lehne et al., 2009; Zander et al., 2009, 2010; Zander and Jatzev, 2012). Given appropriate signal-processing algorithms in the passive BCIs, meaningful information can be directly extracted from the EEGs. For instance, time-domain analysis such as averaging across different channels, moving average with a specific window length, standard deviation, linear correlation and so on are useful approaches to extract information from EEGs (Dong et al., 2011). In a frequency-domain analysis, the short-time Fourier transform (STFT) is often applied to the EEG data to estimate the power spectral density in distinct frequency bands, including delta (1–3 Hz), theta (4–7 Hz), alpha (8–13 Hz), beta (14–30 Hz), and gamma (31–50 Hz). Many studies have shown that the brain dynamics linked to fatigue and behavioral lapses can be assessed by EEG power spectra (Kecklund and Akerstedt, 1993; Makeig and Inlow, 1993; Jung and Makeig, 1995; Makeig and Jung, 1996; Jung et al., 1997; Lal and Craig, 2002; Campagne et al., 2004; Horne and Baulk, 2004; Debener et al., 2005; Peiris et al., 2006; Davidson et al., 2007; Eichele et al., 2010, 2008; Golz et al., 2010; Lin et al., 2010a), combinations of EEG band power (Jap et al., 2011), alpha spindle parameters (Simon et al., 2011) and autoregressive features (Rosipal et al., 2007). These studies provided solid evidence for the neurophysiological correlates of fatigue and behavioral lapses. In short, while the physical- and behavioral symptom-based methods indirectly measure drivers' cognitive states, the neurophysiology-based methods offer a more direct path to assess the brain dynamic linked to fatigue and behavioral lapses with a high temporal resolution.

Efforts have also been made to assist individuals in combating fatigue and/or preventing lapses in concentration. For instance, Dingus et al. (1997) and Spence and Driver (1998) proposed using warning signals to maintain drivers' attention. The types of warning signals could be auditory (Spence and Driver, 1998; Lin et al., 2009), visual (Liu, 2001), tactile (Ho et al., 2005) or mixed (Liu, 2001). Empirical results showed that auditory warning could reduce the number of lapses in sustained-attention tasks (Spence and Driver, 1998), and could help subjects to maintain driving performance (Lin et al., 2009). More recent studies demonstrated that arousing auditory signals presented to individuals experiencing momentarily behavioral lapses could not only agitate their behavioral responses but also change their EEG theta and alpha power in a sustained-attention driving task (Jung et al., 2010; Lin et al., 2010a, 2013). However, the studies also showed that sometimes subjects did not respond to the arousing signals, and more importantly the EEG activity of these non-responsive episodes showed little or no changes following the ineffective warning (Jung et al., 2010; Lin et al., 2010a, 2013). Lin et al. (2013)

later demonstrated the feasibility of using the post-warning EEG power spectra to predict the (in)efficacy of the arousing warning. A caveat of their studies was that the arousing warning was delivered to subjects after they behaviorally failed to respond to lane-departure events. In reality, the delivery of arousing warning could have been too late because the behavioral lapse might have led to catastrophic consequences. A truly EEG-based lapse monitoring system needs to continuously and non-invasively observe EEG dynamics to predict fatigue-related lapses, deliver arousing signal to arouse the user, and assess the efficacy of the arousing signal to trigger a repeated or secondary warning signal if necessary. Furthermore, all of the aforementioned studies were conducted with traditional bulky and tethered EEG systems and were performed in well-controlled laboratories. However, it is argued that there might be fundamentally dynamic differences between laboratory-based and naturalistic human behavior in the brain (McDowell et al., 2013). It thus remains unclear how well the current laboratory-oriented knowledge of EEG correlates of cognitive-state changes can be translated into the highly dynamic real world.

This study aims to extend previous studies to design, develop and test a truly On-line Closed-loop Lapse Detection and Mitigation (OCLDM) System that can continuously monitor EEG dynamics, predict fatigue-related lapses based on EEG signals, arouse the fatigued users by delivering arousing signals, and assess the efficacy of the arousing signal based on EEG spectra. This study hypothesized that (1) EEG spectral values would differ under different arousal states; (2) it is feasible to predict lapses based on the spectral changes in the spontaneous EEG; (3) arousing warning delivered to cognitively challenged subjects would mitigate cognitive lapse, and (4) the rectified performance would be accompanied by the changes in EEG power spectra. This study conducted an off-line experiment to explore the neurophysiological correlates of lapses, which tested the above-mentioned hypotheses and guided the development of a truly OCLDM system. The system was then validated by an on-line driving experiment. Furthermore, to be practical for routine use in a car or workplace by freely moving individuals, the EEG-based lapse monitoring system must be non-invasive, non-intrusive, lightweight, battery-powered, and easily to put on and take off (Lin et al., 2008a,b). This study thus also investigates the feasibility of using a practical, low-density, lightweight dry EEG headgear and a smartphone-based EEG-processing platform (Wang et al., 2012) to build a truly mobile and wireless OCLDM System for real-life applications.

MATERIALS AND METHODS
SUBJECTS

Eleven healthy and naive subjects (10 males and one female) with normal hearing and aged 20–28 years old participated in this study. All of them were free of neurological and psychological disorders. They were introduced how to manipulate the car and practiced ~10 min to get acquainted before the experiment started. None of them worked night shifts or traveled across multiple time zones in the previous 2 months. All participants were asked to read and sign the informed consent form before participating in the studies. After the experiments, subjects were asked to complete the questionnaire for assessing their cognitive states during the experiments.

EXPERIMENTAL EQUIPMENT

Experiments of this study were conducted in an 8-screen and 8-projector immersive virtual-reality (VR) environment that simulates the 1st person view scene of highway driving. This study adapted an event-related lane-departure driving paradigm originally proposed by Huang et al. (2006, 2007a,b, 2009) that allowed objective and quantitative measures of momentary event-related brain dynamics following lane-departure events and driving-performance fluctuations over longer periods. The VR scenes simulated driving at a constant speed (at ~100 km/h) on a highway with the simulated car randomly drifting away from the center of the cruising lane to simulate driving on non-ideal road surfaces or with poor alignment (Huang et al., 2007a,b, 2009; Lin et al., 2008b, 2009). The scene was updated according to the land-departure events and the subject's manipulation. The vehicle trajectory, user's input, and lane-departure events could be accurately logged and time-synchronized to the EEG recordings (Huang et al., 2007a,b, 2009; Lin et al., 2008b). There were no

traffic or distractive objects other than 4-lane roads and dark sky appeared in the VR while the simulated car was cruising on the highway.

Thirty-two channel EEG data were collected from participants by the NuAmp system (32-channels Quick-Cap, Compumedics Ltd., VIC, Australia). The electrodes were placed according to a modified international 10–20 system with a unipolar reference at the right earlobe. The EEG activities were recorded with 500 Hz sampling rate and 16-bit quantization level.

EXPERIMENTAL PARADIGM

Figure 1A shows the experimental paradigm of this study. The simulated car starts cruising at a fixed speed (~100 km/h) on the 3rd lane and drifting to either right or left with equal probability within 8–10 s. Subjects were instructed to steer the simulated car back to the 3rd lane as soon as they noticed the lane drift. The simulated car keeps cruising on the right (or left) most lane if the subjects failed to respond to lane drift. The baseline period of each lane-departure epoch is defined as the 3 s before the onset of a lane-drifting event. The empty circle in **Figure 1A** represents the unexpected lane-departure events marked as the "deviation

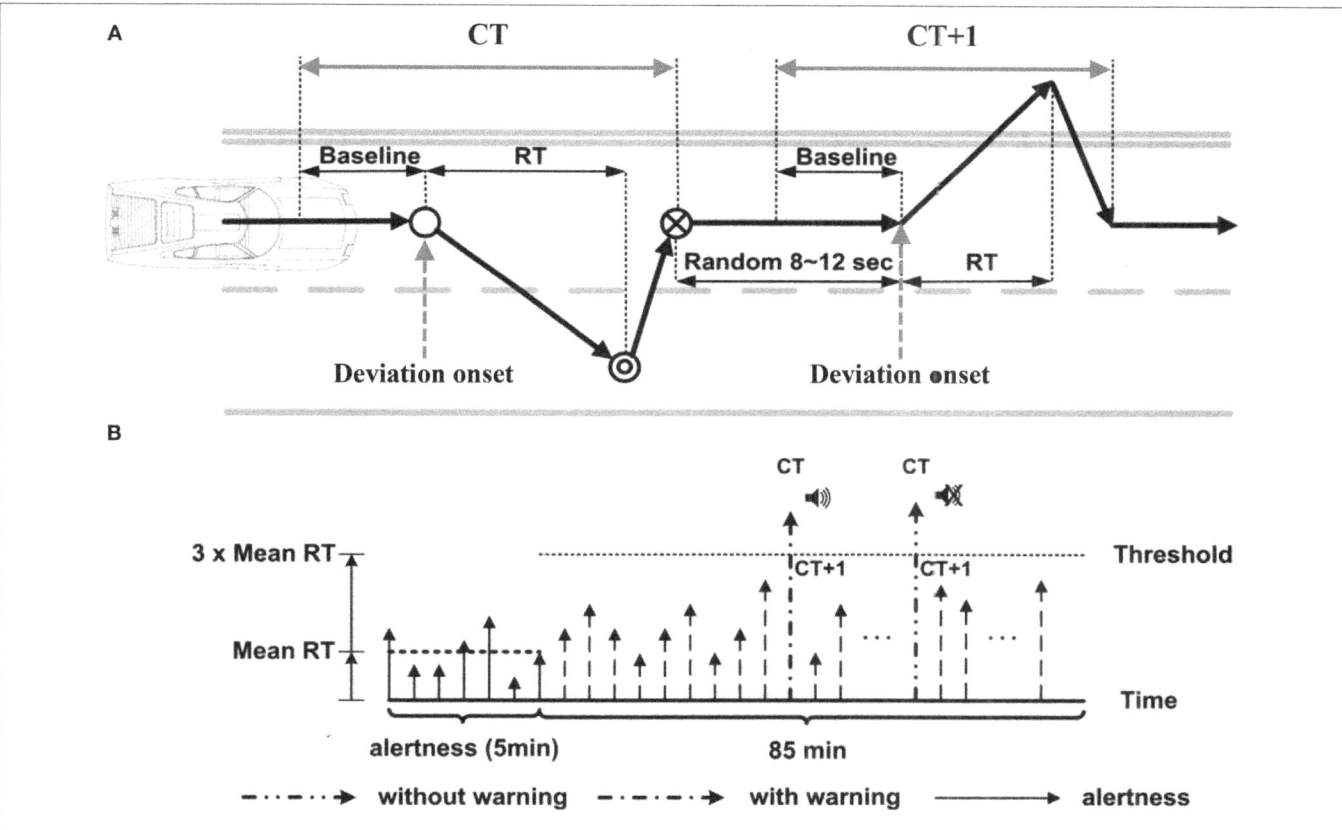

FIGURE 1 | Experiment paradigm. (A) Event-related lane-departure driving tasks. The solid arrows represent the driving trajectory. The empty circle represents the deviation onset. The double circle represents the response onset. The circle with the cross represents the response offset. The baseline is defined as the 3 s period prior to deviation onset. The response time (RT) of a driver is the interval from the deviation (empty circle) to the response onset (the double circle). A trial starts at deviation onset and ends at

response offset (circle with a cross). The next deviation begins 8–12 s after response offset. **(B)** Criterion for delivering auditory warning during driving tasks. The height of an arrow represents the response time in a single trial. The warning was delivered to the subject when the RT in the trial exceeded three times the mean RT of trials in the first 5 min of the task, when the subject was presumably alert and fully attended to lane-departure events. In this figure is adapted with permission from Figure 1 of Lin et al. (2010a).

onset." After the deviation onset, subjects were instructed to steer the simulated car back to the center of the cruising lane immediately (double circle), and the time when the subjects started steering was marked as the "response onset." The moment that the simulated car reached the center of the cruising lane (circle with cross) was marked as the "response offset." A subject's response time (RT) was defined as the time between the deviation onset and the response onset. At the first 5 min of the experiment, subjects were asked to be fully alert, verified by the vehicle trajectory and the video from a surveillance camera, to obtain an averaged alert RT (aRT) for each subject (1.51~2.54 s), which is a threshold for the entire experiment. The entire experiment consisted of 5 min training and 85 min driving periods.

Figure 1B shows the criterion of delivering auditory warnings in the experiment. When a subject failed to respond within three times the aRT, the system treated the trials as a behavioral lapse and triggered a 1750 Hz tone-burst to arouse the subject from fatigue-related lapse in half (50%) of these drowsy trials (marked as the "current trial (CT)" in **Figure 1A**). The very next trial is defined as CT + 1, and so on. The lapse trials that were randomly selected to receive arousing warning were referred to as CT with warning, whereas the remaining half of trials that did not receive auditory warning were referred to as CT without warning. Note that our previous studies showed that in some trials subjects remained non-responsive following the arousing warning, which was analogous to sleeping through an alarm clock (Jung et al., 2010; Lin et al., 2013). If the RT of the following trial (CT + 1) was shorter than the double of the averaged aRT, the warning signal delivered in the CT trial was defined as an "effective warning." On the other hand, if the RT of the CT + 1 trial was longer than triple of the averaged aRT, the warning was defined as an "ineffective warning." This study did not include the trials with RTs between 2 and 3 aRT to define the alert vs. fatigue spectral thresholds because the cognitive states of the subjects during those trials were unclear. Note that, subjects didn't know about the warning before the experiments.

DATA ANALYSIS

The 32-channel EEG data were first down-sampled to 250 Hz, and a low-pass filter of 50 Hz and a high-pass filter of 0.5 Hz were applied. Channels or trials with severe artifacts (such as body movements or muscle activities) were manually removed (less than three channels and 20% trials per subject in general). The remaining EEG data were segmented into several 115 s trials, each of them consisting of 15 s before and 100 s after the lane-deviation onsets. Independent Component Analysis (ICA, Bell and Sejnowski, 1995; Makeig et al., 1997) implemented in EEGLAB (Delorme and Makeig, 2004) was then applied to decompose the ~32-channel EEG into ~32 independent components (ICs), based on the assumption that the collected EEG data from the scalp were a weighted linear mixture of electrical potentials projected instantaneously from temporally ICs accounting for distinct brain sources. The comparable ICs across subjects were grouped into component clusters based on their scalp maps, equivalent dipole locations and baseline power spectra of component activations (Jung et al., 2001; Delorme and Makeig, 2004). Across 11 subjects, there were 155 trials with warning (30 trials

were ineffective and 125 trials were effective) and 192 trials without warning.

Since the RT and EEG power were not normally distributed, non-parametric statistic tests were performed for the data analysis (Delorme and Makeig, 2004). The Wilcoxon rank-sum test (Matlab statistical toolbox, Mathworks) was used to assess the effects of warning on RTs. Bootstrapping (EEGLAB toolbox, University of California, San Diego) was used to test the statistical significance of EEG power changes at specific frequency bins from 2 to 30 Hz with a 0.25 Hz resolution. To test group statistics, the intrinsic inter-subject RT differences were reduced by dividing RTs by the mean RT. The EEG spectra were normalized by dividing the spectral power by the standard deviation of the spectral distribution.

RESULTS: NEUROPHYSIOLOGICAL CORRELATES OF BEHAVIORAL LAPSES

EFFICACY OF AROUSING AUDITORY SIGNALS FOR RECTIFYING LAPSES

This study first explored the efficacy of the delivery of arousing auditory signals by measuring the change in subjects' reaction time. **Figure 2A** shows the boxplots of RTs of three trial groups:

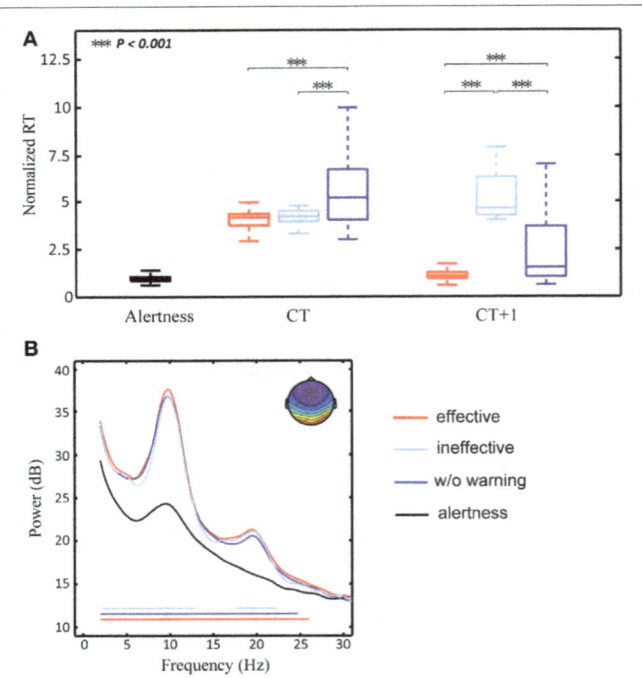

FIGURE 2 | Experiment results. (A) The boxplot for the RT distribution of trials with effective warning, ineffective warning, and without warning among CTs and CTs + 1. Note that middle horizontal line is the median of the distribution, and the top and bottom of the rectangle are the third and first quartile, and the dash line ends are the maximum and minimum after outlier removal. **(B)** The component spectra of the alert CTs (black curve), with an effective warning (red curve), with an ineffective warning (light blue curve) and without warning (dark blue curve). The red, light blue and blue horizontal lines mark the spectral differences between the alert trials and trials with an effective warning, with an ineffective warning, and without warning, respectively. All the spectral plots were calculated from the activity of the bilateral occipital components separated by ICA.

Alertness, CT, and CT + 1 (left to right). The averaged aRT of trials within the Alertness group across 11 subjects was ~676 ms. The RTs of the CT group with arousing warning (red and light blue) were statistically significantly shorter than those of trials without receiving arousing warning (dark blue). The RTs of the CT + 1 group with effective vs. ineffective warning differed while the RTs of the preceding group (CT) were comparable. Even though the subjects responded to the arousing warning by immediately steering the simulated car back to the cruising position, they could well be totally non-responsive to the very next lane-departure event (~10 s later). In other words, the arousing signals reliably rectified human behavioral lapses, but did not guarantee that subjects were fully awake, alert, or attentive. This suggests an analogous regime of snooze after an alarm is turned off.

EEG DYNAMICS PRECEDING BEHAVIORAL LAPSES

Figure 2B shows the mean scalp map of the bilateral occipital cluster (upper-right corner) and its component baseline power of drowsy trials without auditory warning (dark blue), with either effective (red) or ineffective warning (light blue). First, among the resultant ICA clusters, bilateral occipital components exhibited statistically significant spectral differences between trials with and without auditory warning. Second, the component power spectra exhibited tonic increases in theta (4–7 Hz), alpha (8–12 Hz), and beta (13–30 Hz) bands in drowsy trials (red, dark blue, and light blue), compared to the alert trials (black). Horizontal lines mark the frequency bins under which the spectral differences between alert trials and drowsy trials with either (in)effective warning, or without warning were statistically significant (alpha = 0.05, Bonferroni adjusted p-value of 0.05/(112 frequency bins) = 0.0004 for multiple comparisons). Note that

the spectra shown here were calculated from the component activities prior to the lane-deviation onset. The nearly identical pre-lapse spectra of these three groups of non-responsive trials demonstrate the robustness of the broadband spectral augmentation preceding the behavioral lapses, suggesting the feasibility of using theta and alpha power from the lateral occipital areas to predict behavioral lapses in this sustained-attention driving task.

EFFECTS OF AROUSING AUDITORY SIGNALS ON THE EEG

Next, this study explored temporal spectral dynamics preceding, during, and following fatigue-related behavioral lapses and following arousing warning. **Figure 3** shows time courses of spectral changes in the bilateral occipital area following ineffective warning (light blue trace), effective warning (red trace), and without warning (dark blue trace), compared to those of the alert trials (black trace). **Figure 3** shows that both theta- an alpha-band power steadily increased prior to the lane-departure onset (at time 0 s). Again, the trends of steady increasing theta- and alpha-band power leading to behavioral lapses in the three groups of drowsy trials were nearly identical, indicating the robustness of the theta and alpha augmentation preceding the behavioral lapses.

Figure 3 also shows that after the lane-departure onset (at time 0 s), the alpha (top panel), and theta (bottom panel) power abruptly decreased by over 10 and 5 dB to nearly the alert (black trace) baseline, respectively. More importantly, following the subjects' responses, the spectra of trials with ineffective warning (light blue trace) and without warning (dark blue trace) rapidly rose from the alert baseline to the drowsy level in 5–15 s. The theta and alpha power of trials with effective warning, however, remained low for ~40 s. The green horizontal lines mark the time points when the difference between the spectra of trials with

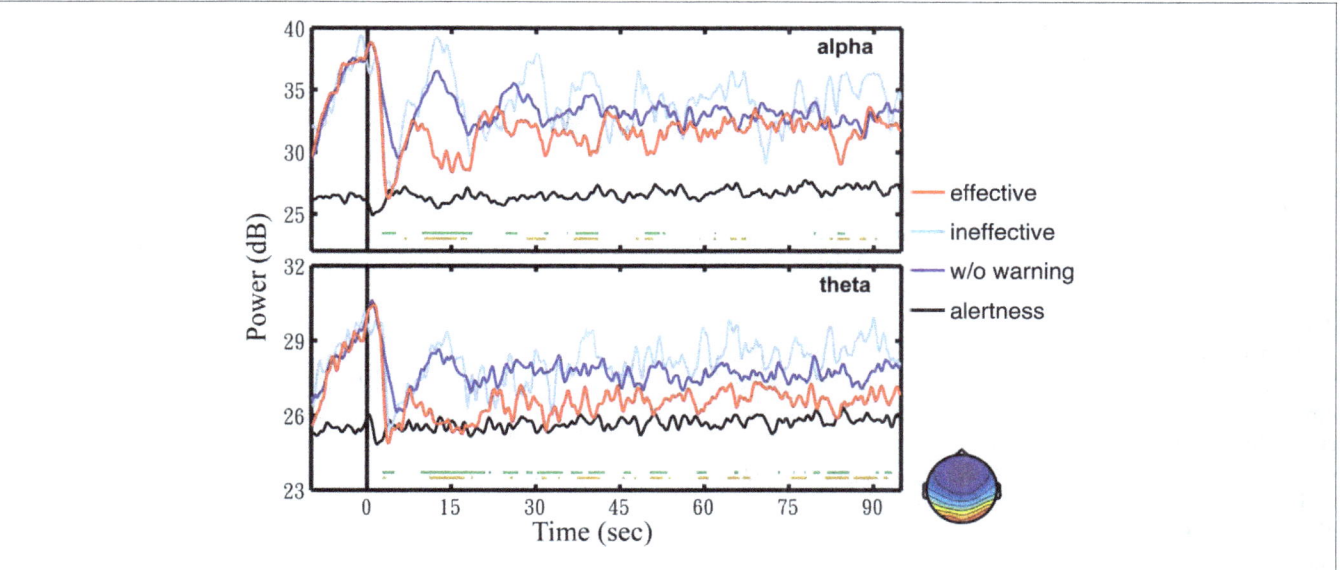

FIGURE 3 | Average component EEG power changes in alpha (top panel) and theta (bottom panel) bands from the bilateral occipital components (lower right corner). All the trials are aligned to the lane-deviation onsets at time 0 s (vertical solid black line). The red, light blue, dark blue, and black traces are the averaged spectra of trials with effective feedback, with ineffective feedback, without feedback, and in alertness, respectively. The green horizontal line indicates the statistically significant differences ($p < 0.01$) between trials with effective feedback and without feedback. The brown indicates the statistically significant differences ($p < 0.01$) between trials with effective feedback and ineffective feedback.

effective warning and without warning were statistically significant ($p < 0.01$). The spectral difference between the trials with effective warning and without warning was significant from 7 to 18 s in alpha band and from 7 to 21 s in the theta band ($p < 0.01$). Furthermore, the spectral difference between the trials with effective and ineffective warning was significant from 7 to 16 s in both alpha and theta bands (brown horizontal lines).

In sum, these results provided invaluable insights into the optimal electrode locations (lateral occipital region) and EEG features (theta- and alpha-band power) for a practical OCLDM system detailed below. The EEG and behavioral data collected from this experiment were used to assess the EEG correlates of fatigue-related lapses and build a lapse prediction model for the second experiment.

DEVELOPING A OCLDM SYSTEM

Our previous study (Wang et al., 2012) proposed a cell-phone based drowsiness monitoring and management system to continuously and wirelessly monitor brain dynamics using a lightweight, portable, and low-density EEG acquisition headgear. The system was designed to assess brain activities over the forehead, detect drowsiness, and deliver arousing warning to users experiencing momentary cognitive lapses, and assess the efficacy of the warning in near real-time. However, the system was not fully implemented nor experimentally validated in humans. Furthermore, according to the neurophysiological results in section Results: Neurophysiological Correlates of Behavioral Lapses, EEG signals collected over the lateral occipital regions were more informative for lapse detection. This study extends the previous work to design, develop, and test an OCLDM System.

SYSTEM ARCHITECTURE

Figure 4A shows the system diagram of the proposed OCLDM System. The system consists of two major components: (1) a mobile platform featuring the OCLDM algorithm, and (2) a mobile and wireless 4-channel headgear measuring EEG signals over the hair-bearing occipital regions with dry EEG sensors (Liao et al., 2011). The OCLDM System was implemented as an App on an Android-based platform (e.g., Samsung Galaxy S3). The smartphone has a Bluetooth module, 16 GB RAM, an ARM Cortex-A9 processor, Android (Ice Cream Sandwich) OS, and other components. When the App is launched, it can automatically search and connect to a nearby EEG headgear to receive data from the EEG acquisition headgear. In the mean time, the App opened an USB port to receive the events from a four-lane highway scene to synchronize the EEG data and scene events. The build-in speaker (or plug-in a ear set) of the smartphone delivers auditory warning signal once the OCLDM System detects that the subject is experiencing a cognitive lapse. Both the EEG data and scene-generated events could be logged onto either smartphone's build-in memory or an external microSD card for further analysis.

The mobile and wireless EEG acquisition headgear features a 4-channel lightweight portable bio-signal acquisition device powered by a 3.7 v Li-ion battery (Lin et al., 2010b). It consists of a TI MSP430 microprocessor, a pre-amplifier, a battery-charging circuit, a 24 bit ADC, a Bluetooth module, and dry spring-loaded

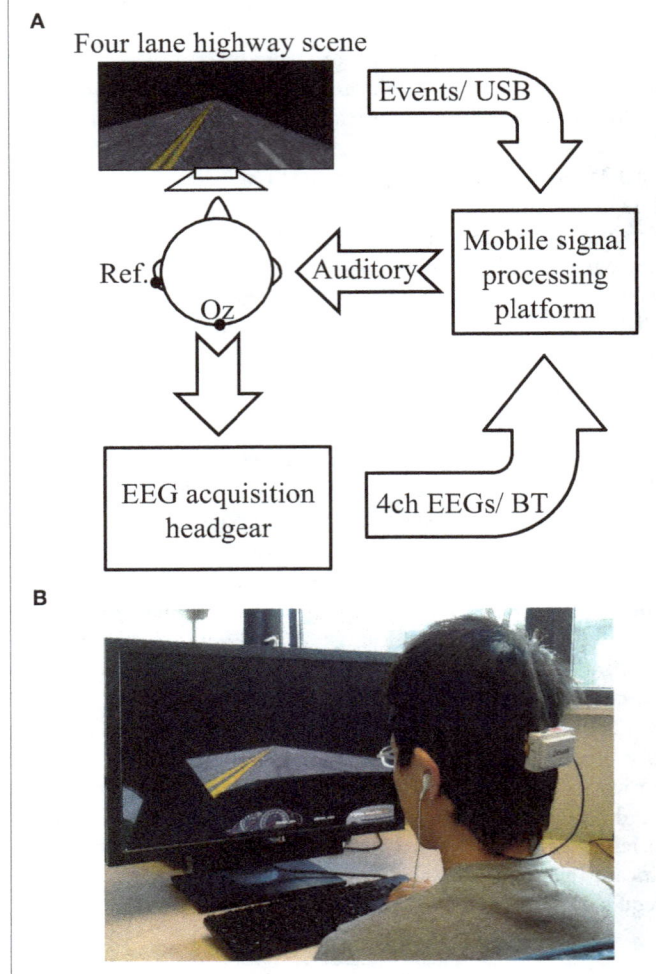

FIGURE 4 | The system diagram of the proposed OCLDM System. (A) The EEG headgear collected 4-channel brain activities from the lateral occipital area while a subject was performing the lane-drifting experiment. The mobile signal-processing platform received the acquired EEG raw data through Bluetooth, and the event markers generated from the lane-departure scene through an USB interface. Finally, the auditory feedback was delivered to the subject when the averaged EEG power across four channels was 3 dB over the alert baseline. **(B)** A photo of a subject performing the on-line driving experiment while wearing a 4-channel EEG headgear (the white small box attached on a flexible band) over the lateral occipital area.

EEG sensors (Liao et al., 2011). The spring-loaded probes of the sensor can penetrate the hair to provide good electrical conductivity with the scalp. The microprocessor controls all the components including the amplifiers, digitizers, and transmits the digitalized EEG data to the Bluetooth module. The 4-channel EEG data are then transmitted to the authorized receiver of the OCLDM System. Depending on the applications, the system's sampling rate can be programmed at 128, 256, or 512 Hz. An experienced subject can easily put on this EEG acquisition device within 1–3 min without any help from a technician. **Figure 4B** shows a photo of a subject wearing a 4-channel EEG headgear and performing the simulated driving experiment.

SYSTEM SOFTWARE DESIGN

Figure 5 shows the program's state diagram of the proposed OCLDM System. Three major states, including Baseline Collecting (BC), Driving Performance Monitoring (DPM), and Warning Efficacy Assessment (WEA), were implemented in the program. When the program is launched, one can modify the parameters in the SETTING page, shown as a square box in the figure. For instance, the parameters can be the duration of baseline data collection, or the threshold of auditory warning delivering for the other two states. Depending on the applications, the lapse threshold in the DPM state can be calculated accordingly. For example, one can use a combination of power of alpha, beta, theta, and delta bands to detect cognitive lapse. The program then enters the next (DPM) state after the Baseline (calibration) data collection has completed. The DPM module continuously monitors the driver's neurophysiological data. The program stays in the DPM state until the lapse threshold is met, which depends on the neurophysiological results as shown in section Results: Neurophysiological Correlates of Behavioral Lapses. For instance, when the subject's power spectrum in alpha band is 3 dB higher than the threshold (alert baseline collected in the BC state), the program delivers an auditory warning to arouse the subject and enters the FEA state. The current value is stored as the lapse reference in the FEA module. The system repeatedly delivers auditory warning until the EEG power decreases to another threshold.

ON-LINE EXPERIMENTAL PARADIGM

Three new male subjects (who did not participated in the first experiment) with normal hearing and aged 25–30 years old participated in the on-line closed-loop lane-departure driving experiments to evaluate the OCLDM System in a more naturalistic setting (in a regular office without any electromagnetic shielding). All of them were asked to read and sign the informed consent form before participating in the studies.

The entire experiment consisted of a 1 min training and a ~60 min driving periods. During the training session, subjects were asked to stay fully alert. The averaged alpha power collected in the BC session was used as an alert baseline to determine whether a subject is experiencing cognitive lapses in the driving task. The subject performed the lane-departure driving experiments following the protocol below:

(1) Subjects seated in an armchair and the driving scene was displayed on a 27″ monitor, placed at ~60 cm in front of the subject.
(2) Subjects used a keyboard to control a vehicle cruising on a high way, i.e., a left key turns the simulated car to the left while a right key turns to the right.
(3) Four electrodes were placed over the lateral occipital area to collect EEG data non-invasively. The data were transmitted to a smartphone for processing via Bluetooth.
(4) When the averaged power spectra in alpha band met a certain criterion, arousing auditory warning (~65 dB 1750 Hz tone-burst) would be delivered in half of these lapse episodes through an ear set to the subjects. Note that, the subjects didn't know the warning before the experiments.
(5) The arousing tone-burst would be continuously delivered to the subjects until the averaged power spectra in the alpha band has dropped 3 dB from the lapse power.

The cognitive lapses were detected when the subject's alpha-band power (Jung et al., 2010; Lin et al., 2010a, 2013), calculated by a moving-averaged STFT with a 256-point sliding window advanced at 1 s step running on the smartphone, was 3 dB over the alert baseline power (Lin et al., 2010a, 2013 and Results in section Results: Neurophysiological Correlates of Behavioral Lapses). This study used the alpha power fluctuations to monitor cognitive lapses because (1) a recent study showed that the alpha augmentation was sensitive to the transition from full alertness to mediate drowsiness, while the theta augmentation was more sensitive to the transition from mediate to deep drowsiness (Chuang et al., 2012); (2) the empirical results of this study showed that the augmentation of alpha-band power changes was greater than that of the theta-band power (**Figure 2**). The system would repeatedly deliver auditory warning until the alpha-band power amplitude has dropped to 3 dB below the power level when the cognitive lapse was identified.

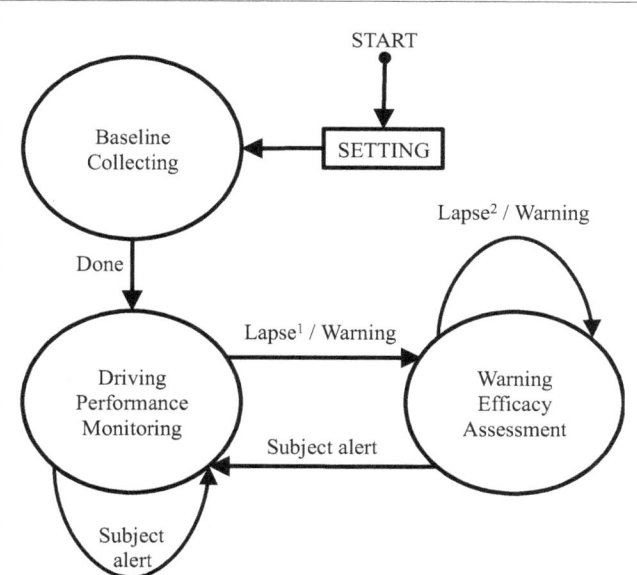

FIGURE 5 | The software state diagram of the OCLDM System. The program first goes through SETTING and Baseline collecting state. Then, the system continuously detects and monitors subjects' driving performance until the EEG spectra indicate cognitive lapse. Note that, Lapse[1] represents the averaged EEG power across four channels is 3 dB over the alert baseline. Lapse[2] represents that the averaged EEG power across four channels has not yet dropped 3 dB from the lapse power.

RESULTS FROM THE OCLDM SYSTEM

The numbers of detected cognitive lapses varied across subjects. **Table 1** lists the numbers of trials with effective, ineffective warning and without warning, respectively. Here, the way we defined the effective trials was based on the RT in response to the lane-departure event immediately following the arousing signal (CT + 1 whose RT was shorter than two times aRT); while the ineffective trials had RT longer than three times aRT.

Table 1 | Number of trials collected from the on-line experiment.

	With auditory warning		Without auditory warning
	Effective	**Ineffective**	
Subject 1	20	2	21
Subject 2	17	1	24
Subject 3	23	0	27

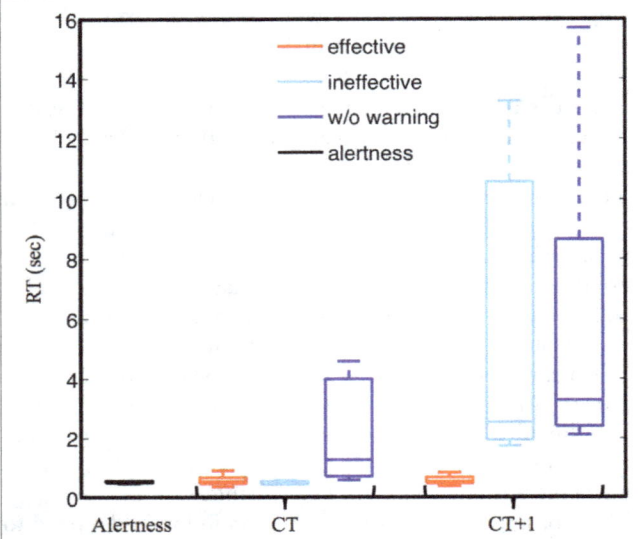

FIGURE 6 | The behavioral performance comparison for the trials of with effective feedback (red), with ineffective feedback (light blue), and without feedback (blue), compared to alert trials (black) after removing the outliers.

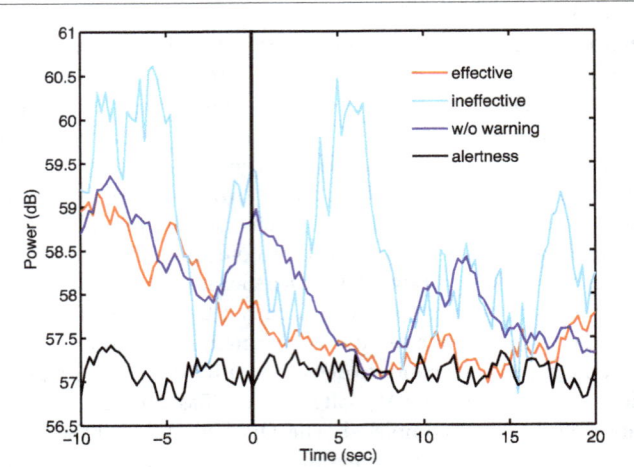

FIGURE 7 | The averaged alpha power time course plotting time-locked to subject response onset (vertical solid line at time 0 s). Averaged alpha power of trials with effective feedback (red trace), with ineffective feedback (light blue), and without feedback (blue trace), compared to trial with aRT (black). The time course of power was estimated by short time Fourier transform with 256 points of time window and 224 points overlapping.

Figure 6 shows the boxplot of behavioral performance (RTs) of trials with effective trials (red), ineffective trials (light blue), and without warning (dark blue), compared to the averaged aRT (black) during the on-line experiments. The effective trials had RTs comparable to the averaged aRT (less than 1 s) in both CT and CT + 1. Note that the RTs of CT + 1 with effective vs. ineffective warning differed largely because that was how the effective and ineffective trials were defined. However, the RTs of CT trials (red and light blue) of these two groups of trials were very comparable. That is, even though the subjects responded to the arousing warning by steering the simulated car immediately back to the cruising position, they could well be totally non-responsive to the very next lane-departure event. This finding is consistent to our off-line study reported in section Results: Neurophysiological Correlates of Behavioral Lapses in which the arousing warning was delivered to the subjects who just had a behavioral lapse.

Figure 7 showed the averaged alpha-band spectral time courses across subjects and trials with effective warning (red trace), with ineffective warning (light blue trace), and without warning (dark blue trace), compared to averaged aRT (black trace). All spectral time courses were aligned to the user response onset (thick vertical black line at time 0 s), and the auditory warning for effective- and ineffective-trials were delivered ∼5 s before

the user response. In the trials following effective auditory warning, the alpha power decreased steadily and reached the averaged aRT in ∼7 s. The power spectra remained as low as that of the alert baseline from 7 to 20 s after response onset. In the trials with ineffective auditory warning, the spectral time series fluctuated fiercely due to the small number of trials. In the trials without warning, the alpha power fluctuated before response onset and steadily dereased until ∼7 s. Thereafter, the alpha power increased again from ∼7 to 13 s, suggesting the subjects might be partially arouse by the lane-departure event and their own bebavioral reposense temportally but returned to the fatigue state rapidly thereafter.

DISCUSSIONS

Many studies have shown that the brain dynamics correlated with behavioral lapses can be assessed from EEG data. Recent studies have also shown auditory signals can arouse drowsy subjects and affect EEG activities (Lin et al., 2010a, 2013). However, in these studies, the arousing warning was delivered to subjects after they displayed behavioral lapses, which in reality may be too late because the behavioral lapse might have already had catastrophic consequences. Therefore, a system that features real-time lapse detection and delivers warnings to the drowsy subjects is desirable in preventing catastrophic incidents while driving.

The first experiment of this study showed that EEG power changes in either alpha or theta band can be used as an indicator for assessing the subjects' fatigue (cf. **Figure 3**), and auditory warning temporarily reduces the alpha and theta band power and mitigates the behavioral lapses (cf. **Figure 2A**). In addition, EEG changes after delivery of auditory warning are a good indicator of the efficacy of arousing warning. More importantly and interestingly, empirical results of the first study showed that arousing auditory signals could always reliably mitigate human behavioral lapses, but these immediate behavioral responses could not guarantee the subjects were fully awake, alert, or attentive, similar to snooze after an alarm is turned off. This finding may open a new research direction of how to accurately confirm a subject's cognitive level for some sustained-attention tasks, such as an aircraft navigator or a long-haul truck driver. In other words, further studies to explore the brain changes in this sleep inertia period may provide valuable insights of brain dynamics during a transitional state of lowered arousal occurring immediately after awakening from sleep. Based on previous studies (Lin et al., 2010a, 2013) and the results of the first experiment, this study further developed a truly OCLDM system to detect/predict cognitive lapse based on the EEG spectra, deliver arousing warning on the occurrence of cognitive lapse, and assess the efficacy of the arousing warning, again, based on the EEG spectra. Most importantly, the EEG spectra changes within ~10 s after delivering arousing warning were closely monitored, such that any false-awake situations could be decreased. This study then documented the design, development, and on-line evaluation of the proposed OCLDM System that featured a lightweight wireless EEG acquisition headgear and a smartphone-based signal-processing platform. Experimental results showed that subjects' EEG power could almost remain at the alert state without bouncing back to the drowsy level (cf. **Figure 7**). These results suggest that the proposed system could prevent potential behavioral lapses based solely on the EEG signals, and this demonstration could lead to a real-life application of the dry and wireless EEG technology and smartphone-based signal-processing platform. An interesting question is if the neural correlates of fatigue could be generalized across different sustained-attention tasks and different recording conditions. In the past few years, we have conducted several sustained-attention tasks, including auditory target detection tasks (Makeig and Jung, 1995, 1996; Jung et al., 1997), visual compensatory tracking tasks (Huang et al., 2008),

and simulated driving tasks (Lin et al., 2005, 2006, 2008b) and found that performance-related EEG dynamics were comparable across tasks (Huang et al., 2007b). Results of these studies also showed the fatigue-related brain dynamics were quite consistent across different recording environments (within a well-controlled EEG laboratory vs. a 6-degree-of-freedom motion platform) and responding methods (using a button press or a steering wheel). Therefore, it is reasonable to believe the methods developed under this study could be translated from laboratory settings to real-world environments.

In sum, this study demonstrated the feasibility of translating a laboratory-based passive BCI system to a neuroergonomic device that is capable of continuously monitoring and mitigating operator neurocognitive fatigue using a pervasive smartphone in real-world environments. The passive BCI technologies might also be applicable to other real-world cognitive-state monitoring, such as attention, distraction, comprehension, confusion, and emotion. We thus believe more real-world passive BCI implementations will emerge in the foreseeable future.

ACKNOWLEDGMENT

This work was supported in part by US Office of Naval Research, Army Research Office (W911NF-09-1-0510), Army Research Laboratory (W911NF-10-2-0022), and DARPA (DARPA/USDI D11PC20183). This work was also supported in part by the UST-UCSD International Center of Excellence in Advanced Bioengineering sponsored by the Taiwan National Science Council I-RiCE Program under Grant Number: NSC-102-2911-I-009-101, and the Aiming for the Top University Plan of National Chiao Tung University sponsored by the Ministry of Education of Taiwan, under Grant Number 103W963. The authors also appreciate Melody Jung's editorial assistance.

REFERENCES

Bell, A. J., and Sejnowski, T. J. (1995). An information-maximization approach to blind separation and blind deconvolution. *Neural Comput.* 7, 1129–1159. doi: 10.1162/neco.1995.7.6.1129

Bergasa, L. M., Nuevo, J., Sotelo, M. A., Barea, R., and Lopez, M. E. (2006). Real-time system for monitoring driver vigilance. *IEEE Trans. Intell. Transport. Syst.* 7, 63–67. doi: 10.1109/TITS.2006.869598

Campagne, A., Pebayle, T., and Muzet, A. (2004). Correlation between driving errors and vigilance level: influence of the driver's age. *Physiol. Behav.* 80, 515–524. doi: 10.1016/j.physbeh.2003.10.004

Chuang, C.-H., Huang, C.-S., Lin, C.-T., Ko, L.-W., Chang, J.-Y., and Yang, J.-M. (2012). "Mapping information flow of independent source to predict conscious level: a granger causality based

brain-computer interface," in *International Symposium on Computer, Consumer and Control (IS3C)* (Taichung: IEEE), 813–816. doi: 10.1109/IS3C.2012.209

Connor, J., Norton, R., Ameratunga, S., Robinson, E., Civil, I., and Dunn, R. (2002). Driver sleepiness and risk of serious injury to car occupants: population based case control study. *BMJ* 324:1125. doi: 10.1136/bmj.324. 7346.1125

Croo, H. D., Bandmann, M., Mackay, G. M., Rumar, K., and Vollenhoven, P. V. (2001). *The Role of Driver Fatigue in Commercial Road Transport Crashes.* Etterbeek: European Transport Safety Council.

Davidson, P. R., Jones, R. D., Peiris, M., and Davidson, T. R. (2007). EEG-based lapse detection with high temporal resolution. *IEEE Trans. Biomed. Eng.* 54, 832–839. doi: 10.1109/TBME.2007.893452

Debener, S., Ullsperger, M., Siegel,

M., Fiehler, K., Von Cramon, D. Y., and Engel, A. K. (2005). Trial-by-trial coupling of concurrent EEG and fMRI identifies the dynamics of performance monitoring. *J. Neurosci.* 25, 11730–11737. doi: 10.1523/JNEUROSCI.3286-05.2005

Delorme, A., and Makeig, S. (2004). EEGLAB: an open source toolbox for analysis of single-trial EEG dynamics including independent component analysis. *J. Neurosci. Methods* 134, 9–21. doi: 10.1016/j.jneumeth.2003.10.009

Dingus, T. A., McGehee, D. V., Manakkal, N., Jahns, S. K., Carney, C., and Hankey, J. M. (1997). Human factors field evaluation of automotive headway maintenance/collision warning devices. *Hum. Factors* 39, 216–229. doi: 10.1518/001872097778543930

Dong, Y., Hu, Z., Uchimura, K., and Murayama, N. (2011). "Driver inattention monitoring system

for intelligent vehicles: a review," in *2009 IEEE Intelligent Vehicles Symposium* (Xi'an), 875–880.

D'Orazio, T., Leo, M., Guaragnella, C., and Distante, A. (2007). A visual approach for driver inattention detection. *J. Pattern Recogn.* 40, 2341–2355. doi: 10.1016/j.patcog.2007.01.018

Eichele, H., Juvodden, H. T., Ullsperger, M., and Eichele, T. (2010). Mal-adaptation of event-related EEG responses preceding performance errors. *Front. Hum. Neurosci.* 4:65. doi: 10.3389/fnhum.2010.00065

Eichele, T., Debener, S., Calhoun, V. D., Specht, K., Engel, A. K., Hugdahl, K., et al. (2008). Prediction of human errors by maladaptive changes in event-related brain networks. *Proc. Natl. Acad. Sci. U.S.A.* 105, 6173–6178. doi: 10.1073/pnas.0708965105

Golz, M., Sommer, D., Trutschel, U., Sirois, B., and Edwards, D.

(2010). Evaluation of fatigue monitoring technologies. *Somnologie Schlafforschung und Schlafmedizin* 14, 187–199. doi: 10.1007/s11818-010-0482-9

Ho, C., Tang, H. Z., and Spence, C. (2005). Using spatial vibrotactile cues to direct visual attention in driving scenes. *Transp. Res. F Traffic Psychol. Behav.* 8, 397–412. doi: 10.1016/j.trf.2005.05.002

Horne, J. A., and Baulk, S. D. (2004). Awareness of sleepiness when driving. *Psychophysiology* 41, 161–165. doi: 10.1046/j.1469-8986.2003.00130.x

Huang, R.-S., Jung, T.-P., Delorme, A., and Makeig, S. (2008). Tonic and phasic electroencephalographic dynamics during continuous compensatory tracking. *Neuroimage* 39, 1896–1909. doi: 10.1016/j.neuroimage.2007.10.036

Huang, R.-S., Jung, T.-P., Delorme, A., and Makeig, S. (2009). "Tonic and pha-sic brain dynamics during responses to simulated driving challenges," in *15th Annual Meeting, Organization of Human Brain Mapping, NeuroImage 47, Supplement 1, S103* (San Francisco, CA).

Huang, R.-S., Jung, T.-P., Duann, J.-R., and Makeig, S. (2006). *Imaging Brain Dynamics during Continuous Driving using Independent Component Analysis, in Human Brain Mapping*. Florence: Wiley Periodicals Inc.

Huang, R.-S., Jung, T.-P., and Makeig, S. (2007a). "Multi-scale EEG brain dynamics during sustained attention tasks," in *Acoustics, Speech and Signal Processing, 2007, ICASSP 2007, IEEE International Conference* (Honolulu, HI), 1173–1176.

Huang, R.-S., Jung, T.-P., and Makeig, S. (2007b). "Event-related brain dynamics in continuous sustained-attention tasks," in *Foundations of Augmented Cognition*, eds D. Schmorrow and L. Reeves (Berlin; Heidelberg: Springer), 65–74.

Jap, B. T., Lal, S., and Fischer, P. (2011). Comparing combinations of EEG activity in train drivers during monotonous driving. *Expert Syst. Appl.* 38, 996–1003. doi: 10.1016/j.eswa.2010.07.109

Jung, T.-P., Huang, K.-C., Chuang, C.-H., Chen, J.-A., Ko, L.-W., Chiu, T.-W., et al. (2010). "Arousing feedback rectifies lapse in performance and corresponding EEG power spectrum," in *Engineering in Medicine and Biology Society (EMBC), 2010 Annual International Conference, IEEE)* (Buenos Aires), 1792–1795.

Jung, T.-P., and Makeig, S. (1995). "Prediction failures in auditory detection from changes

in the EEG spectrum," in *Proceeding of the 17th Annual International Conference of the IEEE Engineering in Medicine and Biology Society* (Montreal, QC), 927–928.

Jung, T.-P., Makeig, S., Stensmo, M., and Sejnowski, T. J. (1997). Estimating alert-ness from the EEG power spectrum. *IEEE Trans. Biomed. Eng.* 44, 60–69. doi: 10.1109/10.553713

Jung, T.-P., Makeig, S., Westerfield, M., Townsend, J., Courchesne, E., and Sejnowski, T. J. (2001). Analysis and visualization of single-trial event-related potentials. *Hum. Brain Mapp.* 14, 166–185. doi: 10.1002/hbm.1050

Kecklund, G., and Akerstedt, T. (1993). Sleepiness in long-distance truck driving: an ambulatory EEG study of night driving. *Ergonomics* 36, 1007–1017. doi: 10.1080/00140139308967973

Lal, S. K., and Craig, A. (2002). Driver fatigue: electroencephalogra-phy and psychological assessment. *Psychophysiology* 39, 313–321. doi: 10.1017/S0048577201393095

Lehne, M., Ihme, K., Brouwer, A. M., van Erp, J., and Zander, T. O. (2009). "Error-related EEG patterns during tactile human-machine interaction," in *Affective Computing and Intelligent Interaction and Workshops, 2009. ACII2009. 3rd International Conference* (Los Alamitos, CA), 1–9.

Liao, L.-D., Wang, I.-J., Chen, S.-F., Chang, J.-Y., and Lin, C.-T. (2011). Design, fabrication and experimental validation of a novel dry-contact sensor for mea-suring electroencephalography signals without skin preparation. *Sensors* 11, 5819–5834. doi: 10.3390/s110605819

Lin, C.-T., Chen, Y.-C., Huang, T.-Y., Chiu, T.-T., Ko, L.-W., Liang, S.-F., et al. (2008a). Development of wireless brain computer interface with embed-ded multitask scheduling and its application on real-time driver's drowsi-ness detection and warning. *IEEE Trans. Biomed. Eng.* 55, 1582–1591. doi: 10.1109/TBME.2008.918566

Lin, C.-T., Huang, K.-C., Chao, C.-F., Chen, J.-A., Chiu, T.-W., Ko, L.-W., et al. (2010a). Tonic and phasic EEG and behavioral changes induced by arousing feedback. *Neuroimage* 52, 633–642. doi: 10.1016/j.neuroimage.2010.04.250

Lin, C.-T., Huang, K.-C., Chao, C.-F., Chuang, C.-H., Ko, L.-W., and Jung, T.-P. (2013). Can Arousing

feedback rectify lapses in driving? Prediction from EEG power spectra. *J. Neural Eng.* 10:056024. doi: 10.1088/1741-2560/10/5/ 056024

Lin, C.-T., Huang, T.-Y., Liang, W.-C., Chiu, T.-T., Chao, C.-P., Hsu, S.-H., et al. (2009). Assessing effectiveness of various auditory warning signals in main-taining drivers' attention in virtual reality-based driving environments. *Percept. Mot. Skills* 108, 825–835. doi: 10.2466/pms.108.3.825-835

Lin, C.-T., Ko, L.-W., Chang, M.-H., Duann, J.-R., Chen, J.-Y., Su, T.-P., et al. (2010b). Review of wireless and wearable electroencephalogram systems and brain–computer interfaces—a mini-review. *Gerontology* 56, 112–119. doi: 10.1159/000230807

Lin, C.-T., Ko, L.-W., Chiou, J.-C., Duann, J.-R., Chiu, T.-W., Huang, R.-S., et al. (2008b). Noninvasive neural prosthesis using mobile and wireless EEG. *Proc. IEEE* 96, 1167–1183. doi: 10.1109/JPROC.2008.922561

Lin, C.-T., Ko, L.-W., Chung, I.-F., Huang, T.-Y., Chen, Y.-C., Jung, T.-P., et al. (2006). Adaptive EEG-based alertness estimation system by Using ICA-based fuzzy neural networks. *IEEE Trans. Circuits Syst. I* 53, 2469–2476. doi: 10.1109/TCSI.2006.884408

Lin, C.-T., Wu, R.-C., Liang, S.-F., Huang, T.-Y., Chao, W.-H., Chen, Y.-J., et al. (2005). EEG-based drowsiness estimation for safety driving using inde-pendent component analysis. *IEEE Trans. Circuits Syst.* 52, 2726–2738. doi: 10.1109/TCSI.2005.857555

Liu, Y.-C. (2001). Comparative study of the effects of auditory, visual and mul-timodality displays on drivers' performance in advanced traveller information systems. *Ergonomics* 44, 425–442. doi: 10.1080/00140130010011369

Makeig, S., and Inlow, M. (1993). Lapses in alertness: coherence of fluctuations in performance and EEG spectrum. *Electroencephalogr. Clin. Neurophysiol.* 86, 23–35. doi: 10.1016/0013-4694(93)90064-3

Makeig, S., and Jung, T.-P. (1995). Changes in alertness is principal component of variance in the EEG spectrum. *Neuroreport* 7, 213–216, doi: 10.1097/00001756-199512000-00051

Makeig, S., and Jung, T.-P. (1996). Tonic, phasic, and transient EEG correlates of auditory awareness in drowsiness. *Brain Res. Cogn. Brain Res.* 4, 15–25. doi: 10.1016/0926-6410(95)00042-9

Makeig, S., Jung, T.-P., Bell, A. J., Ghahremani, D., and Sejnowski,

T. J. (1997).

Blind separation of auditory event-related brain responses into independent components. *Proc. Natl. Acad. Sci. U.S.A.* 94, 10979–10984.

McDowell, K., Lin, C.-T., Oie, K. S., Jung, T.-P., Gordon, S., Whitaker, K. W., et al. (2013). Real-world neuroimaging technologies. *IEEE Access* 1, 131–149. doi: 10.1109/ACCESS.2013.2260791

National Highway Traffic Safety Administration. (2003). *Drowsy Driving and Automobile Crashes*. New Jersey, NJ: N.H.T.S. Administration.

National Sleep Foundation. (2005). *Summary Findings of the 2005 Sleep in America Poll*. Arlington, VA. Available online at: http://sleepfoundation.org/sites/default/files/2005_summary_of_findings.pdf

Peiris, M. T. R., Jones, R. D., Davidson, P. R., Carroll, G. J., and Bones, P. J. (2006). Frequent lapses of responsiveness during an extended visuomotor tracking task in non-sleep-deprived subjects. *J. Sleep Res.* 15, 291–300. doi: 10.1111/j.1365-2869.2006.00545.x

Rosipal, R., Peters, B., Kecklund, G., Akerstedt, T., Gruber, G., Woertz, M., et al. (2007). "EEG-based drivers'drowsiness monitoring using a hierarchi-cal Gaussian mixture model," in *Foundations of Augmented Cognition*, eds D. Schmorrow and L. Reeves (Berlin; Heidelberg: Springer), 294–303.

Simon, M., Schmidt, E. A., Kincses, W. E., Fritzsche, M., Bruns, A., Aufmuth, C., et al. (2011). EEG alpha spindle measures as indicators of driver fatigue under real traffic conditions. *Clin. Neurophysiol.* 122, 1168–1178. doi: 10.1016/j.clinph.2010.10.044

Spence, C., and Driver, J. (1998). Inhibition of return following an auditory cue. The role of central reorienting events. *Exp. Brain Res.* 118, 352–360. doi: 10.1007/s002210050289

The Royal Society for the Prevention of Accidents. (2001). *Driver Fatigue and Road Accidents. A Literature Review and Position Paper*. Birmingham. Available online at: http://www.rospa.com/roadsafety/info/fatigue.pdf

Wang, Y.-T., Cheng, C.-K., Huang, K.-C., Lin, C.-T., Wang, Y., and Jung, T.-P. (2012). "Cell-phone based drowsiness monitoring and management sys-tem," in *2012 IEEE on Biomedical Circuits and Systems Conference (BioCAS)* (Hsinchu), 200–203.

Wolpaw, J. R., Birbaumer, N., McFarland, D. J., Pfutscheller,

G., and Vaughan, T. M. (2002). Brain-computer interfaces for communication and control. *Clin. Neurophysiol.* 113, 767–791. doi: 10.1016/S1388-2457(02)00057-3

Zander, T. O., and Jatzev, S. (2012). Context-aware brain-computer interfaces: exploring the information space of user, technical system and environment. *J. Neural Eng.* 9:016003. doi: 10.1088/1741-2560/9/1/016003

Zander, T. O., and Kothe, C. (2011). Towards passive brain-computer interfaces: applying brain–computer interface technology to human–machine systems in general. *J. Neural Eng.* 8:025005. doi: 10.1088/1741-2560/8/2/025005

Zander, T. O., Kothe, C., Jatzev, S., and Gaertner, M. (2010). "Enhancing human-computer interaction with input from active and passive brain-computer interfaces," in *Brain-Computer Interfaces,* eds D. S. Tan and A. Nijholt (London: Springer), 181–199.

Zander, T. O., Kothe, C., Welke, S., and Roetting, M. (2009). "Utilizing secondary input from passive brain-computer interfaces for enhancing human-machine interaction," in *Foundations of Augmented Cognition. Neuroergonomics and Operational Neuroscience,* eds D. Schomorrow, I. Estabrooke, and M. Grootjen (Berlin; Heidelberg: Springer), 759–771.

Permissions

All chapters in this book were first published in CLANS, by Frontiers; hereby published with permission under the Creative Commons Attribution License or equivalent. Every chapter published in this book has been scrutinized by our experts. Their significance has been extensively debated. The topics covered herein carry significant findings which will fuel the growth of the discipline. They may even be implemented as practical applications or may be referred to as a beginning point for another development.

The contributors of this book come from diverse backgrounds, making this book a truly international effort. This book will bring forth new frontiers with its revolutionizing research information and detailed analysis of the nascent developments around the world.

We would like to thank all the contributing authors for lending their expertise to make the book truly unique.

They have played a crucial role in the development of this book. Without their invaluable contributions this book wouldn't have been possible. They have made vital efforts to compile up to date information on the varied aspects of this subject to make this book a valuable addition to the collection of many professionals and students.

This book was conceptualized with the vision of imparting up-to-date information and advanced data in this field. To ensure the same, a matchless editorial board was set up. Every individual on the board went through rigorous rounds of assessment to prove their worth. After which they invested a large part of their time researching and compiling the most relevant data for our readers.

The editorial board has been involved in producing this book since its inception. They have spent rigorous hours researching and exploring the diverse topics which have resulted in the successful publishing of this book. They have passed on their knowledge of decades through this book. To expedite this challenging task, the publisher supported the team at every step. A small team of assistant editors was also appointed to further simplify the editing procedure and attain best results for the readers.

Apart from the editorial board, the designing team has also invested a significant amount of their time in understanding the subject and creating the most relevant covers. They scrutinized every image to scout for the most suitable representation of the subject and create an appropriate cover for the book.

The publishing team has been an ardent support to the editorial, designing and production team. Their endless efforts to recruit the best for this project, has resulted in the accomplishment of this book. They are a veteran in the field of academics and their pool of knowledge is as vast as their experience in printing. Their expertise and guidance has proved useful at every step. Their uncompromising quality standards have made this book an exceptional effort. Their encouragement from time to time has been an inspiration for everyone.

The publisher and the editorial board hope that this book will prove to be a valuable piece of knowledge for researchers, students, practitioners and scholars across the globe.

List of Contributors

Peter J. Grahn and B. Michael Berry
Mayo Clinic College of Medicine, Mayo Clinic, Rochester, MN, USA

Grant W. Mallory and Jan T. Hachmann
Department of Neurologic Surgery, Mayo Clinic, Rochester, MN, USA

Darlene A. Lobel
Department of Neurosurgery, Cleveland Clinic, Cleveland, OH, USA

J. Luis Lujan
Department of Neurologic Surgery, Mayo Clinic, Rochester, MN, USA

Department of Physiology and Biomedical Engineering, Mayo Clinic, Rochester, MN, USA

JacopoTessadori, Marta Bisio and Michela Chiappalone
Department of Neuroscience and Brain Technologies, Istituto Italiano di Tecnologia, Genova, Italy

Sergio Martinoia
Department of Neuroscience and Brain Technologies, Istituto Italiano di Tecnologia, Genova, Italy
Department of Informatics, Bioengineering, Robotics and System Engineering, University of Genova, Genova, Italy

Yoram Baram
Computer Science Department, Technion – Israel Institute of Technology, Haifa, Israel

Martin Egelhaaf, Norbert Boeddeker, Roland Kern, Rafael Kurtz and Jens P. Lindemann
Neurobiology and Centre of Excellence "Cognitive Interaction Technology", Bielefeld University, Germany

Poramate Manoonpong and Florentin Wörgötter
Bernstein Center for Computational Neuroscience, The Third Institute of Physics, Georg-August Universität Göttingen, Göttingen, Germany

Ulrich Parlitz
Max Planck Research Group Biomedical Physics, Max Planck Institute for Dynamics and Self Organization, Göttingen, Germany
Institute for Nonlinear Dynamics, Georg-August-Universität Göttingen, Göttingen, Germany

Kevin T. Beier and Constance L. Cepko
Department of Genetics and Department of Ophthalmology, Harvard Medical School, Harvard University and Howard Hughes Medical Institute, Boston, MA, USA

Arpiar B. Saunders, Ian A. Oldenburg and Bernardo L. Sabatini
Department of Neurobiology, Harvard Medical School, Harvard University and Howard Hughes Medical Institute, Boston, MA, USA

Jan Müller, Douglas J. Bakkum and Andreas Hierlemann
Bio Engineering Laboratory, ETH Zürich, Basel, Switzerland

Tim Gollisch and Andreas V. M. Herz
Department of Ophthalmology and Bernstein Center for Computational Neuroscience Göttingen, University Medical Center Göttingen, Göttingen, Germany
Department Biology II and Bernstein Center for Computational Neuroscience Munich, Ludwig-Maximilians-Universität München, Munich, Germany

Bryce Beverlin II
Department of Physics, University of Minnesota, Minneapolis, MN, USA

Theoden I. Netoff
Department of Biomedical Engineering, University of Minnesota, Minneapolis, MN, USA

Pedram Afshar, Ankit Khambhati, Scott Stanslaski, David Carlson, Randy Jensen, Dave Linde, Siddharth Dani, Maciej Lazarewicz, Peng Cong, Jon Giftakis, Paul Stypulkowski and Tim Denison
Medtronic Neuromodulation, Minneapolis, MN, USA

Amy L. Orsborn
UC Berkeley - UCSF Joint Graduate Program in Bioengineering, University of California Berkeley, Berkeley, CA, USA

Jose M. Carmena
UC Berkeley - UCSF Joint Graduate Program in Bioengineering, University of California Berkeley, Berkeley, CA, USA
Department of Electrical Engineering and Computer Science, University of California Berkeley, Berkeley, CA, USA
Helen Wills Neuroscience Institute, University of California Berkeley, Berkeley, CA, USA

Yaroslav I. Molkov
Department of Neurobiology and Anatomy, Drexel University College of Medicine, Philadelphia, PA, USA
Department of Mathematical Sciences, Indiana University – Purdue University, Indianapolis, IN, USA

Bartholomew J. Bacak and Ilya A. Rybak
Department of Neurobiology and Anatomy, Drexel University College of Medicine, Philadelphia, PA, USA

Thomas E. Dick
Departments of Medicine and Neurosciences, Case Western Reserve University, Cleveland, OH, USA

Jonathan P. Newman, Riley Zeller-Townson and Steve M. Potter
Laboratory for Neuroengineering, Department of Biomedical Engineering, Georgia Institute of Technology and Emory University School of Medicine, Atlanta, GA, USA

Ming-Fai Fong
Laboratory for Neuroengineering, Department of Biomedical Engineering, Georgia Institute of Technology and Emory University School of Medicine, Atlanta, GA, USA
Department of Physiology, Emory University School of Medicine, Atlanta, GA, USA

Sharanya Arcot Desai
Laboratory for Neuroengineering, Department of Biomedical Engineering, Georgia Institute of Technology and Emory University School of Medicine, Atlanta, GA, USA
Department of Neurosurgery, Emory University School of Medicine, Atlanta, GA, USA
Department of Neurology, Emory University School of Medicine, Atlanta, GA, USA

Robert E. Gross
Department of Neurosurgery, Emory University School of Medicine, Atlanta, GA, USA

Department of Neurology, Emory University School of Medicine, Atlanta, GA, USA
Department of Biomedical Engineering, Georgia Institute of Technology and Emory University School of Medicine, Atlanta, GA, USA

Obaid U. Khurram
Mayo Clinic College of Medicine, Mayo Clinic, Rochester, MN, USA

Allan J. Bieber
Department of Neurologic Surgery, Mayo Clinic, Rochester, MN, USA
Department of Neurology, Mayo Clinic, Rochester, MN, USA

Kevin E. Bennet
Department of Neurologic Surgery, Mayo Clinic, Rochester, MN, USA
Division of Engineering, Mayo Clinic, Rochester, MN, USA

Hoon-Ki Min, Kendall H. Lee and J. L. Lujan
Department of Neurologic Surgery, Mayo Clinic, Rochester, MN, USA
Department of Physiology and Biomedical Engineering, Mayo Clinic, Rochester, MN, USA

Su-Youne Chang
Department of Neurologic Surgery, Mayo Clinic, Rochester, MN, USA

Jacobo Fernandez-Vargas, Hanns U. Pfaff, Francisco B. Rodríguez and Pablo Varona
Grupo de Neurocomputación Biológica, Departamento de Ingeniería Informática, Escuela Politécnica Superior, Universidad Autónoma de Madrid, Madrid, Spain

Yu-Te Wang
Department of Computer Science and Engineering, Jacobs School of Engineering, University of California San Diego, La Jolla, CA, USA
Swartz Center for Computational Neuroscience, Institute for Neural Computation, University of California San Diego, La Jolla, CA, USA

Kuan-Chih Huang, Teng-Yi Huang and Chin-Teng Lin
Department of Electrical Engineering, National Chiao-Tung University, Hsinchu, Taiwan

Chun-Shu Wei
Swartz Center for Computational Neuroscience, Institute for Neural Computation, University of California San Diego, La Jolla, CA, USA
Department of Bioengineering, Jacobs School of Engineering, University of California San Diego, La Jolla, CA, USA

Li-Wei Ko
Department of Biological Science and Technology, National Chiao-Tung University, Hsinchu, Taiwan

Chung-Kuan Cheng
Department of Computer Science and Engineering, Jacobs School of Engineering, University of California San Diego, La Jolla, CA, USA
Center for Advanced Neurological Engineering, Institute of Engineering in Medicine, University of California San Diego, La Jolla, CA, USA

Tzyy-Ping Jung
Swartz Center for Computational Neuroscience, Institute for Neural Computation, University of California San Diego, La Jolla, CA, USA
Department of Bioengineering, Jacobs School of Engineering, University of California San Diego, La Jolla, CA, USA

Center for Advanced Neurological Engineering, Institute of Engineering in Medicine, University of California San Diegc, La Jolla, CA, USA

Index

CPSIA information can be obtained
at www.ICGtesting.com
Printed in the USA
BVHW062124290822
645775BV00003B/73